Pathogenic Microbiology

The Biology and Prevention of Selected Bacterial, Fungal, Rickettsial, and Viral Diseases of Clinical Importance

Vernon T. Schuhardt

Department of Microbiology
The University of Texas at Austin
Austin, Texas

With contributions by:

Thomas W. Huber

Houston Health Department Laboratory and
The University of Texas School of Public Health
Houston, Texas

J. B. Lippincott Company

Philadelphia   New York   San Jose   Toronto

Design and production: Rick Chafian
Project editor: Carl May
Illustrator: Judith McCarty
Copyeditor: Don Yoder
Compositor: Typothetae
Printer: Halliday Lithograph

Library of Congress Cataloging in Publication Data

Schuhardt, Vernon T   1901–
    Pathogenic microbiology.

    Bibliography: p.
    Includes index.
    1. Medical microbiology. 2. Micro-organisms,
Pathogenic. I. Huber, Thomas W., 1942–
joint author. II. Title. [DNLM: 1. Communicable
diseases. 2. Communicable disease control.
WC100 S385p]
QR46.S34   616.01   77-13862
ISBN 0–397–47373–7
ISBN 0–397–47370–2

Contents

PART III. INTESTINAL GROUP DISEASES

Subgroup A: Excreta-Borne Diseases

Bacterial Diseases

Viral and Leptospiral Diseases

Subgroup B: Milk-Borne and Meat-Borne Diseases

Subgroup C: Noninfectious Diseases

PART IV. INOCULATION GROUP DISEASES

Subgroup A: Arthropod Inoculation

Bacterial Diseases

Rickettsial Diseases

Viral Diseases

Subgroup B: Vertebrate Inoculation

Subgroup C: Wound Inoculation

Preface

Since the terminology of medically-related sciences is essentially a foreign language to the average beginning student, I long ago became convinced that the neophyte student of medicine or related health sciences could profit by an introduction to the terminology and principles involved in the biology and prevention of human infectious diseases. Although the approach elaborated in this text is particularly adaptable to microbiology courses for preprofessional students of medicine, medical technology, public health, and related health sciences, it should prove useful and interesting to all students. Everyone confronts pathogenic microorganisms—be it in the clinical laboratory, the hospital, the office, in crowds, or even in the home, preventing communicable diseases is everyone's concern.

During the forty years prior to my retirement from the University of Texas at Austin, I taught a one-semester lecture course in pathogenic microbiology to more than five thousand undergraduate students, most of them interested in careers in the health sciences. Frequently these students, after completing their professional studies, told me how much the preprofessional introduction to this subject matter helped them. These reports have bolstered my conviction of the value of such a course.

Throughout my years of teaching I continually felt the need for an introductory textbook to supplement my lectures. Although an adequate number of both introductory general microbiology and more advanced medical microbiology textbooks were available—several of the latter being listed among the general references at the end of Chapter 1—none dealt with the subject matter at the nonencyclopedic level of complexity nor in the degree of emphasis on prevention that I desired. Consequently, in the hopes that other instructors might desire to supplement their lectures in introductory pathogenic microbiology with such a textbook, I spent the two years following my retirement from teaching in compiling this book.

Infectious diseases for this text have been selected from the realm of bacterial, fungal, rickettsial, and viral etiology to illustrate introductory terminology and principles of pathogenic microbiology. Following the general introductory chapters (Part I), each disease considered in Parts II, III, and IV is discussed in terms of etiology, epidemiology, pathogenic mechanism, clinical symptoms, laboratory diagnosis, prophylactic and therapeutic procedures, control, and prevention. For these discussions, the diseases have been grouped on the basis of the adaptations of their etiological agents to vehicles and modes of transmission from host to host—their epidemiology. However, all of the diseases to be considered are listed alphabetically in Table 1-1 of Chapter However, all of the diseases considered are listed alphabetically in Table 1-1 of Chapter 1. The etiological agent and chapter in which each disease is found is also indicated in Table 1-1.

Laboratory procedures are discussed extensively in the chapters dealing with the individual diseases, even though these discussions may not include the minutiae of technical details that are essential to clinical laboratory work. Such details are found in clinical laboratory manuals, several of which are listed in the general references at the end of Chapter 1. One of these—the *Manual of Clinical Microbiology* by Lennette et al. (1974)—is referred to most frequently for such details. Other manuals, however, can serve equally well to supplement the laboratory information presented in this text. The American Society for Microbiology also publishes a series of updated laboratory procedures, designated *Cumitechs,* which can be consulted by interested readers.

In setting a tone for the writing I kept in mind my major graduate professor, Asa C. Chandler—one of America's great parasitologists—who impressed me with the fact that neither lectures nor textbooks dealing with scientific matter need be dry, humorless, and impersonal compositions. Consequently, I make no apologies for occasional use of the personal pronoun nor for presenting personal experiences, even though they might involve a bit of humor.

The reader may also notice fewer illustrations than are found in many introductory microbiology texts. This is due, in part, to the assumption that undergraduate students enrolling in a course of pathogenic microbiology will have had an introductory laboratory course in general microbiology with an adequately illustrated textbook. Also, professors can be expected to have their own ideas for illustrating their particular lectures and laboratory sections using visual aids. These aids may be provided by the professors themselves in the form of photographic slides or from inexpensive sources for such aids, including (1) the American Society of Microbiology Slide Collection, Washington, D.C., or (2) the Photo-Art Resource Library of the Instructional Media Division, Center for Disease Control, Atlanta.

On the other hand, no attempt was made to avoid figures where they might be helpful and interesting, and the author wishes to express appreciation to the persons and institutions— too numerous to list here—who generously contributed micrographs and other photographic illustrations. These donors are credited by name in the figure legends, and a complete list of illustration credits may be found at the end of the book. Appreciation also is due to the reviewers of a preliminary draft of the text—W. S. Jeter of the University of Arizona, Maryanne McGuckin of the School of Allied Medical Professions, University of Pennsylvania, and Lee Anne McGonagle of the Division of Medical Technology, University of Washington, Seattle. Their critiques and constructive suggestions were helpful in arriving at the final format of the text.

Special appreciation must be expressed to my faculty colleagues in the Department of Microbiology and to my former colleagues and many friends at the Texas State Department of Health Resources, Laboratory Division; both groups have contributed significantly to my teaching efforts. Among my current and longstanding departmental colleagues, I particularly want to thank Professors C. E. Lankford, L. J. Rode, and Orville Wyss for contributions in their areas of expertise. Finally, a colleague most deserving of my appreciation is Professor L. Joe Berry, who not only counseled with me on many aspects of the preliminary manuscript but reviewed the entire final draft—again with helpful suggestions.

Thanks also are due to our departmental secretaries, Mrs. Sudie Campbell and Linda Gaddy, who transcribed much of my handwritten scrawl into readable first draft. Mrs. Gaddy then spent many long weekends in typing a significant portion of the final manuscript. Another departmental employee deserving of my deep appreciation is our electron microscopist and curator of stock cultures (among other responsibilities), Leodocia M. Pope.

Acknowledgements would not be complete without credit to my graduate students, whose thesis and dissertation research frequently provided more to my education than my formal course teaching provided to their's. Among these former graduate students, particular thanks is expressed to Thomas W. Huber for his contribution of two chapters to this text and for proofreading and other forms of assistance.

Lastly, I wish to express appreciation to the personnel of the Center for Disease Control who publish the Morbidity and Mortality Weekly Reports. Without MMWR, keeping a pathogenic microbiology text current would be much more of a chore.

This text is dedicated to my wife, Savannah G. Schuhardt.

Vernon T. Schuhardt

PART ONE

Introduction, History, and Terminology

1

The Parasitic Mode of Life

Parasitism might be defined simply as the practice of one organism (the parasite) living at the expense of another live organism (the host). Since all animals live at the total expense of other live biological species, both plants and other animals, no animal is very far removed from the biological classification of "parasite." However, the parasites with which we will be concerned commonly cause disease symptoms in their hosts as a consequence of, or in association with, their extraction of nutrients from the host's body. An exception to this general rule based on nutrient acquisition is the *ectoparasites:* the bloodsucking arthropods. These ectoparasites cause much discomfort, but rarely by themselves do they cause human disease. They do, however, frequently serve as an excellent mechanism for transmitting other parasitic organisms from host to host.

The organisms with which we are concerned fall into the general category of *endoparasites,* of which there are three basic types. (1) Some endoparasites (certain parasitic worms) may live inside the gastrointestinal tract, either attached to the lining membranes from which they may suck blood or free in the lumen

absorbing food otherwise intended for host nutrition. (2) Other endoparasites may live in close association with the lining membranes of body cavities, including the gastrointestinal tract, where they may produce toxic products that erode the membranes, causing leakage of serous fluids; these fluids may serve as nutrients for the parasites. (3) Yet other endoparasites may invade through the covering or lining membranes of the host and utilize the internal body fluids and tissues as essentials for nutrition, growth, reproduction, and survival as parasitic species. Some of the organisms discussed in this text are type 2, but most of the bacteria and all rickettsiae and viruses are type 3 endoparasites.

EVOLUTION OF THE PARASITIC MODE OF LIFE

Since parasites live at the expense of their hosts, it is obvious that this is an "easy" mode of life; it follows naturally that over evolutionary time many organisms have adapted to the parasitic mode. There was a time on this planet, however, when neither hosts nor parasites nor any form of life, as we know it, existed. It seems rather paradoxical, therefore, that modern studies of our smallest, chemically least complex, and most successful parasitic organisms, the viruses, continue to give background knowledge that is being used by those who are attempting to visualize the origin of life on earth. These viruses are composed of one type of nucleic acid—either deoxyribonucleic acid (DNA) or ribonucleic acid (RNA). In most cases, a protein coat surrounds the viral nucleic acid. Some recently discovered plant viruses (viroids), however, consist only of a naked strand of nucleic acid (RNA). In the environment of the cell cytoplasm of a susceptible host, the viral nucleic acid (the genetic material) can, with the aid of enzymes and other essentials, direct the host cell to synthesize copies of the virus (or viroid) nucleic acid and the virus protein and to assemble these components into new virus or viroid progeny. This replication of the virus structure is viral reproduction, and reproduction is an essential characteristic of all living things. But viruses as we know them today can carry on these reproductive processes only inside living host cells; they all are *obligate parasites,* as are all organisms that can reproduce only in living host tissue.

Various laboratory scientists, using confined atmospheres of water vapor, carbon, hydrogen, and nitrogen compounds comparable to those believed to have existed on earth during prebiotic time, have shown that a variety of amino acids can be produced by electrical discharges (comparable to lightning) into this simulated prebiotic atmosphere. Similar results have been obtained with other physical or chemical procedures. Prebiotic, geosynthesized amino acids could have accumulated in the primitive oceans and under suitable temperature and other physicochemical conditions may have polymerized into a great variety of peptides, proteinoids, and proteins.

The attempted laboratory synthesis of the purine and pyrimidine bases and their conversion to the nucleotide precursors of nucleic acids under simulated prebiotic conditions has been less productive. In 1970 and 1971, however, workers at the Salk Institute and at Texas A & M University, using simulated prebiotic conditions, reported the synthesis of arabinose nucleoside and its conversion into a natural ribose nucleotide. Again such geosynthesized nucleotides may have accumulated in the prebiotic oceans where they were polymerized into a variety of polynucleotides and nucleic acids— none of which was capable of replication, a key characteristic of life. Thus, as millions of years passed, the oceans of this earth, after surface cooling, probably accumulated a soupy mixture of phosphates, carbohydrates, amino acids, polypeptides, proteins, purines, pyrimidines, nucleotides, polynucleotides, nucleic acids, and other essential chemicals, including all the components that a present-day virus might find in the cytoplasm of a live susceptible cell.

Given these prebiotic conditions, it seems reasonable to expect that at least one macromolecule (protein or nucleic acid) might have encountered in its environment the physicochemical ingredients and conditions for self-replication, thereby becoming the prototype molecule of life. Although this protoorganism could have had physicochemical characteristics similar to our obligately parasitic viruses, it could not have been a parasite since there were no prior living organisms for it to exploit. This concept of the origin of life is an example of true *abiogenesis*—the genesis of life from nonliving material—and must have taken place at least once in the geological history of the earth.

Just how long it took this protoorganism to add the necessary genetic coding (the genome) to direct the synthesis of a complex cytoplasm and a retaining cell wall—as well as a mechanism for inherent metabolism and replication comparable to a modern *procaryotic** bacterium—can only be imagined. But, even after this extensive evolution, there is no evidence that these primitive plant cells were parasitic (or predatoristic). The only certainty with regard to the origin of predatorism (the biological equivalent of parasitism) is manifested in the most primitive *eucaryotic†* animal cell: the amoeba.

---

*Genome free in the cytoplasm with no encasing nuclear membrane, among other characteristics.

†Genetic material encased within a nuclear membrane.

This protozoan ingests bacteria and other microscopic life and digests them to provide its nutritive, metabolic, and other requirements. This predatoristic practice probably led to the first instance of infectious parasitism. If a bacterium happened to have evolved a mechanism for resisting digestion by the protozoan, for example, it could be expected to multiply within and to utilize the substance of the predator in its own metabolism. From this small beginning, and over millions of years, there has evolved the parasitic mode of life and the great realm of pathogenic microbiology and parasitology we know today.

THE EPIDEMIOLOGY OF ENDOPARASITES

The parasitic microorganisms of primary concern to us have no inherent means of locomotion to aid in getting from host to host. Yet they must eventually achieve this transition or cease to exist as members of their species. And since organisms that adapt to the parasitic mode of life can rarely multiply effectively in nature outside their hosts, they must adapt to some means of being carried from host to host. The means whereby endoparasites are physically carried *from* the infected host are called *primary vehicles*. These can be generalized as secretions (saliva, mucus), excretions (feces, urine, exudates), or tissues (blood). Therefore each endoparasite must spend some (or all) of its parasitic life in body sites that will enable it to enter one or another of these primary vehicles. Otherwise it will not make the transition to another susceptible host and thereby fail to outlive the original host.

In contagious diseases the primary vehicle from the infected host may carry the parasite directly, by physical contact or its equivalent, to the susceptible host. The site of parasitic invasion of the susceptible host is referred to as the *portal of entry*. Basically, the portals of entry are through the skin or through lining membranes of the gastrointestinal tract or other body cavities. More specifically, the mouth, nose, and eyes are portals through which a parasite might gain entrance to the lining membranes of the respiratory and gastrointestinal tracts. The genital organs are portals of entry to the lining membranes of the urogenital tract.

In many instances the primary vehicle carrying the parasite may contaminate any object in the environment (fingers, flies, food, pencils, books) and these in turn might carry the contaminating parasite to the portal of entry of the susceptible host. Contaminated environmental objects are called *secondary vehicles* and may be good or poor transmitters—a good secondary vehicle is one that is frequently contaminated by primary vehicles and rapidly transports this contamination to the portal of entry of susceptible hosts. A specialized type of secondary vehicle, when infected host blood constitutes the primary vehicle, is bloodsucking (hemophagus) arthropods. These we prefer to call *vectors*. The vectors ingest the parasites along with the blood meal when feeding on the infected host and may transmit the parasite to susceptible hosts during subsequent feeding. In some instances the parasite multiplies extensively in the tissues of the arthropod vector before being transmitted to new human or animal hosts. This generalized epidemiology of communicable diseases is summarized in Figure 1-1.

Figure 1–1. Epidemiology of communicable diseases.

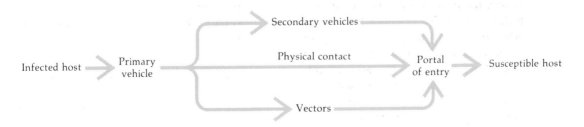

GROUPING OF COMMUNICABLE DISEASES

When called upon to group diseases caused by microorganisms, one usually turns to one of two general types of classification: the "textbook of microbiology" type, wherein the diseases are grouped according to the taxonomic classification of the causative organisms; or the "health officer's manual" type, wherein the diseases are listed in alphabetical order. Neither grouping takes into consideration the fundamental survival adaptations by the parasite to a primary vehicle and, therefore, to a mode of transmission from host to host. Furthermore, these groupings do not provide insight into group rather than individual disease epidemiology.

We, therefore, will group diseases on the basis of the adaptations of the causative organisms to the same primary vehicle and thereby to the same epidemiological pattern, the same mode of transmission. In other words bacterial, fungal, rickettsial, and viral diseases will be grouped together if their modes of transmission from host to host are the same, regardless of the taxonomic or alphabetical classification of the causative organisms or their diseases. Emphasis should be placed upon the fact that some disease organisms have adapted to two or more primary vehicles and, therefore, might fit in more than one of our epidemiological groups. This, however, does not nullify the preventive advantages of knowing the mode of transmission of each group involved. The following outline shows the major communicable disease groups and subgroups:

1. Contact Group
   (a) Respiratory (buccolabial contact) subgroup: diseases for which secretions (saliva or mucus) or exudates of the buccal or respiratory tract serve as primary vehicles. The modes of contact transmission are by kissing or by coughing or sneezing in the immediate proximity of a susceptible host. The diseases in this group frequently are transmitted indirectly by contaminated secondary vehicles. The mucus membranes of the mouth, nose, and eyes constitute the usual portals of entry, and the epidemiology is commonly referred to as "traffic in saliva."
   (b) Genital contact subgroup: diseases in which exudates or secretions from the infected membranes and glands of the urogenital tract constitute the primary vehicle and the common mode of transmission is by sexual intercourse (venereal diseases). In the case of syphilis, infectious lesions may occur in the mouth or on extragenital skin and transmission may result from kissing or other types of contact. The diseases may also be transmitted congenitally from infected mothers to their newborn infants.
   (c) Miscellaneous contact subgroup: conceivably all contagious diseases. However, the group is designed to include only those diseases in which the mode of transmission either is unknown or involves occupational or other unusual types of contact.
2. Intestinal Group*
   (a) Diseases for which intestinal or urinary excreta of humans or animals are the primary vehicle.
   (b) Diseases for which secretions (milk) or tissues (meat) from infected animals serve as the primary vehicles.
   (c) Bacterial food poisoning, including diseases caused by preformed bacterial toxins (enterotoxins) in contaminated food.
3. Inoculation Group†
   (a) Arthropod (ectoparasite) inoculation subgroup: diseases for which blood of the infected host serves as the primary vehicle. The disease organisms are ingested along with the blood meal of the arthropod vector and are transmitted to susceptible hosts during subsequent feedings.

---

*The mouth serves as the portal of entry for all diseases of this group that we will consider.

†The skin serves as the portal of entry for the diseases of this group.

Table 1-1. List of diseases discussed in the text.

Disease	Etiology	Chap.	Disease	Etiology	Chap.
BACTERIAL					
Actinomycosis	*Actinomyces* sp.*	21	Pneumonia	*S. pneumoniae*	7
Anthrax	*B. anthracis*	19	Rat-bite fever	Dual sp.	36
Botulism	*C. botulinum*	28	Relapsing fever	*Borrelia* sp.	30
Brucellosis	*Brucella* sp.	27	Rheumatic fever	*S. pyogenes*	8
Bubonic plague	*Y. pestis*	29	Salmonelloses	*Salmonella* sp.	24
Chancroid	*H. ducreyi*	17	Shigellosis	*Shigella* sp.	23
Cholera	*Vibrio cholerae*	23	Staphylococcal	*Staphylococcus* sp.	20
Diphtheria	*C. diphtheriae*	5	Streptococcal	*Streptococcus* sp.	8
Food poisoning	Multiple	28	Syphilis, bejel	*T. pallidum*	18
Gas gangrene	*Clostridium* sp.	37	Tetanus	*C. tetani*	37
Gonorrhea	*N. gonorrheae*	17	Tuberculosis	*Mycobacterium* sp.	9
Leprosy	*M. leprae*	19	Tularemia	*F. tularensis*	22
Leptospirosis	*Leptospira* sp.	25	Typhoid fever	*S. typhi*	24
Meningitis	*N. meningitidis*	6	Whooping cough	*B. pertussis*	10
Nocardiosis	*N. asteroides*	21	Yaws	*T. pertenue*	19
FUNGAL					
Aspergillosis	*Aspergillus* sp.	21	Dermatophytosis	Multiple	21
Blastomycosis	*Blastomyces* sp.	21	Histoplasmosis	*H. capsulatum*	21
Candidiasis	*C. albicans*	21	Mucormycosis	*Rhizopus* sp.	21
Coccidioidomycosis	*C. immitis*	21	Mycetoma	Multiple	21
Cryptococcosis	*Cryptococcus* sp.	21	Sporotricosis	*S. schenkii*	21
RICKETTSIAL					
Lymphogranuloma	*Chlamydia* sp.	17	Scrub typhus	*R. tsutsugamushi*	32
Ornithosis	*C. psittaci*	19	Spotted fever RMT	*R. rickettsii*	31
Q fever	*Coxiella burnetii*	19	Typhus fever	*Rickettsia* sp.	32
Rickettsialpox	*R. akari*	32			
VIRAL					
Chickenpox	*H. varicellae*	16	Meningitis	Multiple	6
Common cold	*Rhinovirus* st.*	12	Mononucleosis	Epstein-Barr (E-B)	19
Encephalitides	Arboviruses	33	Mumps	*M. parotidis*	15
Hemorrhagic fevers	Multiple	34	Pneumonitis	Multiple	19
Hepatitis	Dual	25	Poliomyelitis	*Poliovirus* st.	26
Herpesvirus	Multiple	16	Rabies	*Rabiesvirus* st.	35
Influenza	*Myxovirus* st.	13	Rubella	Rubella virus	14
Lassa fever	*Lassavirus*	19	Rubeola	*Myxovirus rubeolae*	14
Marburg fever	Marburg virus	19	Smallpox	*Poxvirus variolae*	16
Measles	Dual	14	Zoster (shingles)	V-Z virus	16

*sp. = species; st. = serotypes.

(b) Vertebrate animal inoculation subgroup: diseases transmitted to humans by the bite of vertebrate animals. The buccal secretions of the infected animal serve as the primary vehicle, which is inoculated through the skin during the act of biting.

(c) Wound inoculation subgroup: diseases caused by organisms commonly found in the soil (especially soil contaminated with animal excreta) and inoculated through the skin as a result of traumatic injury.

Table 1-1 lists, in alphabetical order, the diseases to be considered in the text along with the etiological agent and the chapter in which each is discussed. The accepted genus and species designations for the etiological agents are given in the chapter in which each disease is discussed.

GENERAL REFERENCES

These general references contain material applicable to all chapters of the text and are included for those who wish to pursue a more comprehensive coverage of certain aspects of the subject matter. A limited number of literature references are offered at the end of each chapter for the same purpose and also to give credit for sources of specific information.

Medical Dictionary

Stedman's Medical Dictionary. 1972. 22nd ed. Baltimore: Williams & Wilkins.

Laboratory Manuals

Bailey, W. R. and E. G. Scott. 1974. *Diagnostic Microbiology.* 4th ed. St. Louis: Mosby.

Cowan, S. T. 1974. *Cowan and Steel's Manual for the Identification of Medical Bacteria.* 2nd ed. Cambridge: Cambridge University Press.

Lennette, E. H., E. H. Spaulding, and J. P. Truant (eds.). 1974. *Manual of Clinical Microbiology.* 2nd ed. Washington: American Society for Microbiology.

Rose, N. R. and H. Friedman (eds.). 1976. *Manual of Clinical Immunology.* Washington: American Society for Microbiology.

Thompson, R. A. (ed.). 1977. *Techniques in Clinical Immunology.* Oxford: Blackwell.

Antibiotics

Kucers, A. and N. M. Bennett. 1975. *The Use of Antibiotics.* 2nd ed. Philadelphia: Lippincott.

Public Health Manual

Bennenson, A. S. (ed.). 1970. *Control of Communicable Diseases in Man.* 11th ed. New York: American Public Health Association.

Public Health Reports

Morbidity and Mortality Weekly Reports (MMWR). Atlanta: U.S. Public Health Service, Center for Disease Control (CDC).

Taxonomic Manual

Buchanan, R. E. and N. E. Gibbons. 1974. *Bergey's Manual of Determinative Bacteriology.* 8th ed. Baltimore: Williams & Wilkins.

Medical Microbiology Textbooks

Burrows, W. 1973. *Textbook of Microbiology.* 20th ed. Philadelphia: Saunders.

Davis, B. D., R. Dulbecco, H. N. Eisen, H. S. Ginsberg, W. B. Wood, and M. McCarty. 1973. *Microbiology.* 2nd ed. New York: Harper & Row.

Dubos, R. J. and J. G. Hirsch (eds.). 1965. *Bacterial and Mycotic Infections of Man.* 4th ed. Philadelphia: Lippincott.

Horsfall, F. L., Jr. and Igor Tamm (eds.). 1965. *Viral and Rickettsial Infections of Man.* 4th ed. Philadelphia: Lippincott.

Joklik, W. K. and Hilda P. Willett (eds.). 1976. *Zinsser Microbiology.* 16th ed. New York: Appleton-Century-Crofts.

Wilson, G. S. and A. A. Miles. 1975. *Topley and Wilson's Principles of Bacteriology and Immunity.* 6th ed. Baltimore: Williams & Wilkins.

Color Atlases

Gillies, R. R. and T. C. Dodds. 1973. *Bacteriology Illustrated.* New York: Longman.

Olds, R. J. 1975. *Color Atlas of Microbiology.* Chicago: Yearbook Medical Publishers.

Stratford, B. C. 1977. *An Atlas of Medical Microbiology.* Oxford: Blackwell.

2

A Brief History of Medical Microbiology

Since all the diseases of concern to us here are caused by pathogenic microorganisms, we will survey some of the historical developments that led to our current knowledge in this area. Two lines of development—the fields of medicine and microscopy—are obvious precursors to the attainment of knowledge about medical microbiology. Two additional lines of development—studies of fermentation and abiogenesis—at first glance seem to be unrelated to medical microbiology. Since fermentation is a microbiological phenomenon, however, techniques developed for this study proved applicable to studies on the microbiology of disease. Abiogenesis, which, as indicated in Chapter 1, must have occurred at least once on this planet, was looked upon as a common phenomenon by Aristotle, biblical writers, and other thinkers of early civilizations. This belief, insofar as macroscopic organisms were concerned, was no longer accepted by thinking minds by the seventeenth century A.D. Then, in 1676, the discovery of microscopic organisms by Leeuwenhoek revitalized the argument over abiogenesis. Thereafter studies in this area led to the development of techniques that were applicable to studies on the microbiology of disease. Figure 2-1 lists, in chronological order, the names of those who contributed significantly to developments in these four areas of investigation.*

In the field of medicine primitive minds, past and present, have tended to consider disease a supernatural phenomenon. The diseased body either was possessed by devils or was being punished for sin (the demonic theory). Another aspect of this supernatural concept might be illustrated by the classical story of the box containing the ills of mankind; Pandora, in her·curiosity, opened it and thereby liberated a swarm of ills to plague her fellow human beings. Thereafter her father, Aesculapius, son of Apollo and god of medicine, set about with his snake-entwined caduceus and the aid of his daughters Hygeia and Panacea to round up the ills and get them back in the box. Unfortunately for us they did not succeed.

By the fifth century B.C., supernatural concepts of disease were failing to satisfy certain medical minds. Methods of treating disease other than by prayer and supplication—bloodletting, purging, and the like—began to be practiced. One practitioner of that time, who even to this date is recognized as the father of medicine, was Hippocrates (460–377 B.C.). He introduced the scientific method into the study of disease causation and treatment. He regarded disease as natural rather than supernatural and sought to observe and interpret the patient's symptoms as natural phenomena. Hippocrates, and others before him, noted that febrile patients frequently were flushed, had inflamed

---

*The first name or initials of the individuals involved and additional information about the historical microbiological events can be found in the references listed at the end of this chapter.

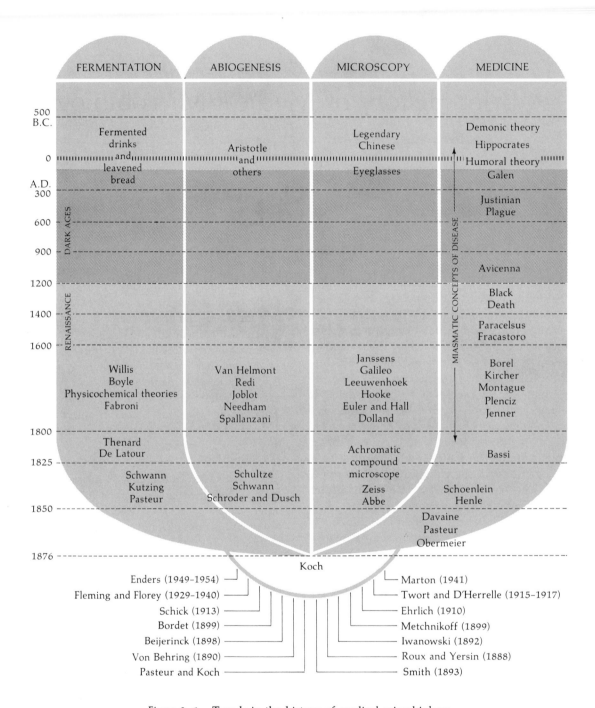

Figure 2–1. Trends in the history of medical microbiology.

membranes or red skin rashes, and had markedly increased pulse rates. This obviously could be interpreted as an excess of blood in the patient, and the obvious treatment was to let out this excess. Hippocrates also established the concept that the "source" of the blood was the heart, but he did not establish the circulation of the blood.

It was Hippocrates' observation that in some diseases copious discharges of phlegm occurred. He therefore concluded that the cause of these diseases was the excess of this normal body fluid. Treatment varied, but one that was recommended was the application of a blistering agent to the nose or throat to draw off the excess phlegm. The Hippocratic concept of the source of the phlegm would be obvious to anyone with a postnasal drip—namely, the brain. To explain cases of jaundice, which undoubtedly occurred then as now, Hippocrates concluded that excess of another normal body fluid, yellow bile, was the cause. The assigned source of this excess was the liver and treatment consisted of purging.

Thus three normal body fluids were postulated to be the cause of a variety of diseases when present in excessive amounts. Yet the number four had significance in Greek mythology—and besides, there was a group of diseases, including black eyes and other bruises, in which the skin of the patient turned black. This necessitated another fluid that, when in excess, could account for this symptom. Hippocrates postulated a black bile, the source of which he decided was the spleen.

The humoral theory of disease, as advocated by Hippocrates and his followers, explained health as the consequence of a proper balance of the four body fluids or humors. Disease, of characteristic symptomatology, occurred when one of these humors got out of balance and became excessive. Disease therapy consisted of efforts to eliminate the excessive humor and thereby restore the normal, healthy balance.

The next great name in the field of medicine was the Greek Physician Galen (A.D. 130–201). Galen was a true and energetic medical scientist and a voluminous writer. He accepted the hu-

moral theory of disease and set about to expand medical knowledge as it related to this theory. His texts included anatomy, pathology, physiology, symptomatology (clinical diagnosis), and therapy. He was particularly expert in human skeletal anatomy, in part due to his discovery, in a mountain pass, of a skeleton which he secretly reassembled and sketched, drawing each articulation as well as the total skeleton. Galen practiced in Rome, and his outstanding ability and reputation resulted in his being appointed court physician. This appointment undoubtedly helped his reputation and the preservation of his writings, which became totally accepted as the infallible medical authority. To oppose Galenism was considered medical heresy.

During and following Galen's lifetime, the historical era known as the Dark Ages set in, a period that defies complete explanation. With the increasing urbanization of the Byzantine, Greek, and Roman city-states and the resultant crowding of human populations, conditions for epidemics of communicable disease were greatly increased. Smallpox could be expected to become epidemic under such conditions, for example, and this disease has been known to kill 50 percent or more of those who contract it. During the reign of the Byzantine emperor Justinian I (A.D. 483–565), one of the three great plagues of history spread over the then known world. This disease—bubonic plague—is estimated to have killed a quarter or more of the human population. It is easy to visualize the effect that such epidemics must have had on the superstitious mentality of the times. Perhaps the gods, displeased with human endeavor, were wreaking their epidemic evidence of this displeasure on the human population. Considering the great strides in art, philosophy, and learning made during Grecian and early Roman times, the most obvious thing for the gods to be displeased with was the human effort to outdo them in learning. This notion could be expected to lead to a mass psychological conclusion that everything worth knowing was already known and that anyone who expressed a new thought was a heretic; penalties for heresy became pretty severe. Such a mass psychology could be expected to put a solid brake on the innovative learning process and could have contributed to the period of history called the Dark Ages. Be that as it may, no real progress was made in any of the areas of knowledge relating to our subject for a thousand years following Galen's contributions. An Arabian physician by the name of Avicenna published medical texts during the late tenth or early eleventh centuries, but his writings and concepts were essentially similar to those of Hippocrates and Galen.

Although the Renaissance of art and literature began in the thirteenth century and was accompanied by new developments in the fields of chemistry and physics, no real progress in the field of medicine occurred for at least another three hundred years. During this time, in the thirteenth century, the second of the three greatest plagues of humanity broke out. This one was called the Black Death and again was mainly bubonic plague. The third pandemic was influenza in 1918 (see Chapter 13). Thus the humoral theory of disease, as propounded by Hippocrates and expanded by Galen (and to a lesser extent by Avicenna), persisted unchallenged for more than seventeen hundred years.

The first medical practitioner publicly to challenge the Galenistic concept (humoral theory) of disease was a character by the name of Paracelsus. The following sketch of this man is found in a footnote published by John Rotheram, M.D., in 1801 in his reprinting of William Cullen's "First Lines of the Practice of Physic*" published in 1789 in Edinburgh:

> The remarkable circumstances in the life of Aureolus Philippus Theophrastus Bombastus Paracelsus de Hohenheim, as he called himself, are too numerous for insertion in the narrow limits alloted to these Notes. He was born in the village of Einfidlen, about two German miles from Zurick in the year 1493. At three years old he was made a eunuch by an accident. He traveled all over the continent of Europe, obtaining knowledge in chemistry and physic and then traveled about the country

practicing what he had learned. His chief remedies were opium and mercury, and his great success increased his celebrity. He cured the famous printer Frobenius of Basil of an inveterate disease; this cure brought him acquainted with Erasmus and made him known to the magistracy of Basil, who elected him professor in 1527. He lectured for two hours every day. While seated in his chair, he burnt with great solemnity the writings of Galen and Avicenna; and declared to his audience, if God would not impart the secrets of physic, it was not only allowable, but even justifiable, to consult the devil. He soon left Basil, and continued to ramble about the country generally intoxicated, and never changing his clothes, or even going to bed. He died after an illness of a few days, in an inn at Saltsburgh, in 1541, in his 48th year, tho' he had promised himself that, by the use of his elixer, he should live to the age of Methusalem.

Thus it is obvious that Paracelsus' influence on his colleagues and superiors was not overwhelming, but at least he should be given credit for initiating a trend away from the humoral theory of disease causation and treatment.

From early Grecian times on through the Roman period and beyond, bad air was believed to be in some way involved in disease causation—the miasmatic concept. Burning of fires all over Athens was once advocated as a means of purifying the air during an epidemic. One of the main diseases so explained was malaria (literally "bad air"). Even nineteenth-century treatises elaborated on the relationship of marsh air to this widespread disease; the authors never recognized that it was the mosquito and not the air that transmitted the disease.

Shortly after the death of Paracelsus, Fracastoro of Verona in 1546 postulated seeds or germs of contagious disease which could be transmitted from case to case by contact, or by fomites (secondary vehicles), or at a distance through the air. Thus was initiated the concept of a contagium vivum: living infectious agents.

A number of developments in our four areas of interest took place during the seven-

---

*Medicine.

teenth and eighteenth centuries. Willis in 1659 advocated the physicochemical concept of fermentation—namely, that fermentation resulted from a spontaneous rearrangement of the unstable molecules in a fermentable fluid, such that the molecular composition changed from the juice state to alcohol and the gaseous (CO_2) state. This concept did not satisfy Robert Boyle, who in 1663 made a prediction which almost came true two hundred years later. Boyle noted the similarities between fermentation and communicable disease: exposure, incubation period with no symptoms, bubbling, temperature changes, symptoms and recovery with resistance to refermentation or to reinfection. He predicted that the person who provided a satisfactory explanation for fermentation would probably be best qualified to explain communicable disease.

During the seventeenth century the physics of magnification and the art and science of lens grinding and mounting resulted in the production of primitive compound microscopes by the Janssen brothers and the telescope used by Galileo in his celestial studies. Unfortunately for the Janssens, the phenomenon of chromatic aberration (the rainbow effect) rendered their instrument and all early compound microscopes practically useless. Borel in 1653, however, using such an instrument, reported seeing eel- and dolphinlike objects in the blood of a sick patient, and Kircher in 1658 examined exudate from the bubo of a bubonic plague victim and reported microscopic worms present. Although Borel and Kircher were not seeing the causative organisms of the diseases they were studying, their reports tended to strengthen the concept of a contagium vivum as the causation of disease.

About this same time Antony van Leeuwenhoek of Delft, Holland, started his hobby of grinding, polishing, and mounting small lenses to obtain maximum magnification by a single lens. He mounted the lens between metal plates below which he suspended a pointer that could be manipulated into focus by thumbscrews (Figure 2-2a). Leeuwenhoek was a secretive Dutchman, and he kept his lens grinding technique to himself. During his lifetime he would not sell even one of the instruments. He had other professional responsibilities in Delft, but he spent as much time as possible looking at all manner of objects (fly legs, wings, eyes, beer, fecal matter, urine, tartar) under his single-lens microscopes. Also, he started the practice of sketching the images of the more interesting magnified objects and sending the sketches along with written descriptions to the Royal Society in London, where they were published in the transactions. His reputation became so great that it is said the czar of Russia, since he could not buy a microscope, came to Delft incognito to look at some of the magnified objects.

On one occasion Leeuwenhoek ground up some peppercorns in rainwater with the objective of trying to see what makes pepper hot. When he mounted a drop of the suspension and looked at it through the lens, however, what he saw did not impress him and he returned to other duties. A few days later he decided to have another look at his ground pepper suspension. This time he found the fluid swarming with motile microscopic organisms, which he called animalculae. He made sketches and sent his report to the Royal Society. One of these sketches, published in 1676, included rodlike organisms that he illustrated as motile by tracing the erratic movements about in the microscopic field (Figure 2-2b). Since Leeuwenhoek's best microscopes would magnify only about 300 diameters, questions have persisted as to how he was able to see the rodlike organisms that his illustrations indicate he undoubtedly saw. In some reports he mentioned using glass capillaries or thin glass plates for mounting fluid specimens; however, he was even more secretive about his method of observation than about his method of lens production. Dobell in 1960 suggested that Leeuwenhoek might have devised some simple method of obtaining darkfield illumination.

Casida (1976) mounted a drop of broth culture of a large motile bacterium commonly found in organic infusions, Bacillus mycoides, between two microcover glasses. When he examined the preparation with a replica of a

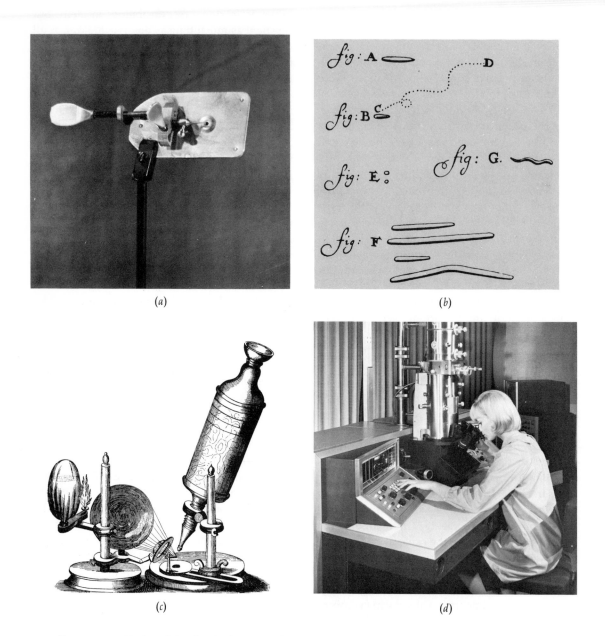

Figure 2–2.   (*a*) A replica of one of Leeuwenhoek's microscopes. The lens is the small, dark circle seen in this photo at the tip of the needle on which the specimen was placed. (*b*) Leeuwenhoek's drawings of bacteria. (*c*) Hooke's own drawing of one of his microscopes. (*d*) Operator at a modern electron microscope. ((*a*) Courtesy of Bausch and Lomb, Rochester, N.Y.; (*c*) The Bettmann Archive, Inc., N.Y.; (*d*) courtesy of Forgflo Corporation, Sunbury, PA.)

Leeuwenhoek microscope, using bright-light illumination, he was unable to see the bacilli. When he illuminated the underside of the preparation with a beam of light at an angle of about 45 degrees, however, he reported seeing the bacilli swimming in and out of the field of vision. They appeared as bright objects in a dark field. This experiment apparently resolves the Leeuwenhoek mystery on the three-hundredth anniversary of its inception. Regardless of how he did it, Leeuwenhoek is given credit for having discovered the first bacterium—thereby becoming the founder of bacteriology.

Robert Hooke, who in 1665 had built a crude compound microscope (Figure 2-2c), was able to confirm the microscopic animalculae described by Leeuwenhoek. In 1762 these discoveries led Plenciz to postulate that these animalculae were the seeds (germs) of disease first proclaimed by Fracastoro. Thus one might say that Plenciz was the first to put forward a germ theory of disease, but he did nothing to prove his theory.

Two developments in immunology were introduced to the English-speaking world during the eighteenth century. The Royal Society in London published an extract from a letter dated December 1713 from Emanuel Timonius, M.D., at Constantinople, indicating the widespread practice of intentional infection with mild smallpox matter to prevent more serious smallpox. In 1718 Lady Mary Montagu, wife of the British ambassador to Constantinople, wrote her kin back home about this practice of inoculation or *variolation* to prevent severe smallpox and reported that she had had her children so inoculated. The basis for this practice rested on two facts: first, smallpox outbreaks could be mild with no mortality, or they could be severe with mortality ranging from a few to 50 percent or more of the cases; and second, the disease always left scars on the faces of recovered patients. Consequently, when an epidemic of the disease spread through the population, it was obvious that those who were not attacked were largely those who showed the scarred-face evidence of a prior attack of smallpox. As a result of these letters, the practice of variolation spread to England and from there to colonial America. This practice, moreover, made possible the experiment leading to the second immunological development.

Late in the eighteenth century Edward Jenner was a practicing physician in the English countryside. He was familiar with the common observation that milkmaids and others who worked with cattle failed to contract smallpox during severe epidemics even though they had no scars to indicate prior smallpox infection. This apparent immunity to smallpox was attributed to contact with cowpox matter from cattle lesions located on the udder of a diseased animal. Jenner decided to test this belief. Consequently when James Phipps was brought to him for variolation, Jenner dipped his lancet into a cowpox lesion on a dairymaid's finger and inoculated James. When the boy developed a typical skin sore at the inoculation site, which healed in due course, Jenner still did not know whether James was immune to smallpox or not. The record merely states that James received follow-up inoculations with variolous matter about 6 weeks later. That may not be the whole story, however. It is reasonable to speculate that Jenner informed Mrs. Phipps the reaction on James' arm was rather small and he was not sure that James was immune to smallpox as a result of the inoculation. He therefore recommended that James be variolated again. He probably informed her that if James was immune, there would not be a second sore, and that if he was not immune, he needed the second variolation. When Mrs. Phipps agreed, Jenner this time dipped his lancet into a skin lesion of a mild case of smallpox and variolated James. When no sore developed after the second inoculation, Jenner concluded that James had been immunized against smallpox by the inoculation of the cowpox matter. Consequently, in 1796, he wrote up his experiment, calling his inoculation *vaccination* (from *vacca,* cow), and sent the report off to the Royal Society for publication. The editors, however, were not convinced that the one experiment justified the conclusions drawn and turned down the manuscript, thereby missing publication of one of the great discoveries of all time.

Jenner was a stubborn type, though. He had the report printed at his own expense and in 1798 distributed the publication widely to the medical practitioners of the area. For a while he regretted his actions because of the vilification heaped upon him, but fortunately he lived long enough to see the acceptance and some of the lifesaving potential of smallpox vaccination.

Van Helmont in 1652 was one of the last scientists to advocate abiogenesis of macroscopic organisms. Up to this time maggots were commonly believed to develop abiogenetically from decaying organic matter. Father Redi in 1653 performed the following simple experiment to disprove this belief. He took a piece of fresh meat and placed one half of it in a glass container with gauze netting tied over the top. The second half he left uncovered. In due course maggots developed in the uncovered meat but not in the covered. Redi correlated the maggot development with the eggs laid by flies on the uncovered meat.

With the discovery of microscopic organisms (animalculae) by Leeuwenhoek, the question of the spontaneous generation of these organisms became the subject of philosophical discussion and some experimental observations. Joblot in 1718 reported the development of microscopic organisms in hay infusions which had been previously boiled. In 1748 Needham reported another of these experiments to the Royal Society in London. He heated a flask up to the neck in glowing ashes, then added some mutton gravy hot from the fire, and immediately closed it with a cork, giving what he considered a hermetic seal. The closed flask was left exposed for several days to the summer heat. When he removed a drop for examination he found the gravy swarmed with microscopic life. He reported that scores of different infusions of both animal and vegetable substances constantly gave the same results. Needham concluded that "there is a vegetative force in every microscopical point of matter . . . whence its atoms may return again and ascend to a new life." This new life, in other words, was the consequence of abiogenetic development from nonliving matter.

Lazaro Spallanzani carried on a large number of experiments on infusions prepared from a variety of beans, lentils, and other seeds. The infusions were placed in glass containers that could be left open to the air, covered with cotton gauze, closed with wooden stoppers, or hermetically sealed with a blowtorch. The containers were either untreated or heated in boiling water for periods varying from $\frac{1}{2}$ minute to 1 hour. In 1754 Spallanzani reported that great numbers of two types of animalculae had developed in all his unheated infusions. Heating for $\frac{1}{2}$ minute or more suppressed the development of the larger animalculae. Longer heating up to 1 hour was required to suppress the development of the smaller animalculae (probably spore-forming bacteria). Many of his hermetically sealed preparations, after heating in boiling water for from 1 to 60 minutes, failed to develop animalculae. Since the heated preparations exposed to open air and some of the stoppered preparations did develop animalculae, Spallanzani concluded that the progenitors of these organisms were seeded into the infusions from the air. The animalculae were not, therefore, developed abiogenetically.

Since oxygen in the atmosphere had been discovered by this time and its essentiality for life established, it did not take much imagination to extend Needham's concept of a "vegetative force" in atoms of matter to a concept of a "vital force" in the atmosphere. Those favoring abiogenesis of microscopic organisms contended that Spallanzani had heated his infusions long enough to destroy the vital force and had sealed his containers too quickly and too tightly for reentry of vital force from the atmosphere—therefore, he could not expect to obtain abiogenetic development of microorganisms. And there the question of abiogenesis versus biogenesis of microorganisms rested for another 25 to 50 years.

By the end of the eighteenth century the crude microscopes of the time were being used to study many things, including fermenting fluids. Brewer's yeast was well known, but its nature and exact relationship to the phenomenon of beer fermentation were not established. Organic chemists knew that the sugar in grape juice was the component that was converted to alcohol and carbon dioxide, but the mechanism of this conversion had not been established. Fabroni in 1787 reported that the glutinous material in fermenting fluids was composed of yeastlike particles. Thenard in 1803 reported that all natural sugar juices when undergoing fermentation gave a deposit which had the appearance of brewer's yeast and which, like brewer's yeast, could initiate fermentation of pure sugared water. No further developments in the field of fermentation occurred until improvements were made in the compound microscope.

In about 1733 a Swiss mathematician by the name of Euler and an English barrister named Hall are credited with theorizing that the chromatic aberration of the simple lens could be corrected if the lens were constructed of two glasses of different refractive indices. In 1759 John Dolland fashioned an achromatic objective for a telescope by combining two lenses made of glasses with different indices of refraction and thereby proved the Euler-Hall theory. Achromatic lenses were not adapted to the compound microscope until the first quarter of the nineteenth century, however, and even these early achromatic lens microscopes suffered from spherical aberration. In 1833 Carl Zeiss and Ernst Abbe solved the basic problems of both chromatic and spherical aberration of lenses and produced a compound microscope with optical properties similar to those of modern light microscopes. With these new improved microscopes available, rapid developments in the various fields of microbiology took place.

In the field of fermentation three workers, Cagniard de Latour in 1826, Theodor Schwann in 1837, and Frederick Kutzing in 1837, independently came to the conclusions that yeasts were living vegetable matter and were responsible for alcoholic fermentation. In 1839, however, two great chemists, Baron Liebig and Wohler, ridiculed this biological concept of fermentation, contending that the yeasts were just another product of fermentation and not its primary cause. The sheer weight of Liebig's repeated objections tended to delay acceptance of the biological concept of fermentation until after studies reported by Louis Pasteur.

Pasteur took his doctorate degree at age 25 from the *école normale* in Paris in 1847. He presented his thesis in two parts: in the chemistry of arsenous oxide and in the physics of optical rotation of liquids. His first publication, in 1848, resolved the problem of the left and right deviation of polarized light by crystals of otherwise identical salts of tartaric acid (tartrates). He showed that an optically inactive solution consisted of an equal (racemic) mixture of levo- and dextrorotary components that could be separated into their individual optical types. From this point on, Pasteur turned his attention to biochemical, microbiological, and immunological phenomena. He reported studies on the optical activity of amyl alcohol derived from beet sugar fermentation, on lactic acid derived from lactose fermentation, and particularly on butyl alcohol and other compounds from butyric acid fermentation. He noted that morphologically different microorganisms predominated in different types of fermentation. In butyric acid fermentation he noted the requirement for strict anaerobic conditions: The rod-shaped microorganisms responsible for the fermentation were killed by the presence of free oxygen. He showed that by adequate dilution of a fermenting fluid he could obtain a pure culture of the predominant microorganism present. Using such pure cultures, he could obtain the specific type of fermentation he desired. Thus Pasteur is given credit for being the first to prove the *germ theory* of fermentation and for introducing pure culture techniques for microbiological study.

With progress in resolving the controversy over abiogenesis of microorganisms stymied by the question of vital force, Schultze in 1836 and Schwann in 1837 carried out experiments designed to reaerate their flasks of heat-sterilized media and reported no growth after subsequent incubation. Their methods of aeration (drawing

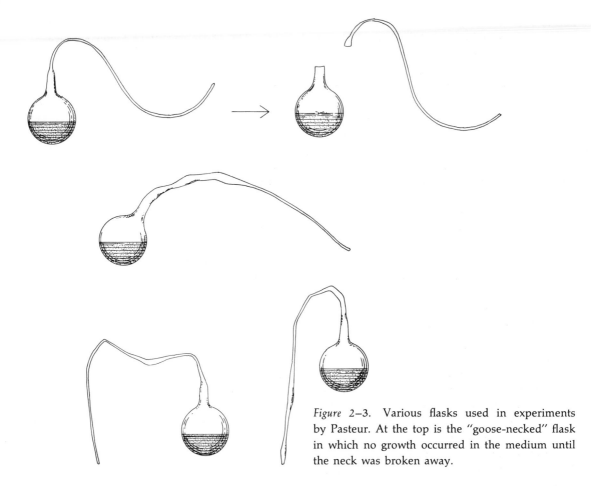

Figure 2–3. Various flasks used in experiments by Pasteur. At the top is the "goose-necked" flask in which no growth occurred in the medium until the neck was broken away.

the air into the flask through red hot tubing or bubbling the air through strong acid or alkali), however, were even more harsh than the boiling used to sterilize the infusions. Consequently, these microbiological methods did not influence the thinking of the vital force adherents. The methods were modified in 1859 by Schroder and Dusch, who drew the air into their sterile infusion through a tube stuffed with cotton. When they reported no growth in such reaerated infusions, the vital force argument was dealt a death blow, and the use of cotton plugs to prevent contamination of tubed culture media was initiated. Pasteur in 1860 reported the results of extensive additional experiments, including his famous gooseneck flask experiment (Figure 2-3). The neck of a flask containing a sterile beef infusion was drawn out in the shape of a gooseneck with the lower end left open to allow free exchange of air, "vital force," or any other normal atmospheric components but restricting the entrance of dust particles. He showed that although dust might accumulate in the lower bend of the glass tubing, no growth occurred in his medium. If he broke off the neck, however, or tilted the flask so that the broth ran into the area of the dust and then tilted it back so that the dust-contaminated fluid ran back into the bulk of the medium, growth of microorganisms occurred within a short period of time. He then exposed identical open flasks of sterile medium in the dusty streets of Paris, in the dustfree countryside, and on top of Mont Blanc—and noted that the time required for seeding the broth for growth of microorganisms bore a reverse correlation with the amount of dust in the atmosphere. He also noted, as had others, that some of the rod-shaped microorganisms contained refractile granules and that these (spore-formers) were more resistant to heat than the vegetative (non-spore-forming) cells. Thus studies in fermentation and abiogenesis gave rise to microbiological methods, including preparation and sterilization of media, protection against contamination, and the use of pure cultures. These developments were later applied to studies on the microbiological aspects of disease.

After Fracastoro in 1546 initiated the concept of living infectious agents, and Borel and Kircher had reported the presence of motile, microscopic organisms in blood and exudates of patients, the concept of a contagium vivum was further extended in 1762 by Plenciz and his advocacy of the germ theory of disease based upon Leeuwenhoek's microscopic animalculae. This concept then lay dormant until Bassi in 1834–1837, using an improved compound microscope, reported the presence of refractile granules in diseased silkworms and their absence in healthy ones. He concluded that they were the cause of the silkworm disease. Schoenlein in 1839 reported a fungus associated with the falling hairs of the human scalp disease favus. Since he failed to find the fungus on hairs of healthy scalps, he concluded that the fungus was the cause of the disease.

J. Henle was a professor of anatomy at Göttingen, where Robert Koch was one of his medical students. As professor of anatomy Henle manifested little interest in the developing field of microbiology until 1840, when he published "Pathological Investigations." In this treatise he made it clear that he was familiar with the repeated claims that certain microscopic organisms were the cause of associated diseases. He postulated that to prove this etiological relationship to a specific disease (1) the agent must be found in the host in every case of the disease, (2) the agent must be isolated, and (3) the isolated agent must be shown to be capable of producing the disease. Henle failed to follow through insofar as establishing the etiology of any disease, but his student Koch must have

been inspired by his teachings. Some 10 or more years after graduation Kock applied Henle's postulates to the disease anthrax.

In 1863, Davaine reported finding rod-shaped microorganisms in the blood of animals sick or dying with anthrax and none such in healthy animals. He passed the disease to healthy animals by inoculation of blood containing the organisms. Davaine was convinced that these organisms were the cause of anthrax, but he failed to use the isolated culture technique to prove his conviction. By this time a silkworm epizootic was threatening to destroy the silk industry in southern France, and Pasteur was called upon to investigate the problem. He responded that he had never seen a silkworm and hardly felt qualified to undertake such a task. Previously, however, he had resolved an industrial problem in the field of his expertise, alcoholic fermentation. He found that contaminating microorganisms were carrying on undesirable fermentations following completion of the alcoholic fermentation. Among other things, he advocated heating the finished alcoholic product sufficiently to destroy the undesirable microorganisms without affecting the taste of the beer or wine. Thereby he introduced the principle of disinfection, which we now call pasteurization. The industrial response to Pasteur's pleading of ignorance relative to the silkworm problem was that this ignorance might be beneficial—at least he would start with no preconceived ideas.

Pasteur took his microscope with him to the south of France and soon made two significant observations: microorganisms ("corpuscles") were found in the bodies of sick silkworm moths and silkworms that were not present in healthy animals; moreover, these microorganisms were observed on the exterior of eggs laid by the infected silkworm moths. Pasteur advocated the isolation of each newly mated female moth along with the eggs that she produced. If, on microscopic examination, the moth showed the presence of the infectious corpuscles, she and the eggs were destroyed, whereas the eggs from noninfected moths were allowed to hatch. This simple method enabled the silk growers to obtain healthy broods of silkworm moths that were kept healthy by this microbiological prevention of infection. Also, he demonstrated that eggs showing external corpuscles could be disinfected by weak solutions of carbolic acid. These disinfected eggs then yielded healthy silkworms. Thus Pasteur, who had solved the nature of fermentation, almost fulfilled in 1865 the prophecy of Robert Boyle in 1663 by coming ever so close to discovering the nature of infectious disease.

Obermeier in 1873 was the first to report a microorganism (spirochete) in the blood of human patients, an organism that later became accepted as the cause of the disease relapsing fever. Unfortunately for Obermeier, the spirochete could not be isolated in pure culture and, in fact, only recently (1971) has one strain of the relapsing fever spirochete been cultivated outside the body of infected hosts.

The rod-shaped organisms reported by Davaine were found in the blood of all animals that were examined while suffering from anthrax. This tended to fulfill the first requirement postulated by Henle for establishing the etiology of a specific disease. It remained for Robert Koch in 1876 to report his studies on the isolation and cultivation of the anthrax bacilli in sterile drops of beef serum or, preferably, aqueous humor from the eyes of freshly slaughtered cattle or sheep. These drops were placed on sterile microscopic slides, inoculated with blood or spleen fragments from infected animals, and covered with sterile cover glasses. The preparations were kept in moist chambers to prevent drying and were examined microscopically at intervals to note purity, growth, morphological changes, spore formation, and other cultural characteristics of the microorganisms. These isolated cultures satisfied Henle's second requirement for etiology determination. Both the infected tissue material and the isolated cultures were shown to be capable of infecting and causing disease in experimental animals (mice in this case) when inoculated under the skin. Thus Henle's third requirement for the establishment of etiology was satisfied. Koch then carried his experiments further and showed

that he could reisolate identical microorganisms from the experimentally infected animals and that the disease could be passed serially through at least 20 animals by the inoculation of infected spleen material from each preceding case. Koch in 1876 thus became the first to apply Henle's postulates by establishing the etiology of anthrax. He thereby proved the germ theory of infectious disease. Since Koch performed the experiments and added to Henle's requirements, many workers have designated these etiology requirements as the Koch postulates. But in deference to professors who teach, it would be more appropriate to designate them the Henle-Koch postulates.

Following Koch's report, the bacterial etiology of many human diseases was rapidly established. W. Bullock in his history of bacteriology designated the period 1876–1880 as "the heyday of bacterial aetiological discovery." There are some pathogenic bacteria (leprosy bacilli and syphilis spirochetes and others), however, which have never been cultivated in their virulent form free of host tissue. Therefore diseases caused by these and other obligate parasites (rickettsia and viruses) cannot have their etiology established by the Henle-Koch requirement for isolation in pure culture. Other methods, including immunological procedures, have been adapted to establish the etiology of diseases caused by these obligate parasites.

Many new developments of historical significance in medical microbiology have taken place since 1876. We will mention only a few. Pasteur continued his work in the microbiology of diseases and by chance propelled himself into research on immunology. Working with a bacterial disease of chickens commonly called chicken cholera, he used a culture of the cholera bacillus that routinely infected and killed exposed chickens. While Pasteur was absent from his laboratory for a period of months, the chicken cholera culture dried out somewhat but did not die. When he returned to his studies and inoculated chickens with progeny of the dried culture, the chickens failed to die. For the ordinary microbiologist that would have been the end of that experiment, and both the culture and the chickens would have been discarded. But not for Pasteur. He isolated a fresh strain of the chicken cholera bacillus from a sick chicken and proved its virulence for other chickens. He then inoculated the freshly isolated, virulent strain into the previously inoculated chickens and they survived the inoculation, although control chickens were killed by the same inoculum. In other words, the chickens that survived the previous inoculation of organisms from the old culture had been rendered immune. Pasteur in 1880 reported the results of this experiment; in the report he went on to establish the lengths of time required for the progressive diminution of the virulence and finally the death of the bacterial culture. These studies convinced him that the best vaccines for animal immunization could be produced by weakening the virulence of the pathogen to the point where it would not cause disease even though it was still a living microorganism. This immunological philosophy guided his subsequent contributions to the immunoprophylactic control of anthrax and rabies in animals and immunotherapy in human rabies (see Chapter 35). Koch made major contributions in the field of tuberculosis; they are discussed in Part II.

Friedrich Loeffler (Löffler), in studies of diphtheria reported in the mid-1880s, visualized a toxin produced by the diphtheria bacilli at their localized site of infection as the cause of the major systemic pathology of the disease. Roux and Yersin in 1888, however, were the first to demonstrate that the diphtheria bacillus could produce, in a broth culture, a toxin (exotoxin) that, when freed of the diphtheria bacilli by filtration and injected into susceptible animals, produced the generalized pathology of diphtheria.

Shortly after the report by Roux and Yersin, a German worker by the name of Emil Von Behring in collaboration with a Japanese worker named Kitasato in 1890–1892 reported one of the truly great discoveries of early medical history. They noted that if they gave repeated sublethal injections of either tetanus or diphtheria toxin to animals, the animals not only developed immunity to the respective toxins but

the serum of the immunized animal would neutralize the respective toxins and would protect other animals against lethal doses of the toxins. The responsible serum component, called *antitoxin*, was recognized as not only the first but the only specific therapy for these diseases (and it continues to be so to date).

Chamberland in 1884 reported the invention of a filter designed to remove bacteria from water, and this was the filter used by Roux and Yersin to obtain diphtheria toxin. In 1892 a Russian named Iwanowski (Ivanowski) reported that the sap of tobacco leaves infected with mosaic disease retained its infectious properties after filtration through Chamberland filters even though no bacteria could be found in the filtrate. Iwanowski was reluctant to come to the right conclusion in interpreting his results, and their significance went unnoticed by the scientific world. In 1898, however, two independent studies were reported that did indicate the significance of Iwanowski's results. Loeffler and Frosch showed that lymph from vesicles of foot-and-mouth disease of cattle and hogs was infectious both before and after filtration through Chamberland filters. Again, however, these workers were more concerned with establishing that the filter-passing agent was not a toxin, rather than discovering its true nature. Beijerinck, that same year, reported extensive studies on the filterability and diffusibility of the infectious agent of tobacco mosaic disease. He came to the conclusion that the infectious agent of this disease was a "living liquid virus." Thus was the significance of viruses in plant, animal, and later human disease first recognized.

Theobald Smith was born in Albany, New York, and received his medical training at Albany College and graduate training at Cornell University. He joined the newly organized U.S. Bureau of Animal Industry, and in 1889 he and F. L. Kilborne began studying a disease called Texas cattle fever. Within three years Smith and his associate had established that the disease was caused by microorganisms found in the red blood corpuscles of sick animals that were transmitted from animal to animal by cattle ticks. In 1893 these workers published an extensive bulletin on this disease, providing one of the earliest studies to focus attention upon the transmission of disease by bloodsucking ecto-parasites—arthropod vectors. These studies led to the extensive cattle dipping program that eventually eliminated the disease from the Texas herds.

Elie Metchnikoff in 1899, after studies on the water flea *Daphnia* infected with yeast cells, reported the phenomenon of phagocytosis, which was soon observed in white blood cor-puscles and other animal phagocytic cells. Metchnikoff advocated the concept that the extent of symptoms and final outcome of any disease was the consequence of the competition between the pathogenic microorganisms and the host phagocytic cells. Others reported that blood serum free of phagocytic cells, and partic-ularly the serum of immune animals, could destroy pathogenic microorganisms. After Von Behring and Kitasato reported the antitoxic activity of serum from immunized animals, a number of investigators reported evidence of the development of other types of antibody in the sera of immunized animals. One of the first to advance both the theoretical and the applied aspects of this new science of serology was Jules Bordet. Between 1895 and 1899 at the Pasteur Institute in Paris and later at his own institute in Brussels he discovered the immunocidal and immunolytic properties of a labile component of fresh normal serum which he called "alexin," but which Paul Ehrlich later designated *comple-ment.* He noted that the complement (alexin) was fixed by antigen-antibody reaction complexes regardless of whether the antigen was a living or dead organism or a soluble antigen. This led him and his colleague to develop the complement fixation test, which is used widely in the sero-diagnosis of disease.

Paul Ehrlich started working with Von Behring on diphtheria toxin-antitoxin produc-tion and standardization and advocated immu-nological theories, some aspects of which still stand. However, his greatest contribution to medical microbiology was his initiation of the synthetic chemotherapeutic approach to the healing of disease. He searched for a "magic bullet" to heal disease. Ehrlich and his col-leagues in the chemical industry synthesized hundreds of chemical compounds that were routinely tested for toxicity in normal animals and therapeutic efficacy in infected animals. Some of his organic arsenicals showed evidence of therapeutic value against animals infected with trypanosomes (African sleeping sickness) and one (number 606, an arsphenamine) proved effective in the treatment of syphilis.

F. W. Twort in 1915 reported a filterable agent that, when added to a vigorously growing young culture of micrococci, brought about the rapid disintegration and death of the bacterial cells. In 1917 Felix d'Herrelle rediscovered Twort's filterable, bacteriolytic agent and desig-nated it bacteriophage. His strain of the lytic agent was active against Shiga dysentery bacilli. D'Herrelle published extensively and gained quite a reputation for his research on bacterio-phage. He visualized the possibility that the outcome of a bacterial disease could depend upon whether the bacterium or the specific bacteriophage got the upper hand in the infected host. He advocated treating bacterial diseases with specific bacteriophages. Unfortunately, bacteriophages that were effective in test tubes showed no therapeutic value in patients. Bac-teriophages have, however, become one of the favorite tools for the study of genetic phenom-ena, a usage that has resulted in the award of several Nobel prizes. Moreover, they are used for identifying subgroup biotypes (phage types) of several pathogenic bacterial species.

Alexander Fleming in 1929 reported the production by a species of the fungal genus *Penicillium* of a soluble substance that was highly bactericidal for staphylococci, streptococci, and certain other pathogenic bacteria. He called the substance penicillin and reported that it was relatively nontoxic in experimental animals. Among other uses, he suggested that penicillin might be effective in the treatment of diseases caused by organisms that were susceptible to it. There the matter stood until Florey and his group at Oxford undertook further studies in the late 1930s. They grew large quantities of the mold in broth cultures and developed methods of concentrating and partially purifying the penicillin. They proved the nontoxicity of large doses in experimental animals and the therapeutic efficacy of the penicillin in animals infected with species of bacteria that were susceptible to the drug *in vitro*. In 1941 they used their still limited supply of penicillin to treat a case of streptococcal septicemia in a human patient. The clinical response to the treatment was good, but the supply of penicillin was inadequate to produce a cure. Since Great Britain was then involved in World War II, Florey came to America and enlisted the help of the drug industry in the mass production of penicillin. Thus began the extensive search for and discovery of antibiotics for disease therapy. Fleming, Florey, and Chain later shared a Nobel prize in medicine.

After an experimental model of the electron microscope had been produced in Germany, L. Marton of the Radio Corporation of America in 1941 published a description of the first commercial electron microscope. This instrument (see Figure 2-2*d*) provided a tremendously higher magnifying power as compared to the best light microscopes and, if the reader will permit a personal aside, thereby made a poor prophet out of my old professor of physics. As a freshman in 1920, I remember his solemnly assuring us that we were seeing images of the smallest objects that would ever be seen. He was a world authority on light and magnification and noted that the wavelength of light was a fixed entity and could not be changed. He also noted that lenses had been ground as small and as perfectly as possible and therefore could not be made to yield greater magnification. The principles on which he based his prediction were sound at that time. He simply did not know about electron beams that could be bent by electromagnets and focused on suitable screens, resulting in the formation of images of infinitely smaller objects than were possible to visualize with the light microscope. We are now commonly seeing images of formerly "submicroscopic" viruses and even some large molecules.

Evidence of the *in vitro* culture of animal tissue (corneal epithelium) and the infection of these cultured tissue cells with vaccinia virus was reported as early as 1913. However, active development of *in vitro* tissue culture media and procedures was delayed until the 1930s and 1940s. One of the early adaptations of the animal tissue culture technique to the propagation of a virus (*Poliovirus*) was that of John Enders in 1949. His report led to the development of mass propagation of poliovirus in monkey kidney tissue culture and made possible the development of the Salk and later Sabin vaccines for the prevention of the crippling disease poliomyelitis. Enders received the Nobel prize for this discovery. In 1954 Enders and Peebles propagated a strain of measles (*Rubeola*) virus in tissue culture and made possible the production of measles vaccine. Additional discoveries of historical significance will be presented as they relate to the individual bacterial, fungal, rickettsial, or viral disease to be considered in subsequent sections of this book.

REFERENCES

Brock, T. 1962. *Milestones in Microbiology.* Washington: American Society for Microbiology.

Bullock, W. 1938. *The History of Bacteriology.* London: Oxford University Press.

Casida, L. E., Jr. 1976. Leeuwenhoek's observation of bacteria. *Science* 192:1348–1349.

Coxe, J. R. 1846. *The Writings of Hippocrates and Galen.* Philadelphia: Lindsay and Blakiston.

Lechevalier, H. A. and M. Solotorovsky. 1965. *Three Centuries of Microbiology.* New York: McGraw-Hill.

Vallery-Rabot, R. 1919. *The Life of Pasteur.* Translated by Mrs. R. L. Devonshire. London: Constable.

3

Principles of Infection

The term *infection* is defined as the invasion, by living organisms, of a part of the body where the conditions are favorable for their growth and possible resultant injury to the tissues. In order of increasing size, the organisms involved in infections range from the smallest viruses (about 10 nanometers) to the rickettsiae, other bacteria, fungi, and protozoa to the largest helminths (parasitic flat- and roundworms), some of which range up to several feet in length. All members of the viruses and rickettsiae (with one possible exception) are *obligate parasites*—that is, they require living host tissues for reproduction. Some of the bacteria, fungi, and protozoa also are obligately parasitic microorganisms, but many are *facultative parasites*—they can grow and reproduce on nonliving culture media. Cultivation on such media is commonly used for

isolation, propagation, identification, and other purposes in clinical and public health laboratories. In all these groups, with the exception of the viruses and rickettsiae, we find many nonparasitic species. Their life-style is *saprophytic.* Saprophytes live on and decompose dead organic matter, either free in nature or within the intestinal tracts or other body cavities of animals. Some microorganisms that commonly lead a saprophytic existence may, however, under special circumstances, infect and cause damage to host tissues. As previously indicated, we will confine our discussions to selected diseases from four of the groups of parasitic microorganisms: bacteria, fungi, rickettsiae, and viruses.

The causative organism of an infectious disease is known as the *etiological agent* of that disease. As noted in Chapter 2, Robert Koch in

1876 was the first to determine the etiology of a bacterial disease when he applied the Henle-Koch postulates to the disease anthrax. Since the second postulate requires the isolation of the infectious organism in pure culture, only diseases caused by facultative parasites can have their etiology established by these postulates. The etiology of viral and other diseases caused by obligate parasites must be established by modifications of the Henle-Koch postulates, including considerable dependence on immunological procedures.

Students who use this book are presumed to have had at least an elementary course in laboratory microbiology. As a consequence, they should be familiar with (1) the inoculation and cultivation of bacteria in at least the simplest sterile nutrient broth media (beef extract, peptone, and water—sterilized at 121°C for 15 minutes) and such a medium solidified with agar; (2) using a sterile bacteriological loop to streak the surface of a nutrient agar plate for isolated colony growth (see Figure 3-1); (3) transplanting such growth from a single colony to tubed broth or agar-slant media for pure

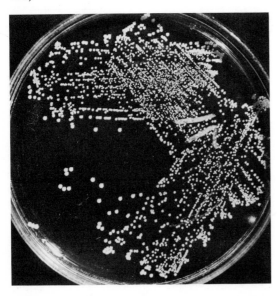

Figure 3–1. Colonies of staphylococci streaked on agar. Note isolated colonies arising from single cells. (Courtesy of the Center for Disease Control, Atlanta, GA.)

culture studies; and (4) preparing smears on microslides, staining (gram stain) these smears, and examining them with the oil-immersion objective of a compound microscope. Just as a reminder, gram-positive cells retain the purple color of the crystal violet, whereas gram-negative cells do not, but stain red with the usual counterstain, safranin or basic fuchsin (see Figure C on the back cover). For the formulation and preparation of the more complex media that will be mentioned in Parts II, III, and IV of this book, see Vera and Dumoff (1974). For the preparation of reagents and stains, and for miscellaneous test procedures advocated for the identification of microorganisms, see Paik and Suggs (1974).

ENDOGENOUS AND COMPROMISED HOST INFECTIONS

Figure 1-1 might give the impression that all infections are *exogenous*—that the causative agent is carried by a primary vehicle from an infected host either directly or indirectly to the susceptible host. Although this usually is true, there are increasing numbers of human infections wherein one of the organisms constituting the extensive microflora of the normal human body is able to change its life-style from saprophytic to parasitic, to invade host tissue, and to cause endogenous infection (see Isenberg and Painter 1974).

These endogenous infections bring into focus another potential misinterpretation of Figure 1-1: the fact that not all susceptible human hosts exhibit the same degree of natural susceptibility or resistance to infection. Human hosts who appear normal may have their resistance to infection compromised in a variety of ways. Individuals designated agammaglobulinemic are inherently unable to produce gamma globulin antibody (see Chapter 4). Consequently they are more susceptible than normal persons to diseases that are suppressed by that antibody. Some human hosts have their normal resistance to infection compromised by chemotherapy, which tends to destroy the normal bacterial flora of the intestinal tract. This permits endogenous yeasts that are not destroyed by the therapy (but are suppressed by the normal intestinal bacteria) to flourish and cause a serious fungal infection of the gastrointestinal tract. Severely burned patients frequently suffer serious infections with normally saprophytic species of the bacterial genera *Pseudomonas* and *Proteus*. Finally, the increasing practice of human-organ transplants has necessitated efforts to suppress the immunological rejection of the transplant by the recipient. Unfortunately this immunosuppression involves a concurrent suppression of the patient's immune response to infection. Consequently the patient may retain the transplanted organ only to succumb as a result of either an endogenous or exogenous infection.

VIRULENCE

The pathology of a disease involves evidence of the structural or functional damage done to tissues of the infected host. Different strains of the same disease-causing organism can vary in their capacity to produce pathological effects. These differences in pathogenicity tend to correspond to the relative *virulence* of the strains of the infectious agent. Different strains of the same pathogenic species can range from highly virulent to weakly virulent to avirulent. The practice of variolation (Chapter 2), using matter from a mild case of smallpox, was based on this natural variation in the virulence of different strains of the smallpox virus. The clinical symptoms of an infectious disease depend upon the site and extent of pathological damage caused by the infectious organism.

The pathogenic organisms produce pathological effects almost invariably by means of chemical poisons known as *toxins*. Two types of bacterial toxins have long been established— they originally were designated *exotoxins* and *endotoxins* according to the ease with which they could be separated from live bacterial cells by the filtration of broth cultures of the producing organisms. Classic examples of exotoxins are those involved in diphtheria and tetanus. Endotoxins are not found in broth culture filtrates

unless many of the cultured cells have undergone death and disintegration prior to filtration. Typhoid and diseases produced by many other gram-negative organisms involve endotoxins in their pathogenicity. There are more significant differences between these two types of toxin than ease of separation from the cells. Exotoxins in general are simple proteins, whereas endotoxins are lipopolysaccharide complexes. This chemical difference would be of little pathological significance if it were not for the more fundamental immunological differences. Both types of toxin, upon repeated sublethal injections into animals, will stimulate the production of serum antitoxins. The antitoxins can be demonstrated by their neutralization of homologous (but not heterologous) toxin; that is, diphtheria toxin is neutralized by diphtheria antitoxin but not by tetanus antitoxin and vice versa. However, the really fundamental difference between the two types of toxin is the fact that exotoxins can be totally neutralized (in multiple proportions) by homologous antitoxin, whereas endotoxins are only partially (about 80 percent) neutralized by their antitoxins. Thus 1, 10, 100, or more lethal doses of an exotoxin can be neutralized by corresponding increases in the amount of antitoxin used. A lethal dose is defined as the smallest amount of the toxin that will kill the test animal. Since about 20 percent of the toxicity of an endotoxin is not neutralized by homologous antitoxin, however, only one to four lethal doses can be neutralized to the extent of preventing death of the test animal. When the amount of toxin exceeds five lethal doses, no amount of antitoxin will prevent death of the test animal.

Exotoxins frequently show specific tissue toxicities. Diphtheria toxin, for example, interferes with the capacity of susceptible cells to synthesize proteins. One tetanus toxin is a neurotoxin. Some exotoxins are cardiotoxic; others (hemolysins) attack erythrocytes. Some certainly are enzymes such as the lecithinases of the histiolytic anaerobic bacteria of Chapter 37. These enzymes attack the lecithin component of muscle cell membranes, thereby causing necrosis (death and disintegration) of the tissues.

There are many other enzymes produced by disease organisms, some of which may participate in the overall pathology of the diseases: proteinases, hyaluronidase, fibrinolytic and other kinases, nucleotidases (leucocidins), reductases, and deoxyribonucleases (see Chapter 8). Some noninfectious bacteria and fungi produce *enterotoxins* that cause food poisoning (see Chapter 28).

Another factor that has been correlated with virulence is the capsule that surrounds some pathogenic organisms. Encapsulated pneumococci (Chapter 7), for example, are highly virulent for experimental animals, whereas the same strain of pneumococcus without these surface structures is relatively avirulent. Moreover, the presence or absence of certain surface antigens (see Chapter 4)—commonly designated the Vi antigen—is correlated with strain virulence or avirulence. Typhoid bacilli tend to show this correlation. Invasiveness likewise constitutes a factor in the virulence and pathogenicity of disease organisms. Lack of this factor may prevent an otherwise highly virulent (toxigenic) organism from penetrating or eroding surface or lining membranes, thereby preventing pathogenic disease in the host. Such organisms may be carried on mucus or other membranes for prolonged periods. The mechanism whereby each pathogenic organism produces its pathology, if known, is discussed with the individual diseases in Parts II, III, and IV of this book.

SYNERGISTIC PATHOLOGY

In the early 1930s R. E. Shope reported that two organisms (a virus and a bacterium) could produce a serious disease in swine (swine influenza) whereas neither organism alone produced the typical disease. Since the capacity of two organisms to bring about a reaction that neither alone can accomplish is known as synergism, we may designate this phenomenon *synergistic pathology*. There are no proved instances of synergistic pathology in humans, but many human infections predispose the patient to more serious complicating infections with other pathogenic organisms. The mechanisms whereby these predispositions or synergisms are brought about are not understood.

MEASURING VIRULENCE

The ease or difficulty of measuring the virulence of an isolated organism depends upon the pathogenic mechanism of the isolate. If most or all of the damage in the infected host is due to an exotoxin produced by the organism, the capacity of the isolated organism to produce this exotoxin can be measured with ease. Such laboratory procedures—toxigenicity or virulence tests—are commonly called for in determining the time of release of patients from quarantine in diphtheria. If the disease organisms produce the pathological effects by means of endotoxins or by unknown mechanisms, about the only way of establishing the virulence of the isolated organism is by determining the *average infectious dose* (ID/50) of the isolate for a susceptible host animal. This requires the determination of the smallest quantity of the culture (the number of cells) required to infect 50 percent or more of the experimental animals receiving that dose. This procedure is rarely used except in research experiments.

INTENTIONAL REDUCTION OF VIRULENCE

In developing live-organism vaccines for animal or human immunization, it frequently has been necessary to start with a virulent pathogen from a case of the disease and by various types of treatment to diminish the virulence to the point where, even though the organism infects and grows in the tissues of the host animal, it does not cause serious disease. Pasteur, for example, found that aging his broth cultures of organisms causing chicken cholera did not kill them but weakened them to the point where they would stimulate an immune response without causing disease. He showed that growing anthrax bacilli at temperatures above or below optimum tended to produce similar results. In developing his rabies vaccine, he dried the rabbit spinal cord containing the virulent virus and thereby weakened the virus. Passing infectious organisms from natural to unnatural hosts, or culturing the organisms on suboptimum media, has also, on occasion, resulted in depressed virulence for disease organisms. These practices are restricted to the activities of research scientists in their attempts to develop new vaccines or immunogens for disease prevention.

VARIATIONS OF VIRULENCE

Natural variation in the virulence of infectious organisms, as previously indicated, is known to occur. In some instances these variations are correlated with visual or other easily demonstrable changes in isolated pure cultures of the organisms. One of these virulence changes is associated with the colony characteristics of the isolate when grown on agar media. The colony of a virulent typhoid bacillus shows a smooth (S) glistening surface, for example. When this organism loses virulence, the colonies may show a rough (R) nonglistening surface. Beta-hemolytic streptococci give almost the reverse of these appearances; colonies of these virulent organisms show a matted, nonglistening appearance, whereas colonies of nonvirulent streptococci show a glistening surface. Thus by merely looking at the colonies of such organisms conclusions can be drawn relative to the virulence or avirulence of the strain represented by that colony. Also, as indicated above, capsules can be demonstrated on virulent pneumococci and Vi antigen is found on virulent typhoid bacilli. Moreover, organisms that depend upon exotoxin or enzyme production for their virulence become avirulent if they lose the capacity to produce these toxins or enzymes. For recent developments in the areas of microbial toxins, virulence, and pathogenic mechanisms, see Schlessinger (1975).

EPIDEMIOLOGY OF DISEASE-CAUSING ORGANISMS

Although parasitic microorganisms may survive for varying periods of time outside the bodies of infected hosts, very few retain the capacity to grow and reproduce in such environments. Therefore the major ultimate sources of exoge-

nous parasitic microorganisms are infected hosts. Exceptions to this rule are found among the pathogenic fungi (Chapter 21) and the spore-forming anaerobes (Chapter 37). Obligate parasites and others that will reproduce only in host tissues or laboratory media are carried from the infected host by one or more of the primary vehicles: secretions (saliva, milk, mucus); excretions (feces, urine); exudates (pus, serous fluids); or infected tissue (blood, meat). These infected primary vehicles may carry the infectious agents directly to the portal of entry of the susceptible host by physical contact (for example, by kissing, by coughing and sneezing in immediate proximity, or by sexual intercourse). The infected primary vehicles, however, particularly saliva, excreta, and exudates, might contaminate many types of environmental objects such as fingers, food, eating utensils, water, flies, or toys. These contaminated secondary vehicles may then carry the infectious agents to the portal of entry of susceptible hosts. As previously stated, good secondary vehicles are environmental objects that are frequently contaminated with primary vehicles and that rapidly pass on the contamination to the portal of entry of the susceptible host. The bloodsucking (hemophagus) arthropod ectoparasitic vectors are ideal secondary vehicles.

Parasitic organisms tend to develop a variety of specific adaptations to hosts, host tissues, and vectors. An essential survival adaptation on the part of the parasite is invasion of tissues that either will serve as the primary vehicle or will permit the shedding of the parasite into a primary vehicle. All such organisms for which blood serves as the primary vehicle, for example, must spend part or all of their parasitic existence in the bloodstream. Other pathogens may never or may only transiently penetrate the bloodstream. Although many species of ectoparasites may ingest blood containing organisms of a given disease, these organisms frequently adapt to only one or a few species of these ectoparasites, which thereby become the specific vectors of that disease. The *Anopheles* mosquito, for example, is the major vector of *Plasmodium* species that cause human malaria. For a more detailed discussion of the principles of epidemiology of infectious diseases, see Anderson (1965).

TAXONOMY OF DISEASE-CAUSING ORGANISMS

Parts II, III, and IV give the taxonomic designations for the causative organisms of individual infectious diseases in terms of the accepted genus and species names. In technical writing, the first letter of the name of the genus is always capitalized and the name is spelled out the first time it is used. Afterwards it can be abbreviated by using the capitalized first letter only. The species name is always spelled out with all letters lowercase. Also, both the genus and species names are italicized in printed text. In typed or written manuscripts, the need for italics can be indicated by underlining the names of the genus and species—for example, Salmonella (S.) typhi.

It is beyond the scope of this book to give even a detailed outline of the taxonomic classification of all the pathogenic organisms to be considered. Such a classification of division II (bacteria and rickettsia) of the kingdom Procaryotae can be found in *Bergey's Manual* and in the medical microbiology textbooks listed in the general references at the end of Chapter 1. Although the taxonomic classification of the viruses has made significant advances during the past few decades—due largely to the efforts of the International Committee on the Taxonomy of Viruses (ICTV)—no complete taxonomic code of the viruses is yet available. See Fenner (1976) and other references at the end of Chapter 11 for the current status of viral taxonomy. For aspects of the taxonomy of the pathogenic fungi, see references at the end of Chapter 21.

All microbial taxonomists classify the pathogenic microorganisms into phyla, subphyla, classes, orders, families, subfamilies or tribes, genera, and species. Some of these groupings have characteristic suffixes. Orders, for example, always end in the suffix -ales— Eubacteriales, Rickettsiales, Spirochaetales, Haplovirales. Bacterial, fungal, and rickettsial families always end in the suffix -aceae—Bacillaceae, Enterobacteriaceae, Rickettsiaceae. Viral families, however, end in the suffix -adae—

Adenoviridae, Picornaviridae, Poxviridae. A most helpful recommendation of the ICTV was that all virus genus names end in the suffix -virus—Herpesvirus, Influenzavirus, Poliovirus, Poxvirus, Rabiesvirus. Thus many of the names commonly used in the past only as descriptive designations—polio virus, rabies virus, and others—now assume the formal status of generic designations.

A taxonomic species frequently is divisible into strain differences. If the strain differences within the species are demonstrable by serological reactions (see Chapter 4), the strains are called *serotypes*. If the differences are demonstrated by other biological phenomena (not serological), the strains that subdivide the species may be designated *biotypes*. A good example of the proper approach to serotype differentiation and designation is found in Chapter 7: The single species *Streptococcus pneumoniae* has been gradually expanded from the originally recognized 3 to a current 92 serotypes, each dependent upon the synthesis of chemically distinct capsules. Thus we have *S. pneumoniae* types 1, 2, 3, . . ., 92. By contrast, an example of the improper taxonomic use of serotype designation is found in Chapter 24 dealing with serotypes of the genus *Salmonella*. Prior to the introduction of serotype procedures, members of this genus were given medically significant species designations such as *S. typhi, S. paratyphi, S. enteritidis, S. typhimurium, S. cholerasuis,* and others. Thereafter, each newly discovered serotype strain of the genus was given a comparable species-type name, not a number designation as was the practice with serotypes of *S. pneumoniae*. Consequently we have many hundreds of designated species of the genus *Salmonella*, a great many of which do not justify distinct species status.

A good example of biotype strain differences within species is found in the area of susceptibility to bacteriophages (phage typing). Different virulent (Vi) strains of the *Salmonella typhi* species, for example, are susceptible to attack and lysis by certain phages and not others that attack different phage types of *S. typhi*. The same situation is true for the taxonomic species *Staphylococcus aureus* and for other taxonomic species. One biotype of *S. aureus*, phage type 80/81, some years back became a serious problem in hospital-associated infections (see Chapter 20). Another common biotype differential within species is strain differences in susceptibility or resistance to antibiotics or other chemotherapeutic agents. Biotyping and serotyping of isolated pathogenic organisms mainly are helpful to the epidemiologist involved in tracking down sources of infection.

TYPES OF INFECTION

The site and extent of tissue damage caused by an infectious organism determine the symptoms, if any, of the disease and the ultimate consequences of the infection. The possible types of infection relative to pathology and symptomatology are summarized below.

Symbiotic infections are infections in which both the host and the "parasite" benefit. There are no known examples of this type in the animal kingdom, but such infections do occur in leguminous plants. Bacteria of the genus *Rhizobium* infect the root hairs of the plant, stimulating a typical hypertrophy of tissue response comparable to an infectious wart. However, the resulting nodule provides housing and nutrient for the infecting bacteria. The bacteria, in return, can fix atmospheric nitrogen (which the plants cannot do) and turn it over to the host plant in the form of nitrates. Although commensal associations beneficial to both the bacterium and the animal host are well known (for instance, bacteria in the gut that produce vitamin K), these are not true infections.

Subclinical infections involve true tissue invasion and possible multiplication of the infectious agent, but pathological damage, if any, is insufficient to be recognized as symptoms of disease. Some such infections are called latent or quiescent infections. When subclinical infections occur repeatedly, they may stimulate an immune response in the absence of disease symptoms; if they occur in an immune individual, they may boost the level of that person's immunity. This phenomenon has been called *herd immunization*. The causative organisms of a subclinical infection in one individual may cause clinical disease if passed to other susceptible hosts. Subclinical infections, however, differ from the carrier state, which generally does not involve true infection. In carriers the disease organisms usually are carried in body cavities or ducts rather than within the body tissues. The carrier usually is immune to that disease.

Clinical infections are infections in which the resulting damage to the host is sufficient to cause recognizable symptoms of disease. Following the penetration of the infectious agent into one or more tissues, there is an incubation period of variable duration for different diseases, during which time the organisms multiply in the tissues until there is sufficient accumulation of toxic products to result in the onset of the disease symptoms. This onset of symptoms may be sudden, reaching a maximum level within a few hours' time; or the onset may be gradual, reaching a serious level only after days, weeks, or months. In many instances, the onset (*prodromal*) symptoms are too vague and indefinite (nausea, headache, malaise, slight fever, vague aches and pains, loss of appetite) to aid the clinician in making a diagnosis. If the prodromal symptoms are not indicative of the seriousness of the disease, they might be characterized as an *insidious onset*. The major symptoms may be typical or atypical of a disease, depending upon the location and extent of tissue damage caused by the pathogen.

The severity and duration of clinical infections may range from a barely recognizable change from the normal healthy state to severe or even rapidly fatal pathological effects. Some clinical infections are called *chronic* if there are low-grade symptoms over a prolonged period of time. Clinical infections may reach an *acute*, or life-threatening, stage after either a short or long (chronic) duration of symptoms. Other clinical infections may progress with such intensity that they result in overwhelming damage leading to death within a few hours or days without the usual clinical symptoms of the disease. Such infections are called *fulminating*.

A clinical infection that results in a recognizable lesion such as an abscess or other tissue degeneration at the site of invasion is called a *local infection*. If a localized lesion occurs at a tissue site away from the site of invasion, it is called a *focal infection.* Some clinical infections do not result in localized lesions but, instead, spread throughout the tissues; these are termed *generalized infections.* When the organisms causing a local or focal infection break away and spread through the lymphatic or blood channels with the subsequent establishment of multiple foci of infection, the process is termed *metastasis.*

Pathogenic organisms are sometimes transiently carried but do not multiply in the bloodstream—a situation termed a *bacteremia* or *viremia* depending upon the nature of the organism. If the organisms persist or multiply in the bloodstream, the result is a *septicemia.* Bacteremias, viremias, or septicemias can only be established by demonstrating the presence of the pathogen in the blood by culture techniques or by inoculation of the blood specimen into a susceptible animal or tissue culture. If organisms at the site of local infections produce toxins that are disseminated through the bloodstream, the resulting damage and symptoms are those of a *toxemia.*

DIAGNOSIS OF INFECTIOUS DISEASES

The diagnosis of clinical infections depends upon one or more of the following: the recognition of clinical symptoms; laboratory demonstration of the presence of the causative organism; and serological evidence of the immune response of the patient to the infection (see Chapter 4). A *specific diagnosis* is made when the causative organism is definitely identified. An *idiopathic diagnosis* can be made when the cause of the clinical symptoms is unknown and the symptoms might be caused by a variety of different organisms—for example, the broad clinical designation "meningitis," meaning inflammation of the meningeal membranes that envelop the brain and spinal cord, with symptoms that can be caused by many different pathogens. Idiopathic was formerly defined in *Stedman's Medical Dictionary* as "a high flown term for concealed ignorance." A former professor of pathology at a medical school in Texas is reputed to have defined it as "idio—I don't know, and pathic—I don't give a damn."

A term related to diagnosis is *prognosis.* This involves an effort by the attending physician to evaluate the seriousness of the disease in the patient. If the prognosis is good, the physician probably will use only supportive therapy such as bed rest, diet, control of constipation, and an aspirin or two. If the prognosis is bad, the physician is justified in using intensive or heroic therapy such as higher than normal doses of drugs or heart or kidney transplants. The prognosis is always bad for heart patients who need heart transplants. Unfortunately, until the problem of foreign tissue rejection is solved, the prognosis is still bad after the therapy.

Any clinical diagnostician has to make extensive use of the suffix *-itis,* which merely means inflammation or irritation. The clinician can couple this suffix with the designation for organs at the anatomical site of the irritation and give idiopathic designations for dozens of diseases. Starting in the head region we can have an encephalitis, an encephalomyelitis, or a meningitis; an otitis or mastoiditis of the ear region; an iritis or conjunctivitis of the eye; a naritis or lingitis or nasopharyngitis, a parotitis, a tonsilitis, laryngitis, bronchitis, or pneumonitis of the buccal or respiratory region. Moving on down the gastrointestinal tract we can have an oesophagitis, a gastritis, a duodenitis, an ileitis, an appendicitis, a colitis, a proctitis, or an anitis. In the abdominal area we can have a hepatitis, or cholecystitis of the liver, a nephritis or a glomerulonephritis of the kidney, a pancreatitis of the pancreas, or a peritonitis. In the urogenital tract we can have a urethritis, a cystitis, a prostatitis, an orchitis, a vaginitis, a salpingitis, or an ovaritis. When the patient describes symptoms, the clinician can come up with a technical designation for the disease or diseases that might involve organs in the area of irritation and satisfy the patient regarding the doctor's competence. Thereby the clinician gains the necessary time to perform tests and observe additional symptoms necessary for arriving at the *specific* diagnosis often needed for specific therapy.

CHEMOPROPHYLAXIS AND CHEMOTHERAPY

The term *prophylaxis* implies efforts to prevent the development of clinical disease, whereas therapy implies efforts to cure existing clinical disease. Chemoprophylaxis and chemotherapy involve the use of chemical drugs, including antibiotics, in the prevention or cure of infectious diseases. Immunoprophylaxis and immunotherapy involve immunological procedures that are discussed in Chapter 4.

Hippocrates and Galen compiled a pharmacopoeia of herbs, extracts, and various concoctions they believed to be effective in purging or otherwise eliminating the excess humors they considered responsible for human diseases. Paracelsus, in the sixteenth century, added the chemicals mercury and morphine to the medical pharmacopoeia. After the discovery and exploration of the Americas, the Peruvian Indians were found to be using the bark of the cinchona tree to treat malaria successfully. Since this disease was widespread throughout the tropical and temperate areas of the world, and since the etiology of all febrile diseases was unknown prior to the late nineteenth century, the "Peruvian bark" became the drug of choice for treating all fevers, particularly the intermittent fevers. It was effective, however, only in malaria, and this was due to the alkaloid quinine among its other components.

Among the greatest of the contributions to the field of medicine during the twentieth century has been the discovery and production of chemotherapeutic drugs that are effective in preventing and curing infectious diseases. As indicated in Chapter 2, Paul Ehrlich, around the turn of the twentieth century, initiated the synthetic chemical approach to the search for chemotherapeutic agents. His greatest success was his six hundred and sixth test chemical, arsphenamine. This organic arsenical, and modifications of it, remained the drug of choice for the treatment of syphilis and other spirochetal infections until the 1940s.

In the mid-1930s, workers in Germany and France reported that sulfanilamide, a cleavage product of the dye prontosil, was effective in the treatment of a variety of bacterial diseases. D. D. Woods, in 1940, reported that the antibacterial activity of sulfanilamide was due to its interference with the chemically related, essential growth factor para-aminobenzoic acid (PABA). Thus he introduced the concept of chemical-analog competitive inhibition to explain the mode of action of the drug. In other words, the chemical structures of sulfanilamide and PABA are so similar that the bacteria, which required the latter for metabolic survival, were tricked into accepting the therapeutic concentration sulfanilamide, which failed to supply the PABA metabolic requirement. Conversely, the therapeutic efficacy of the sulfanilamide could be reversed by high concentrations of PABA. This concept then led to the synthesis of many modifications of sulfanilamide (the sulfonamides) and to the discovery of other drugs that act as metabolic inhibitors.

During World War II, the sulfonamides, which are effective when taken by mouth, were used extensively by military personnel for the chemoprophylactic suppression of respiratory and other infections that might interfere with the war effort. When one of these sulfonamides, sulfathiazole, proved effective in the treatment of the venereal disease gonorrhea, prostitutes began taking sulfathiazole tablets daily to prevent infection. Within a very few years, the undesirable aspect of this form of chemoprophylaxis became apparent: All gonococci became resistant to sulfathiazole, and clinical cases of gonorrhea could no longer be cured by sulfathiazole therapy. Fortunately, other therapeutic drugs proved to be effective in treating this disease. For a detailed consideration of these and more modern synthetic chemotherapeutic drugs, see Kucers and Bennett (1975).

Webster's dictionary defines *antibiosis* as an antagonistic association between living organisms to the detriment of one of them. I. M. Lewis, the author's first bacteriology professor, demonstrated antibiosis between *Pseudomonas* and other bacterial colonies on agar plate cultures to his classes in the early 1920s. Alexander Fleming in 1929 reported antibiosis between a

Penicillium mold colony and surrounding *Staphylococcus aureus* growth on a nutrient agar plate. When he suggested that the antibiotic product of the mold, which he isolated and called penicillin, might have therapeutic value, the antibiotic era in chemotherapy was conceived. It took a gestation period of another dozen years, however, before the studies of H. W. Florey and his colleagues actually proved the therapeutic efficacy of penicillin and thereby gave birth to the antibiotic era in infectious disease therapy (see Chain 1972). When penicillin production was first started here in the United States, the mold *Penicillium notatum* was grown in flasks, milk bottles, or any containers in which quantities of culture medium could be sterilized, inoculated, and incubated. At this time the crude product was almost prohibitively expensive. The drug industry, however, rapidly adapted volume fermentation procedures involving fermenters with capacities of 100,000 gallons or more, lowering the cost of the product spectacularly. Figure 3-2 illustrates a bank of fermenters currently used in antibiotic production.

The penicillin discovered by Fleming appeared as golden yellow droplets on the surface of the *P. notatum* colony. When harvested, this penicillin was a mixture containing pigment and other impurities as well as four different penicillins, designated F, G, X, and K. When these were separated, penicillin G proved to be the most satisfactory; but when this was purified to the crystalline form, it proved to be a rather unstable acid. When the acid was converted to either the sodium or potassium salt, however, the crystalline sodium or potassium penicillin not only became more stable but was completely soluble in water. Two additional salts of penicillin G, procaine and benzathine, also were stable but far less soluble in water. When these latter crystalline penicillins were suspended and injected intramuscularly, the crystals dissolved slowly in the tissue fluids, providing long-lasting (about 24 hours) therapeutic concentrations of the drug in the blood and tissues of the patient. A number of additional modifications of penicillin G, some semisynthetic, have been developed: One, ampicillin, is widely used and is claimed to have a broader antibacterial spectrum than penicillin G. Some bacteria, particularly staphylococci, tend to develop resistance to penicillins. This resistance frequently is asso-

Figure 3-2.   Worker at the top of a commercial antibiotic fermentation tank. The entire tank is four stories high and has a 150,000-liter capacity. (Photo courtesy of The Upjohn Company.)

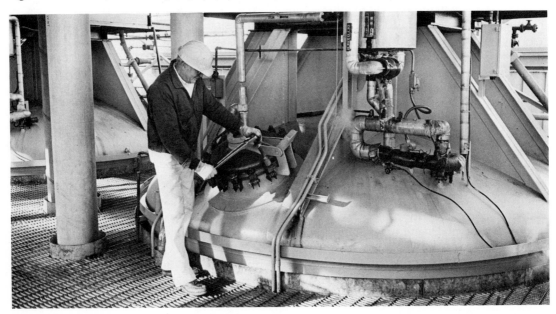

Table 3-1. Antibiotics: source and mode of action.

Antibiotic	Source*	Mode of Action
ANTIBACTERIAL		
Penicillins	M	Inhibit cell-wall synthesis
Cephalosporins	M	Same as penicillins
Aminoglycosides		Inhibit bacterial protein synthesis
Streptomycin	S	
Kanamycin	S	
Gentamycin	B	
Chloramphenicol (chloromycetin)	S syn.	Inhibits bacterial protein synthesis
Clycoserine	S	Interferes with cell-wall synthesis (but differs from action of penicillin and cephalosporins)
Fucidin	M	Inhibits bacterial protein synthesis
Lincomycin	S	Inhibits bacterial protein synthesis
Clindamycin	S	Inhibits bacterial protein synthesis
Macrolides		Interfere with bacterial protein synthesis at ribosomes
Erythromycin	S	
Oleandomycin	S	
Novobiocin	S	Inhibits bacterial cell-wall and nucleic acid synthesis
Polymyxins	B	Damage bacterial plasma membrane
Rifamycins	S	Inhibit bacterial RNA synthesis by binding to DNA-dependent RNA polymerase
Rifamide		
Rifampin		
Spectinomycin	S	Inhibits bacterial protein synthesis
Tetracyclines	S sp.	
Oral (9)		Inhibit bacterial protein synthesis
Parenteral (6)		Broad antibacterial spectrum
Vancomycin	S	Inhibits bacterial cell-wall synthesis
ANTIFUNGAL		
Amphotericin B (fungizone)	S	Interferes with permeability of plasma membrane osmotic barrier
Griseofolvin	M	Unknown—probably interferes with normal DNA replication
Nystatin (topical only)	S	Damages plasma membrane like amphotericin B
Natamycin (topical or oral)	S	Probably similar to amphotericin B

*M = mold; S = streptomyces; B = bacterium; sp. = species; syn. = synthetic.

ciated with the capacity of the bacterium to produce the enzyme penicillinase, which destroys the penicillin.

Following the discovery of penicillin, a worldwide search for other organisms that produce antibiotic substances was initiated. Most of the antibiotic producers were isolated from soil samples. Table 3-1 lists most of the commonly used antibiotics along with their source and mode of antibiotic action. With increasing knowledge of the chemical structure of some of these antibiotics, either partial synthetic chemical modifications (penicillins) or complete chemical synthesis (chloromycetin by Parke Davis) have been achieved. For more detailed considerations of other aspects of the usage of these antibiotics, see Kucers and Bennett (1975). Some of these usages will be discussed as they apply to the individual diseases in Parts II, III, and IV.

ANTIVIRAL DRUGS

In the early 1960s, two synthetic agents were found to exhibit chemoprophylactic activity against viral infections: N-methylisatin-B-thio-semicarbazone (Methisazone), active in preventing smallpox infections; and amantadine hydrochloride (Symmetrel), a preventive of influenza A_2. Neither of these drugs was therapeutically effective once clinical symptoms of the diseases developed.

Walwick et al. in 1959 synthesized a pyrimidine nucleoside analog (Cytarabine—CTB) that was introduced for the treatment of the blood cancer leukemia, and it continues to be a potent drug for this therapy. Cytarabine and another pyrimidine nucleoside analog (Idoxuridine—IDU) were found to inhibit certain DNA viruses both in tissue cultures and in experimental animals. Human eye, skin, and mucus membrane infections caused by Herpesvirus species, cytomegalovirus, and vaccinia virus have been treated topically with both CTB and IDU. The latter drug also has been used parenterally for the treatment of viral encephalitis and other serious systemic diseases caused by the DNA viruses. Nolan et al. (1970), for example, reported good results in the treatment of six cases of Herpesvirus hominis encephalitis parenterally with IDU. Nahmias (1970) advocated the use of IDU for the treatment of DNA virus infections of compromised hosts. Although toxic effects have been encountered in the parenteral use of IDU, the poor prognosis particularly in viral encephalitis (lasting brain damage and high mortality) justifies its use until safer drugs are found.

A purine nucleoside analog (adenine arabinoside—Ara-A) was synthesized in 1960, again as a potential anticancer drug. Ara-A was found to be less toxic than the pyrimidine nucleoside analog and to have a somewhat broader antiviral spectrum. Although diseases caused by these DNA viruses have been primarily involved in Ara-A therapy, the drug has been claimed to be active against one RNA virus, that causing Rous sarcoma. In 1969 Ara-A was found to be a naturally occurring product in cultures of Streptomyces antibioticus, thereby becoming the first potential antiviral antibiotic. See Bauer (1973) for a review of the first decade of antiviral chemotherapy.

REFERENCES

Anderson, G. W. 1965. The principles of epidemiology as applied to infectious diseases. Chapter 38 in Bacterial and Mycotic Infections of Man, 4th ed., R. J. Dubos and J. G. Hirsch (eds.), Philadelphia: Lippincott.

Bauer, D. J. 1973. Antiviral chemotherapy: the first decade. Brit. Med. J. 3:275–279.

Chain, E. 1972. Thirty years of penicillin therapy. J. Roy. Coll. Phycns. 6:103.

Isenberg, H. D. and B. G. Painter. 1974. Indigenous and pathogenic microorganisms of man. Chapter 5 in Manual of Clinical Microbiology.

Kucers, A. and N. M. Bennett. 1975. The Use of Antibiotics. 2nd ed. Philadelphia: Lippincott.

Nahmias, A. J. 1970. Disseminated herpes simplex virus infections. New Eng. J. Med. 282:684–685.

Nolan, D. C., M. M. Carruthers, and A. M. Lerner. 1970. Herpesvirus hominis encephalitis in Michigan: report of thirteen cases, including six treated with idoxuridine. New Eng. J. Med. 282:10–13.

Paik, G. and M. Suggs. 1974. Reagents, stains, and miscellaneous test procedures. Chapter 96 in Manual of Clinical Microbiology.

Schlessinger, D. (ed.). 1975. Microbiology—1975. Washington: American Society for Microbiology.

Vera, Harriette D. and M. Dumoff. 1974. Culture media. Chapter 95 in Manual of Clinical Microbiology.

4

Principles of Immunology and Serology

The science of immunology grew out of the recognition that individuals who had recovered from a disease resisted infection during subsequent exposures to that disease—they were immune. The early awareness of this fact involved the disease smallpox, the scars of which left clear evidence of past infection on the faces of those who recovered and who failed to contract the disease during subsequent epidemics. The field of serology grew out of observed changes in the reactivity of the blood serum of immune individuals, the most spectacular of which was the discovery of diphtheria antitoxin in the serum of immunized animals by Von Behring and Kitasato in 1890. This led to devel-

opments in the science of serology that, in many ways, have outstripped those of the parent science immunology. See Burnet (1976) for a semitechnical overview of the fields of immunology and serology.

TYPES OF IMMUNITY

There are two general types of immunity (resistance to infection). Type 1 is designated *natural immunity* and is based on genetic mechanisms—that is, the genetics of the host and the genetic adaptations of the parasite. Type 2 immunity is designated *acquired immunity* and is based either directly or indirectly on antigenic mechanisms.

37

For the present discussion, antigens may be defined simply as components or products (toxins, enzymes) of disease organisms that stimulate immune responses.

In natural immunity, the genetics of the host determines the chemical makeup of the tissues of that host species. When a parasitic organism undergoes genetic adaptations to survival in the tissues of a host, these adaptations may be specific for the biochemistry of that host and render the parasite incapable of infecting other potential host species. Although humans and dogs are frequently exposed to each other's respiratory diseases, dogs do not contract the humans' common cold and humans do not contract the dogs' distemper. It should be emphasized, however, that many other parasites can infect more than one host species. In fact, one of the parasites that we will consider later (*Francisella tularensis*) is quite cosmopolitan in its ability to infect a variety of both host and vector species. Moreover, there are well-documented instances of natural racial immunities in both the plant and the animal kingdoms. These have been utilized in crossbreeding experiments in plant and animal husbandry. Although claims have been made for racial, family, and individual natural immunities to infectious human diseases, these are difficult to authenticate.

There are two types of acquired immunity: active and passive. In actively acquired immunity, the penetration of the antigen (disease organism or its products) into the animal's tissues stimulates the immune response. The antigen may get into the tissues as a result of a natural infection, wherein the immune response, if adequate, will terminate the infection. Or the antigen (*immunogen* or *vaccine*) in a safe form may be administered orally (live vaccines) or inoculated into the tissues by hypodermic injection. Actively acquired immunity by either mechanism takes weeks or months to acquire; but, once acquired, it usually lasts for months to years. Because of these time relationships, artificial active immunization almost invariably is used prior to exposure to disease. (It is prophylactic or preventive, generally, not curative immunization.) As a result of active immunization, antibodies (globulin molecules with specific re-

active capacity for the antigen) usually appear in measurable amounts in the blood serum of the immunized individual. Some of these antibodies (for example, diphtheria antitoxin) have immunological significance; others do not but may have serodiagnostic significance.

Passively acquired immunity results when serum antibodies, with immunological significance, are introduced into the tissues of previously nonimmune individuals. The tissues of the recipient, therefore, have nothing to do with the production of the immune state but passively accept the preformed antibody immunity. The two ways whereby such antibodies can get into the tissues of the recipient are (1) by passage through the placenta of an immune human mother into the bloodstream of the fetus *in utero* or (2) by artificial inoculation. In cattle the antibodies do not pass the placental barrier but are shed into the colostrum. When the calf ingests this first milk, the antibodies pass the gastrointestinal barrier into the bloodstream. Thus the recipients, at or shortly after birth, are immune to diseases for which their mothers possessed immunologically significant serum antibodies at the time of birth. This immunity lasts for several (2 to 4) months. When antibodies are inoculated for passive immunization, the resulting immunity is available to all body tissues within minutes to hours, depending upon the route of inoculation. This passive immunity, however, lasts a relatively short time, only 2 to 3 weeks, if foreign (horse) serum antibodies are involved. Since this type of immunity is acquired almost immediately upon antibody inoculation, it is commonly used for treatment after the onset of disease symptoms (passive immunotherapy). Unfortunately, relatively few diseases can be cured by this type of therapy. A prognostically serious case of diphtheria, however, can only be cured by passive (antitoxin) immunotherapy.

ANTIGENS, ANTIBODIES, AND THEIR REACTIONS

As stated above, all disease-causing organisms possess antigenic components and many produce soluble antigens such as toxins or enzymes.

In reality practically all foreign proteins, some complex polysaccharides, and some lipopolysaccharide complexes can function as antigens whether or not they are components of pathogenic organisms. In other words, all living things are composed, in part, of antigens that do not function as such in self but will stimulate an immune response in other (nonself) animal species. Thus a general definition of an antigen is any substance that, upon penetration into the tissues of a suitable animal, will stimulate an immune response, frequently resulting in the production of antibodies that will react specifically with that antigen. In addition to antibodies, antigenic stimulation may result in the production of antigen-specific lymphocytes that are involved in a nonantibody type of immune phenomenon—cell-mediated immunity.

As just indicated, antibodies result from antigenic stimulation. Since all antibodies are globulin molecules of one type or another, a general definition of an antibody is a globulin molecule that (1) is produced, in quantity, as a result of the antigenic stimulation of suitable animal tissues and (2) will react specifically with the antigen involved in its production. Electron micrographs (Figure 4-1) indicate that one of the major antibody molecules (7s or IgG) is Y-shaped. The arms of the Y are hinged to the base, however, making it possible for the molecule to assume a variety of angles including a T configuration. Additional considerations of antigen and antibody structure and functions are discussed later in the chapter.

The preceding definitions indicate that homologous antigens and antibodies will react with each other specifically. In fact, the way one can prove that a substance is an antigen is to demonstrate its capacity to stimulate the production of and reaction with homologous antibodies. And the only way that one can establish the presence of a specific antibody in an animal serum is to demonstrate the capacity of that serum to react specifically with a given antigen. These antigen-antibody reactions may be used in the serological diagnosis of disease. In such usage, one principle is paramount: The antigen must be known to be specific for the suspected disease. The patient's serum is the

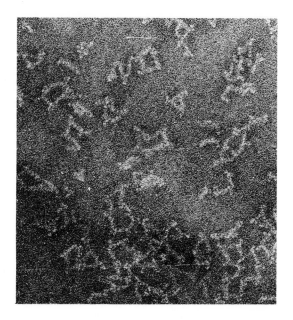

Figure 4–1. Electron micrograph of polymers of the Y-shaped antibody molecule IgG. The ends of the "arms" of a given molecule in this preparation are attached to the arms of other molecules by small, divalent haptens, and the "bases" of the Y's project from the corners of the polygons thus formed. The angle between the arms of the IgG molecules varies from dimer to trimer to tetramer, making it obvious there must be flexible "hinge" regions at the intersection of arms and base. ×400,000. (Courtesy of N.M. Green, National Institute for Medical Research, London.)

unknown in serodiagnosis; the presence of antibody, resulting from the infectious antigen of the suspected disease, is determined by a positive serodiagnostic test. Also, antigen-antibody reactions may be used in the taxonomic identification of an isolated microorganism, which is the unknown antigen for the test. In such usage, the following principle must be observed: The antibody (antiserum) must be known to react specifically with the species of organism the unknown antigen is suspected to be. A positive test result gives serotaxonomic confirmation of the suspicion; for example, an anti—*Salmonella typhi* antiserum is used to give serotaxonomic aid in the identification of an organism suspected to

Table 4-1. Commonly observed antigen-antibody reactions.

GA Reaction Phenomena	Designations		Antigenic Test Material
	Antibody (A)	Antigens (G)	
Agglutination	Agglutinin	Agglutinogen	Cellular antigens
Precipitation or flocculation	Precipitin	Precipitinogen	Soluble antigens
Complement-dependent			
Lysis	Bacteriolysin		Some bacteria
	Hemolysin		Erythrocytes
Death	Bactericidin		Live: bacteria
			Viruses
	Cytotoxic		Tissue cells
Complement fixation			Most antigens
Opsonization	Opsonin		Bacteria
Neutralization	Antitoxin		Toxins
	Antiviral		Viruses
Hypersensitivity			
Immediate	Reagin (IgE)	Allergen	Proteins, pollen, foods, others
Delayed*	No A		Tuberculin, others
Fluorescence	Fluorescent antibody (FA)		Bacteria, rickettsia, fungi, viruses.
Direct test	F-antiorganismal A		Unknown organisms
Indirect test	F-antiglobulin		Known organisms

* Cell-mediated immunity phenomena.

F = fluorescent.

be *S. typhi*. Table 4-1 summarizes the commonly observed antigen-antibody (GA) reaction phenomena and related terminology.

The site on the antigen with which the antibody reacts is designated the *determinant* site; the homologous reactive site on the antibody is designated the *receptor* site. The highly specific primary reaction between these two sites binds the antigen and antibody together and must take place prior to any of the secondary GA reaction manifestations listed in Table 4-1. These secondary phenomena, resulting from reactions between homologous GA mixtures, are discussed below. In serodiagnostic test procedures, including blood typing, the antibody specific for the determinant sites of the known antigen occasionally may be present and react with these sites without manifesting the expected GA reaction phenomenon (for example, agglutination). Such antibody is designated *incomplete* for that particular reaction. Incomplete antibody reacts with and blocks the determinant sites of the antigen and consequently may be designated *blocking* antibody. If suspected, following a negative test result, the presence of blocking antibody in the test serum can be demonstrated by either one of two procedures. The first procedure is to add known complete antibody specific for the test antigen to the negative test preparation and to a tube of untreated test antigen as a control. If, after incubation, the test preparation continues to yield negative results, whereas the control is positive, procedure 1 proves the presence of incomplete (blocking) antibody in the original test serum. Procedure 2 was designed by Coombs and is called the antiglobulin test. Since antibody globulin molecules are proteins, they possess species-specific antigenic determinant sites (located on the base of the Y) in addition to their antibody receptor sites (located at the ends of the arms of the Y). Antiglobulin antibody, therefore, can be produced by immunizing rabbits or other animals with heterologous (for example, human) serum globulin. The antiglobulin antibody will react with determinant sites of homologous species globulin whether the globulin molecules are free in solution or attached as antibody to an antigen (see Figure 4-2). If the negative serodiagnostic test involved a cellular test antigen and homologous incomplete antibody (iA), the iA molecules will be attached to the cells. The cell–iA complex can be sedimented, washed, and resuspended in saline

solution with the iA remaining attached. The addition of homologous antiglobulin will result in a positive agglutination test. If the antiglobulin test is negative, it indicates that there was no iA in the original test serum.

AGGLUTINATION AND PRECIPITATION

When cellular antigens are aggregated as a result of their reaction with homologous antibody, the GA reaction is designated *agglutination.* When the antigen, in a soluble or colloidal state, is aggregated it is designated *precipitation* or *flocculation.* These reactions require the presence of electrolyte, usually isotonic saline (0.85 percent NaCl in water). The agglutination tests may

Figure 4–2. Schematic illustration of Coombs antiglobulin test to determine presence of incomplete (blocking) antibody in human serum.

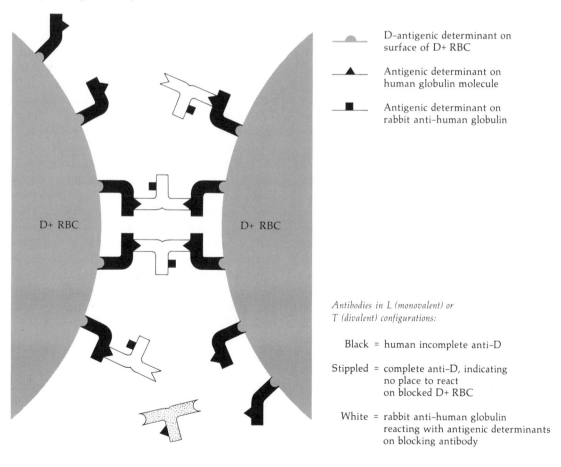

D-antigenic determinant on surface of D+ RBC

Antigenic determinant on human globulin molecule

Antigenic determinant on rabbit anti-human globulin

D+ RBC

D+ RBC

Antibodies in L (monovalent) or T (divalent) configurations:

Black = human incomplete anti-D

Stippled = complete anti-D, indicating no place to react on blocked D+ RBC

White = rabbit anti-human globulin reacting with antigenic determinants on blocking antibody be performed in test tubes, on glass microslides, or on glass or clear plastic plates; the aggregates may be observed macroscopically or microscopically. Precipitation reactions may be performed in small test tubes or in glass capillary tubes. In the latter, rings of precipitate develop at the interface where antigen and antibody meet. Precipitation tests also may be performed in clear agar gels after allowing the antigen and antibody to diffuse toward each other through the gel. In this test, lines of precipitate develop where the two reagents meet in suitable concentrations. These are designated *gel precipitation* tests.

COMPLEMENT-DEPENDENT GA REACTIONS

Cellular antigens may be lysed and living organismal antigens may be killed as the result of GA reactions if complement (C') is present to result in a GAC' reaction complex. Lytic (bacteriolytic or hemolytic) reactions require that the cellular antigens be suspended in an isotonic solution and that in addition to specific antibody, complement must be present. Complement is a very complex (at least nine components), labile entity of fresh normal serum. Guinea pig serum usually is used as complement in serological testing procedures. A positive GAC' lytic reaction is indicated by disintegration of the cells. If the cells are erythrocytes (red blood cells), the reaction is designated *hemolysis.* Lysis of living cell antigens (bacteriolysis), of course, results in their death. However, some live bacteria and viruses may be killed by homologous antibody and complement without undergoing microscopically visible lysis. To determine a positive bactericidal reaction, without lysis, one must demonstrate either immobilization of motile organisms or failure of the test organisms to grow on suitable culture media. Virucidal reactions may be performed by demonstrating the incapacity of the virus–antibody–complement mixture to infect susceptible animals or tissue cultures, whereas control mixtures without antibody prove infective.

The GA reaction complex of practically any antigen, after reacting with homologous antibody, will fix (tie up) complement present in the reaction environment. Since this fixation of complement may not give visible evidence of a positive GA reaction, Bordet and his colleagues devised a complement fixation test involving two GA systems. The test system consists of a mixture of antigen and antibody—one of which must be of known identity. The tube containing the test G and A then receives a suitable aliquot of C' and the mixture, along with the necessary controls, is placed at 4–6°C for about 17 hours. If at the end of this time no visible evidence of a GAC' reaction can be observed, an indicator GA system is added to the tube containing the test system. The indicator G usually is a suspension of sheep red blood cells (RBC). The indicator A (hemolysin) is the serum from a rabbit that has been "immunized" with sheep RBC and which, in a control, can be shown to contain antibody that reacts with the RBC and C' to give visible hemolysis. This fivefold test mixture and the necessary control mixtures are incubated at 37°C for 1 hour. If the test system (which includes the only unknown) consists of a homologous GA mixture, the GA complex will fix C' during the 4–6°C incubation and free C' will not be present to react with the indicator system. Therefore there will be no hemolysis of the sheep RBC, a result that indicates a positive (reactive) test (see Figure A on the front cover). If the test system does not contain homologous G and A, there will be no GA reaction and no C' fixation during the 4–6°C incubation. Therefore the C' will be present to enter into the indicator GAC' reaction and cause hemolysis of the sheep RBC. This hemolysis indicates a negative (nonreactive) test system result. For a comprehensive discussion of complement, including both its beneficial as well as detrimental participation in immunological phenomena, see Bellanti (1971) and Hobart and McConnell (1975).

OPSONIC GA REACTIONS

After Metchnikoff demonstrated the phenomenon of phagocytosis (the ingestion of bacteria and other organisms by phagocytic cells, including white blood corpuscles) others observed that the rate of phagocytosis could be increased significantly, *in vitro*, if antibody specific for the bacteria was added to a mixture of bacteria and phagocytic cells. Moreover, the addition of complement further enhanced the rate of phagocytosis. To perform the test, the three- or fourfold test mixture and a two- or threefold (no antibody) control mixture in separate equal-volume preparations are incubated for equal times at 37°C. Each mixture is then spread and fixed on separate microslides; after drying, each is stained with a polychromatic (Wright or Giemsa) stain and examined microscopically. The deeply stained bacteria can be seen and counted in the lightly stained cytoplasm of the phagocytic cells (usually polymorphonuclear leucocytes). If the test serum contained antibody specific for the test antigen (bacterial cells), a significantly greater number of bacteria will be ingested per leucocyte in the test mixture as compared to the control mixture. At least 100 leucocytes from each mixture must be counted. This GA test is rarely used in routine clinical laboratory procedures.

GA NEUTRALIZATION REACTIONS

As previously stated, Von Behring and Kitasato were the first to show that immune serum antibody (antitoxin) would neutralize homologous toxin. If the indication of toxicity is death of the test animal or of cultured tissue cells, suitable amounts of the antitoxin will neutralize the toxin and prevent death. If the indication of toxicity is an inflammatory skin reaction, this reaction can be prevented by the use of homologous antitoxin. If the indication of toxicity is hemolysis of certain animal erythrocytes, this hemolysis can be prevented by homologous antitoxin. These reactions are used extensively in the commercial production of antitoxins and other immunobiological products and, to a lesser but significant extent, in public health and clinical laboratory work.

The capacity of viruses to infect experimental animals or tissue culture cells can be neutralized (inhibited) by homologous antiviral antibody. If the virus infection in control animals results in death, the survival of the test animals that receive the antibody is evidence of the neutralization of the virus. An *in vitro* manifestation of the presence of certain viruses in test specimens was observed by G. K. Hirst in 1941. He reported that influenza virus, in infected chick embryo fluid, agglutinated chicken erythrocytes. This reaction is designated *viral hemagglutination* (HA). Homologous antiviral antibody added to the virus prior to adding the red blood cells will neutralize (inhibit) the capacity of the virus to cause HA. This GA reaction is designated *hemagglutination inhibition* (HI).

HYPERSENSITIVITY

Tissues of an individual may become hypersensitive to a great variety of antigens as a consequence of repeated superficial exposures (pollens, foods, drugs), a single parenteral inoculation (foreign antiserum), microbial infections, or organ transplants. The antigen involved in these hypersensitivities is designated *allergen.* These hypersensitivities have long been known as either *immediate type* (ITH) or *delayed type* (DTH) on the basis of the time required for the onset of the reaction following exposure of the hypersensitive tissues to the allergen. As implied, the allergic reaction in ITH occurs within minutes; that in DTH usually requires 24 to 48 hours or longer following exposure to the allergen. Individuals classed as ITH have small quantities of a special type of antibody (reagin or IgE) in their sera that tends to attach to and to sensitize the tissues to the homologous allergen. In contrast, no serum antibody is demonstrable in the DTH individual. The hypersensitivity that develops in a clinical case of tuberculosis is the classic example of DTH. Although there is no humoral antibody, lymphoidal cells from the DTH individual can passively transfer this type of hypersensitivity to a nonhypersensitive recipient. During the past decade this DTH has been expanded to include a number of immunological phenomena classified as cell-mediated immunity, which is discussed later in the chapter.

FLUORESCENT ANTIBODY REACTIONS

A. H. Coons and his associates in 1941 reported that a fluorescent dye (fluorescein isothiocyanate) could be coupled to specific antibody globulin without affecting the capacity of the antibody to react with its homologous antigen. To perform the test, a smear of an organismal antigen is fixed on a glass microslide and allowed to react with a known fluorescent antibody (FA). After washing and drying, the preparation is examined with an ultraviolet-light microscope. If the FA is specific for the antigen, the GFA complex will fluoresce as a result of the GA reaction. If the antigen is not specific for the FA, no GA reaction will occur and the antigen will not fluoresce under ultraviolet light. This test can be done directly, as described here, using a known antibody (FA) to identify an unknown organismal antigen. This is FA serotaxonomy.

In FA serodiagnosis, an indirect test is used. As in all serodiagnostic tests, the patient's serum is tested for the presence or absence of antibody resulting from a suspected disease. The test organismal antigen known to be specific for the patient's suspected disease, is spread and fixed on a microslide, the patient's serum is added, and time is allowed for a GA reaction to take place. The excess serum is washed off and the antibody globulin, originally in the serum, will be attached to the surface of the antigen on the slide. However, this cannot be observed under either bright-light or ultraviolet-light microscopic examination. Therefore, to determine whether or not antibody specific for the test antigen was present in the patient's serum and is attached to the test antigen, the preparation is flooded with fluorescent anti–human globulin. This antibody will react with human globulin even though the latter is attached as antibody to the test antigen. After a suitable time for the FA reaction, the preparation is washed, dried, and examined with an ultraviolet-light microscope. If there was homologous antibody in the patient's serum, the antigen will fluoresce under the ultraviolet light; if not, there will be no fluorescence. Since the fluorescent anti–human globulin is an anti–"*auntibody*," some wits have chosen to call it an "unclebody."

IMMUNOBIOLOGY OF ANTIGENS

Antigens can stimulate animal tissues to produce homologous antibodies with which the antigen will react in one or more of the GA reactions described above. Such antigens are designated *complete* antigens. Biologically, they must be foreign to the animal's tissues; chemically, they are either proteins, complex polysaccharides, or lipopolysaccharide complexes. They all are macromolecules of greater than 5,000 to 10,000 molecular weight.

Another group of compounds is known that fit only the reactivity portion of the antigen definition. These substances, when not part of a complete antigen, will not stimulate animal tissues to produce antibodies. If antibodies are produced by a complete antigen composed in part of the partial antigen, however, the latter by themselves will react with the antibodies. K. Landsteiner coined the term *hapten* for such a partial antigen (a polysaccharide), which he isolated from the capsules of pneumococci. When intact pneumococcal cells were used to immunize rabbits, antibodies were produced that reacted with the capsular polysaccharides whether attached to or separated from the pneumococcal cells. When Landsteiner injected the purified capsular polysaccharides into rabbits, no antibody was produced. A few years later, O. T. Avery and W. F. Goebel confirmed Landsteiner's findings insofar as the rabbit was concerned. However, these workers showed that the purified polysaccharides would stimulate antibody production in mice and humans and in some other animals. In other words, the polysaccharides were haptenic in rabbits but completely antigenic in certain other animals.

Sites on the antigen molecule that are involved in antigenic stimulation of antibody production and in the reaction with such antibody molecules are called determinant sites. There may be a few or many such sites on molecularly dispersed antigens, depending upon the size of the molecules, whereas there may be many thousands of determinant sites on the surface and within cellular antigens. Each surface determinant site is capable of reacting with and binding one homologous antibody molecule. Each molecule of diphtheria toxin, for example, is capable of binding eight molecules of diphtheria antitoxin—indicating the presence of eight determinant sites on the surface of the toxin molecule. Small synthetic haptens may have only one or two determinant sites (mono- or divalent haptens).

Cellular antigens must be processed by macrophages of the *reticuloendothelial system* (RES) prior to exerting their antigenic stimulation of the lymphoidal tissues involved in the immune response. This processing (including enzymatic liberation of antigenic molecules) tends to make internal as well as surface G determinants of the cells available for participation in the immune response. Even soluble antigens such as toxoids or albumins may require or benefit by RES processing. The nature of such processing, however, is poorly understood.

In intact cells, however, only G determinants located at the surface are available for reaction with homologous antibody. The distribution of such surface determinants is referred to as the *antigenic mosaic* of the cell. Human erythrocytes offer a good example of this mosaic concept. There are numerous antigenic types of human red blood cells (A, B, M, N, S, C, D, E, and many others), each represented by corresponding determinant sites distributed over a significant portion of the surface of the RBC (see D sites in Figure 4-2). Antibody specific for any one of these sites (monospecific antibody) will give a GA reaction indicating the presence of an adequate distribution of that particular determinant on the test cells. Monospécific anti-A antibody, for example, will identify the presence of the A determinants on the RBC by a positive agglutination test.

The same antigenic mosaic concept holds for bacterial cells, with the additional presence of anatomical structures over which the determinant sites may be distributed. A motile bacterium may possess somatic (body) antigens that differ from the flagellar antigens. These are designated O and H antigens, respectively, because the antigenic differences were reported by German workers studying two colony types of a species of *Proteus* bacilli. One colony produced a spreading (*H*auch) type of growth on the surface of agar media, whereas the other produced a circumscribed colony without spreading (*O*hne Hauch). The O type was later found to be a nonmotile variant of the motile H type, and the antigenic difference between the two strains was located on the flagella of the H type. Some bacteria produce surface antigens (Vi) that are indicative of their virulence and that may mask other O antigens. Others, like the pneumococcus, produce distinctive capsular antigens that cover and mask the cell somatic antigens.

Bacteria frequently undergo either genetic or phenotypic variations in their antigenic structure. Many of these variations are of the loss type. Motile bacteria may have either a transient or a permanent loss of the capacity to produce flagella. This results either in a temporary or a permanent OH→O type of antigenic variation. Cells may lose the capacity to produce the Vi antigen—a Vi→non-Vi antigenic variation. Likewise the capacity to produce capsular antigens may be lost temporarily or permanently. Antigenic variations of bacteria may be induced in the laboratory by genetic *transformation.* This phenomenon provided the first evidence that deoxyribonucleic acid (DNA) was genetic material. This is considered in greater detail in Chapter 7, which deals with *Streptococcus pneumoniae,* the causative organism of a type of pneumonia. Also, variations in the antigenic structure or metabolic capacity of a bacterial cell can be brought about by bacteriophage *transduction.* A unique example of phage modification, if not transduction, will be considered in detail in Chapter 5 dealing with *Corynebacterium diphtheriae,* the causative organism of diphtheria. An interesting type of antigenic variation is observed in the flagella of some members of a large group of pathogenic organisms belonging to the genus *Salmonella.* In the diphasic members of this group, the flagellar antigens may show phase 1⇌phase 2 reversible antigenic variation. Since phase 1 antigens differ from phase 2 antigens, antisera for both phase antigens must be available for serotaxonomic identification of these strains.

Disease-causing organisms or their products serve as the antigens (immunogens) for active immunization. This active immunization may involve animals (horses, rabbits, or others) for the production of antisera of known specific reactive capacity for (1) use in passive immunoprophylaxis or immunotherapy or (2) use in serotaxonomy. Active immunization may involve humans or animals in the process of active immunoprophylaxis (preventive immunization). Probably the most extensive active immunization, however, involves the antigenic stimulation resulting from natural infections, with recovery. The practice of active immunoprophylaxis depends upon the availability of safe and effective immunogens. Although smallpox immunoprophylaxis—first in the form of variolation and then, after Jenner, vaccination—has been practiced for centuries, most of the safe and effective immunogens for other diseases have been developed during the twentieth century; and the search for new ones continues.

There are three types of immunogens in common use in immunoprophylaxis: killed disease organisms; living but weakened disease organisms; and detoxified toxic products of disease organisms (toxoids). The type of immunogen, if any, used to prevent specific diseases will be considered in detail during the discussion of the diseases in Parts II, III, and IV. A substance that, when added to immunogens, tends to enhance the antigenicity of the immunogen is designated an *adjuvant.* Adjuvants may or may not be antigenic on their own, but their antigenicity is not a factor in their adjuvanticity. The usage of adjuvants will be considered during the discussions of human disease immunoprophylaxis.

IMMUNOBIOLOGY OF ANTIBODIES—IMMUNOGLOBULINS

Antibodies are globulin molecules that react specifically with the determinant site of the antigen involved in their production. The sites on the immunoglobulin responsible for the GA reaction are designated *receptor sites.* Whereas all antibody globulins must have the capacity to react with homologous antigen, they may be quite heterogeneous in other characteristics. The immunoglobulin designations and some of

Table 4-2.   Designations and characteristics of human immunoglobulins.

Designation	Approximate Molecular Weight	Sedimentation Coefficient	Biological Functions
IgG	150,000	7s	Humoral immunity; complement fixation; aggregation; transplacental immunity
IgA	170,000	7–14s*	Secretory antibody
IgM	900,000	19s†	Early immune response; complement fixation; avid agglutination
IgD	150,000	7s	? Found in penicillin hypersensitivity
IgE (Reagin)	196,000	8s	Immediate-type hypersensitivity; does not fix complement

Ig = Immunoglobulin.

* 7s dimer attached by a secretory factor.

† 7s pentamer.

their important characteristics are listed in Table 4-2. Additional characteristics of these immunoglobulins are summarized below:

1. Complete antibodies
   (a) IgG type
       (1) Are stable to heat at 56°C for 1+ hour.
       (2) Give all the expected GA reactions.
       (3) Pass the human placenta.
       (4) Are not fixed at and do not sensitize the site of intradermal inoculation.
   (b) IgA and IgM types
       (1) Same as IgG except for failure to pass the human placenta.
       (2) IgA and some IgG are secreted through lining membranes.
2. Incomplete antibodies: IgG, IgM, and IgA types—same as above except for failure to give one or more of the expected GA reactions
3. Reagin antibodies: IgE type
       (1) Reactivity is destroyed by heat at 56°C for 1 hour.
       (2) Usually fail to give one or more of the expected GA reactions.
       (3) Do not pass the human placenta.
       (4) Are fixed at and sensitize the skin at the site of inoculation.

A significant aspect of any GA reaction is the exquisite specificity of the primary reaction between the G-determinant and the A-receptor sites. For example, chicken and duck egg albumins can be distinguished by their reactions with homologous antibody, but not by any reasonable chemical method. As previously indicated, this specificity was first recognized in the neutralization of diphtheria toxin by diphtheria antitoxin but not by tetanus antitoxin and vice versa. This discovery led to the notion of biological species specificity in GA reactivity. This concept holds true in human and animal immunization against disease. However, different biological species soon were shown capable of producing cross-reacting antigens. Also, as indicated above for *S. pneumoniae,* different members of the same species may produce different antigens. These observations introduced the twofold concept of biological heterogeneity of GA relationships.

Extensive studies with haptens of *known chemical structure* that were coupled to proteins (carrier antigens) and used to "immunize" animals yielded antibodies specific for the haptens and resulted in convincing evidence that all primary GA reactions are chemically specific. This evidence explained the biological heterogeneity of different GA relationships by indicating that different biological species might synthesize chemically identical G determinants and different members of the same species can synthesize chemically different G determinants. The specificity of the primary GA reaction commonly is visualized as resulting from complementary distributions of reactive forces on complementary topographies at the determinant and receptor sites of the homologous antigen and antibody molecules—the "hand in glove" or "key in lock" concept.

There are two additional phenomena in antibody production, following the injection of antigens, that must be taken into consideration in any theory designed to explain the mechanism of antibody synthesis. The first of these is the fact that, under normal circumstances, self-antigens (proteins and others) do not stimulate an immune response in self whereas biologically foreign antigens do. The second is the fact that secondary antigenic stimuli, at suitable time intervals, produce much greater amounts of antibody than does the equivalent primary antigenic stimulus. The latter phenomenon has been designated the secondary or *anamnestic response* to antigenic stimulation.

Starting with the side-chain theory of Paul Ehrlich in 1900, a number of hypothetical mechanisms for antibody synthesis have been advocated (see Lachmann 1975a). Only two of these, however, adequately explained the essential aspects of GA reaction phenomena and received persistent scientific support. The first was advocated by Horowitz, Mudd, and others early in the twentieth century and was designed primarily to explain the exquisite specificity of GA reactions. It has been referred to as the *antigenic template* or *instructive* hypothesis of immune antibody synthesis. It postulated a genetic mechanism in animals for the production of "normal" globulin molecules without antibody reactivity. If the antigen was present at the site of this normal globulin synthesis, reactive forces present on the G-determinant site would react with and hold complementary reactive forces on the developing polypeptide of the immature globulin molecule. This reaction could be expected to result in the development of a complementary force distribution and topographic site—the receptor site—on the globulin molecule. The remainder of the polypeptide then coils in normal globulin fashion as a consequence of inherent forces of attraction. After dissociation from the antigen, this modified globulin molecule could be expected to exhibit antibody reactivity for other homologous antigen molecules. As indicated, this theory offers a simple physicochemical explanation for the exquisite specificity of GA reactions. One of the strongest advocates of this theory was Linus Pauling, who reported that he accomplished the *in vitro* conversion of partially denatured "normal" globulin into antibody globulin. He received a Nobel prize.

The antigenic template theory, however, cannot explain the nonantigenicity of self-antigens or the anamnestic response to secondary antigenic stimuli in immune antibody synthesis. No polypeptide or immature globulin molecule can be conceived as having the capacity to reject the myriad determinant sites of self-antigen molecules in its environment while accepting the globulin-modifying determinant sites of the less prevalent foreign antigen. Furthermore, since the antigenic template theory requires physical contact between each antigen and new antibody molecule, only a finite number of globulin molecules could be modified into antibody molecules by a given number of antigen molecules. This finite number of antibody molecules should be the same whether it results from a primary or a secondary antigenic stimulus. Consequently the maximum increase in antibody concentration following the secondary antigenic stimulus could be twice that from the primary stimulus. In reality, however,

the secondary response to the same dose of antigen given in the primary injection results in antibody concentrations many times greater than that of the primary stimulus—the anamnestic response.

These inconsistencies of the antigenic template theory led Burnet (1959) to propose the second major theory designed to explain immune antibody synthesis: the *clonal selection* theory. Burnet made use of background information provided by Jerne, Good, and others which indicated that lymphoidal tissue and plasma cells were involved in antibody production. Of significance also was the observation by Medawar and his colleagues that when persistent foreign antigens, such as heterologous skin transplants, were introduced during the embryonic stage they were accepted as self-antigens. The recipient then remained nonresponsive to those antigens when they persisted or were reintroduced postnatally. Medawar called the phenomenon *immune tolerance.* For a comprehensive discussion of the current complex aspects of immunological tolerance, see Lachmann (1975b).

The basic postulate of the clonal selection theory is that during cellular differentiation from the zygote stage throughout the fetus' embryonic life at least one lymphocyte is produced with genetic coding for the production of globulin molecules with receptor sites capable of reacting with *one* of any possible variety of antigenic determinants. Since there have been reports of 2×10^9 or more lymphocytes in the body of a medium-sized dog, this number was considered adequate to meet the needs of the theory. Each lymphocyte was visualized as having surface receptors homologous with the receptor sites of the globulin it was coded to produce. The function of the antigen in this theory was to locate and react with the homologous lymphocyte. If this reaction took place prenatally, as will all *self-antigens + homologous lymphocyte* reactions, the lymphocyte was eliminated or permanently repressed (see self-G coded lymphocytes in Figure 4-5). Since there would be no such lymphocytes to function postnatally, this would account for both the

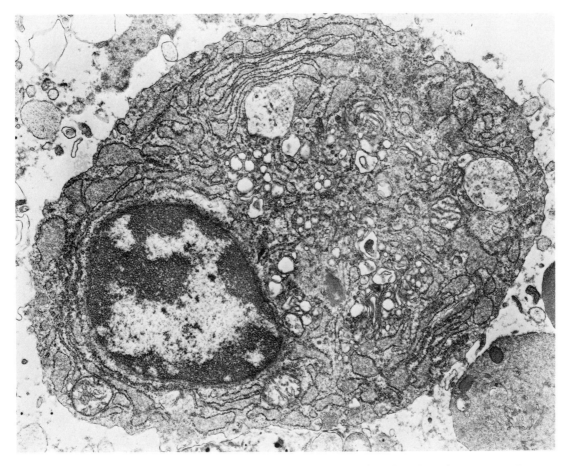

Figure 4–3. Electron micrograph of a plasma cell from a human axillary lymph node. 17,800×. (Courtesy of T. A. Barber.)

postnatal nonantigenicity of self-antigens and the immune tolerance observed by Medawar.

If the reaction between the antigen and its homologously coded lymphocyte first occurs postnatally, the lymphocyte is stimulated to divide rapidly, leading to a large clone of homologous lymphocytes. Some of these then differentiate into plasma cells that 'produce the antibody globulin. Figure 4-3 is an electron micrograph of a plasma cell showing the highly reticulated endoplasm, characteristic of cells involved in active protein synthesis. The undifferentiated clonal lymphocytes serve as persistent memory cells, each of which, upon secondary postnatal antigenic stimulation, can go through the same response procedure and pro-

duce correspondingly larger numbers of clonal lymphocytes, plasma cells, and larger yields of antibody—the anamnestic response to secondary antigenic stimulation (see Figure 4-4). Although the clonal selection theory as propounded by Burnet has been modified and extended, the basic concepts still hold true. Burnet received a Nobel prize in 1960.

T AND B LYMPHOCYTES

Karl Landsteiner and Merrill Chase in 1940 demonstrated that tuberculin hypersensitivity (DTH), which did not involve humoral (serum) antibody, could be transferred to nonsensitive individuals by the inoculation of lymphoidal

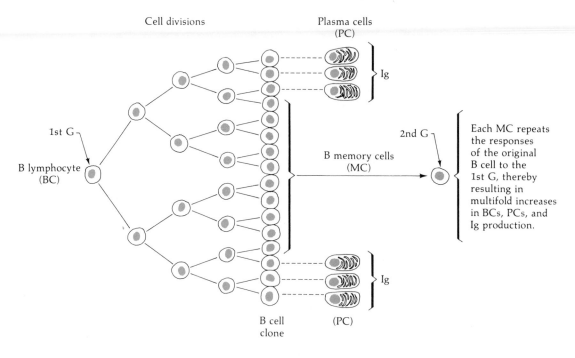

Figure 4–4. Clonal selection mechanism of postnatal immunoglobulin production. (Ig = immuno-globulin specific for G determinant.) After antibody production, the plasma cells die.

Figure 4–5. Production, processing, and differentiation of lymphocytes in humans and other mammals.

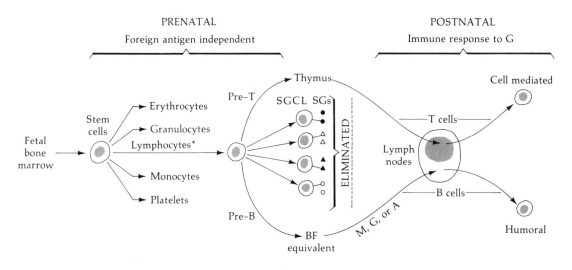

SGCL = self-antigen-coded lymphocytes
   SGs = self-antigens
     BF = bursa of Fabricius
   Pre- = precursor
M, G, or A = commitment to produce IgM, IgG, IgA

*Genetically coded for G recognition

cells from a hypersensitive person. Later reports indicated that emulsified spleen (lymphoidal) cells, from an antigenically stimulated rabbit, would produce antibody specific for the antigen when the cells were inoculated to normal rabbits. Moreover, workers reported the absence of plasma cells in individuals who could not produce antibody in response to antigenic stimulation (agammaglobulinemic individuals). These lymphoidal tissue discoveries and Burnet's clonal selection theory led to intensive studies of lymphocytes in animal and human immune phenomena.

Studies on such phenomena in baby chicks indicated that two types of lymphocytes were involved. One type was dependent upon the presence of an active thymus gland (thymic-dependent) and designated T lymphocytes, thymocytes, or T cells. The other type, which did not require participation of the thymus, was designated thymic-independent lymphocytes. Since the latter, in chicks, were found to require the bursa of Fabricius (BF), a lymphoidal structure associated with the posterior gut of the chick, they were designated B lymphocytes. The B lymphocytes were established as the cells responsible for the production of plasma cells, which in turn were responsible for the production of humoral antibodies. The T lymphocytes were found to be responsible for DTH and other, nonantibody, immune phenomena that are now designated cell-mediated immunity. For a comprehensive discussion of T and B lymphocytes, see Greaves et al. (1973) and McConnell (1975).

Humans and other mammals do not possess a BF, and the primary site (BF equivalent) of processing B lymphocytes in mammals is not established with certainty. Two candidates for this processing in mammals are (1) fetal liver and (2) gut-associated lymphoidal tissue (Galt), namely Peyer's patches, appendix, and submucus and mesenteric lymph nodules. All human lymphocytes and other hematopoietic cells (erythrocytes, granulocytes, monocytes, and platelets) develop from stem cells that arise in bone marrow. Both the thymus and the BF-equivalent tissues appear to support the extensive proliferation and differentiation of the precursor T and B lymphocytes from the bone marrow into functional T and B lymphocytes respectively. A number of workers have reported a hormone derived from the thymus (thymopoietin) to be the inducer of the differentiation of precursor T cells into thymic (T) lymphocytes. Brand et al. (1976) reported that a similar hormone from the BF of chicks appears to be responsible for inducing the differentiation of precursor B cells into functional B lymphocytes. They suggested the name *bursapoietin* for this hormone. The B lymphocytes then differentiate into IgM, IgG, or IgA producers. After differentiation, the T and B lymphocytes enter lymph channels and travel through regional lymph nodes to begin their circulation in the lymphatic and blood channels and colonization of lymphoidal organs. Postnatally they become immunocytes capable of reacting with homologous foreign antigen and producing their individually committed type of immune phenomena. Figure 4-5 gives a diagrammatic summary of the prenatal events that lead to the postnatal functioning of T and B lymphocytes in humans and other mammals.

Since lymph nodes have both afferent and efferent blood vessels as well as lymph channels, the inactive immunocytes traveling the bloodstream can pass through the walls of the blood capillaries within the nodes and enter the efferent lymph channels. Lymph nodules intersect the lymphatic channels throughout the body, particularly in the submucus tissues of the respiratory, gastrointestinal, and genitourinary tracts. Many of the lymphoidal tissues possess phagocytic cells (macrophages) in addition to lymphocytes. Thus the lymphatic system serves as the first line of defense against pathogens that penetrate the covering or lining membranes of the body. The lymphocytes traveling the lymph channels eventually reach the thoracic duct in the neck region, which empties into the bloodstream. Thus these inactive immunocytes continue to circulate, ever available for contact activation by homologous foreign antigen and the initiation of their committed immune responses.

The B lymphocytes, in addition to their inherent commitment to produce immunoglob-

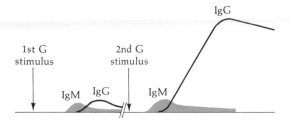

Figure 4–6. IgM and IgG responses to primary and secondary antigenic stimuli. (Both IgM and IgD have been reported being produced by progeny of the same B lymphocyte. The IgG, IgA, and probably IgE antibodies are produced by individually committed B lymphocyte progeny.)

Figure 4–7. Rosettes consisting of sheep RBC's attached to T lymphocytes (400×). Such rosettes are termed E (erythrocyte) rosettes and serve in enumeration of T lymphocytes. Inset: scanning electron micrograph of an E rosette showing several sheep RBC's attached to a rough-surfaced T lymphocyte (2690×). (Courtesy of R. M. Albrecht and S. D. Horowitz.)

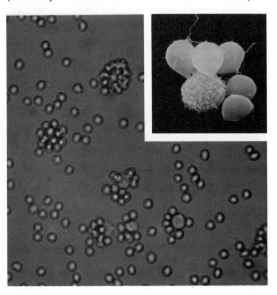

ulin specific for a particular antigen, undergo an antigen-independent differentiation in the BF or its equivalent, resulting in commitments to produce IgM, IgG, or IgA immunoglobulins. Studies of time-related Ig responses to G stimulation have indicated that IgM is produced first. The IgG production is significantly higher, however, particularly in response to the secondary antigenic stimulation (see Figure 4-6). Serum IgA and IgE antibodies are more difficult to quantitate because of the secretory nature of IgA and the tendency of IgE to attach to tissue surfaces. The clonal memory cells, produced as a result of postnatal G stimulation of B lymphocytes (Figure 4-4), have a long life span, whereas the half-life of the plasma cells, which produce the antibody, is measured in days.

The IgA immunoglobulins frequently are found on the surface of mucus or other lining membranes or in body cavities. Such antibodies in the gut formerly were known as copra antibodies. A number of workers have reported IgA in the salivary secretions of the parotid gland. Crawford et al. (1975), however, reported consistently higher concentrations of IgA in the secretions of the labial minor salivary (LMS) glands than in the secretions of the parotid glands of the same individuals. They reported IgA concentrations (in micrograms per milliliter of secretion) from the LMS glands, in four individuals, ranging from 262 to 731 percent of those found in the parotid gland secretions.

Neiburger et al. (1976) reported their results of quantitative studies on the distribution of T and B lymphocytes in lymphoidal tissues from normal and from diseased infants and children. The tissues included thymus, spleen, lymph nodes, and appendix, all of which were obtained during elective surgery. Single cell suspensions were obtained by forcing the mascerated tissue through stainless steel mesh, followed by gradient centrifugation. Stained smears of the selected cell layers revealed 98 percent concentrations of lymphocytes. The T lymphocytes in the suspensions were identified by their reaction with sheep RBC to form rosettes consisting of three or more RBC surrounding the lymphocyte (see Figure 4-7). The B lymphocytes were identified by direct fluorescent anti-B cell antibody techniques. These studies are cited as evidence of the ability to obtain and identify human lymphocytes for further research. Hudson and Hay (1976) used such procedures for establishing the following percentages of T, B, and N (neither) lymphocytes in the lymphoidal organs of 8-week-old BALB/c and CBA mice: thymus T—97 percent, B—1 percent; N—2 percent; lymph node T—77 percent, B—18 percent, N—5 percent; spleen T—35 percent, B—38 percent, N—27 percent; blood T—24 percent, B—70 percent, N—6 percent; thoracic duct lymph T—80 percent, B—19 percent, N—1 percent.

CHEMICAL STRUCTURE OF IgG

The treatment of diphtheria antitoxin with the proteolytic enzyme pepsin has been practiced since it was introduced by C. G. Pope in 1939. This treatment reduced the size of the antitoxin molecule about 30 to 40 percent, giving it a greater diffusion capacity without affecting its toxin neutralizing capacity. R. R. Porter in 1958 reported that the enzyme papain split rabbit IgG into three fragments—two subsequently designated Fab and one Fc. The Fab fragments are identical and each retains one receptor site— they are monovalent, incomplete antibody molecules. Each will react with homologous antigen and block the determinant sites but will not cause aggregation of the antigen or complement fixation by the GA complex. The Fc fragment has no antibody reactivity but is essential in the intact IgG molecule for complement fixation and certain other characteristics.

Edelman, Porter, Nisonoff, Mandy, and others, using mild reducing agents, were able to disassociate the IgG antibody molecule into four polypeptide chains; two, with higher sedimentation coefficients, were designated H (heavy) type and the other two the L (light) type. The Fab fragments were shown to consist of all of one L polypeptide and a portion of one H polypeptide held together by one disulfide linkage. The receptor site of this monovalent antibody was found to be at the aminoterminal end of the two polypeptides involved. Amino acid (AA) analyses of the H and L polypeptides from antibody molecules with different receptor site reactivities indicated a constant AA structure for both H and L polypeptides of all IgG molecules tested except for the aminoterminal areas in the vicinity of the receptor sites. In these areas, the AA composition differed (was variable) for each antibody molecule of different GA reactivity. In other words, the variability of the amino acids accounts for the specificity of the receptor site. From these and other studies there evolved a diagrammatic visualization of the IgG antibody molecule as indicated in Figure 4-8. Porter and

Figure 4–8. An IgG antibody molecule.

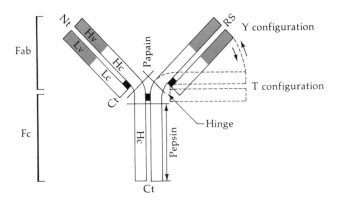

H = heavy polypeptide
L = light polypeptide
v = variable amino acids
c = constant amino acids
■ = disulfide (—S≡S—) bridges
Nt = aminoterminus of polypeptides
Ct = —COOH terminus of polypeptides
RS = receptor site
—— = enzyme cleavage sites

Edelman, after completing their studies of the sequence of the 1,320 amino acids that constitute the myeloma IgG molecule, were jointly awarded the 1972 Nobel prize for physiology and medicine.

Other studies on the digestion of IgG by pepsin indicated that this enzyme attacks the COOH-terminal portions of the two H polypeptides posterior to the disulfide linkage that binds them together (see Figure 4-8). This digestion yields one $(Fab')_2$ fragment and oligopeptides. Since the $(Fab')_2$ fragment retains both receptor sites, it remains a divalent antibody in its GA reactivity. It will give aggregation, neutralization, and other (but not C' fixation) GA reactions. Therefore, it is another example of an incomplete antibody but not so incomplete as the Fab. Thus the mechanism whereby the diphtheria antitoxin molecule was reduced in size but not in toxin neutralizing capacity, by treatment with pepsin, finally has been explained.

CELL-MEDIATED IMMUNE PHENOMENA

This chapter has dealt almost exclusively with antibody-mediated immune phenomena; the distinctions between antibody (ITH) and cell-mediated (DTH) hypersensitivity, other than the onset of reaction times, have not really been discussed. The first recognition of a cell-mediated immune phenomenon was the transfer of DTH from a tubercular patient to a nonhypersensitive person by Landsteiner and Chase using lymphoidal cells, but not when using serum antibodies, from the patient. By contrast, serum antibody transfer of ITH from a hypersensitive donor to a nonsensitive recipient had been demonstrated earlier in this century by Prausnitz and Küstner.

One of the most serious forms of ITH was discovered and named by Portier and Richet while they were immunizing dogs with sublethal doses of a toxic product of sea anemones. After several innocuous injections, the dogs would suddenly suffer a severe to fatal shock reaction following an intravenous injection. Since the objective of the immunological procedure had been prophylaxis, its failure prompted Portier and Richet to designate the shock phenomenon *anaphylaxis*. Subsequently anaphylaxis has been studied extensively in animals by using a variety of nontoxic soluble antigens, including ovalbumin and purified serum proteins. Anaphylactic hypersensitivity can be a problem in passive human immunotherapy using horse or other animal antisera, particularly when administered intravenously. See Chapter 5 for precautions in immunotherapy.

The mechanism of anaphylactic and other forms of ITH involves the reaction of the allergen with IgE antibody attached to basophilic leucocytes or other tissue cells. These GA reactions result in the liberation of vasoactive amines (including histamine), especially from the basophilic (mast) cells. The amines produce a variety of pharmacological reactions including increased permeability of blood capillaries (resulting in leakage of fluid) and spastic contractions of smooth muscle tissue. Because such tissues surround the bronchioles in the lung of the guinea pig, anaphylaxis in this animal results in death from asphyxiation within a few minutes after administration of the allergen. In different animal species, the vasoactive amines exert their damaging effects on different organ tissues. Since antibodies are involved, the ITH phenomena are considered in the realm of B-lymphocyte induction. It is possible, however, that T lymphocytes may cooperate in these as they do in other antibody-induced phenomena. The allergens in ITH include plant pollens, fungus spores, organic substances in house dust, feathers, animal dander, some drugs, milk, eggs, other foods, and foreign antisera. Common ITH diseases include hay fever (iritis and rhinitis), asthma, urticaria and other types of skin rash, and allergic gastroenteritis. Anaphylactic shock resulting from intravenous inoculation of antisera or antibiotics (penicillin), although not so common, is the most serious of the ITH diseases.

Robert Koch, after he established the etiology of tuberculosis, noted that a protein extracted from the tubercle bacilli would yield a skin reaction in tubercular patients 24 to 36 hours after inoculation. He designated the protein *tuberculin,* and this tuberculin test—the first recognized DTH phenomenon—continues to be the earliest possible means of diagnosing tubercular infections. Other examples of T-cell-mediated DTH are the poison oak or ivy types of contact dermatitis, the immune response to smallpox vaccination, some drug hypersensitivities, and skin or organ graft rejections.

Human graft rejection results from the presence of a large number (about 40) of *histocompatibility antigens* that are genetically controlled and shared in variable ratios by different individuals. Grafts transplanted from one site to another on the same individual (such as skin grafts) are designated *autografts.* Since the donor and recipient sites of these grafts possess the same histocompatibility antigens, autografts usually succeed. The same is true for identical twin donor and recipient grafts, which are designated *syngenic* grafts. *Isogenic* grafts involve tissues from genetically similar but not identical donors and recipients, whereas *allografts* involve genetically dissimilar donors and recipients of the same species. Isogenic grafts and allografts usually are rejected by the recipient unless immunosuppressive measures are undertaken.

As a result of the increasing practice of human organ transplants, two new practices have been added to the armamentarium of the surgical laboratory. First, since autografts cannot be involved in such transplants and since identical twin donors are rarely available, the practice of histocompatibility matching of potential isogenic donors with the recipient's tissues is increasing rapidly. This might be conceived as a more complex extension of the long practiced typing and cross-matching of donor and recipient blood cells prior to blood transfusions. The nearer the histocompatibility antigens match, the more likely the grafted tissue will be retained. Second, since the recognition of the fact that the graft rejection is a T-lymphocyte-mediated phenomenon, the production and use of anti–T cell antiserum as an immunosuppressive agent has been advocated. If graft rejection or even DTH were the only T-cell-mediated phenomenon, this would be the ideal immuno-suppressive procedure. However, T-cell-mediated immune phenomena are much broader and more essential to human well-being than these potentially adverse reactions would indicate. For example, T-cell-mediated immunity is functional in both facultative and obligate intracellular infections wherein antibody (B-cell-mediated immunity) may not function. These include tuberculosis, brucellosis, typhoid and other bacterial infections, viral and rickettsial disease infections, and certain fungal and protozoal infections. Consequently immunosuppression of T lymphocytes can render the patient more susceptible to a considerable variety of serious infections. Even the DTH and graft rejection phenomena appear to be unfortunate extensions of the desirable aspects of T-cell immunity in tuberculosis and other microbial diseases and in the suppression of malignant cells—cancer immunity.

As indicated in Figure 4-4, circulating B lymphocytes begin replicating immediately after activation by contact with homologous antigen. This replication leads directly to the production of plasma cells yielding their soluble product (antibody) and a clone of memory cells. The T lymphocytes also replicate after activation by contact with homologous antigen—but not immediately. Both the initial T cell and its clonal memory cell progeny undergo a latent period, after G activation, prior to onset of replication. During this latent period the activated T cells produce soluble products with physiological or pharmacological functions—somewhat comparable to the production of histamine by mast cells as a consequence of antigen reaction with the attached homologous IgE antibody.

Dumonde et al. (1969) coined the term *lymphokines* to include all the biologically active soluble factors, other than antibodies, that can be detected in cell-free supernatants of G-activated lymphocytes. Among the lymphokines produced by T lymphocytes are:

1. *Chemotactic factors* that attract phagocytic cells to the site of release of the factor.

2. *Migration inhibitory factor* (MIF), which inhibits the migration of wandering macro-

phages—possibly tending to concentrate these phagocytic cells at the site of tissue damage.

3. *Transfer factors* that are capable of transferring DTH to nonsensitive individuals. They have been reported to be effective in treating systemic mycoses in T-cell-deficient children.

4. *Cytotoxicants* that may destroy target cells, such as malignant cells.

5. *Interferon,* which inhibits viral replication.

Following lymphokine production and the replication of activated T lumphocytes, the clonal progeny persist as inactive memory cells awaiting secondary antigenic activation and a cell-mediated anamnestic response. For a comprehensive discussion of cell-mediated effector mechanisms, see Valdimarsson (1975).

CLINICAL APPLICATIONS OF ANTIGENS AND ANTIBODIES

The most extensive antigenic stimuli are those resulting from naturally occurring infections. As a general rule it takes 10 days to 2 weeks or more following onset of symptoms for the immune response to result in measurable amounts of antibody in the serum of the patient. If a serodiagnostic test is performed during the first week (acute phase) of clinical symptoms, no antibody resulting from the current infection should be expected. However, serum antibodies from past infections or immunizations might be present. If the onset symptoms indicate the possibility of any one of several diseases, baseline concentrations of antibodies to antigens for each of these diseases should be established during the first week. Both these onset and later serodiagnostic tests should be performed on serial dilutions (1:10, 20, 40, . . . , 320) of the patient's serum (quantitative tests). The highest dilution of the serum that yields a positive test result is the antibody *titer* of the serum for that antigen. A negative onset titer to the antigen responsible for the current disease is more indicative of the disease than are positive titers at that stage. Antibody present at onset of infection, as stated, is the result of past infec-

tions or antigenic stimuli. Onset antibody titers should remain constant throughout the course of the current infection. In contrast, antibody to the antigen responsible for the current disease should begin to appear in the serum early in the second week of symptoms and thereafter should show a continuously rising titer, even into the convalescence. Therefore a *rising antibody titer,* which involves at least two quantitative tests on serum specimens spaced 1 to 2 weeks apart, is much more significant in serodiagnosis than a stationary or a single test titer. Such serodiagnosis can never result in early diagnosis.

In serotaxonomy, morphologically and stainingly similar organisms, either pathogenic or saprophytic, may share antigens with the pathogen one is trying to identify. Therefore the antiserum, prepared by immunizing an animal (rabbit) with the pathogen, may contain antibodies that will react with both the pathogen and other organisms possessing the shared antigens. If the pathogen possesses unshared antigen specific for that species only, however, the cross-reacting antibodies can be absorbed onto the bodies of the organisms that possess shared antigens and be removed by centrifugation. Such highly specific antisera may be produced by laboratory personnel or purchased from commercial laboratories.

Immunoprophylaxis (preventive immunization) usually involves the injection of specific disease antigens—prior to exposure to the disease. Passive (antibody) immunoprophylaxis can be used, but the immunity is short-lived and, if a foreign (horse) antiserum is used, the recipient will be rendered hypersensitive (ITH) to the proteins of that serum. This hypersensitive state will persist for months to a year or more beyond the duration of the passive immunity.

In contrast to immunoprophylaxis, immunotherapy involves the injection of preformed antibodies specific for the disease. The earlier in the course of the disease this therapy is used, the more likely it is to be effective. Once diphtheria toxin has been absorbed by susceptible tissues, for example, no amount of diphtheria antitoxin will neutralize its pathological effect. Foreign (horse) antisera may be injected with safety into nonsensitive patients for a week to 10 days or so before the patient begins to develop hypersensitivity to that serum. If antiserum from other animal species (cows, rabbits, goats) is available, it may be substituted for the one to which the patient is hypersensitive.

If we define therapy as treatment of a patient already showing disease symptoms, there are few diseases for which active immunotherapy is justifiable. Usually disease symptoms indicate that the patient has more toxic antigen in his tissues than can be accommodated and there is no justification for injecting more. However, human ITH allergies are treated by active immunotherapy using repeated injections of *subreactional* doses of the allergens to which the patient is hypersensitive. This treatment is visualized as *desensitization* therapy and possibly is explainable by the stimulation of IgG or IgA antibodies that may accumulate in secretions from the hypersensitive membranes and coat the allergen with bland human globulin before the allergen comes into contact with the sessile IgE antibody responsible for the hypersensitivity of the tissues. In chronic or prolonged diseases (for example, whooping cough) in which the causative organisms do not penetrate but do damage the lining membranes, supplemental antigenic stimulation (active immunotherapy) may speed recovery and prevent complications. One disease in which the designation of prophylactic or therapeutic immunization may be equivocal is rabies. Here active immunization, introduced by Pasteur, is practiced after infection (the bite of a rabid animal) but before onset of symptoms. This is possible because the incubation period is long—usually a month or more—and the time of exposure can be pinpointed as the time the animal bit the patient. See Chapter 35 for current modifications of this therapy. The applications of immunological and serological procedures to human disease are considered in Parts II, III, and IV.

REFERENCES

Bellanti, J. A. 1971. *Immunology.* Philadelphia: Saunders.

Brand, A., D. G. Gilmour, and G. Goldstein. 1976. Lymphocyte-differentiating hormone of bursa of Fabricius. *Science* 193:319–321.

Burnet, F. M. 1959. *The Clonal Selection Theory of Acquired Immunity.* Nashville, Tenn.: Vanderbilt University Press.

———. 1976. *Immunology: Readings from Scientific American.* San Francisco: Freeman.

Cherry, W. B. and M. D. Moody. 1965. Fluorescent-antibody techniques in diagnostic bacteriology. *Bacteriol. Rev.* 29:222–250.

Collins, F. M. 1974. Vaccine and cell mediated immunity. *Bacteriol. Rev.* 38:371–402.

Cooper, M. 1975. B lymphocyte differentiation. Chapter 13 in Hobart and McConnell (1975).

Crawford, J. M., M. A. Taubmen, and D. J. Smith. 1975. Minor salivary glands as a major source of secretory immunoglobulin A in the human oral cavity. *Science* 190:1206–1209.

Dumonde, D. C., R. A. Wotstencroft, D. S. Panayi, M. Mathew, J. Morley, and W. T. Howson. 1969. Lymphokines. Nonantibody mediators of cellular immunity generated by lymphocyte activation. *Nature* (London) 224:38–42.

Edelman, G. M. 1973. Antibody structure and molecular immunology. *Science* 180:830–840.

Greaves, M. F., J. J. T. Owen, and M. C. Raff. 1973. T and B lymphocytes, origins, properties, and roles in immune responses. *Excerpta Medica, Amsterdam.* New York: American Elsevier.

Hobart, M. J. and I. McConnell (eds.). 1975. *The Immune System.* Oxford: Blackwell.

Hudson, L. and F. C. Hay. 1976. *Practical Immunology.* Oxford: Blackwell.

Lachmann, P. J. 1975a. Theories of antibody formation. Chapter 9 in Hobart and McConnell (1975).

———. 1975b. Immunological tolerance and unresponsiveness. Chapter 10 in Hobart and McConnell (1975).

McConnell, I. 1975. T and B lymphocytes. Chapter 7 in Hobart and McConnell (1975).

Neiburger, J. B., R. C. Neiburger, S. T. Richardson, J. L. Grosfeld, and R. L. Baehner. 1976. Distribution of T and B lymphocytes in lymphoid tissue of infants and children. *Infect. Immunity* 14: 118–121.

Valdimarsson, H. 1975. Effector mechanisms in cellular immunity. Chapter 12 in Hobart and McConnell (1975).

PART TWO

Contact Group Diseases

Subgroup A: Respiratory (Buccolabial) Contact

The primary vehicles of all respiratory contact diseases are secretions or exudates of the respiratory tract and the buccal region of infected hosts. Although mucus secretions or exudates from the posterior nasopharynx, bronchi, or lungs may be the true primary vehicles, these always pass through the buccal area where they are mixed with saliva. Since saliva is the best-known secretion of this area, the epidemiology of the respiratory diseases is commonly designated "traffic in saliva." The usual portals of entry of the disease organisms of this subgroup are the mucus membranes of the mouth, nose, and eyes of susceptible hosts. The mode of transmission that justifies placing the respiratory diseases in the contact group is the direct transmission of saliva during the act of kissing or coughing or sneezing in the immediate proximity of a susceptible host. Secondary vehicles frequently are contaminated with salivary discharges, however, and these provide indirect (noncontact) modes of transmission for these

diseases. In some of these diseases, moreover, exudates from skin or other lesions may function as additional primary vehicles and must be considered in the overall epidemiology of those particular diseases. The major epidemiology of the traffic-in-saliva aspect of the respiratory diseases is summarized in Figure II-A.

The respiratory subgroup includes many of the most prevalent and highly contagious diseases of human beings. No preventive measures, other than active immunization, have been effective in controlling the diseases of this subgroup. Diseases from this and the other groups have been selected for discussion on the basis of past or present significance to humans or because of interesting or unique aspects of their host-parasite biology. The emphasis is on measures applicable to the prevention of the diseases, including laboratory diagnostic procedures that frequently are essential to the application of specific control measures. The bacterial diseases of the respiratory subgroup are considered first, followed by a consideration of the viral diseases. For more detailed discussions of laboratory techniques, culture media, reagent preparations, and staining procedures for these and other diseases, see the clinical laboratory manuals listed in the references at the end of Chapter 1.

Figure II–A. Major modes of transmitting respiratory diseases of the contact group.

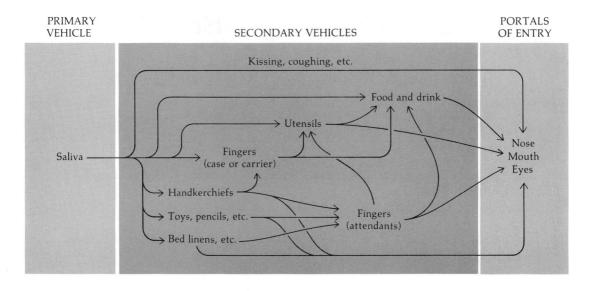

5

Diphtheria

The disease diphtheria has been described in the literature under a variety of names. In the time of Hippocrates, two designations are believed to be synonyms for diphtheria: *Malum aegyptiacum* in Syria and *Ulcus syriacum* in Egypt. The symptomatic disease diphtheria also has been designated membranous croup and membranous laryngitis because of membranous lesions in the throat region. It has also been called malignant angina and, by the Spaniards, *garotillo* (the strangler) because of the interference by the membranous lesion with respiration. Breton-neau in 1821 reported the differences between the angina of scarlet fever and that of malignant angina (and membranous croup), indicating that the latter two were identical. For these two he coined the term "diptherite" (from the Greek word for leather), which subsequently was converted to "diphtheria."

THE ETIOLOGICAL AGENT

The causative organism of diphtheria was first described by E. Klebs in 1883 and was first cultivated in 1884 by F. A. Loeffler, who applied the Henle-Koch postulates. Although it is commonly referred to as the diphtheria bacillus, the proper taxonomic designation is *Corynebacterium diphtheriae.*

When observed in smears of lesion exudate or of early primary culture, *C. diphtheriae* is a nonmotile, non-spore-forming, drumstick-shaped bacillus. In old cultures, particularly 7-day-old broth cultures used for toxin production, the organisms may grow as short or long filaments intermingled with large spherical structures. When young diphtheria bacilli reproduce, they tend to remain attached and rotate at the site of division, giving rise to V, N, M, W, or palisade configurations. When stained with polychrome stains, the cells show the presence of deeply stained granules in the differentially stained cytoplasm of the cell. These are called *metachromatic granules,* and a number of stains have been formulated for their demonstration. A very satisfactory metachromatic granule stain is Loeffler's alkaline methylene blue. The organisms are gram-positive (purple), but this stain masks the metachromatic granules (see Figure D on the back cover).

It is possible to cultivate *C. diphtheriae* on a variety of solid media. The most extensively used is Loeffler's coagulated serum medium: a mixture of two parts of a peptone-glucose-beef-infusion broth and one part of beef or horse serum. The liquid mixture is dispensed into test tubes that are slanted to give a large surface area of the medium in the tube. The preparations are then heat-coagulated and sterilized in this slanted position. This medium can be prepared in screw-capped tubes by laboratory personnel or it can be bought in hermetically sealed tubes from clinical laboratory commercial sources.

If isolated colonies of *C. diphtheriae* are desired, the culture specimen may be streak-inoculated onto a petri plate of sterile peptone, glucose, beef infusion, blood or serum (7–10 percent), and agar (1.5 percent). The peptone, infusion broth, and agar mixture is sterilized in an autoclave at 121°C for 15 to 20 minutes, at which temperature the agar is melted. The mixture is then cooled to 50°C and the sterile

beef or other blood or serum is added. The mixture is then poured into sterile petri plates where the agar solidifies into a gel at temperatures below 45°C. The culture specimen is streaked onto the surface of the agar medium with the aid of a bacteriological loop of platinum or nichrome wire (2 inches long) mounted in a suitable handle. The loop is heated to incandescence to sterilize it before and after use. The objective of the streaking is to disperse the bacteria so that single cells will be deposited at well-separated sites on some area of the plating medium (see Figure 3-1). The streaked plates are incubated at 37°C in an inverted position to prevent drops of condensation water on the glass surface from falling onto the medium. During the period of incubation the isolated single cell grows into a macroscopic colony. The colony represents a population of cells that are the progeny of the original single bacterium deposited at that site. This streak inoculation, for pure culture isolation, is much simpler and more reliable than the dilution method described by Pasteur. It is widely used in bacteriological studies and requires a bit of practice to become proficient.

Anderson et al. (1931) reported a potassium tellurite, chocolate-blood agar medium that selectively favored the growth of *C. diphtheriae* while suppressing the growth of most of the other bacteria commonly found in the throat region. The medium consists essentially of the same peptone, glucose, infusion, and agar medium described above with the addition of potassium tellurite. After sterilization, the agar base medium is cooled to 75°C, at which temperature the blood is added. After a few minutes at 75°C, the color of the blood medium changes from brilliant red to chocolate brown. The medium is then poured into sterile petri plates and allowed to solidify.

In their report of this medium, Anderson et al. noted that *C. diphtheriae* from different patients could be divided into three varieties (biotypes) on the basis of colony appearances on the tellurite medium. One biotype, commonly isolated from mild cases of diphtheria, gave a glistening black, bonbon-shaped colony. They designated this biotype *C. diphtheriae mitis.* A second biotype, commonly isolated from severe cases of diphtheria, gave a grayish, flattened colony with a central papilla and striations from the center to the periphery of the colony (a daisy-head colony). They designated this biotype *C. diphtheriae gravis.* A third biotype, isolated from both mild and severe cases of diphtheria, gave rise to colonies intermediate in color and morphology between the *mitis* and *gravis* biotypes. They designated this biotype *C. diphtheriae intermedius.*

Upon reading their publication, the author was impressed with the potential prognostic significance of the biotype observations. If a laboratory technologist, on the basis of a culture isolate, were able to inform the clinician not only of the presence of a morphologically typical *C. diphtheriae* but also of the potential danger of that infection to the patient, it obviously would be most helpful. Consequently, considerable effort was concentrated on isolating and identifying these biotypes of *C. diphtheriae.* Unfortunately, it soon became obvious that it took 48 hours or more to get typical colony growth of *C. diphtheriae* on the tellurite medium, and even after this length of time the biotype distinctions frequently were equivocal. By 48 hours after onset of symptoms, the clinician knows whether or not he has a severe case of diphtheria. If he delayed antitoxin therapy long enough to get this information from the laboratory, he probably would have a fatal case of diphtheria before the information reached him. Furthermore the correlation between biotype and virulence is not as strict as first visualized. The tellurite medium is rarely used for the cultivation of *C. diphtheriae,* but it can be helpful in a search for carriers of diphtheria bacilli wherein relatively few organisms are expected to be present and time is of little concern. For characteristics of other pathogenic *Corynebacterium* species, see Hermann and Bickham (1974).

Nonpathogenic species of the genus *Corynebacterium* are frequently found in the throat. These may have similar, if not identical, morphologies and staining characteristics as those of *C. diphtheriae.* Because of their relative numbers, they rarely lead to confusion in the laboratory diagnosis of a case of diphtheria. They can, however, become a problem in establishing the termination of the carrier state that is required for the release from quarantine of a recovered case. These saprophytic species of *Corynebacterium* are designated diphtheroids.

PATHOGENIC MECHANISM

Roux and Yersin reported that the cell-free filtrate of a broth culture of *C. diphtheriae* would cause the same systemic symptoms and death when inoculated into experimental animals as would the inoculation of a pure culture of the live organisms. This was the first demonstration of a soluble bacterial exotoxin.

Diphtheria toxin is a thermolabile (75°C for ±10 minutes) unstable protein of about 62,000 to 65,000 molecular weight. Fortunately the toxin is antigenically homogeneous; that is, all isolates of *C. diphtheriae* produce the same antigenic type of toxin, which can be neutralized by any diphtheria antitoxin. The toxin selectively attacks a variety of tissues, the most vital being the striated muscles of the heart and diaphragm. Once the toxin is absorbed by susceptible tissues, its slow, degenerative pathology cannot be reversed by antitoxin.

Paul Ehrlich in 1895, while studying diphtheria toxin filtrates stored at 4–6°C, noted that the filtrate gradually lost some of its toxicity over a period of a year or so without losing significant antigenicity. Even though he could not separate the nontoxic but antigenic fraction of the filtrate from the residual toxin fraction, he designated the former fraction *toxoid.* Some years later, G. Ramon reported that adding a small amount of formaldehyde to a diphtheria toxin filtrate and storing the mixture at 39°C resulted in complete detoxification in 2 to 3 months without significant loss of antigenicity. Ramon designated his nontoxic, but antigenic, material *anatoxine.* Ehrlich's toxoid and Ramon's anatoxine are considered to be identical, and the priority of Ehrlich's designation is generally accepted. These changes in diphtheria toxin filtrates are illustrated diagrammatically in Figure 5-1. Diphthe-

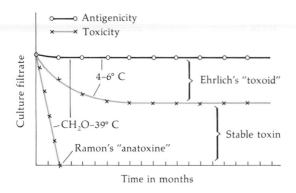

Figure 5–1. Time-correlated changes in diphtheria toxin filtrate.

ria toxin becomes stable toxin after about a year at 4–6°C. The ratio of toxin to toxoid in the stable toxin filtrate does not change over a period of months.

Freeman (1951) reported a unique requirement for toxin production by *C. diphtheriae.* Although it had been known for some time that different isolates of *C. diphtheriae* were either toxigenic or nontoxigenic, no prior explanation for these differences was reported. Freeman discovered the presence of small amounts of bacteriophage (phage) in the culture filtrates of all toxigenic strains of *C. diphtheriae.* This phage (designated *beta*) would infect and cause lysis of nontoxigenic strains. When he subjected the toxigenic cultures to ultraviolet-light irradiation, all the cells were lysed by the phage, resulting in the production of large quantities of the phage. He concluded that all toxigenic strains of *C. diphtheriae* were lysogenized with phage DNA. He also showed that nonlysogenic strains of *C. diphtheriae* were nontoxigenic. When these non-toxigenic cultures were exposed to the phage, most of the cells were attacked and lysed by the phage infection. In one in a billion or so cells, however, the infecting phage DNA, instead of causing lysis of the cell, associated itself with the DNA (genome) of the host cell—it lysogenized the cell. The lysogenized cell was immune to further attack by the phage and grew into a colony in the presence of the phage. This colony was shown to consist of toxigenic cells of *C.*

diphtheriae. In other words, the phage DNA had converted the nontoxigenic strain and all its progeny into lysogenic and toxigenic strains of *C. diphtheriae.* Other workers have shown that the gene for diphtheria toxin production is located on the DNA of the beta phage responsible for the lysogenization of *C. diphtheriae.* Uchida et al. (1971) and Gill et al. (1972) used mutants of such beta phages to show that the tox$^+$ phage gene can result in toxin production whether or not it is integrated into the bacterial genome and replicated as prophage (lysogen) or nonintegrated and nonreplicated.

Much effort has gone into attempts to explain the mechanism of the degenerative pathology caused by diphtheria toxin. A significant breakthrough was reported by Strauss and Hendee (1959), who noted that the addition of diphtheria toxin to an actively growing culture of HeLa (human carcinoma tissue) cells resulted in virtually immediate cessation of protein synthesis in the cell culture. A. M. Pappenheimer and his group at Harvard conducted experiments on HeLa cell cultures and on cell-free systems which (1) confirmed the findings of Strauss and Hendee; (2) indicated that the effect on protein synthesis resulted from blockage of a step in the transfer of amino acids from soluble RNA to the growing polypeptide in the ribosome; and (3) that the action of diphtheria toxin was neutralized by prior treatment with diphtheria antitoxin. They reported that the inhibition of amino acid transfer by the toxin required the presence of the cofactor nicotinamide-adenine dinucleotide (NAD) and that the toxin inactivated one of the two supernatant transfer factors while not affecting the other. Additional studies indicated that it was the enzyme transferase II (T-II) which was inactivated by the covalent attachment of the ADP-ribose moiety of NAD. A formulation, by Goor and Maxwell (1970), of the mode of activity of diphtheria toxin is:

$$NAD^+ + T\text{-}II \xrightleftharpoons{\text{toxin}} ADP\text{-}ribose\text{-}T\text{-}II$$
$$\text{(active)} \qquad\qquad \text{(inactive)}$$
$$+ \text{ N (nicotinamide)} + H^+$$

Thus the current concept of the mode of action of diphtheria toxin, in the degenerative pathology of the disease, is the blocking of protein synthesis by ADP-ribosylation of the soluble enzyme transferase II. Diphtheria toxoid does not cause this reaction. Transferase II, however, is now designated elongation factor 2. For additional aspects of the structure and mode of action of diphtheria toxin, see Uchida et al. (1972), Pappenheimer and Gill (1973), and Collier (1975).

CLINICAL SYMPTOMS

Diphtheria is a rapidly developing, acute, febrile infection, frequently with insidious onset and tending to involve both local and systemic pathology. The local lesion usually is found in the upper respiratory tract and involves necrotic injury to the epithelial cells. As a result of this injury, blood plasma leaks into the area and the fibrinogen is precipitated into a fibrin network. This network interlaced with rapidly growing *C. diphtheriae* tends to form a membranous covering over the site of the local lesion—the *pseudomembrane*. This local lesion may be a small structure a few millimeters in diameter; or it may cover extensive areas of the nasopharyngeal, laryngeal, or bronchial region. When located at or below the larynx, the pseudomembrane may block respiration (malignant angina or garotillo.) Figure 5-2 illustrates a preserved pseudo-

membrane that is a cast of the bronchial tree including branches into the larger bronchioles; this pseudomembrane was coughed up by an infant just before death. Local lesions occasionally involve cells of the conjunctiva or skin. Skin diphtheria is particularly liable to occur in the tropical areas of the world, where respiratory diphtheria is rare.

The diphtheria bacilli do not tend to invade tissues below or away from the surface epithelial cells at the site of the local lesion. At this site, they produce the toxin that is absorbed and disseminated through lymph channels and blood to the susceptible tissues of the body. Degenerative changes in these tissues—striated muscles, peripheral nerves, adrenals, kidney, liver, and spleen—result in the systemic pathology of the disease. The fatal degeneration of heart muscle may result in a structure that is little more than a mass of jelly. Microscopic hemorrhages in the adrenals may result in these glands assuming a cherry red color. This is one of the diagnostic manifestations of experimental diphtherial toxemia in the guinea pig.

COMPLICATIONS AND SEQUELAE

A respiratory tract infection, such as diphtheria, is liable to be complicated by a concomitant infection with streptococci or other potential pathogens commonly found in this area. Whereas antitoxin therapy may be expected to

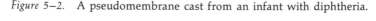
Figure 5–2. A pseudomembrane cast from an infant with diphtheria.

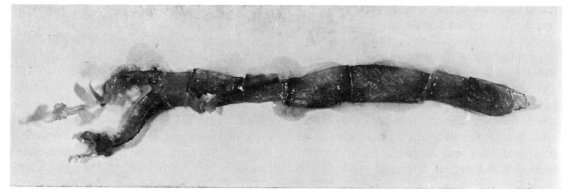

cure most early cases of diphtheria, it will have no effect on complicating infections. Suitable antibiotic or chemotherapeutic agents should be used to supplement the antitoxin therapy whether or not bacterial complications are suspected.

Paralyses may be an early (first week after onset) or late (to ninth week after onset) sequel following symptomatic recovery from diphtheria. Local paralyses usually occur between the first and fourth week after the onset of symp-• toms and may involve (1) the muscles of the palate, resulting in a nasal voice and difficulty in swallowing; (2) the ciliary muscles of the eye; or (3) any localized muscle that absorbs a sufficient quantity of the toxin. Paralyses may result if peripheral nerve endings that control the muscles are damaged. These local paralyses usually occur in younger children and in individuals who receive antitoxin late (fourth day after onset or later).

General paralysis may develop as late as the ninth week after onset and 6 to 8 weeks after apparent recovery from the clinical symptoms of diphtheria. Since these paralyses may result in heart or respiratory failure, the postrecovery precautions following a severe case of diphtheria should be comparable to those following a heart attack.

MORBIDITY AND MORTALITY STATISTICS

Diphtheria is worldwide in distribution, but the respiratory form of the disease is rare in the tropics. Carriers of toxigenic C. diphtheriae can be found in most areas of the world, and the respiratory form of the disease is endemic in most larger nontropical cities. There is convincing evidence that the disease could be eliminated by the immunization of all preschool children. The fact that this desirable situation has not been realized, even in many communities in the United States, is indicated by recent epidemics. Since all of them could have been prevented, they indicate the price we pay for ignorance and neglect. Localized epidemics of

diphtheria have been reported in *Morbidity and Mortality Weekly Reports (MMWR)* from Austin, Texas (1969), with 62 cases and 2 deaths; Dade County, Florida (1969), with 22 cases and 4 deaths; Chicago, Illinois (1970), with 16 cases and 2 deaths; and San Antonio, Texas (1970–1971), with 201 cases and 4 deaths. In general, most diphtheria cases occur in children under 5 years of age. In 1971, however, 5 of 17 cases reported in Washington state were in adults. In 1970, 3 cases were reported in Portland, Oregon, in adults 56, 59, and 64 years old; the latter was fatal. The 13 October 1973 issue of *MMWR* reported an outbreak of 44 cases of diphtheria on or near the Navajo Indian Reservation in Arizona and New Mexico. The 44 cases followed reports of 10 cases in 1970, 30 cases in 1971, and 20 cases in 1972. Immunization histories on 28 of the 44 cases in 1973 indicated that 6 had been fully vaccinated against diphtheria. Fourteen had been incompletely vaccinated and 8 had no history of immunization.

SUSCEPTIBLE ANIMAL SPECIES

Naturally occurring diphtheria is restricted to the human species. The occasionally recovered diphtheria bacilli from cats, horses, or cows are not believed to be of epidemiological significance. In other words, there are no nonhuman animal reservoirs of infection. Experimental animals, however, are extremely important in the bioassay and standardization of immunobiological products for diphtheria prophylaxis and therapy. The animal of choice, and of legal requirement in antitoxin standardization, is the guinea pig. Rabbits are preferable for some preliminary bioassay procedures. Dogs, cats, horses, and birds are susceptible to diphtheria toxin. Monkeys are relatively resistant, and mice and rats are highly resistant to diphtheria toxin. These resistances to diphtheria toxin are not due to the presence of diphtheria antitoxin in the tissues of the resistant animals. They must be explained as some form of tissue immunity. Possibly the transferase II of these resistant species is not inactivated by diphtheria toxin.

EPIDEMIOLOGY

For all practical purposes, human cases and carriers are the ultimate source of diphtherial infections. The primary vehicle is exudate from the local lesion usually admixed with saliva. The respiratory epidemiology is illustrated diagrammatically in Figure II-A. In the relatively rare cases of skin or other nonrespiratory lesions, the exudate of these lesions constitutes another possible primary vehicle. No epidemics of such forms of diphtheria have been reported.

A case of diphtheria usually shows onset of sore throat symptoms after a short (2–5 day) incubation period. Communicability of the infection begins at or shortly before the onset of symptoms. The patient continues to be capable of transmitting the disease to others until toxigenic (virulent) diphtheria bacilli have disappeared from the upper respiratory tract. This disappearance can be established by swabbing the nose and throat area and inoculating the swab specimen to a tube of Loeffler's coagulated serum medium and incubating at 37°C overnight. Generally the release of a patient from quarantine requires that two such cultures, taken at least 24 hours apart, must be negative for diphtheria-form bacilli when stained smears are examined microscopically. This rarely takes more than 2 weeks following symptomatic recovery. If diphtheria-form bacilli persist longer than 2 weeks, a virulence (toxigenicity) test should be performed.

LABORATORY DIAGNOSIS

Because of the need for early antitoxin therapy in cases of diphtheria, the laboratory should only be used to confirm a clinical diagnosis. If the clinician has immediate access to a clinical laboratory, however, he or she may be able to swab the area of the pseudomembrane and inoculate the swab specimen to a tube of Loeffler's medium; moreover, the technologist can prepare a smear of the swab specimen on a microslide, stain, and examine the smear microscopically. This much probably can be done before the antitoxin is ready for injection. If large numbers of diphtheria-form bacilli (see Figure D on the back cover) are present in the smear from the swab, this can give the physician added confidence in his or her clinical diagnosis. A negative or questionable result should not, however, be allowed to shape clinical judgment. If the physician is convinced the patient has clinical diphtheria, the antitoxin should be administered immediately.

The inoculated tube of Loeffler's medium should be incubated at 35–37°C for 8 to 16 hours before preparing a smear of the growth on a microslide. The smear should be stained with a metachromatic granule stain and examined microscopically. Again, the finding of typical diphtheria-form bacilli should serve only to confirm the clinical judgment of the physician in charge.

The laboratory technologist should remember that typical diphtheria-form bacilli can be (1) toxigenic *C. diphtheriae,* (2) nontoxigenic (avirulent) *C. diphtheriae,* or (3) diphtheroids. Consequently, the observations resulting from the microscopic examination of a stained smear from a swab or a culture should be reported merely as the presence or absence of diphtheria-form bacilli—not *C. diphtheriae.* This is particularly true when cultures are taken to determine the time for release of a recovered case from quarantine. The collection of specimens for this latter purpose should include swabbing the nasal passages as well as the throat, since this practice has been shown to give a significantly higher yield of isolations of *C. diphtheriae* than swabbing the throat only.

The only way to establish the virulence of a diphtheria-form bacillus is to isolate the bacillus in pure culture and do a toxigenicity test. This test may be done by a bioassay method or by an *in vitro* procedure. The bioassay usually involves the use of two guinea pigs, one of which (the control) receives an injection of 500 units of diphtheria antitoxin. The pure culture (12–18 hour) of the bacillus, usually growing on a Loeffler medium slant, is suspended in 1–2 milliliters of sterile saline (0.85 percent NaCl). Equal amounts (0.5 milliliter) of the bacillary suspension are injected subcutaneously into both the test and the control pigs. If the isolate is a toxigenic *C. diphtheriae*, the unprotected test animal will die in 36 to 72 hours, whereas the antitoxin-protected control animal will survive. If the isolate is a nontoxigenic *C. diphtheriae* or a diphtheroid, both animals will survive the injections. If both animals die, the isolate is virulent for guinea pigs but is not *C. diphtheriae*. Toxigenicity testing generally is the responsibility of public health laboratories.

An *in vitro* toxigenicity test was first described by Elek (1948). It requires having known toxigenic (tox$^+$) and nontoxigenic (tox$^-$) strains of *C. diphtheriae* in addition to the pure culture of the unknown test organism. For the test a 0.5-inch-wide strip of sterile filter paper, saturated with diphtheria antitoxin, is embedded in serum-enriched peptone infusion agar.

To perform the test, the tox$^+$ strain is streak-inoculated to the surface of the agar medium at right angles to and across the filter paper near one end. The tox$^-$ strain is similarly inoculated across the filter paper near the other end of the strip. The unknown (tox$^?$) isolate is inoculated across the filter paper near the center of the strip. The preparation is then incubated at 35–37°C for 24 to 48 hours. The three cultures grow along the streaks of inoculation, and the tox$^+$ strain produces toxin that diffuses into the agar. This gives a gradient of toxin concentrations in the agar from the edges of the growth outward. At the same time the antitoxin diffuses from the filter paper, giving a gradient of antitoxin concentrations in the agar from the edges of the filter paper outward. Visible lines of precipitate develop where the concentrations of toxin and antitoxin meet in equivalent proportions. Thus the tox$^+$ control culture will give four lines of precipitate radiating in two V configurations from the edges of the filter paper at the intersections of the tox$^+$ culture growth. The tox$^-$ control culture gives no such lines of precipitate. If the unknown (tox$^?$) test culture gives lines of precipitate comparable to the tox$^+$ culture, it is a toxigenic *C. diphtheriae*. If not, it is a nontoxigenic diptheria-form bacillus. See Olds

(1975) for an excellent photographic illustration of an Elek test plate. Toxigenicity tests are never used to aid in the diagnosis of diphtheria, but they may be required to permit the release of a recovered case of diphtheria from quarantine.

TOXIN AND ANTITOXIN ASSAY

Diphtheria toxin is produced commercially by growing a toxigenic strain of *C. diphtheriae* (usually the Park and Williams No. 8 strain) in a suitable broth medium. After an adequate incubation period (6–7 days), the toxin (antigen) concentration in the broth can be measured by the *in vitro* flocculation test, first described by Ramon. The test is performed by placing varying amounts of diphtheria antitoxin (30–120 units at intervals of 10, each in 1-milliliter volume) in a series of 10 small (0.5-inch-diameter) tubes. Each tube then receives 1 milliliter of clear toxin broth and the mixtures are incubated at 50°C in a water bath. Within 5 to 30 minutes one or more of the tubes will develop a floccular precipitate. The tube in which the first floccules develop contains an equivalent (optimum proportion) mixture of toxin and antitoxin. The number of units of antitoxin in that tube indicates the Lf/ml ± 5 (in this example) of toxin antigen in the broth culture. If the tubes containing 80 and 90 units of antitoxin flocculated first, the exact LF/ml value of the toxin would be between 80 and 90. If a more exact Lf/ml value is needed, the test may be repeated using smaller differences in the number of units of antitoxin per tube until an exact Lf/ml value is established. Since this test is merely the measure of the antigenicity of the toxin broth, it can be used on either toxin or toxoid. Diphtheria toxoid used for human immunization must contain a specified minimum Lf/ml of antigen.

When a commercial batch (say 100 liters) of diphtheria toxin is harvested, the diphtheria bacilli are filtered out and the sterile filtrate represents a crude mixture of toxin, unmodified and modified broth ingredients, and soluble metabolic products of the diphtheria bacilli. A small quantity (100 milliliters) of this toxin filtrate usually is stored at 4–6° for a year or more to become stable toxin for future bioassay use (see Figure 5-1). The remainder of the crude toxin is converted to toxoid by adding formaldehyde and incubating at 39°C. This toxoid is used for both human and animal (horse) immunization. Stable toxin is composed of a mixture of toxin and toxoid, neither of which changes in relative concentration over a period of months. Different batches of diphtheria toxin, however, tend to stabilize at different toxin/toxoid concentration ratios. Stable diphtheria toxin is required for the biological standardization of diphtheria antitoxin.

Diphtheria antitoxin is produced by immunizing horses (or occasionally other animals) with repeated injections of diphtheria toxoid. Earlier, Von Behring and others used repeated, sublethal injections of diphtheria toxin. When it became obvious that antitoxin would be an effective treatment for diphtheria, Ehrlich proceeded to establish means of standardizing this horse serum product. He established the minimum lethal dose (MLD) of a batch of stable diphtheria toxin for guinea pigs. His arbitrary requirements for this dose were: the guinea pigs must weigh 250 grams; the toxin must be injected subcutaneously; and the guinea pig must die exactly 96 hours after injection. (Currently, an average lethal dose or LD/50 is considered more accurate than the older MLD.) Having established the quantity of his stable toxin, which represented one MLD, Ehrlich arbitrarily chose 100 times this quantity of the toxin (100 MLD) for use in the first standardization of his horse serum antitoxin. After preparing dilutions of his antitoxin serum in 1-milliliter quantities, he added 100 MLD of toxin to each dilution and injected each mixture subcutaneously into a 250-gram guinea pig. The smallest amount of the antitoxic serum that completely neutralized the 100 MLD of toxin was designated *one unit* of antitoxin. Thus Ehrlich intended that stable diphtheria toxin should be the test material with which all antitoxin would be standardized. When he added 100 MLD of other stable diphtheria toxins to his originally standardized antitoxin, however, he found that one unit of the latter either overneutralized or underneutralized the 100 MLD of toxin. This we now recognize as being due to the different ratios of toxin to toxoid in different batches of stable diphtheria toxin. Whatever the cause, these results negated the reuse of the 100 MLD of toxin method of standardizing the unit value of subsequent antitoxins.

Since the serum antitoxin proved to be quite stable in its toxin neutralizing capacity, Ehrlich designed a second method for establishing the unit value of antitoxic horse serum while he still had a supply of his first antitoxin. This method was based on the use of the original unit quantity of his original horse serum antitoxin, as determined by the 100 MLD of toxin method. In other words, this original antitoxic serum became the first *standard antitoxin*, and a known quantity of it constituted one unit of standard antitoxin. Ehrlich then proceeded to establish an "L+ dose" of stable diphtheria toxin by mixing varying amounts of the toxin each with one unit of his standard antitoxin. Each mixture was injected subcutaneously into a 250-gram guinea pig. The mixture, which resulted in the death of the guinea pig at exactly 96 hours, contained the L+ dose of diphtheria toxin. This dose can be determined using any stable diphtheria toxin regardless of toxin/toxoid ratios in the toxin. Since this dose (quantity) of the stable toxin was established in the presence of one unit of standard antitoxin, it became the means of measuring one unit of antitoxin in any immune serum. For example, 1-milliliter aliquots of suitable dilutions of the immune serum each receive one L+ dose of the stable diphtheria toxin and each mixture is injected subcutaneously into a 250-gram guinea pig. The mixture that results in death of the guinea pig at 96 hours must contain one unit of antitoxin. The reciprocal of the serum dilution in that mixture, therefore, indicates the number of units of antitoxin per milliliter of undiluted serum.

When individuals in other countries began producing diphtheria antitoxin, they first turned to Ehrlich for standard antitoxin. With this they could establish the L+ dose of their own stable diphtheria toxin and use it to standardize the unit value of their antitoxic horse serum. The U.S. National Institutes of Health in Bethesda, Maryland, maintain standard diphtheria antitoxin for use in this country. Since each new antitoxic serum is standardized against a prior batch of antitoxin, all the way back to Ehrlich's original antitoxin, the unit of diphtheria antitoxin may be defined today as the quantity of any antitoxic serum that has the same toxin neutralizing capacity as Ehrlich's original unit.

Since even guinea pigs of the same weight vary somewhat in natural susceptibility or resistance to diphtheria toxin, lethal dose (LD/50 or L+ dose) determinations usually involve the injection of three or more animals with each test amount of the toxin. For example, the LD/50 of the toxin would be the amount that resulted in death at 96 hours of 50 percent or more of the animals that received that dose. The L+ dose would be determined similarly by multiple animal injections for each amount of toxin tested. Further, the standardization of diphtheria antitoxin requires multiple animal injections with each dilution of horse serum tested. Since lethal end-point assays require one animal for every test mixture, the number of 250-gram guinea pigs required for such assays can become quite large.

The L+ dose method is required for the final determination of the unit value of diphtheria antitoxin for human use. However, preliminary skin reaction tests in guinea pigs or rabbits or *in vitro* flocculation tests can be used to approximate the unit value of an antitoxic serum and thereby save the lives of many guinea pigs. For example, 1-milliliter aliquots of diphtheria toxin or toxoid of known Lf value (say 50 Lf/ml) can be placed in each of 10 tubes. Each tube then receives 1 milliliter of a dilution of the antitoxic serum ranging, say, from 1:5 to 1:14 and the mixtures are incubated at 50°C in a water bath. The first mixture to develop a floccular precipitate would indicate the presence of about 50 units of antitoxin in that tube. By multiplying the reciprocal of the dilution of the serum in that tube by 50, the approximate number of units of

antitoxin per milliliter of the undiluted serum can be established. To arrive at this approximation of the unit value by the L+ dose technique would require many guinea pigs.

Diphtheria toxin will cause an inflammatory reaction in susceptible animals when very small amounts (the skin test dose) are injected intracutaneously. This reaction in human skin was first reported by Béla Schick in 1913 when he devised the Schick test to measure susceptibility or immunity to the disease diphtheria. Others adapted this skin reaction to the assay of antitoxin. The Lr dose of stable diphtheria toxin may be defined as the amount of toxin that, when mixed with one unit or some fraction of a unit (for example, 0.01 unit to give an Lr/100 dose) of standard diphtheria antitoxin and 0.1 milliliter of the mixture is injected intracutaneously, will result in an inflammatory reaction 1 centimeter in diameter. The depilated skin on the back and flanks of guinea pigs or rabbits may be used for these titrations. The skin is marked into approximately 1-inch squares and a map of the area is prepared to identify the mixture injected at each site. For the assay of horse serum antitoxin the principle is the same as that for the L+ dose technique except that approximately 40 mixtures of the Lr dose of the toxin plus suitable dilutions of the serum antitoxin may be tested on one rabbit, rather than the 40 or more guinea pigs required by the L+ dose procedure. Again the Lr dose technique is used only for the preliminary approximation of the unit value of the antitoxic serum.

Schick designed his test as a means of determining susceptibility or immunity to diphtheria in human beings. The Schick test dose (STD) of stable diphtheria toxin is approximately one-fiftieth of an LD/50 (for the guinea pig) contained in 0.1 milliliter. The toxin is diluted to this STD in buffers that stabilize it at this level for 6 months or more. Since the Schick toxin contains broth culture ingredients in addition to the diphtheria toxin, and since some persons give inflammatory skin reactions to any injection, the Schick test should include both a test and a control injection. The Schick control involves an aliquot of the same diluted toxin as that used in the test. The control toxin, however, is heated at 75°C for 10 minutes to destroy the toxicity without altering the other (nontoxic) ingredients of the filtrate involved in both the test and control injections.

Both the Schick test and the control involve intracutaneous injections of 0.1 milliliter of the respective preparations into the flexor surfaces of the forearms. A positive Schick test reaction may range from a slight inflammatory flush to a severe inflammatory burn with blistering. These reactions are in every way comparable to a localized site of sunburn. The reaction begins 36 to 48 hours after injection and may persist for a week or more, followed by brownish pigmentation that may persist for months. If blistering occurs, indicating extreme susceptibility to the toxin, peeling and even slight scar formation may result. The four possible combinations of reactions or no reactions at the sites of the test and control injections are listed below:

1. Negative test—no reaction at either the test or control site. Interpreted as immune to diphtheria.

2. Positive test—a reaction at the test site but no reaction at the control site. Interpreted as susceptible to diphtheria.

3. Pseudopositive test—equal reactions at both the test and the control sites. Interpreted as immune to diphtheria but sensitive to the nontoxic ingredients present in both the test and the control injections.

4. Combined positive test—reactions at both injection sites but a greater or more persistent reaction at the test site. Interpreted as susceptible to diphtheria and sensitive to the nontoxic control ingredients.

Of 1,050 young adults who were Schick-tested in our immunology classes, 95 (9 + percent) gave pseudopositive reactions whereas only 5 (0.47 percent) gave combined positive test results. Obviously the latter Schick test result is relatively rare. The Schick test results in these 1,050 students were correlated with their serum antitoxin concentrations as determined by the Lr/500 dose of toxin technique. No student with

0.01 unit or more of antitoxin per milliliter of serum gave a positive Schick test. Eighty-five (55.5 percent) of 153 students with $> 0.002 < 0.01$ units/milliliter of serum antitoxin gave positive Schick tests, whereas 68 (44.5 percent) with this amount of antitoxin were found to be Schick-negative. Moreover, 261 of 275 students with < 0.002 units/milliliter of serum antitoxin gave positive Schick test results (95 percent). The remaining 14 students in this group, who were Schick-negative (resistant to diphtheria toxin) although their serum showed no antitoxin, are interesting. This result can be interpreted as cellular or natural immunity. The class, however, facetiously accused them of being of closer kin to the rat than their fellow students. Again, it would be interesting to determine whether or not such individuals possessed a transferase II that resisted inactivation by diphtheria toxin.

IMMUNOPROPHYLACTIC MEASURES

Active immunization of human beings has been practiced since the second decade of the twentieth century. Park and his colleagues at the New York City Health Department prepared diphtheria toxin-antitoxin (TAT) mixtures that were practically neutral as demonstrated by animal inoculations. When TAT was injected, even though the toxin was neutralized, it exerted an immunogenic effect in the recipient. This immunogenic response was first measured in animals by assaying the serum antitoxin produced. Subsequently it was measured in humans by means of noting the conversion of the Schick positive state prior to injection to Schick negativity following the injections. For some years this was the only means of active immunization against diphtheria for human beings. The TAT, however, had two undesirable characteristics. First, the diphtheria toxin used was highly pathogenic and the quantity injected in the mixture, if not neutralized by the antitoxin or if the neutrality was reversed, could result in a fatal toxemia. Second, the antitoxin in the mixture was horse serum, which tended to sensitize the recipient, and this hypersensitivity to horse serum tended to persist for 6 months or more. If the hypersensitive recipient needed horse serum antibody for therapy in a case of diphtheria or other disease contracted during the hypersensitive state, the serum therapy might result in an anaphylactic shock reaction more dangerous than the disease itself.

When Ramon demonstrated the conversion of diphtheria toxin into its nontoxic but antigenic equivalent by using formaldehyde (see Figure 5-1), he provided humanity with one of the safest and surest immunogens of all time—diphtheria toxoid. This toxoid rapidly displaced TAT for human immunization and sublethal injections of toxin for animal immunization.

Subsequently two modifications of the original crude toxoid have been shown to have adjuvant effects on the fluid immunogen. A. T. Glenny, in England, reported that precipitating the toxoid antigen with aluminum potassium sulfate (alum) not only eliminated much of the nonantigenic ingredients that remained in the discarded supernatant fluid but also enhanced the immunogenicity of the floccular precipitate after resuspension in sterile saline. Wells and Havens of the Alabama Department of Health Laboratory then proved the safety and the adjuvant immunogenicity of the alum-precipitate toxoid for human beings. The second adjuvant modification of fluid toxoid was noted when killed *Bordetella pertussis* cells (whooping cough vaccine) were suspended in the fluid diphtheria toxoid to give a divalent (DP) immunogen. Not only did the *B. pertussis* cells immunize the recipient against whooping cough (pertussis), but their presence at the injection site enhanced the immunogenicity of the fluid toxoid. Currently a trivalent immunogen DPT is available, consisting of a mixture of the fluid toxoids of diphtheria and tetanus in which are suspended killed *B. pertussis* cells. Injection of DPT results in immunity to diphtheria, whooping cough, and tetanus.

Health authorities recommend that all infants 2 to 3 months of age be actively immunized against diphtheria and pertussis—these diseases are particularly dangerous for young children.

Since the trivalent immunogen DPT contains these antigens plus that for tetanus, and since no more injections or reactions are involved, the trivalent DPT is the immunogen of choice. The immunization involves three injections spaced 4 to 6 weeks apart. A single booster injection of DPT should be repeated after 5 or 6 years to maintain immunity.

Passive immunoprophylaxis involves the injection of 1,000 units of diphtheria antitoxin into susceptible individuals who have been in contact with a case of diphtheria. Since this injection provides immunity for only 2 or 3 weeks and sensitizes the recipient to horse serum for 6 months or more, it rarely is justifiable. A preferable procedure is to start active immunization and keep close surveillance on all susceptible contacts. If symptoms of diphtheria develop in the contact, a therapeutic injection of antitoxin can be given. This step will eliminate unnecessary sensitization of noninfected contacts.

IMMUNOTHERAPY

When Emil von Behring, at a scientific meeting in Europe in 1890, reported the prophylactic and therapeutic efficacy of diphtheria antitoxin in experimental diphtheria, the audience stood and cheered. Dr. Park, the director of the New York City Health Laboratories, attended the meeting and is reputed to have cabled his superiors to buy him some horses so he could start diphtheria antitoxin production. Since his superiors had never heard of such a thing, they must have decided that Dr. Park had been imbibing too freely of the good European ferments. By 1895, however, antitoxin therapy for diphtheria had become universal practice. Diphtheria mortality rapidly dropped from 30–60 percent to 2–10 percent after its inception.

The earlier the antitoxin is administered after onset of symptoms, the more certain it is to be effective. Once diphtheria toxin is absorbed by susceptible tissues, it cannot be neutralized regardless of the amount of antitoxin present. Diphtheria mortality statistics (two different surveys), correlated with the day of illness on which antitoxin was administered, are summarized in Table 5-1. These figures show that a 24-hour delay in administering antitoxin resulted in a 3 to 4 percent increase in deaths that could have been avoided by administering antitoxin on the first day of illness. These results indicate why the clinician cannot afford to wait on any laboratory results that take more than a few minutes before deciding whether or not to administer antitoxin.

The dosage of antitoxin in diphtheria immunotherapy may vary from 20,000 to 100,000 units or more, depending upon the patient's age or weight, or the time since onset of symptoms. The routes of injection are either intramuscular or intravenous. The former requires 12 hours or more for absorption and dissemination of the antitoxin to all body tissues. When administered intravenously, the antitoxin is distributed to all body tissues within minutes. Intravenous injections of foreign substances, however, are more dangerous than intromuscular. Since streptococci or other bacteria might complicate the diphtheria infection, penicillin or other antibiotic therapy should supplement the antitoxin therapy.

POSTRECOVERY PRECAUTIONS

Following recovery from a severe case of diphtheria there is the chance that toxin was absorbed by heart muscle prior to the administration of antitoxin. The resultant degenerative heart pathology may or may not be recognized. If it is, the postrecovery precautions are obvious. If not, however, the potential danger requires that the patient be treated as a heart case and confined to practical bed rest for a couple of months. In other words, overexertion might bring on heart failure. The damaged heart tissue can be regenerated within the two months of rest.

ANTITOXIN PRECAUTIONS

Horse serum antitoxin or any foreign serum poses a potential threat to life, particularly when it is administered intravenously. Since diphthe-

Table 5-1. Initiation of diphtheria antitoxin therapy versus mortality.

Day of Illness Therapy Begun	Percent Mortality
1st	0—1.62
2nd	4.2—4.73
3rd	10.37—11.1
4th	15.51—17.3
5th or later	18.7

ria requires more such foreign serum therapy than any other disease, these precautions are summarized here. However, they are equally applicable to passive immunotherapy in tetanus, gas gangrene, and other diseases. The precautions are:

1. Elicit a history of possible hypersensitivity, especially to horse proteins (horse asthma), and prior foreign serum prophylaxis or therapy (sensitivity develops in 7 to 10 days after such serum administration).
2. Test for hypersensitivity.
   (a) Eye test: Place a drop of normal horse serum diluted 1:10 into the conjunctival sac of one eye. Itching, watering, and diffuse inflammation will develop within 30 minutes in hypersensitive persons. A drop of a 1:1,000 dilution of epinephrine or a drop of antihistamine then will control severe reactions.
   (b) Skin test: Inject 1/40 milliliter of saline intracutaneously into the flexor surface of one arm as a control. Into the other arm inject an equal amount of normal horse serum diluted 1:100 in saline. A genuine urticarial wheal with surrounding erythema in 5 to 20 minutes is positive. Pseudopodia formation indicates greater danger.
3. Classify the risk of serum treatment.
   (a) Patients liable to more than the usual risk:

(1) Those with family or personal history of asthma, hay fever, eczema, urticaria, or angioneurotic edema.
(2) Those who have had a previous administration of horse serum.
(3) Those giving a mildly positive reaction to the intradermal test.
(b) Patients to whom the serum should not be given:
  (1) Those with history of asthma or vasomotor rhinitis under exposure to emanations from the animal species from which the serum was obtained.
  (2) Those giving a positive reaction to an eye test or a strongly positive reaction to the intradermal test.
  (3) Those *in extremis*.
  (4) Those who have received serum injections several days to several months (roughly 7 days to 6 months) previously.
(c) Patients for whom serum treatment should be discontinued: those having had a severe shocklike reaction, an asthmatic attack, an urticarial rash, or an alarming thermal reaction following the first or any subsequent injection.

SERUM SICKNESS

Symptoms of serum sickness develop in about 10 percent of nonsensitive persons who receive an injection of foreign serum. These symptoms usually appear within a week to 10 days after the administration of the serum. They consist of an urticarial rash, intense itching, pain in the joints and sometimes swelling, and fever. The symptoms of serum sickness are disconcerting but not serious. They indicate that the involved tissues of the originally nonsensitive person developed hypersensitivity to the foreign serum before all the serum antigens were eliminated from the body. The only treatment indicated is that designed to alleviate allergic reactions. Even if untreated, the symptoms usually do not last for more than a few days.

CONTROL AND PREVENTION

Diphtheria, like all respiratory subgroup diseases, can only be prevented by immunoprophylactic procedures. Although passive immunization with 1,000 units of horse serum antitoxin will prevent the disease in nonimmune contacts, this immunoprophylaxis is rarely justifiable. This is due to the short (2 to 3 weeks) duration of the passive immune state and the prolonged sensitization of the recipient to horse serum. The effective immunological and epidemiological control measures are:

1. Immunize all children during the first 2 or 3 months of life with diphtheria toxoid. The immunogen recommended is DPT because, in addition to diphtheria, it provides immunity to pertussis and tetanus.

2. Quarantine all cases of diphtheria until they can be demonstrated to be free of toxigenic *C. diphtheriae* by two negative cultures taken at least 24 hours apart. If the cultures continue to be microscopically positive, perform a toxigenicity test on the isolated diphtheria-form bacillus.

3. Start active immunization and daily surveillance of all susceptible individuals who have been in contact with a case of diphtheria.

4. Disinfect all primary and secondary vehicles of the respiratory diseases (see Figure II-A) during and after a case of diphtheria.

REFERENCES

Anderson, J. S., F. C. Happold, J. W. McLeod, and J. G. Thompson. 1931. On the existence of two forms of diphtheria bacillus—*B. diphtheriae gravis* and *B. diphtheriae mitis*—and a new medium for their differentiation and for the bacteriological diagnosis of diphtheria. *J. Path. Bact.* 35:667–681.

Barksdale, L. 1970. *Corynebacterium diphtheriae* and its relatives. *Bacteriol. Rev.* 34:378–422.

Collier, R. J. 1975. Diphtheria toxin: mode of action and structure. *Bacteriol. Rev.* 39:54–85.

Elek, S. D. 1948. The recognition of toxicogenic bacterial strains in vitro. *Brit. Med. J.* 1:493–496.

Freeman, V. J. 1951. Studies on the virulence of bacteriophage-infected strains of *Corynebacterium diphtheriae. J. Bacteriol.* 61:675–688.

Gill, D. M., T. Uchida, and R. Singer. 1972. Expression of diphtheria toxin genes carried by integrated and nonintegrated phage. *Virology* 50:664–668.

Goor, R. S. and E. S. Maxwell. 1970. The diphtheria toxin-dependent adenosine diphosphate ribosylation of rat liver aminoacyl transferase II. *J. Biol. Chem.* 245:616–623.

Hermann, G. J. and S. T. Bickham. 1974. *Corynebacterium.* Chapter 12 in *Manual of Clinical Microbiology.*

Olds, R. J. 1975. *Color Atlas of Microbiology.* Chicago: Yearbook Medical Publishers.

Pappenheimer, A. M., Jr. and M. Gill. 1973. Diphtheria. Molecular mechanisms involved in its pathogenesis. *Science* 183:353–358.

Strauss, N. and E. D. Hendee. 1959. The effect of diphtheria toxin on the metabolism of HeLa cells. *J. Exper. Med.* 109:145–163.

Uchida, T., D. M. Gill, and A. M. Pappenheimer, Jr. 1971. Mutation in the structural gene for diphtheria toxin carried by the temperate phage. *Nature* (London) *New Biology* 223:8–11.

Uchida, T., A. M. Pappenheimer, Jr., and A. A. Harper. 1972. Reconstitution of diphtheria toxin from two nontoxic crossreacting mutant proteins. *Science* 175:901–903.

6

Meningococcal Meningitis

The term *meningitis* is a good example of the idiopathic use of the suffix *-itis*. Pathology in the meninges of the brain or spinal cord can be caused by a number of different bacteria and viruses. This pathology, regardless of the etiology, tends to result in similar or identical symptoms that justify the designation of the disease as meningitis. If the etiological agent is identified by laboratory procedures, a specific type of meningitis, such as meningococcal meningitis, can be designated. Although meningitis can be caused by a variety of cocci (streptococci, staphylococci, pneumococci), these are not called meningococci. This term is restricted in its usage to a gram-negative, coffee-bean-shaped (flattened on adjacent edges) diplococcus, which frequently is involved in the epidemic form of meningitis.

Marchiafava and Celli in 1884 were the first to report the presence of these gram-negative diplococci in the meningeal exudate of fatal cases of meningitis. In 1887, Weichselbaum isolated the organisms from six cases of menin-

gitis and established the isolates as a distinct species. Later the isolates were established as the etiological agents of one type of meningitis by the Henle-Koch postulates (using monkeys).

THE ETIOLOGICAL AGENT

The taxonomic designation for the causative organism of this disease is *Neisseria meningitidis;* the common designation is the meningococcus. The organism tends to occur intracellularly in the cytoplasm of polymorphonuclear leucocytes (see Figure E-1 on the back cover). Since these leucocytes are attracted to the site of irritation in the meninges, the infection is called pyogenic (pus-forming).

Neisseria meningitidis can be cultivated on a peptone-infusion agar medium enriched with blood or serum. All media should be warmed to 37°C prior to inoculation. The organism is extremely susceptible to temperatures above or below 37°C. This latter susceptibility is relatively unique among bacteria. Also, the organism tends to undergo rapid autolysis after death due to the presence of a thermolabile, autolytic enzyme. Recognition of these characteristics is important to the laboratory personnel responsible for isolating and identifying this organism. The meningococci are found in the spinal fluid of a patient, and this is the specimen used for cultural isolation for a specific diagnosis. The organism also tends to colonize the posterior nasopharyngeal mucus membranes in carriers and in the early stage of an infection prior to the invasion of the meninges. The route of invasion to the meninges appears to be via the bloodstream. This meningococcemia, however, may develop without invasion of the meninges, in which case the symptoms are distinct from those of meningitis. A blood culture is necessary for establishing the diagnosis of a case of meningococcemia or any other bacteremia or septicemia.

Most individuals in close contact with a case of meningococcal meningitis become carriers of meningococci. This carrier rate can reach 20 percent of a contact group by the time the first case is recognized, and it may reach 80 percent or more at the height of an epidemic. Since the meningococci tend to colonize the posterior nasopharynx, a swab of mucus from this area is the specimen necessary for the isolation of meningococci from carriers. To prevent contamination of the swab with mucus from the uvula, fauces, tonsils, and tongue, a West tube can be a simple but valuable aid. This tube is a piece of $\frac{1}{4}$-inch glass tubing about an inch shorter than the handle of the swab. The ends of the West tube should be fire-glazed to avoid sharp edges. The sterile cotton swab is inserted into the sterile West tube, which is then inserted past the uvula and fauces to the posterior nasopharyngeal region. While the glass tube is held in place, the swab is pushed forward out of the tube and the nasopharyngeal membranes are swabbed. The swab is then pulled back into the glass tube before removing it and the swab from the mouth. A plate of blood-agar medium at 37°C should be inoculated immediately with the swab and then the plate returned to a 37°C incubator for 18 to 24 hours. Special selective media have been formulated to suppress the growth of gram-positive organisms that com-

monly inhabit the throat region. All cultures for meningococci should be incubated in a moist chamber containing 5 to 10 percent added CO_2. For this purpose a large-mouth glass jar containing a moistened filter paper, a small, no-smoke candle, and an airtight lid can be used. After placing the cultures in the jar, the candle is lighted and the lid is closed. As the flame burns itself out, enough CO_2 will be produced to meet the needs of the meningococci.

Saprophytic species of gram-negative diplococci (*Neisseria* sp.) may be found on the nasopharyngeal or buccal mucus membranes. These are practically never found in spinal fluid. The isolation of a gram-negative diplococcus from the posterior nasopharynx, therefore, necessitates additional taxonomic testing before concluding that it is *N. meningitidis.* Although biochemical tests on the isolated culture can be used, the quickest taxonomic differentiation of *N. meningitidis* from saprophytic *Neisseria* sp. is a serological agglutination test using polyvalent antiserum specific for all known antigenic serogroups of *N. meningitidis.* For this test, a saline suspension of the isolated organism (the test antigen) should be heated at 65°C for 10 to 15 minutes to destroy the autolytic enzyme (if the organism should be *N. meningitidis*). Since some strains of the saprophytic *Neisseria* sp. tend to autoagglutinate in saline or normal serum, a control, using a saline dilution (1:10) of normal serum from the same animal species from which the antiserum was obtained, should be included with the antiserum agglutination test. The meningococci generally do not autoagglutinate.

Different isolates of *N. meningitidis* have been shown to differ significantly in antigenic structure. This phenomenon of *antigenic heterogeneity* within a species will be found to occur to a greater or lesser extent as we consider other disease organisms. The phenomenon has a marked effect on serodiagnostic, serotaxonomic, and immunological practices. By 1953, four antigenic types (serogroups) of *N. meningitidis* were generally accepted and designated groups A, B, C, and D (Branham 1953). Group D meningococci are rarely found in the United States. Additional antigenic types of *N. meningitidis* (X, Y, Z, and two others) have been isolated occasionally from cases of the disease. With the possible exception of Y, however, they appear to be of little significance in the etiology of epidemic meningitis. A polyvalent antiserum, containing antibodies specific for four of the antigenic groups, will give a positive agglutination test result for a majority of N. meningitidis isolates regardless of its antigenic serogroup. If the individual group (A, B, C, or Y) of the isolate is desired, four agglutination tests may be needed, using antisera specific for each of the serogroups.

The mechanism whereby N. meningitidis produces its pathology was quite controversial at one time. One group of workers found toxin in the filtrate of broth cultures of the organism and claimed it to be an exotoxin. Another group found the washed meningococcal cells to be toxic for experimental animals. Further studies indicated that both the washed cells and the culture filtrates were antigenic and when animals were immunized with each, the reactivity of the antibodies, including the antitoxins, was identical. The explanation for these observations was the fact that during incubation many meningococci in the broth cultures underwent autolysis, thereby liberating all their body antigens including toxins into the broth. These soluble antigens then passed through the filter into the filtrate. More recent studies have indicated that the major toxin of the meningococci is a lipopolysaccharide and that the pathogenic mechanism is endotoxic.

Since roughly only one case of meningococcal meningitis occurs out of every twenty carriers of meningococci, N. meningitidis is considered to be low in invasive capacity. However, meningococcal meningitis can be one of the most fulminating of all infectious diseases. Death may occur in a few hours after onset. Consequently the low invasiveness is not a true measure of the potential virulence or pathogenicity of N. meningitidis.

CLINICAL CRITERIA

Meningococcal meningitis usually has a sudden onset of meningeal symptoms following a transient rhinopharyngitis. When tested by blood culture at this prodromal stage, a meningococcemia usually can be demonstrated. Following the short prodromal period, the patient may vomit and develop a fever and an agonizing headache. At this stage, the patient will develop a positive Kernig's sign—the inability to straighten the lower leg when the thigh is flexed at a right angle to the trunk. The patient may also develop a positive Brudzinski sign—coincident flexure of the ankle, knee, and hip when the neck is bent forward. Later the patient may develop a spasm of the trunk muscles leading to opisthotonos—the body bends backward and becomes rigid. These symptoms are not restricted to meningitis caused by N. meningitidis but may be observed to a greater or lesser extent in meningitis caused by any etiological agent, such as other bacterial species or viral (aseptic) meningitis. During the first 26 weeks of 1975, for example, 196 cases of meningitis caused by Haemophilus influenzae were reported in the United Kingdom (MMWR, 11 June 1976).

A case of meningococcal meningitis may be complicated by kidney damage (nephritis) or by cranial nerve involvement. Moreover, the disease may result in changes in the permeability of the meninges leading to hydrocephalus in infants.

PREVALENCE AND EPIDEMIOLOGY

There are no geographical limitations to the incidence of meningococcal meningitis, although such limitations may be observed relative to the serogroup of the organism causing meningitis in different areas of the world. Serogroup-A meningococci, for instance, were not found in cases of meningitis in North America for approximately 30 years prior to 1970. During this time, however, serogroup-A meningitis was quite prevalent in Africa. In January 1970 a case of serogroup-A meningococcal meningitis was identified in northern Manitoba, Canada. During the following 13 months, 107 cases of meningococcal disease were reported from this province; of the 61 typed isolates from these cases, 38 proved to be serogroup-A. Subsequently cases of serogroup-A meningococcal meningitis have been identified in other provinces in Canada and in New Hampshire, Massachusetts, Washington (state), and Illinois in the United States. Serogroup-A meningococci appear to be unique in their ability to cause widespread epidemics. This has been related to a higher ratio of cases to carriers of serogroup A than that found in other meningococcal serogroups (Aycock and Mueller 1950). Another interesting aspect of serogroup-A meningococci is the fact that practically all isolates tested have been found to be susceptible to sulfonamides, whereas many serogroup B and C isolates have been found to be resistant to these drugs. A total of 1,478 cases of meningococcal infection were reported to the National Center for Disease Control (CDC) in Atlanta during 1975 (see *MMWR* annual supplement, August 1976). De Morais et al. (1974) reported 2,005 cases of serogroup-C meningococcal meningitis during 1971–1972 in São Paulo, Brazil.

The mortality rate in untreated meningococcal meningitis has ranged from 25 to 90 percent with an average of about 50 percent. Immunotherapy first tended to cut this mortality rate, but with the discovery of the therapeutic efficacy of sulfonamides, penicillin, and other antibiotics, immunotherapy has been displaced by treatment with these more effective drugs.

Meningococcal meningitis frequently has been a health problem among armed forces personnel, especially new recruits. Since fatigue and crowding have been established as factors influencing infection in this disease, the armed forces, particularly during wartime emergencies, could be expected to be a high-risk group. During World War I, a study of the relationship between bed spacing and the meningococcal carrier rate in barracks during outbreaks of meningitis yielded the results presented in Table 6-1. Findings such as these resulted in the practices of alternating head and foot orientation of cots in crowded barracks and interposing a triangular sheet of canvas between beds in crowded hospital wards. These practices were designed to decrease the spread of respiratory diseases in general.

Meningococcal meningitis is a disease of humans only. Experimental inoculation of meningococci into the spinal cord or brain of mon-

Table 6-1. Relationship between bed spacing and meningococcal carrier rates.

Bed Spacing (inches)	Carrier Rate (%)
9	30+
12	20+
16	9+
30	5+
36	2

keys produces a disease similar to meningitis in humans. Mice, guinea pigs, rabbits, dogs, and horses can be killed by suitably large injections of meningococci. These inoculations, however, appear to be lethal toxic doses rather than true infections. Consequently, the source of human infection is cases of human meningitis or asymptomatic carriers of meningococci. The primary vehicle is rhinopharyngeal mucus exudate admixed with saliva. Because of the high carrier/case ratio, the epidemiology of meningococcal meningitis is preeminently carrier transmission by the respiratory mode summarized in Figure II-A. Secondary vehicles, however, are of lesser importance here than in most respiratory group diseases because of the high susceptibility of *N. meningitidis* to conditions outside the body of the human host.

LABORATORY DIAGNOSIS

For a specific diagnosis of a case showing symptoms of meningitis, the specimen required is spinal fluid. A plate of a suitable enriched medium such as Mueller-Hinton agar (see Vera and Dumoff 1974) should be warmed to 37°C and brought to the bedside of the patient at the time the physician plans to do the spinal tap. A few drops of spinal fluid should be allowed to fall directly from the tap needle onto the surface of the agar. The plate should be tilted to spread the spinal fluid over the surface and placed immediately in the CO_2 jar in the 37°C incubator. An additional 5 to 10 milliliters of spinal fluid should be collected in a sterile screw-cap tube and kept at 37°C for a stained smear and additional culture and other testing procedures.

If the spinal fluid in the tube is crystal clear or only slightly turbid, it should be centrifuged before preparing a smear of the sediment for staining. Also, a second plate of agar medium should be inoculated with sediment from the clear spinal fluid and then incubated along with the originally inoculated plate of medium. The smear, on a microslide, should be allowed to dry and then be fixed by heat or methanol before staining by the gram method. Finding gram-negative, coffee-bean-shaped diplococci (see Figure E-1 on the back cover) in the spinal fluid, either intracellularly (in the leucocytes) or extracellularly, is about as diagnostic of meningococcal meningitis as any microscopic demonstration of an organism can be for any disease. Except for the occasional presence of N. gonorrhoeae, other gram-negative diplococci are found so rarely in spinal fluid that they can, for all practical purposes, be disregarded.

The plate culture after overnight incubation at 37°C in an added CO_2 atmosphere, should be examined for evidence of bacterial growth. If no growth is present, the plate should be returned to the 37°C incubator for an additional overnight incubation. If growth is present, a smear of the growth should be prepared on a microslide, fixed, and stained by the gram method. If typical gram-negative diplococci are found, they can be assumed to be meningococci. If their serogroup (A, B, C, or Y) is desired, some of the growth can be suspended in saline, heated at 65°C for 10–15 minutes to inactivate the autolytic enzyme, and tested for agglutination in antisera specific for each of the four groups. The group antiserum (anti-A, -B, -C, or -Y), which causes agglutination of the isolated bacterial cell suspension, identifies the serogroup of the isolate. A normal serum control, which receives the same amount of the bacterial suspension as the test preparations, should be included to rule out autoagglutination of the unknown test suspension.

Whereas the determination of the serogroup of a meningococcus isolate or the species of other bacterial isolates from the cerebrospinal fluid (CSF) of cases of meningitis may be important to the epidemiologist, the clinician is more interested in determining the susceptibility or resistance of the isolate to potential therapeutic drugs. Although a number of assay methods are available (see Sabath and Matsen 1974), the agar diffusion (disc) testing method of Bennett et al. (1968) is recommended for N. meningitidis and other bacterial species that require high concentrations of CO_2 for growth.

If meningococcemia is suspected, the specimen for the laboratory diagnosis is 5 to 10 milliliters of the patient's blood. This should be withdrawn aseptically from a vein and inoculated to a container of suitable broth medium at 37°C and placed in a CO_2 jar in the 37°C incubator immediately. After overnight incubation, the cellular elements (erythrocytes and leucocytes) of the blood will have sedimented leaving a clear broth-serum supernatant. Usually, if there is bacterial growth, this supernatant fluid will show some degree of turbidity. If sufficiently turbid, a gram-stained smear of the supernatant fluid will show the presence of typical gram-negative diplococci if the patient has a meningococcemia. If no evidence of growth is found, the broth culture should be incubated at 37°C for an additional overnight period and reexamined. If there is still no evidence of growth, some of the culture fluid should be inoculated to the surface of a plate of blood-agar medium and incubated in a CO_2 jar at 37°C overnight before concluding that the test is negative.

As indicated, N. meningitidis tends to colonize the posterior nasopharynx of carriers. Consequently, a swab specimen of rhinopharyngeal mucus is essential for the laboratory diagnosis of the carrier state. Also, as indicated above, a West tube is a simple and easily prepared aid for preventing contamination of the swab with mucus and bacteria from the buccal region. Again a plate of blood-agar medium should be warmed to 37°C before collecting the swab specimen. For best results in carrier diagnosis, a selective medium might be preferred (see Catlin 1974). The mucus specimen on the swab should be inoculated to a small area on the edge of the warm agar surface. Then, with a sterile bacteriological loop, the bacteria in this inoculum are dispersed (streaked) over the surface of the agar and the plate is immediately placed in a CO_2 jar in the 37°C incubator. After overnight incubation, the plate is examined for small transparent colonies typical of *N. meningitidis.* If such are found, they are encircled on the bottom of the plate for subsequent identification. A portion of each colony is fished by touching the edge with a sterile loop, and a smear is prepared in a tiny drop of water on a microslide. Smears from several colonies can be placed on one microslide and all stained by the gram method at the same time. If one or more of the colonies are composed of gram-negative diplococci, the organisms may be *N. meningitidis* or they may be saprophytic *Neisseria.*

Each colony of typical gram-negative diplococci should be fished from the agar plate and inoculated to a warm agar slant of the same enriched medium as that used in the petri plate. These agar slant tubes are incubated as described above. The growth on each of these slants is rechecked to be sure it is composed only of gram-negative diplococci. Some of the typical growth from each agar slant is suspended, to desirable turbidity, in 5 to 10 milliliters of sterile saline. The suspensions are heated at 65°C for 10 to 15 minutes and are used as the unknown antigens in serotaxonomic agglutination tests using each of the four serogroup (A, B, C, Y) antimeningococcal antisera. A normal serum control should be included for each bacterial antigen tested. If the control shows agglutination, comparable results with the antiserum have no taxonomic significance. If one of the serogroup antisera causes agglutination of the unknown bacterial cells and these are not agglutinated in the normal serum control, the cells are identified as *N. meningitidis* of the same serogroup as that of the positive test antiserum. Biochemical tests (see Catlin 1974) are available for the taxonomic differentiation of the various *Neisseria* species; but in the author's experience they are hardly worth the effort.

Because of the availability of chemotherapy for bacterial but not for viral infections, a significant laboratory contribution to the diagnosis of meningitis involves this etiological differential. If no bacteria are isolated from cultures of the cerebrospinal fluid (CSF), the usual practice is to designate the symptomatic disease as viral or aseptic meningitis. If antibiotics have been administered prior to collecting the CSF specimen from bacterial cases, however, or for other reasons, the culture may yield a false negative result.

At the Ninth International Congress of Chemotherapy in London, Controni and his colleagues of Washington, D.C., reported a rapid method of distinguishing between bacterial and nonbacterial (viral?) meningitis. Prior investigators had reported higher than normal (upper limit of normal is 20 milligrams/100 milliliters) concentrations of lactate in the CSF of cases of meningococcal and other bacterial meningitis. Controni's group studied CSF from 200 cases of clinical meningitis, 21 of which were diagnosed by culture as bacterial—*Streptococcus pneumoniae, Hemophilus influenza*, group B *Streptococcus, Klebsiella pneumoniae,* and *Listeria monocytogenes.* They established the lactate levels of the CSF by means of gas liquid chromatography (GLC), which required only 15 to 20 minutes per test. Cerebrospinal fluid from all 21 bacterial cases yielded significantly elevated levels of lactate, whereas all the 179 nonbacterial (viral) cases yielded normal levels. The authors contend that their GLC lactate method not only leads to a rapid differential diagnosis between viral and bacterial meningitis but also can serve as a means of monitoring the efficacy of chemotherapy in bacterial meningitis.

Serodiagnostic tests (testing the patient's serum for antibodies specific for meningococci) have no practical value in the laboratory diagnosis of meningitis. Moreover, no skin tests, either for diagnosis or for evidence of susceptibility or immunity, are available for use in this disease.

IMMUNOLOGICAL MEASURES

Since 1971 two meningococcal cell-wall polysaccharide vaccines have been licensed for selective use in the United States. These consist of purified polysaccharide antigens of serogroups A and C and may be obtained as monovalent (A or C) or divalent (A-C) vaccines. The vaccines have been proved safe for human use, and serogroup-A vaccine has been evaluated as highly effective in 62,000 Egyptian schoolchildren aged 6 to 15 years. Serogroup-C vaccine has been administered to some 500,000 military recruits and to infants and preschool and school-age children in America. On the basis of antibody response, the vaccine appears to be effective in individuals more than 2 years of age. Routine vaccination of civilians, however, is not recommended (see *MMWR*, 8 November 1975).

Immunotherapy with antimeningococcal antisera from horses was first used around the turn of the twentieth century. Evidence indicated that this treatment decreased the mortality rate to some extent. The belief grew that the antiserum exerted an opsonic effect, thereby increasing the rate of phagocytosis of the meningococcal cells and decreasing the pathology caused by these organisms. With the discovery of sulfonamides, the therapeutic efficacy of these drugs (sulfadiazine and sulfisoxazole) proved to be significantly greater than immunotherapy. Then penicillin proved effective in treating meningococcal meningitis. Consequently, immunotherapy in this disease has been completely displaced by drug therapy.

CONTROL AND PREVENTION

Meningococcal meningitis patients are quarantined for 14 days or until negative cultures are obtained from the posterior nasopharynx. In view of the high carrier rates among contacts in this disease, however, directing the control measures at cases alone can be expected to have little effect on the spread of the disease.

Chemoprophylaxis in contact groups (a sulfonamide tablet every day) has been practiced, particularly by the armed forces during wartime. This policy may have been effective on a short-term basis, but it probably is responsible, in part at least, for the development of sulfonamide-resistant strains of *N. meningitidis*. Such resistant strains of serogroup B and C

meningococci were isolated from carriers at Fort Ord, California, in 1963–1964 and at Fort Wood, Missouri, in 1970. If sulfonamide therapy is considered for treating a case of meningococcal meningitis, it is becoming increasingly important to determine whether the strain of meningococcus causing the infection is susceptible or resistant to these drugs. Fortunately, meningococci have not yet developed significant resistance to the penicillins.

Household contacts of a case of meningococcal disease are generally accepted as probable carriers of meningococci, as are comparably close contacts in other groups. Carrier surveys among contacts in such groups, therefore, are considered unnecessary; and surveys among larger groups are impractical. Since sulfonamide-resistant meningococci are becoming more prevalent, the Food and Drug Administration has approved two additional drugs, rifampin and minocycline, for use in eradicating the carrier state in adults. Minocycline has been reported to cause vestibular reactions in recipients, however. If it is used, recipients should be warned against driving an automobile (see *MMWR*, 11 January 1975 and 13 February 1975).

The greatest hope for the prevention of meningococcal meningitis, at present, is that the meningococcal vaccines now being tested will prove to be effective.

REFERENCES

Aycock, W. L. and J. H. Mueller. 1950. Meningococcus carrier rates and meningitis incidence. *Bacteriol. Rev.* 14:115–160.

Bennett, J. V., H. V. Camp, and T. C. Eickhoff. 1968. Rapid sulfonamide disc sensitivity test for meningococci. *Appl. Microbiol.* 16:1056–1060.

Branham, S. E. 1953. Serological relationships among meningococci. *Bacteriol. Rev.* 17:175–188.

Catlin, B. W. 1974. *Neisseria meningitidis* (Meningococcus). Chapter 10 in *Manual of Clinical Microbiology*.

De Morais, J. S., R. S. Mumford, J. B. Risi, E. Antezena, and R. A. Feldman. 1974. Epidemic disease due to serogroup-C *Neisseria meningitidis* in São Paulo, Brazil. *J. Infect. Dis.* 129:568–571.

Sabath, L. D. and J. M. Matsen. 1974. Assay of antimicrobial agents. Chapter 47 in *Manual of Clinical Microbiology.*

Vera, H. D. and M. Dumoff. 1974. Culture media. Chapter 95 in *Manual of Clinical Microbiology.*

7

Pneumococcal Pneumonia

Pneumonia (pneumonitis), like meningitis, is an idiopathic designation for an anatomical (lung) disease that can be caused by a variety of bacteria, viruses, and rickettsiae. Also like meningitis, pneumonia can be caused by a variety of coccus forms of bacteria, but the designation pneumococcus is reserved for just one of these: a gram-positive, encapsulated, lancet-shaped diplococcus. The disease pneumonia is commonly divided into two anatomical forms, bronchial pneumonia and lobar pneumonia. Bronchial pneumonia is more prevalent in infants, young children, and the aged. It tends to occur as a diffuse lobular involvement of alveoli contiguous to the larger bronchioles of the bronchial tree. It can be caused by a variety of bacteria, including pneumococci, and by viruses, rickettsiae, or fungi. Lobar pneumonia is more prone to occur in young adults. It tends to involve part or all of a single lobe of the lungs, although more than one lobe may be involved. A majority (80 to 90 percent) of the cases of lobar pneumonia are caused by *Streptococcus (Diplococcus) pneumoniae*. In lobar pneumonia the entire area of involvement tends to become a consolidated mass, in contrast to the spongy texture of normal lung tissue. Pasteur in France and Sternberg in the United States were the first to describe pneumococci, although they did not relate the organism to pneumonia. Independent studies by Frankel and by Weichselbaum between 1884 and 1886 established the pneumococcus as the most frequent cause of pneumonia in humans. This chapter deals with pneumonia caused by the pneumococcus, primarily lobar pneumonia.

THE ETIOLOGICAL AGENT

The generally accepted taxonomic designation for the pneumococcus in America prior to the eighth edition of *Bergey's Manual* (1974) was *Diplococcus pneumoniae*. Since the British and now the American taxonomists do not recognize the legitimacy of the genus *Diplococcus*, however, the current name is *Streptococcus pneumoniae.* The diplococcal form of this organism is a pair of gram-positive, encapsulated, lancet-shaped cocci (elongated cocci with slightly pointed outer curvature). The pneumococci, however, may occur as single, paired, or short-chain forms within the characteristic capsules. It is the diplococcal form that tends to predominate in most infections.

Streptococcus pneumoniae can be cultivated at 37°C on a blood or serum-enriched peptone (neopeptone, Difco) infusion agar medium (pH 7.4) or in such broth without the agar. For best results, the agar plate cultures should be incubated in 5 percent added CO_2 (see the candle jar technique described in Chapter 6). On blood-agar medium the pneumococci tend to produce a greenish discoloration immediately surrounding the growing colonies. This is designated *alpha hemolysis* and results from the conversion of the hemoglobin of the red blood cells to methemoglobin. Certain strains of other streptococci (alpha hemolytic or viridans) also produce these changes when grown on blood agar.

Pneumococci will not withstand drying, but otherwise they are not as susceptible to environmental conditions as the meningococci. One function of the blood in the culture medium is to provide catalase to prevent the accumulation of hydrogen peroxide (H_2O_2) to which pneumococci are highly susceptible. Whereas 0.5 percent glucose in the culture medium actively stimulates growth of pneumococci, the glucose is rapidly converted to lactic acid, which tends to suppress growth of the organisms. If a means of maintaining the pH of a broth medium above 7.0 is utilized, glucose in the medium can result in a tenfold increase in the pneumococcal cell yield over the same medium without glucose. Pneumococci frequently die out during serial culture, probably as a result of failure to control the H_2O_2 production and the pH of the medium. For the growth of small inoculae of pneumococci, the broth medium must be in a reduced state. This can be brought about by heating to a boil and rapidly cooling the broth just prior to inoculation.

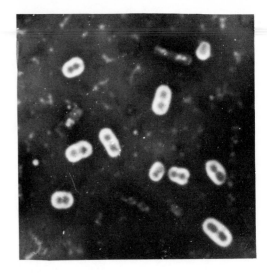

Figure 7–1.   A combination negative-positive stained smear of encapsulated pneumococci.

Pneumococcal cells produce the best-developed and most easily demonstrable capsules of any of the pathogenic bacteria we will consider (see Figure 7-1). The capsules are produced best in host tissues and are readily demonstrable in mucoid exudate coughed up from the lungs of human patients or in the exudate from the peritoneal cavity of experimentally infected mice. They can be demonstrated on young cultures in serum-enriched peptone-infusion broth but are much more poorly developed and more poorly demonstrable in cells grown on agar media. The capsules are composed of complex polysaccharides.

F. Neufeld first reported immunological differences in different cultures of pneumococci. A. R. Dochez and L. J. Gillespie in 1913 classified the pneumococci into antigenic types (serotypes) 1, 2, 3, and a heterogeneous group IV. Prior to 1940, serotypes 1 and 2 pneumococci were found to cause about one-half of the cases of pneumococcal pneumonia. Dochez and Avery in 1917 found a *soluble specific substance* (SSS) in the blood and urine of patients with pneumococcal pneumonia. This SSS gave a precipitation reaction with antiserum specific for the serotype of pneumococcus (1, 2, or 3) causing the disease in the patient. This SSS was later established to be carbohydrate in nature and was found to be produced and liberated from the pneumococci during capsule synthesis. The capsules are composed of the same type of carbohydrate (polysaccharide) material and are responsible for the serotype specificity of the pneumococci.

As early as 1902, Neufeld reported that when pneumococci were placed in the antiserum of a rabbit that had been immunized with the pneumococci, the capsules underwent a "quellung" or swelling reaction (see Figure 7-2). This observation had no practical value at the time. During the 1920s and early 1930s, however, when pneumococcal pneumonia became one of the major causes of human mortality and when specific immunotherapy was the only method of treatment, the Neufeld test was revived for quick serotype diagnosis. First the additional 29 antigenic serotypes, comprising the then known members of group IV pneumococci, were identified. Immune sera (horse or rabbit) for each of the 32 serotypes were then made available for immunotherapy. Yet even at this stage the antigenic heterogeneity (which now has reached 82 serotypes) was too great for the use of polyvalent antiserum for therapy. Consequently the serotype of the pneumococci

Figure 7–2. Demonstration of a positive Neufeld quellung test on *Streptococcus pneumoniae.* Capsules around the pairs of cells are swollen following treatment with specific antiserum. (Courtesy of R. Austrian.)

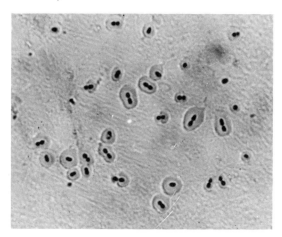

in the sputum of the patient had to be established quickly in order to permit specific therapy. For this purpose the Neufeld test was selected and the 32 serotype antisera were grouped into six groups of 3 to 6 antisera each. Preparations consisting of a bacteriological loop of sputum, a loop of group (pooled) antiserum, and a loop of methylene blue were mixed on a microslide and covered with a microcoverslip. If needed, comparable preparations were made for each of the other group antisera. The group preparation, which showed capsule swelling of the pneumococci in the sputum, reduced the serotype possibilities from 32 to 3, 5, or 6. Individual tests with these 3 to 6 monotypic antisera then pinpointed the serotype of the pneumococcus responsible for the infection. A competent technologist could, by the Neufeld testing procedure, report the serotype (if one of the 32) of the pneumococcus causing the infection within 30 to 60 minutes after receiving the sputum specimen. The patient then could be treated with antiserum specific for that serotype. At about the time (mid-1930s) these diagnostic and treatment procedures were receiving general acceptance by the medical profession, sulfonamides and then penicillin were found to be effective in the treatment of pneumococcal pneumonia regardless of serotype, and both serotyping and immunotherapy were displaced by drug therapy.

Pneumococcal typing antisera for the first 33 serotypes still are available commercially in the pooled (group) form in the United States. The 33 monotypic antisera are produced by the National Center for Disease Control (CDC) in Atlanta and are made available to public health laboratories and to certain research workers. Monotypic antisera for all 82 pneumococcal serotypes, now known, may be purchased from the Statens Seruminstitut, Copenhagen, Denmark. The Seruminstitut also produces a highly concentrated antiserum, "omniserum," which is claimed to react with all 82 pneumococcal capsular types (see Lund and Rasmussen 1966). This antiserum permits the identification of a suspect organism as a pneumococcus by a single Neufeld test, regardless of serotype.

Table 7-1. Physicochemical properties of capsular polysaccharides from serotype 1, 2, and 3 pneumococci.

Serotype	Optical Rotation	Molecular Weight	Percent Nitrogen	Hydrolytic Constituents
1	+265 to +270	171,000	4.6	Galacturonic acid, N-acetylglucosamine, acetic acid
2	+60	504,000	0.2*	D-glucose, D-glucuronic acid, L-rhamnose
3	−33 to −37	141,000	0.05	Glucuronic acid, glucose

* Approximate.

Examples of the physicochemical differences in the capsular polysaccharides are listed for serotype 1, 2, and 3 pneumococci in Table 7-1. The sequence and variety of the simple sugars, sugar acids, and aminosugars in the polysaccharide determine the antigenic specificity of the capsule of that serotype. The synthesis of these polysaccharides is under genetic control so that the progeny of a given serotype normally produce the same type of capsular polysaccharides. The somatic (cell body) antigens of pneumococci differ from the serotype capsular antigens. They appear to be relatively, but not completely, homogeneous in their antigenic composition, regardless of capsular serotype.

DNA TRANSFORMATION OF PNEUMOCOCCAL SEROTYPES

Griffith (1928) injected a mixture of live, nonencapsulated (R), type 2 pneumococci and killed type 3 pneumococci into the peritoneal cavity of a mouse. When he autopsied the mouse and cultured the peritoneal exudate, he was able to demonstrate the presence of live type 3 pneumococci. Control mice, the ones that received the killed type 3 pneumococci only, were not infected. Avery, MacLeod, and McCarty (1944) showed that pneumococcal transformation, comparable to that reported by Griffith, could be effected by purified preparation of deoxyribonucleic acid (DNA) in place of the killed pneumococci. This transformation was demonstrated both in mice and in broth culture preparations. Not only the transformed pneumococcus but all its progeny synthesized capsules of the same serotype as that from which the DNA was obtained. These and related studies provided the first evidence that DNA constitutes the genetic material of the cell.

PATHOGENIC MECHANISM

Extensive efforts have been made to determine the mechanism whereby *S. pneumoniae* produces its pathological effect on the host. No significant toxins have been detected and no necrosis of the involved lung tissue occurs. The organism is highly invasive, and large numbers are found in the tissues and exudates at the site of involvement. That the capsules of the pneumococci are in some way involved in pathogenicity is indicated by the fact that although one to five encapsulated pneumococci of a given serotype will cause a fatal infection in a mouse, 1 to 2 × 10^8 nonencapsulated organisms of the same genetic serotype are required for a fatal mouse infection. Moreover, MacLeod and McCarty, in 1942, noted that type 14 pneumococci are avirulent for the mouse. When nonencapsulated pneumococci of type 14 were exposed to DNA from mouse-virulent type 2 pneumococci, however, the transformed (type 14 to type 2) pneumococci were highly virulent for the mouse. The reciprocal of this experiment also was demonstrated. Obviously other genetic factors may have been involved in these transformations, but only the capsular changes could be related to the virulence of the pneumococci.

Regardless of the mechanism, the gross pathology of pneumococcal lobar pneumonia involves edema of the alveolar walls and leakage of plasma and red blood cells into the alveoli. Precipitation of the plasma fibrin (clotting) in the air sacs leads to the consolidation of the area of involvement. Also, polymorphonuclear leucocytes migrate to the area in large numbers. These components plus mucus compose the highly tenacious, red-tinged or rusty brown sputum coughed up from deep in the bronchial tree of lobar pneumonia patients.

CLINICAL CRITERIA AND PREVALENCE

Pneumococcal pneumonia rarely is a primary human infection. It usually follows viral infections such as the common cold, influenza, or measles. Another predisposing factor is damage to the respiratory mucosa caused by toxic gas inhalation. Just how these predisposing factors influence the invasion by pneumococci is not known. In experimental pneumococcal pneumonia infections in monkeys and dogs, depression of respiration and the cough reflex by the administration of narcotics proved essential to success. In dogs, it was necessary to block off air exchange (atelectasis) at the site in the lungs where the virulent pneumococci were introduced. Whether or not these predisposing factors tend to produce a localized state of atelectasis at the site of initiation of pneumococcal infection in humans has not been established.

The onset of lobar pneumonia is characteristically sudden, usually involving a chill followed by high fever and coincident pain in the chest or side. During deep coughing spasms, a bloodstained or rust-colored tenacious sputum is raised. This usually contains large numbers of pneumococci and is the specimen submitted for laboratory diagnosis. Untreated, the symptoms usually last 5 to 10 days with dramatic recovery if the crisis is passed successfully. Following the crisis, the area of involvement in the lung clears rapidly with no necrosis, scar tissue, or permanent damage. A patient who on one day is near death may feel inclined to get up and proceed with normal activity the next.

Pleurisy is a common complication of pneumococcal pneumonia. If the pleural inflammation extends to the lining membranes of the chest cavity, the two sites may form adhesions as they heal, resulting in a very painful sequel that may necessitate surgery to remedy. Another complication of pneumonia is *empyemia*—pus in the pleural cavity that may necessitate tapping. A complication with prognostic significance is a persistent pneumococcal bacteremia (*pneumococcemia*). Two independent studies yielded a combined mortality rate of 60.7 percent in 173 cases of pneumonia showing a persistent pneumococcal bacteremia, whereas the mortality rate in 382 cases not showing such a bacteremia was only 8.6 percent. Both the incidence of complications and the mortality rates for all cases of pneumococcal pneumonia have been drastically lowered by the availability of antibiotic and other drug therapy.

Pneumococcal pneumonia occurs in all areas of the world, particularly where changeable, inclement weather prevails. Since the viral diseases that predispose patients to pneumococcal pneumonia generally are cold weather diseases, the morbidity rates for pneumonia are higher during the cold weather months and particularly during epidemics of these viral diseases. Cases of pneumococcal pneumonia do occur during all seasons of the year, however. Also, some serotypes of *S. pneumoniae* are significantly more virulent for humans than others. In one study of 3,713 cases, 81 percent were caused by types 1, 2, and 3.

EPIDEMIOLOGY

Streptococcus pneumoniae is a common inhabitant of the nasobuccal region of normal, healthy human beings. Studies on such individuals have yielded carrier rates of 40 to 60 percent, depending upon (1) the season of the year, (2) known contact by the individual with a case of the disease, or (3) culturing during the presence of other respiratory infections in the individuals. This high carrier incidence raises the question of whether the source of the pneumococci that cause pneumonia in a given individual is exogenous or endogenous. Evidence favoring the exogenous source is the following:

1. Whereas pneumococci of types 1 and 2 cause around 40 percent of the cases of pneumococcal pneumonia, they are among the less frequently found serotypes in carriers, except in known contacts with such cases.

2. The incidence of homologous carrier types of pneumococci has been observed to rise in groups in contact with a case or cases of pneumococcal pneumonia.

3. The carrier state in an individual is intermittent, involving carrier-free periods and changes in carrier types.

Although the ultimate source of the pneumococci causing a case of pneumonia appears to be exogenous, there is fairly convincing evidence for a more immediate endogenous source. For example, the pneumococci that a normal healthy person is carrying when he contracts a predisposing infection would seem to be the most likely candidates for invasion to the lungs. Moreover, epidemics of pneumococcal pneumonia are extremely rare, although some have been reported in relatively closed groups. In fact, two concomitant cases of pneumococcal pneumonia in the same family are relatively rare. Thus it appears that the epidemiology of pneumococcal pneumonia involves the presence of virulent pneumococci on the upper respiratory membranes when a predisposing factor lowers the normal resistance of these membranes to invasion by the endogenous pneumococci. The longer that virulent pneumococci are carried on these membranes, the greater the chance that their presence and the predisposing infection will occur simultaneously. There is no doubt, however, that pneumococci from cases or carriers are spread by the respiratory modes of transmission presented diagrammatically in

Figure II-A. The question of the period of communicability of a case of pneumococcal pneumonia, therefore, is not given serious concern. Undoubtedly the case can transmit the virulent pneumococci to others as long as these pneumococci persist in the respiratory tract. However, the rarity of case-to-case or epidemic transmission rules against the need for quarantine and related control measures in this disease.

Although humans constitute the major host for pneumococci, guinea pigs, monkeys, and rats have been reported to suffer natural infections with these organisms. Epizootics of pneumococcal pneumonia have been reported among monkeys in captivity. Pneumococci have been reported, moreover, as the cause of one of the most frequent and fatal epizootic diseases of guinea pigs. These animal infections appear to have little importance insofar as reservoirs for human disease is concerned, however. Although dogs, monkeys, and rabbits have been used as experimental animals for studying pneumococcal disease, the white mouse is the animal of choice for most clinical and public health laboratory work.

LABORATORY DIAGNOSIS

At least one blood culture, using a suitable broth medium, should be performed on every case of suspected pneumococcal pneumonia. If pneumococci are isolated, they have both diagnostic and potential prognostic significance. In such cases, one or more subsequent blood cultures should be performed to establish the prognostic significance of a persistent versus a transient pneumococcal bacteremia. It should be remembered, however, that blood cultures are rarely positive in pneumonia patients who have received chemotherapy.

The laboratory should also receive a sputum specimen coughed up from deep in the bronchial tree. This highly tenacious, frequently rusty brown specimen can be homogenized in a petri plate by adding an equal volume of saline and drawing the mixture into a hypodermic syringe (with no needle attached) and repeatedly expelling it back into the plate. A bacteriological loop may then be used to prepare a smear of the homogenized specimen on a microslide. After fixation, the smear should be stained by the gram method and examined microscopically. If the patient has pneumococcal pneumonia, large numbers of typical gram-positive, encapsulated diplococci usually will be found. If such organisms are not observed, a loop of the specimen should be streaked to the surface of a freshly poured blood-agar plate. The plate culture should be incubated overnight at 37°C in a CO_2 jar. If pneumococci are present in the sputum, they will develop into small colonies surrounded by greenish discoloration (alpha hemolysis) on the blood medium. Other alpha-hemolytic streptococci, which may be present in saliva from the buccal region, will develop into alpha-hemolytic colonies indistinguishable from those of the pneumococci, however. Among the several biochemical tests that may be used to distinguish between pneumococci and other alpha streptococci (see Austrian 1974), we will discuss only one—bile solubility. For such tests, it is best to transplant the alpha-hemolytic colony from the plate to a blood-agar slant to obtain an adequate supply of pure culture growth for testing.

Pneumococci generally are soluble in ox bile or bile salts due to the fact that these agents activate an autolytic enzyme in the cells. Other alpha-hemolytic streptococci generally are not bile-soluble. The bile solubility test should be performed on a fresh culture suspension of live cells at neutral pH. A small amount (1 milliliter) of this slightly turbid suspension should be placed in each of two small (0.5-inch-diameter) test tubes. A few drops of a 10 percent solution of the bile salt sodium deoxycholate are added to the suspension in one tube and an equal amount of sterile saline to the other (the control). The tubes are placed in a 37°C water bath. If the cells are pneumococci, the tube containing the bile salt should lose turbidity within 15 minutes. The incubation should be continued for 1 hour before calling the test negative, however.

A small amount (0.5 milliliter) of the homogenized sputum or of the culture suspension described above may be inoculated intraperitoneally into a white mouse. Eighteen to 96 hours later, the mouse, if still alive, may be sacrificed and autopsied.

The surest and quickest way of identifying a gram-positive coccus as *S. pneumoniae* is the Nuefeld quellung test (see Figure 7-2). However, since antisera (either group or monospecific) for only 33 of the 82 or more known serotypes are available in the United States, only pneumococci belonging to one of these serotypes can be so identified. If the "omniserum" of the Statens Seruminstitut in Denmark becomes widely available at a reasonable price, it should prove to be the ideal reagent for the serotaxonomic identification of an organism suspected to be *S. pneumoniae.* The Neufeld test should be performed on organisms present in the patient's sputum or on organisms in the peritoneal exudate from an infected mouse.

Kronvall (1973) has described a rapid coagglutination test for the identification of pneumococcal serotypes using a strain (Cowan) of *Staphylococcus aureus* with the antipneumococcal IgG absorbed (by the Fc portion) to the protein A coat of the *S. aureus* cells. This unique coagglutination test procedure also has been advocated for the identification of beta-hemolytic streptococci (see Chapter 8). Because of the large number of pneumococcal serotypes, however, the test, although rapid, unique, and serologically sound, is impractical.

Serodiagnostic tests using the patient's serum are not advocated in pneumococcal pneumonia. Patients do develop antibodies specific for the serotype of the pneumococcus causing the infection, but significant titers are reached only following recovery. Since some antibody to the various pneumococcal serotypes is commonly found in sera from normal, healthy individuals, a rising antibody titer in sera collected early in the infection and again after the crisis would be essential to provide even epidemiological significance. Since by the time the second serum specimen is needed the patient is well and happy, neither he nor his physician is interested in this method of post facto diagnosis.

IMMUNOLOGICAL CONSIDERATIONS

Animals can be actively immunized by injections of killed, virulent, encapsulated pneumococci. The immunity is type-specific but does not last more than a few months. There also is evidence that booster injections of the same serotype antigens do not maintain the immunity.

In human pneumococcal pneumonia, there is convincing evidence that recovery is associated with the appearance of type-specific antibody in the patient's serum. The immunity appears to be short-lived, however. MacLeod et al. (1945) conducted carefully controlled active immunization experiments on an armed forces group of human volunteers. They used a polyvalent vaccine consisting of purified polysaccharides from four of the six virulent pneumococcal types known to be prevalent in the group. One-half of the volunteers received no vaccine. The authors reported no cases of pneumonia in the immunized group caused by the four pneumococcal serotypes used in the vaccine. Cases of these and other types of pneumococcal pneumonia continued to occur in the nonimmunized controls. The incidence of the two types of pneumonia, caused by pneumococcal types not included in the vaccine, remained the same in both groups. These studies, performed more than 30 years ago, seem to provide convincing evidence that humans can be immunized against pneumococcal pneumonia. However, no such vaccines are available for human immunization today. Undoubtedly the extent of the antigenic heterogeneity (82 serotypes) among pneumococci is in part responsible for this lack of practical immunoprophylaxis. Probably other factors, such as the short duration of immunity, also enter into this lack of a practical means of preventive immunization against pneumococcal pneumonia.

Specific immunotherapy was the only method of treating pneumococcal pneumonia prior to the discovery of the sulfonamides and antibiotics. Now antibody therapy has been completely displaced by drug therapy. The efficacy of drug therapy in this disease is fortunate because no practical means of prevention have been discovered.

REFERENCES

Austrian, R. 1974. *Streptococcus pneumoniae* (Pneumococcus). Chapter 9 in *Manual of Clinical Microbiology.*

Avery, O. T., C. M. MacLeod, and M. McCarty. 1944. Studies on the chemical nature of the substance inducing transformation of pneumococcal types. Induction of transformation by a deoxyribonucleic acid fraction isolated from Pneumococcus type III. *J. Exper. Med.* 79:137–158.

Fleming, A. 1941. Some uses of nigrosin in bacteriology. *J. Path. Bact.* 53:293–296.

Griffith, F. 1928. The significance of pneumococcal types. *J. Hyg.* 27:113–159.

Kronvall, G. 1973. A rapid slide-agglutination method for typing pneumococci by means of specific antibody absorbed to protein A-containing staphylococci. *J. Med. Microbiol.* 6:187–190.

Lund, E. and P. Rasmussen. 1966. Omniserum. *Acta Pathol. Microbiol. Scand.* 68:458–460.

MacLeod, C. M., R. G. Hodges, M. Heidelberger, and W. G. Bernhard. 1945. Prevention of pneumococcal pneumonia by immunization with specific capsular polysaccharides. *J. Exper. Med.* 82:445–465.

8

Streptococcal Diseases

Streptococci are gram-positive, spherical or ovoid organisms that occur in chains of varying length (see Figure 8-1). Although the early observations of these organisms were in association with human disease (Rosenbach: *Streptococcus pyogenes*), many strains are now known to be either nonpathogenic or pathogenic for animals but not for humans. Some strains of streptococci are always found in the nasobuccal region of normal healthy human beings. Although these (alpha) streptococci are considered to be part of the normal saprophytic flora of this region, they can on occasion invade and cause infectious diseases ranging from simple nasopharyngitis or sinusitis to subacute bacterial endocarditis. Other strains of streptococci are highly virulent for humans and can cause a variety of serious disease symptoms and postrecovery sequelae of considerable importance (see Wannamaker and Matsen 1972).

Figure 8–1. Chains of *Streptococcus pyogenes.* (Courtesy of Center for Disease Control, Atlanta.)

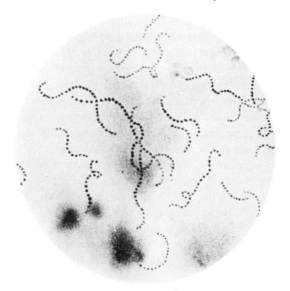

93

CLASSIFICATION

Many early efforts to classify streptococci into taxonomic species led to utter confusion, and this situation has not been completely resolved as yet. The requirement for enriched (blood) agar media for cultivation led to the discovery of the earliest differential characteristics among streptococci. Some strains produced colonies with a zone of greenish discoloration of the blood agar, whereas others produced a zone of complete clearing of the medium surrounding the colony. As noted for the pneumococci, the greenish discoloration is designated alpha hemolysis, although it appears that no true hemolysis of the blood erythrocytes occurs (the hemoglobin is converted to methemoglobin). These streptococci are designated alpha-hemolytic (or alpha type) streptococci and also have been called *viridans* streptococci. Those streptococci that cause complete clearing of the medium surrounding the colony are designated beta-hemolytic (or beta type) streptococci, and the clearing is the result of true hemolysis of the erythrocytes in the medium. Alpha hemolysis and beta hemolysis are shown in Figure F on the back cover. Colonies of other strains of streptococci produce no visible changes in the blood-agar media. Some authors designate these strains as gamma-type streptococci; others prefer to call them nonhemolytic streptococci.

The beta-hemolytic streptococci include most of the strains that cause acute disease in humans and animals. Early efforts at classification involved naming species after the disease from which the streptococci were isolated—such as *Streptococcus scarlatinae* or *Streptococcus erysipelatis*. This approach to streptococcal taxonomy, however, broke down with the recognition that the same strain could cause a variety of different disease symptoms in different individuals.

Efforts to classify beta-hemolytic streptococci into species on the basis of biochemical characteristics, although still practiced, are fraught with many instances of equivocal results. Early efforts at serotaxonomy, using intact streptococcal cells as the unknown antigen in agglutination tests with known antistreptococcal antisera, also were frequently confusing. The results of these initial attempts at taxonomic classification of the streptococci prompted an eminent Harvard bacteriologist, Hans Zinsser, to remark in the early 1930s that efforts to classify the streptococci had led to a maze of complex and shifting relationships of little value.

Beta-hemolytic streptococci from human disease tend to produce three commonly recognized colony types on blood agar. On fresh isolation from the patient, the young colony tends to be mucoid in consistency with a glistening surface. The cells of this type of colony can be shown to possess capsules composed of hyaluronic acid. These capsules are not as stable, as easily demonstrated, or as immunologically significant as the capsules of the pneumococci. As the mucoid colonies age (16–24 hours), they tend to dry down to more flattened colonies with wrinkled and frequently cross-striated (matted), nonglistening surface appearances. Such colony forms may dissociate into cells which produce stable glossy colonies that fail to manifest the matted surface appearance. These stable glossy colonies are composed of avirulent cells, whereas the mucoid and matted colonies are composed of virulent streptococci.

Rebecca Lancefield (1928; 1933) reported the first taxonomic subgrouping of the beta-hemolytic streptococci, which continues to have practical significance. She prepared various extracts of streptococcal cells and used them as the unknown antigen in precipitin tests with antisera specific for known-source streptococcal isolates. She reported that hot N/5 hydrochloric acid (HCl) extracts of the hemolytic streptococci from human disease (after neutralization) gave precipitates with antisera specific for these strains and not for antisera specific for the animal strains tested. The animal strains yielded comparable extracts that gave precipitates with antisera specific for the animal isolates. These extracts were found to be carbohydrate in nature and were designated streptococcal C substance. By 1962 some 18 antigenically distinct C substances had been reported from different streptococcal isolates. The streptococci yielding these group-specific antigens have been placed in Lancefield groups A through T, omitting groups I and J (see Slade and Slamp 1962; Slade 1965). Lancefield's group A streptococci cause the great majority of cases of beta-hemolytic streptococcal diseases of humans. The type species of group A is *Streptococcus pyogenes.*

Lancefield group C and G streptococci, however, have been found in human streptococcal disease. Moreover, Wilkinson et al. (1973) reported a total of 898 group B streptococci isolated from a variety of human clinical sources over a 5-year period. The infections included respiratory tract, genital tract, septicemias, meningitis, and others. Additional studies by CDC epidemiologists indicated that some of the group B cases of neonatal meningitis were acquired in the hospital nursery—they were

nosocomial cases. Thus it appears that group B streptococci are a more frequent cause of human disease than previously thought. Table 8-1 summarizes the isolation sources of the Lancefield group streptococci.

OTHER EXTRACTABLE ANTIGENS

Antigenic M proteins are extractable from the walls of group A streptococci that demonstrate the mucoid or matted colonies but not from glossy colony cells. These antigens are soluble in boiling water at low pH (2–3). Their presence is associated with the virulence of the streptococci and are the immunologically significant antigens (see Fox 1974). Unfortunately the M proteins of different *S. pyogenes* isolates are quite heterogeneous antigenically (more than 50 M serotypes

Table 8-1. Major sources of isolation of Lancefield Groups of streptococci.

Group	Animal Source	Type Species
A	Humans (many diseases)	S. pyogenes
B	Cattle and humans	S. agalactiae
C	Many animals and humans	S. equi (S. animalis)
D	Animals and humans (GI tract)	S. fecalis*
E	Cattle (milk) and swine	
F	Humans (no disease)	
G	Dogs and humans	
H	Humans (no disease)	
I, J	No longer recognized	
K	Humans (no disease)	
L	Dogs	
M	Dogs	
N	Dairy products	S. lactis*
O	Humans (no disease)	
P		
Q		
R		
S		
T		

* No beta hemolysis.

were reported prior to 1970). However, a number of workers have reported cross-reactivity between several of these M serotypes. This heterogeneity of the immunologically significant M serotypes accounts for the fact that human beings can suffer repeated attacks of group A streptococcal (*S. pyogenes*) infections.

Antigenic T and R proteins also are extractable from group A streptococcal cells. These antigens are more or less heat-labile at acid pH, and the T proteins are relatively resistant to proteolytic enzymes that may destroy M and R proteins. The T and R antigens (like the C substance) have no immunological significance, but they do participate in agglutination and other serological reactions with specific antisera.

SIGNIFICANT SOLUBLE PRODUCTS

Streptococcus pyogenes produces a number of significant soluble products, including toxins, hemolysins, and enzymes. These substances may not be produced simultaneously or by all strains, but when produced they may result in pathologically or immunobiologically significant manifestations of such streptococcal infections.

Erythrogenic toxin was established by George and Gladys Dick of Chicago as the cause of the skin (scarlatinal) rash in scarlet fever. Its production has been reported to be associated with lysogeny of the streptococcal cells by certain temperate bacteriophages (Zabriski 1964). It is an unusual exotoxin when compared to that of *C. diphtheriae*, however. It is heat-stable and appears not to be toxic for infants, even in the absence of antitoxin from the mother. This observation has raised the question of whether or not the scarlatinal rash of scarlet fever is a toxicity or a hypersensitivity manifestation of the erythrogenic toxin. For example, the erythrogenic toxin skin test may (1) be negative in an infant, (2) become positive in the same child who develops hypersensitivity resulting from *S. pyogenes* infections, and (3) become negative again as the result of an immune response such as that involved in an attack of scarlet fever. Although certain rabbits have been used in bioassays of erythrogenic toxin, the definitive

assays have been performed on human volunteers by determining the smallest amount of the toxin that will cause a minimal inflammatory reaction when 0.1 milliliter (the skin test dose, STD) is injected intradermally. In addition to this skin reactivity, the erythrogenic toxin results in a number of other pathogenic manifestations. Also, the erythrogenic toxin cannot be converted to toxoid. The majority of group A streptococci produce a single antigenic variety of erythrogenic toxin, although three additional antigenic varieties of the toxin have been reported from occasional strains of these streptococci. Since the erythrogenic toxins are immunogenic, the heterogeneous strains probably account for the occasional second attacks of scarlet fever. The second attack would be expected to involve a different M protein and a different erythrogenic-toxin-producing strain of *S. pyogenes* from that involved in the first attack.

Two hemolysins are produced by group A streptococci. One of these, *streptolysin O*, is antigenic; the other, *streptolysin S*, is not. Streptolysin O is oxygen-labile and, therefore, is hemolytic only in the reduced state. Both hemolysins could be expected to cause *in vivo* pathology due to hemolysis of host erythrocytes. However, streptolysin O has been shown to be toxic for heart tissues both in experimental animals and in cultured human heart tissue. Although streptolysin S has been shown to be highly pathogenic for experimental animals, it has not been sufficiently purified to differentiate its hemolytic activity from other toxic manifestations. Streptolysin S is liberated from the streptococcal cells only in the presence of serum or ribonucleic acid, whereas streptolysin O can be found in broth culture filtrates that are free of serum and RNA. The zones of beta hemolysis surrounding *aerobic* surface colonies of *S. pyogenes* on blood-agar plates are produced by streptolysin S. If the streptococcal cells are seeded into melted blood agar and the mixture is poured into a petri plate, however, both streptolysin O and streptolysin S will participate in the production of beta hemolysis around the embedded colonies. Moreover, streptolysin O will participate in the production of the zone of hemolysis around surface colonies if the blood-agar plates are incubated in an anaerobic environment.

Streptokinase (SKase), a fibrinolytic enzyme, is produced by some strains of Lancefield groups A, C, and G streptococci. This enzyme conceivably could be a virulence factor in that it would enable the streptococci that produce it to break out from entrapment in a fibrin clot and spread from a local or focal lesion. The enzyme has been isolated from streptococcal cultures and used as a fibrinolytic agent in human embolism therapy.

Another enzyme produced by certain strains of group A streptococci is *diphosphopyridine nucleotidase* (DPNase). This enzyme apears to be the cause of leucotoxicity in phagocytic cells that ingest these strains of streptococci.

All group A streptococci as well as some other (C and G) strains produce a variety of serologically (antigenically) distinct *deoxyribonucleases* (DNAses). A high percentage of patients infected with *S. pyogenes* produce antibody specific for one of the serotypes of this enzyme, DNAse B. These enzymes can cause a rapid depolymerization of deoxyribonucleic acid. Since there is no evidence that the DNAses attack living cells, however, the question of their pathological significance remains open.

Some strains of group A streptococci produce large quantities of the enzyme *hyaluronidase* (HDase). Since this enzyme attacks hyaluronic acid, it is either not produced by encapsulated strains or it is produced under growth conditions that are not conducive to capsule production. The rarity of laboratory evidence of HDase production by group A strains of streptococci is offset by the fact that practically every infection with any strain of these streptococci results in the production of a rising titer of anti-HDase antibodies. These are true antibodies, distinct from the nonspecific inhibitors of HDase found in some normal sera.

Another enzyme produced by group A streptococci is *streptococcal proteinase* (SPase) and its inactive precursor. The precursor can be converted autocatalytically to active SPase in culture media if the redox potential is not allowed to fall or if reducing agents are added to

solutions of the crystalline enzyme. Traces of the active enzyme or small amounts of trypsin seem to be essential for initiation of the autocatalytic conversion. Growth of the streptococci under conditions that allow the production of active SPase in the medium can affect other biological properties of the streptococci. The SPase may destroy the M proteins in the cell walls of the streptococci, for example, making it impossible to type these strains with anti-M antibody. Other extracellular protein products such as streptokinase or hyaluronidase may be destroyed by SPase. The extent to which this enzyme is involved in streptococcal pathology is not clear. Although precipitating antibodies to the crystalline enzyme can be produced by immunizing animals, inhibitory antibodies are rarely demonstrable in the sera of patients following group A streptococcal infections. However, a passive hemagglutination technique, wherein the enzyme is attached to red blood cells, has produced evidence of such antibody in a large proportion of patients following *S. pyogenes* infections.

Finally, another enzyme produced by group A streptococci is a *nicotinamide adenine dinucleotide glycohydrolase* (NADase or NADGase). Although the function of this enzyme in the pathology of these streptococci is not clear, antibodies specific for the enzyme have been found in the serum of patients following recovery from *S. pyogenes* infections.

DISEASES CAUSED BY GROUP A STREPTOCOCCI

The following list indicates the variety of pathological manifestations in humans that can result from *S. pyogenes* infections. Occasionally, some of these diseases may be caused by Lancefield group B, C, or G streptococci.

1. Skin: ulcerative dermatitis, lymphangitis, impetigo, erysipelas
2. Respiratory tract: nasopharyngitis, tonsilitis, peritonsillar abscesses, sinusitis, lympadenitis, otitis media, mastoiditis, laryngitis, bronchitis, pneumonitis (pneumonia)

3. Systemic: septicemia, septic arthritis, scarlet fever, puerperal fever, peritonitis, endocarditis (acute), meningitis, acute nephritis (usually a delayed sequel)

IMMUNOBIOLOGY

After it was established that erythrogenic toxin (ET) caused the skin rash of scarlet fever, a minor mystery developed relative to the fact than an individual could suffer repeated infections with strains of *S. pyogenes* that produced ET and yet suffer only one attack of scarlet fever. This mystery was resolved by the discovery of the antigenic heterogeneity (50+) of the immunologically significant M-protein serotypes of *S. pyogenes* and the practical homogeneity of the ET antigen. Eighty percent or more of the toxigenic strains of group A streptococci produce the same antigenic toxin. Therefore an attack of scarlet fever can be expected to provide lasting immunity to the M-protein and ET serotypes of the strain of *S. pyogenes* causing the infection but no immunity to the 49 or so additional M-protein and 3 rare ET serotypes of *S. pyogenes*. A second attack of scarlet fever would only be expected to occur in the rare instances when the recovered individual was subsequently infected with another M-protein serotype of *S. pyogenes* that also produced one of the rare heterologous ET serotypes. As in any immune response, however, there is the possibility that an individual might lose the antitoxic immunity from the first attack and suffer a second attack caused by the same ET. This possibility, in scarlet fever, is very remote, however, because of the frequent subclinical infections with the major toxigenic strains of *S. pyogenes*, each of which would exert a booster effect on the antitoxic immunity.

There are three types of delayed sequelae following symptomatic recovery from group A streptococcal infections in humans. These sequelae, which appear to be based on immunobiological phenomena, are (1) erythema nodosum, (2) acute glomerulonephritis, and (3) rheumatic fever. Sequelae (1) and (3) are prone to recur following subsequent *S. pyogenes* infections, whereas (2) generally is a nonrecurrent sequel. The time of appearance of these poststreptococcal disease sequelae coincides with the time at which the antibody response to *S. pyogenes* antigens reaches its maximum. The mechanism of the delayed pathology in these sequelae has not been clarified, however.

Erythema nodosum is characterized by the occurrence of inflamed, tender, nodular swellings, usually on the extremities. Associated symptoms of fever and general toxemia may occur. When this sequel results from a prior streptococcal infection, the symptoms may recur following subsequent *S. pyogenes* infections. Thus it would appear that as a result of the original streptococcal infection, localized sites become hypersensitive to some of the persistent antigens of *S. pyogenes*. Reaction between the hypersensitive tissue sites and these residual antigens results in the first attack of erythema nodosum. Following recovery, these sites appear to retain (or other sites develop) their state of hypersensitivity. Therefore, when antigens from a subsequent *S. pyogenes* infection are absorbed and disseminated to the sensitive sites, the erythema nodosum symptoms recur. More research is needed to establish or disprove this hypothesis.

Poststreptococcal acute glomerulonephritis (AGN) is characterized by the usual symptoms of kidney disease: albuminuria or hematuria, edema, and hypertension. Usually the period between the streptococcal infection and the onset of AGN is shorter than that in erythema nodosum or in rheumatic fever. Recurrence of AGN following subsequent *S. pyogenes* infections is rare, and there is little evidence of permanent kidney damage following recovery. Rammelkamp and Weaver (1953) and Lindberg and Vosti (1969) have published evidence that only certain nephritogenic strains of *S. pyogenes* are capable of causing AGN. The latter workers used an experimental rat model in their studies. The streptococci used were *S. pyogenes* serotype M-12N, the nephritogenic strain, and *S. pyogenes* serotype M-12, the nonnephritogenic strain. The former strain, but not the latter, caused

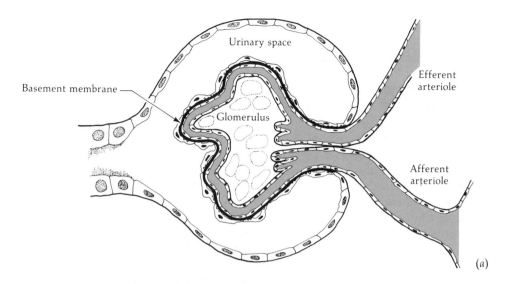

Urinary space

Efferent
arteriole

Basement membrane ———

Glomerulus

Afferent
arteriole

(a)

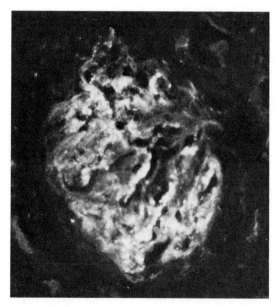

(b)

Figure 8–2. (a) Diagram of a section through a
kidney glomerulus. Note the location of the basement membrane. (b) Fluorescent antibody stain
showing distribution of streptococcus antigen-antibody complexes on the outer surface of glomerular
basement membranes. (Courtesy of H. Bauer.)

typical AGN in the rat. Other M serotypes of *S. pyogenes* also failed to cause AGN in the rat model. Lindberg and Vosti were able to elute IgG antibody globulin specific for M-12 protein from the glomeruli of rats infected with *S. pyogenes* M-12N, but not from rats exposed to *S. pyogenes* M-12. Antibody specific for M-12 protein was found in the serum (but not the kidney tissue) of the latter rats. (Figure 8-2 presents a diagram of a glomerulus and a micrograph showing streptococcus antigen-antibody complexes on the outer surface of the glomerular basement membrane.) Thus it would appear that the nephritogenic strain of *S. pyogenes* stimulated the production of homologous anti-M antibody that was fixed by glomerular tissue, whereas the anti-M antibody stimulated by the nonnephritogenic *S. pyogenes* was not so fixed. When the fixed-tissue anti-M antibody reacted with circulating homologous M protein, the resulting pathology gave rise to the AGN symptoms. It is possible that the failure of AGN to recur during subsequent *S. pyogenes* infections may be the consequence of the limited number of M serotypes of *S. pyogenes* that are nephritogenic.

Rheumatic fever (RF) is the most common and most important poststreptococcal disease sequel. The classic symptoms of RF are fever and migratory polyarthritis with a tendency toward the development of recurrent carditis. The time of onset of the symptoms, following an *S. pyogenes* infection, is variable but averages about 3 weeks. Streptococci are not found in the arthritic joint fluids or in the heart tissue. However, all the heart tissues appear to be subject to inflammatory damage due to some product of the predisposing *S. pyogenes* infection. Inflammatory foci in the heart tend to result in unique myocardial lesions known as *Aschoff bodies*. In contrast to acute glomerulonephritis, rheumatic fever apparently can be caused by any one of the 50 or more M serotypes of *S. pyogenes*. Furthermore, subsequent infection with other M serotypes may cause a recurrence of the RF symptoms resulting in recurrent carditis and leading perhaps to permanent heart damage. Involvement of the endocardium may lead to scarring of the heart valves and chronic valvular disease.

There appears to be a host factor in the tendency to develop rheumatic fever, since only a small percentage of those suffering acute *S. pyogenes* infections develop this disease sequel. Moreover, there appears to be a positive correlation between the duration of the streptococcal infection and the tendency both to develop rheumatic fever and to suffer recurrence. These tendencies have led to two preventive measures. First, the state of Wyoming in 1956 instituted the practice of checking elementary school children daily to determine whether or not they had a sore throat. If the answer was yes, the child was sent to a central medical office for examination and penicillin treatment if streptococci was the cause of the sore throat. The Wyoming Health Department reported that recognized cases of rheumatic fever decreased from 302 in 1956 to 37 in 1968. Second, the child who has suffered an attack of rheumatic fever should be checked routinely for the onset of an upper respiratory infection (sore throat). If the infection is due to *S.*

pyogenes, the child should be treated immediately and adequately to eliminate the infection and, hopefully, to prevent a recurrent carditis. Under such a regimen, the child may outgrow the hypersensitivity, or whatever it is, that causes the recurrent tendency of this heart-damaging disease.

LABORATORY DIAGNOSIS

Two of the diseases caused by *S. pyogenes* involve clinical symptoms that are recognizable and generally do not require laboratory aid for a specific diagnosis: scarlet fever and erysipelas. In the latter disease, streptococci can be demonstrated in fluid aspirated from the advancing edge of the cutaneous edema. Cultural isolation and identification of streptococci are required for a specific diagnosis in most cases of streptococcal disease. The specimen required for such laboratory diagnosis depends upon the site of involvement. In streptococcal meningitis, it would be spinal fluid. In streptococcal septicemia, endocarditis, or puerperal fever, it would be blood, and in the latter disease also uterine exudate. In septic arthritis, it would be joint fluid. In ulcerative lesions of the skin or any upper respiratory lesions, it would be exudate from the site of involvement collected on a sterile swab. Such swabs should be inoculated immediately to the surface of a freshly poured plate of 5 percent blood (sheep or rabbit) agar (pH 7.8). If there is to be a 2-hour or more delay in inoculating the swab exudate to the blood agar, the swab should be placed in a small amount of sterile broth (Todd and Hewitt 1932) and cultured at 37°C for 2–4 hours before inoculation to the blood-agar plate. The plates should be incubated at 37°C for 18–24 hours, preferably in an anaerobic environment.

The inoculation of exudate from a streptococcal lesion to the surface of blood agar must take several factors into consideration. To obtain well-isolated colonies, the swab should be roll-inoculated onto the agar at one edge of the plated medium. Then, with a sterile inoculating loop, the exudate at the swabbed surface should be streaked over approximately one-half of the agar surface. After the loop has been sterilized, the exudate should be cross-streaked repeatedly to the opposite side of the plate without reentering the swab-inoculated area. After each cross-streaking, the loop should be stabbed through the medium to provide subsurface growth. Since streptolysin O is oxygen-labile and will not participate in the production of beta hemolysis around aerobic surface colonies, the stab inoculations enhance the chances of observing beta hemolysis around strains of *S. pyogenes* that do not produce streptolysin S.

Another procedure to increase the chances of obtaining beta hemolysis by streptococcal colonies is a combination poured and streak-inoculated plate. For this combination, the swab should be incubated for 1 to 2 hours in a small amount of broth. Twenty milliliters of nutrient agar should be melted and cooled to 45−50°C and 1 milliliter of sterile defibrinated blood added. The swab should be removed from the broth, drained against the inside of the tube, and placed in an empty sterile tube. A sterile bacteriological loop is then charged with the broth, drained against the inside of the tube, and inoculated to the melted blood agar. The inoculated tube should be rotated between the hands to mix and the contents poured into a sterile petri plate. After the agar has solidified, the swab should be roll-inoculated and streaked onto the surface of the blood agar as described above, omitting the stab inoculations. After incubation the surface colonies may show beta hemolysis due to the production of streptolysin S, whereas the subsurface colonies may show beta hemolysis due to the production of streptolysin S, streptolysin O, or both. If the blood-agar plates are incubated anaerobically, however, streptolysin O will participate in the production of beta hemolysis by surface colonies.

SEROTAXONOMIC TESTS

If large numbers of beta-hemolytic streptococci are present on the swab, the chances are good that they represent the etiological agent of the disease. This does not prove them to be members of the Lancefield group A strain (*S. pyogenes*),

however, because other group (B, C, and G) strains of beta-hemolytic streptococci cause occasional cases of human disease. Nevertheless, since group A (*S. pyogenes*) strains are the major cause of acute human streptococcal disease, and particularly the serious sequel, rheumatic fever, the laboratory may be called upon to identify the group polysaccharide produced by the isolated streptococci. Briefly this involves growing a sufficient quantity (30−40 milliliters) of broth-cultured cells, sedimenting, resuspending in saline (0.9 percent NaCl) and washing them by centrifugation, then re-resuspending the cells in 0.2 N HCl and holding them in a boiling water bath for 10 minutes. After cooling, the extract should be neutralized with 0.2 N NaOH and centrifuged.

The precipitin test for group A streptococcal C substance in this extract requires antiserum specific for Lancefield group A polysaccharide and a capillary tube open at both ends. The capillary tube is barely dipped into the antiserum and a column approximately 1 centimeter long is drawn into the tube by capillary attraction. The tube is removed, held in a vertical position, and the lower end wiped clean with absorbent tissue, being careful not to allow the entrance of air into the tube. The tube is then dipped into the streptococcal extract until an equal volume (about 1 centimeter) is drawn in. The surfaces of the antiserum and the extract must be in physical contact (no air bubble). Otherwise the tube should be discarded and the test restarted. The lower end of the tube containing the two reagents should be wiped clean and jabbed into a block of plasticine to plug the opening. The tube should then be inverted and the open end jabbed lightly into plasticine to hold it in a vertical position. If the extract contains group A polysaccharide (from *S. pyogenes*), a white ring of precipitate will develop at the interface between the extract and the antiserum within 5 to 30 minutes. The preparation should be examined at 5-minute intervals because positive reactions become more difficult to read with the passage of time.

If an ultraviolet-light microscope is available, a highly specific and rapid fluorescent antibody (FA) technique for differentiating group A, C, and G streptococci has been devised by Smith (1965). Antisera from separate rabbits immunized with either group A, C, or G streptococci were pooled into corresponding groups. Each group antiserum was rendered partially more specific by absorbing cross-reacting antibodies onto cells of each of the other two group streptococci and removing them by centrifugation. The remaining specific antibody globulin from each group antiserum was then isolated and tagged with fluorescein isothiocyanate. To reduce cross-reactions further, small amounts of untagged antibody specific for the other two streptococcal group antigens were added to each fluorescent antiserum (FA). These untagged antibodies could be expected to react with and block the cross-reacting antigenic determinants on the streptococcal cells. The cells for this FA procedure were obtained by fishing beta-hemolytic colonies from 18–24-hour blood-agar cultures, inoculating to 10 milliliters of Todd-Hewitt broth, and incubating at 37°C for 4 hours. The young streptococcal cells were sedimented and resuspended in saline to a desired turbidity. Four smears were prepared on separate microslides, air-dried, and fixed for 1 minute with 95 percent ethyl alcohol. Smear 2 was pretreated with nontagged group A antiserum to block *all* antigenic sites and then washed and dried. Smears 1 and 2 were then treated with anti-A FA, smear 3 with anti-C FA, and smear 4 with anti-G FA. After washing and drying, all four smears were examined with the ultraviolet-light microscope. If only smear 1 gave typical greenish fluorescence of the streptococcal cells, they were identified as group A streptococci (*S. pyogenes*). If smear 3 or 4 was the only one in which the streptococci fluoresced, they were identified as group C or G streptococci, respectively.

A rapid and unique serotaxonomic test for the identification of Lancefield groups of beta-hemolytic streptococci was described by Christensen et al. (1973). This test is based on the fact that certain strains of staphylococci (*S. aureus* Cowan) produce a protein (protein A) at the surface of their cell walls that reacts with and

binds the Fc portion of immune gamma globulin (see Figure 4-8). Christensen et al. conceived the idea of reacting Lancefield group-specific IgG to formaldehyde- and heat-treated (80°C) *S. aureus* Cowan cells, thereby leaving the receptor sites of the IgG free to react with the homologous group C substance of the isolated streptococcal cells.

For testing, cells from a beta-hemolytic colony on a blood-agar plate were fished to a tube of Todd-Hewitt broth and incubated at 37°C. When sufficient growth appeared, the cells were sedimented and the supernatant fluid discarded. The cell pellet was suspended in 0.5 milliliter of 0.2 M Tris buffer (pH 8.0), and 1 milliliter of trypsin solution (5 mg/ml) was added. The trypsin-treated cells were incubated at 37°C for 1 hour to remove the M, R, and possibly other protein antigens from the surface of the streptococci. No further treatment was necessary.

To perform the test, one drop of Lancefield group-specific staphylococcal reagent was added to one drop of the trypsinized streptococci and the mixture was spread over an area of about ¾-inch diameter on a glass slide. A control preparation, consisting of one drop of trypsinized streptococci mixed with one drop of staphylococci coated with normal rabbit IgG, was placed on the same slide. The two preparations were observed with the naked eye while tilting the slide gently to and fro for 1 minute. Aggregation of the cells in the test mixture (usually within 30 seconds), but not in the control, constituted a positive test. Hahn and Nyberg (1976) compared the staphylococcal coagglutination technique for identifying 150 group A, B, C, and G streptococcal isolates with the Lancefield precipitation technique. The isolates included 87 from humans, 56 from animals, 1 source unknown, and 6 laboratory reference strains. Hahn and Nyberg found the trypsination of the streptococcal cells, advocated by Christensen et al., unnecessary. However, they reported cross-reactions in isolates that were tested for more than 1 minute. They concluded that because of its being rapid, simple, and reliable, the coagglutination test is a valuable alternative to the precipitin method of Lancefield.

SERODIAGNOSTIC TESTS

A number of specific serodiagnostic tests have been advocated for aid in the diagnosis of *S. pyogenes* infections. As in all serodiagnostic tests, the demonstration of a rising antibody titer in the patient's serum is more significant than a single titer. This necessitates two or more serum specimens, one collected early in the acute state of the infection and one collected 7 to 10 days or more later. Since only the second serum would be expected to have antibodies resulting from the current disease, no serodiagnostic test can be expected to yield an *early* diagnosis.

The most commonly advocated serodiagnostic test for *S. pyogenes* infections is the antistreptolysin O (ASO) test. Streptolysin O, incorporated in a suitable reducing substance, can be purchased from commercial supply houses and will cause hemolysis when added to a suspension of red blood cells. When red blood cells constitute a test or indicator reagent in a serological test, blood must be collected from an appropriate animal (in this case a rabbit) and immediately defibrinated or added to an isotonic saline solution (0.9 percent NaCl) containing a suitable concentration of an anticoagulant. The blood should be strained through two layers of gauze to remove clots. The red blood cells are washed free of serum by repeated centrifuging, removing the supernatant fluid, and resuspending them in saline. After the third washing, they are packed by centrifugation in a calibrated centrifuge tube, the volume of packed cells is noted, and the supernatant saline is removed. The red blood cells are then suspended in a sufficient volume of saline to give the desired v/v percent concentration of the red blood cells (3 or 5 percent in different ASO tests).

The ASO test is performed by preparing serial double dilutions from 1:8 through 1:1,024 or more of the heat (56°C) inactivated serum from the patient. A control (no. 1) containing an equal volume of saline but no serum, a control (no. 2) containing an equal volume of serum 1:8 but no streptolysin O, and a control (no. 3) containing only saline should be included in the titration. A predetermined quantity of streptolysin O is added to all preparations except controls 2 and 3. After a brief (30 minute) period to allow ASO, if any, in the patient's serum to react with the streptolysin O, a suitable amount of the rabbit RBC suspension is added to all tubes and thoroughly mixed; then the preparations are incubated at 37°C for 1 hour. The streptolysin O control (no. 1) should show complete hemolysis of the red blood cells. The serum and the saline controls (2 and 3) should show no hemolysis. The highest dilution of the patient's serum that completely prevents hemolysis of the red blood cells constitutes the ASO titer. If acute-phase serum and 7–10-day postacute serum from the patient are tested, a rising titer (threefold or more) constitutes strong evidence for a diagnosis of *S. pyogenes* infection. Normal individuals may show constant ASO titers up to 1:200, however, whereas others may suffer *S. pyogenes* infection without developing ASO antibodies.

The ASO test has been advocated to aid in the diagnosis of rheumatic fever. Eighty percent or more of such patients show high (1:250 to 1:500+) ASO titers. If the predisposing *S. pyogenes* disease was scarlet fever, however, or if it involved the sequel acute glomerulonephritis, a high ASO titer could be expected to persist for several months with or without the development of rheumatic fever, thereby negating the value of the ASO test for the diagnosis of the rheumatic fever sequel in these patients. Another serological test advocated as an aid in the diagnosis of rheumatic fever is the *C-reactive protein* (CRP) test. C-reactive protein is an abnormal protein that appears in the serum of rheumatic fever patients. Its presence in the serum can be demonstrated by a precipitin test comparable to the capillary tube technique described above. Specific anti-CRP antiserum, which can be purchased commercially, will yield a precipitate when layered in contact with a patient's serum that contains CRP. Unfortunately, CRP appears in the serum of patients suffering *any* inflammatory disease. Consequently, if the patient is suffering any inflammatory disease other than rheumatic fever, the value of the test for diagnosing rheumatic fever is negated.

Since strains of group A streptococci differ in their capacity to produce streptolysin O and other antigenic substances, no single-antigen serodiagnostic test is liable to be effective in diagnosing all cases of *S. pyogenes* infection. An exception to this conclusion would appear to be a test for antibodies that are reactive with group A polysaccharide. Although such antibodies are known to be produced, and to persist for a year or more in rheumatic fever patients with vascular disease (Dudding and Ayoub 1968), significant titers are usually slow in developing and generally are low compared to those for other streptococcal antigens. There are other streptococcal-disease serodiagnostic tests more or less comparable to the ASO tests: the antihyaluronidase (AHDase test); the antistreptokinase (ASKase) test; the antideoxyribonuclease B (ADNAse B) test; and the antinicotinamide adenine dinucleotide glycohydrolase (ANADase or ANADGase) test. Each of these tests requires standard test reagents that can be purchased from commercial sources (for greater detail see Klein 1976). As in all serodiagnostic tests, acute and postacute serum specimens should be available for each test so that rising antibody titers to each antigen may be established. A combination of the four tests mentioned here and the ASO test has been claimed to give 90+ percent positive serodiagnostic results in proved cases of *S. pyogenes* disease. Some of these tests are complicated and difficult to read, however. Furthermore, performing five such titrations in duplicate consumes considerable time and a considerable amount of test reagents.

A single, 2-minute serodiagnostic test incorporating all five of the preceding streptococcal antigens was reported by Dr. I. Ofek at a meeting of the American Heart Association at Dallas in 1972. The polyvalent test antigen is prepared by conjugating SO, HDase, SKase, DNAse B, and NADGase on aldehyde-treated sheep red blood cells. The test is known as the streptozyme test, and the antigen in liquid form can be purchased under the trade name of Streptozyme Test Reagent. The reagent is claimed to have a refrigerator shelf life of at least 16 months. The test is performed on microslides or on glass plates etched into 1-inch squares. The patient's serum is diluted and a designated amount is pipetted to the center of the test area. A drop of the Streptozyme Test Reagent is added, and the serum and reagent are mixed with a toothpick and spread over an area approximately ¾ inch in diameter. The preparation is then tilted back and forth for 2 minutes and examined for agglutination of the red blood cells. If antibody to one or more of the five streptococcal antigens on the red blood cells is present in the patient's serum, agglutination will occur. Rising antibody titers to the Streptozyme Test Reagent can be established by testing serial dilutions of both acute and postacute serum specimens from the patient. If multiple serum dilutions are being tested, each dilution is placed in a row of etched squares, a drop of test reagent is added to each, and, beginning with the highest serum dilution preparation, each is mixed with the same toothpick and spread as indicated above. After 2 minutes of tilting, the highest dilution that shows agglutination of the red blood cells constitutes the antibody titer of that serum. A rising titer is indicated by a significantly higher titer in the postacute serum than in the acute serum. This test needs further research before general acceptance. Nevertheless, the serological principles involved are legitimate, the speed and simplicity of the test are ideal, and reported studies justify further consideration (see Klein and Jones 1971; Collins 1972). For additional details of the laboratory diagnosis of streptococcal infections, see Facklam (1974).

IMMUNOPROPHYLAXIS AND IMMUNOTHERAPY

There are no immunological procedures of practical value in the prevention or treatment of diseases caused by *S. pyogenes*. Erythrogenic toxin and antitoxin were formerly advocated for the prevention and treatment of scarlet fever, but the toxin could not be converted to toxoid and antitoxin therapy has been displaced by chemotherapy, primarily penicillin therapy.

CONTROL AND PREVENTION

Since the development of immunoprophylactic measures does not appear probable, the greatest hope for the control and prevention of group A streptococcal diseases and their serious sequelae is for *early* diagnosis and adequate chemotherapeutic treatment of cases of these diseases. Since serodiagnosis is never early diagnosis, the causative streptococci must be isolated and identified as *S. pyogenes* and the patient must be treated promptly. The use of this regimen for preventing recurrent carditis in rheumatic fever patients has already been discussed.

REFERENCES

Christensen, P., G. Kahlmeter, S. Jonsson, and G. Kronvall. 1973. New method for the serological grouping of streptococci with specific antibodies adsorbed to protein-A containing staphylococci. *Infect. Immunity* 7:881–885.

Collins, O. D. 1972. Antistreptolysin-O determination by sheep cell agglutination. *J. Clin. Path.* 57:598–602.

Dudding, B. A. and E. M. Ayoub. 1968. Persistence of Group A antibody in patients with rheumatic vascular disease. *J. Exper. Med.* 128:1081–1098.

Facklam, R. R. 1974. Streptococci. Chapter 8 in *Manual of Clinical Microbiology.*

Fox, E. N. 1974. M proteins of group A streptococci. *Bacteriol. Rev.* 38:57–86.

Hahn, G. and I. Nyberg. 1976. Identification of Streptococcal groups A, B, C, and G by slide coagglutination of antibody-sensitized protein A containing staphylococci. *J. Clin. Microbiol.* 4:99–101.

Klein, G. C. 1976. Immune response to streptococcal infection. Chapter 33 in *Manual of Clinical Immunology.*

Klein, G. C. and W. L. Jones. 1971. Comparison of the streptozyme test with the antistreptolysin-O, antideoxyribonuclease-B, and the antihyaluronidase tests. *Applied Microbiol.* 21:257–259.

Lancefield, R. C. 1928. The antigenic complex of *Streptococcus haemolyticus.* I. Demonstration of a type specific substance in extracts of *Streptococcus haemolyticus. J. Exper. Med.* 47:91–103.

———. 1933. A serological differentiation of human and other groups of hemolytic streptococci. *J. Exper. Med.* 57:571–595.

Lindberg, L. H. and K. L. Vosti. 1969. Elution of glomerular bound antibodies in experimental streptococcal glomerulonephritis. *Science* 166:1032–1033.

Rammelkamp, C. H., Jr. and R. S. Weaver. 1953. Acute glomerulonephritis. The significance of the variations in the incidence of the disease. *J. Clin. Invest.* 32:345–358.

Slade, H. D. and W. C. Slamp. 1962. Cell wall composition and the grouping antigens of streptococci. *J. Bacteriol.* 84:345–351.

Slade, H. D. 1965. Extraction of cell-wall polysaccharide antigen from streptococci. *J. Bacteriol.* 90:667–672.

Smith, T. B. 1965. Clinical application of immunofluorescence I. Grouping beta-hemolytic streptococci. *J. Bacteriol.* 89:198–204.

Todd, E. W. and L. F. Hewitt. 1932. A new culture medium for the production of antigenic streptococcal haemolysin. *J. Path. Bact.* 35:973–974.

Wannamaker, L. W. and J. Matsen. 1972. *Streptococci and Streptococcal Diseases.* New York: Academic Press.

Wilkinson, H. W., R. R. Facklam, and E. C. Wortham. 1973. Distribution of serological type of group B streptococci isolated from a variety of clinical material over a five year period (with special reference to neonatal sepsis and meningitis). *Infect. Immunity* 8:228–235.

Zabriski, J. B. 1964. The role of temperate bacteriophage in the production of erythrogenic toxin by Group A streptococci. *J. Exper. Med.* 119:761–780.

9

Tuberculosis

Tuberculosis (TB, consumption, phthisis) has been manifested by a wide variety of lesions and clinical symptoms in humans and animals throughout medical history. Prior to the late nineteenth century the disease was considered to be hereditary because of the high incidence of tuberculosis in family environments. Villemin in 1865 demonstrated that exudate from a human tuberculous lung could produce tuberculosis in rabbits. Robert Koch in 1882 was the first to demonstrate tubercle bacilli in human lesions. Later he isolated and established the etiological relationship of tubercle bacilli to the human disease.

In Koch's time, the annual human death rate from tuberculosis was around 200 per 100,000 population. Fifty years later, as a result of educational campaigns (financed in the United States by the sale of Christmas seals), the death rate from this dread disease had declined to around 40 per 100,000 population (80 percent), even though no chemotherapeutic, antibiotic, or widely used immunoprophylactic agent had been provided during this time. This was the first example of what education of both the medical profession and the general public could do to facilitate the control of a communicable disease. Now, with both antibiotic and synthetic therapeutic drugs available, the death rate has declined to less than 3 per 100,000 population. This spectacular decline in death rate, however, still leaves 7,000 to 9,000 deaths per year in the United States.

ETIOLOGY

The organism isolated by Koch is designated *Mycobacterium tuberculosis.* The genus *Mycobac-*

terium, however, includes a number of organisms pathogenic for humans or animals, and some are nonpathogenic. All possess a unique staining characteristic designated *acid-fast.* The mycobacteria cannot be differentially stained by the gram-staining technique. The most widely used acid-fast staining procedure, developed by Ziehl and Neelsen, consists of flooding a microslide smear of the specimen containing the organisms with carbol fuchsin and heating to steaming (but not boiling) for 5 minutes. This procedure drives the stain through the waxy coats of the mycobacteria and stains the whole preparation, including non-acid-fast bacteria, mucus, and leucocytes, an opaque red. The preparation is then destained by dropping an acid-alcohol mixture on the smear until it yields no further red color. The smear is then counterstained with a weak solution of methylene blue or other stain that tints the non-acid-fast bacteria and mucus a light blue or green without masking the retained red stain of the mycobacterial cells (see Figure G-1 on the back cover).

In addition to *M. tuberculosis,* the genus *Mycobacterium* includes *M. leprae,* the causative organism of leprosy, and the other pathogenic mycobacteria listed in Table 9-1. Whereas *M. tuberculosis* causes 98 percent of the cases of human tuberculosis in the United States, other species may cause localized outbreaks here and

elsewhere in the world (see Uganda Buruli Group 1971). Note that neither of the two species listed in Table 9-1 that cause skin tuberculosis, *M. ulcerans* and *M. marinum,* will grow at temperatures of 37°C or above. Also, *M. avium,* which causes bird tuberculosis, is the only species listed that will grow at 45°C. Our discussion will concentrate on tuberculosis caused by *M. tuberculosis* and to a lesser extent by *M. bovis.* These organisms are slender rods, straight or irregularly curved. Colony growth of these two mycobacteria on solid media usually can be distinguished; however, experimental animal susceptibility, niacin production (see Kilburn et al. 1968a and 1968b), drug susceptibility, or other taxonomic tests may be required if there is reason to distinguish among the various mycobacterial species. Such identification should be left to laboratory personnel thoroughly trained in safety precautions and working in laboratories safely equipped for this type of work.

CULTIVATION

Two types of media have been widely advocated for use in the cultivation of mycobacteria: egg-base media and mineral-base media. An example of the former is the Lowenstein-Jensen (L-J) medium composed of eggs, potato flour, bone

Table 9-1. Pathogenic *Mycobacterium* species that may cause disease in humans.

Species	Growth (in weeks) at			Experimental Animal Pathogenicity			
	30°C	37°C	45°C	Guinea Pig	Chicken	Rabbit	Mouse
M. tuberculosis	0	2–4	0	+ +	0	0–±	+ +
M. bovis	0	2–4	0	+ +	0	+ +	+ +
M. avium	0	3–4	2–3	0	+ +	+ +	+ +
M. ulcerans	3–5	0	0	0	0	0	0
*M. marinum**	1–2	0	0	0	0	0	0
*M. kansasii**	2–3	2–3	0	0	0	0	+ +
Others	2–4	2–4	0	0	0	0	0–+ +

* Produce pigment when grown in the light (not in the dark).

marrow infusion, sodium pyruvate, citrate, glycerol, and asparagin, with either malachite green, penicillin, or nalidixic acid added to restrict the growth of possible contaminants. Because of the eggs, such media coagulate during heat sterilization. The tubes or vials containing such media, therefore, are placed in a slanted position in the heat sterilizer. An example of a mineral-base medium is the Middlebrook 7H-10 medium or the Dubos-Middlebrook (D-M) medium. These media consist of nutrient mixtures of minerals, a nitrogen source (ammonia, glutamate, or asparagin), glucose or glycerol, serum albumin, fatty acid (usually oleic), or a synthetic, nontoxic, water-soluble ester of fatty acids (Tween). Such media may be sterilized and used as liquid media; or agar may be added before sterilization and the sterile product, while still hot (above 50°C), may be dispensed into tubes, plates, or vials. The tubes or vials are then placed in a slanted position while the medium cools and the agar solidifies. For details of preparing these media, see Vera and Dumoff (1974).

Due to the hydrophobic nature of the waxy coats of M. tuberculosis, the cultured cells tend to grow in large clumps or heaped-up masses on the surface of solid media and as pellicles on the surface of liquid media. In liquid media containing surface wetting agents, however, such as the Tweens, dispersed growth of the cells can be obtained. This is significant in research requiring cell counts or other needs for dispersed cells in the culture medium.

Mycobacterium tuberculosis and other mycobacteria grow best in an atmosphere of 5 to 10 percent added CO_2. They also require normal concentrations of atmospheric oxygen, however, so the candle jar method of obtaining the added CO_2 cannot be utilized. Since the mycobacteria may be slow-growing (2 to 4 weeks), the cultures must be protected from drying without sealing out the exchange of atmospheric oxygen and the added CO_2. This can be accomplished by dispensing the solid culture media into small screw-capped vials or tubes. After inoculation, the screw cap can be loosened slightly and the culture placed in the atmosphere of increased CO_2 in the incubator at 35–37°C. If plates are used in a CO_2 incubator, they must be enclosed in a plastic bag that is permeable to the O_2 and CO_2 but not to water vapor. The culture may need to be incubated for 3 or 4 weeks before discarding as negative.

Young cultures of virulent strains of M. tuberculosis and M. bovis tend to produce a unique colony growth appearance known as "serpentine cords" (see Figure G-2 on the back cover). Completely avirulent strains of these two mycobacteria, and even virulent strains of other Mycobacterium species, fail to produce this cord type of colony growth. A unique lipid known as "cord factor" can be extracted from cord-producing cultures.

Although extensive studies on the chemical composition of cultured M. tuberculosis and other mycobacteria have indicated the presence of a variety of lipids, carbohydrates, and proteins, these studies have yielded little of practical significance except for the proteins known as tuberculins. These tuberculoproteins are antigenic, and there is considerable cross-reactivity between those from different mycobacterial species. A tubercular infection in a human or animal (guinea pig) will sensitize the infected host to the homologous tuberculoprotein. Such sensitized individuals will give a positive tuberculin test when a small amount of the protein is administered intradermally. The injection of the isolated protein (tuberculin) will not, however, sensitize an experimental animal.

PATHOGENESIS

Again, although extensive studies have yielded much information relative to the mechanism whereby tubercle bacilli produce pathology in the host, a clear concept of the mechanism is still not apparent. There is some evidence that the toxic lipids, associated with serpentine cord formation by virulent tubercle bacilli, immobilize phagocytic leucocytes. Virulent tubercle bacilli tend to multiply rapidly in the infected phagocytic cell, eventually resulting in its disintegration and the liberation of tubercle bacilli to infect neighboring phagocytic cells. This primary involvement of phagocytic cells in a localized lesion may result in the development of tremendous numbers of tubercle bacilli with little or no evidence of clinical disease. However, the tuberculoproteins, and possibly other components of these tubercle bacilli, begin to exert their allergenic effect and by the fourth to sixth week after infection the host becomes hypersensitive to the tuberculoproteins. This sytemic hypersensitivity is believed to play a significant part in the subsequent pathology and clinical course of the disease.

CLINICAL TUBERCULOSIS

Around 98 percent of clinical tuberculosis in the United States is caused by *M. tuberculosis.* In the past in the United States (and at the present time in other parts of the world), *M. bovis* from infected cattle was a common etiological agent in human tuberculosis. These two species of *Mycobacteria* frequently have involved different anatomical organs in humans: *M. tuberculosis* tends to involve the lungs and cause pulmonary tuberculosis, whereas *M. bovis* tends to involve the intestines and related viscera. These different organ involvements are believed to be due to the aerogenic (respiratory droplet) spread of *M. tuberculosis* from human lung lesions in contrast to the milk-borne spread of *M. bovis* from infected cows. Yet *M. bovis* has been known to cause pulmonary tuberculosis in human infections, as has *M. kansasii.* Also, *M. tuberculosis* can cause visceral lesions. Other less well classified mycobacteria have been reported as the cause of cases of pulmonary tuberculosis in humans. In numerous cases of skin tuberculosis, *M. ulcerans* and *M. marinum (balnei)* have been established as the etiological agents. Furthermore, *M. marinum* infections have been associated with swimming pools (Philpott et al. 1963) and other swimming environments—one such environment is the upper Mobile Bay (see *MMWR,* 11 October 1969). Chronic granulomas of the elbows or knees have occurred in children who suffered skin abrasions while swimming in the salt water of Mobile Bay in the vicinity of Daphne, Alabama. The granulomas caused by M. *marinum*

have been designated *Daphne sores.* Other anatomical sites of tubercular infection are lymphoidal tissues (tubercular lymphadenitis), the meninges (tubercular meningitis), the kidneys (tubercular nephritis), bones (tubercular osteitis or osteomyelitis), and practically any other body tissue.

Pulmonary tuberculosis, however, is the most common and most serious form of human TB. This form can result from the inhalation, deep into the air passages of the lung, of respiratory droplets containing one or more tubercle bacilli. Such bacilli are taken up by a fixed mononuclear phagocyte where intracellular reproduction results in the initiation of the primary focus of infection. Following this primary focus, different types of tubercular lesions may develop. The lesion from which the disease derived its name is the *tubercle.* This lesion, at first only microscopic in size, may grow or coalesce into a macroscopically visible tubercle that will cast a shadow on an X-ray film (Figure 9-1). It may be months or longer, however, before such lesions develop, whereas the hypersensitivity to the tuberculoproteins produced by the growing tubercle bacilli in these primary foci, as stated above, occurs within 4 to 6 weeks. Pulmonary X rays have their place in diagnosis and prognosis in tuberculosis, but they should be preceded by tuberculin testing for *early* evidence of TB infection.

The tubercle bacilli in the primary tubercle may be destroyed there and, if calcium is deposited at the site, this calcified tubercle, indicating the past infection, may be the only residual physical evidence that the individual has had tuberculosis. The tubercle bacilli in the primary tubercle may continue to multiply, however, with resulting central necrosis of the lesion. The necrotic material has the consistency and appearance of cheese (*caseation necrosis*). The necrosis may continue to expand, resulting in cavity formation. As long as the tubercle is walled off and does not involve air passages, the patient is considered a *closed case* and is not capable of transmitting the disease to others. If the necrosis breaks into a bronchiole or larger air passage, however, tubercle bacilli can be dis-

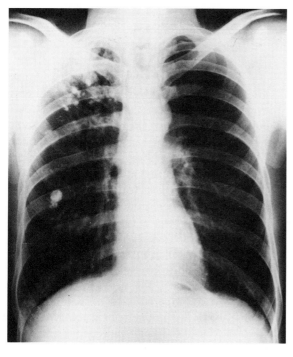

Figure 9–1. Adult pulmonary tuberculosis. X-ray shows a large calcified tubercle in the mid-right lung and smaller tubercles plus infiltration in the apex of the right lung. The left lung is normal. (Courtesy of R. B. Morrison.)

charged into the environment and the patient becomes an *open case* able to transmit the disease to others. When the necrosis breaks into air passages or blood vessels, the area of lung involvement can be extended along these channels. Eventually a cavity may involve the whole of that lobe of the lung. When the tubercle bacilli break out of walled-off lesions in lymph nodes or gain entrance to the bloodstream, they may be dispersed widely and establish multiple new foci of infection. This metastasizing tendency is a common characteristic of tubercular infection in experimental animals and may occur in humans, resulting in *miliary* tuberculosis.

EPIDEMIOLOGY

Pulmonary tuberculosis frequently is a disease of alternating periods of active pathology and quiescence. There are records of apparent quiescence or latency lasting for years without complete healing of the lesions. Then, as a result of unknown physiological factors, the disease becomes active, resulting in renewed progres-

sive pathology. Because of the alternating periods of walled-off (closed) and progressive (open) lesions, the longer a case and susceptible contacts remain in close association, the more likely the susceptibles are to contract the disease. This is the major factor in the tendency toward family outbreaks of the disease. Even so, very brief or even a single close exposure to an open case can result in transmission of the infection.

An outbreak of tuberculosis was described in 1968 (see *MMWR* 20 July 1968), that illustrates a number of the significant factors in the epidemiology of this disease. In January of that year, "far advanced" pulmonary tuberculosis was diagnosed by chest X ray in a 32-year-old woman. Subsequently both stained smears and cultures of her sputum were found to be positive for *M. tuberculosis* (characteristics of an open case). The woman had been employed since September of the preceding year as a teacher's assistant in two classes of 3- to 5-year-old children in a church school. This illustrates the insidious nature of the onset of this form of tuberculosis. Undoubtedly the case had been active for a considerable period of time to have developed the cavitation involved in "far advanced" pathology. The patient had not been incapacitated by the disease, however. In fact, she had felt well enough to accept the teaching position and had performed her duties for several months (until 21 December 1968) before resigning because of her illness.

The woman was in contact with 55 students in two classes. In addition to assisting the teaching of the children, she supervised their play and aided with their meals. After tuberculosis was diagnosed in the teacher, all 55 students, 9 adult school personnel, 4 church employees, 21 additional close contacts, and 14 casual contacts outside the school were tuberculin-tested. Of the 111 contacts (79 close), 28 gave a positive tuberculin test reaction. Chest X rays of the 28 tuberculin-positive individuals revealed 8 new active cases of primary tuberculosis. Two of these were documented *tuberculin converters* (negative to positive) within the year— the conversion from the prior negative tuberculin test being an indication of recent tubercular infection. Four additional tuberculin converters, however, gave negative chest X-ray results. The remaining 22 tuberculin-positive contacts gave no history of a prior tuberculin test and were X-ray negative. All 8 of the new cases of tuberculosis were considered close contacts, 3 being the teacher's own children. One or more such localized outbreaks of tuberculosis in the United States have been reported in *MMWR* every year since 1968. During 1975, 33,989 cases of tuberculosis were reported in the United States (see *MMWR*, 16 July 1976). An outbreak of tuberculosis comparable to that described here was reported from Maryland (see *MMWR*, 2 April 1976). For 1976 a provisional total (awaiting corrected case data) of 32,549 cases was reported to CDC.

The incubation period in the type of tuberculosis described above is difficult to establish. In another type of tuberculosis (some cases of which are called "galloping consumption"), the onset of severe pathology and incapacitation and even death may occur within a relatively short time following infection. In this form of tuber-culosis, tubercle formation and caseation necrosis of the lung tissue may not develop.

TUBERCULIN

The tuberculin test gives the earliest possible evidence of TB infection. And as revealed in the outbreaks cited above, the infection indicated by a positive tuberculin test, even the tuberculin converter, does not always lead to progressive disease. The individual giving a positive tuberculin test should have at least one and preferably several chest X-ray examinations before pulmonary tuberculosis is ruled out. The chest X ray will not, of course, rule out tubercular involvement of other organ sites.

Although the tuberculin test is not a clinical laboratory function, the production and standardization of tuberculin is a commercial or public health laboratory responsibility. Robert Koch produced the first tuberculin, and essentially the same culture and primary laboratory procedures are still used. A virulent strain of *M. tuberculosis* is inoculated to containers of a suitable broth medium (for example, 7H-10). The cultures are incubated for 4 to 6 weeks and then steamed at 100°C, or otherwise heated, for several hours to kill the cells and to extract the heat-stable tuberculoproteins from the cell mass. The dead cells are filtered out either before or after evaporating the culture medium to one-tenth the original volume. The sterile filtrate constitutes the old tuberculin (OT) described and used by Koch. Efforts to separate the active tuberculin protein from inactive components in the OT have resulted in a *partially purified protein derivative* of tuberculin commonly designated PPD. Although PPD contains fewer nonessential extractives than OT, it still contains inactive polysaccharides and other extraneous material. The PPD can be converted to a dry powder, however, which is more stable than the liquid OT.

Either OT or PPD must be standardized for biological activity prior to use in human tuberculin testing. This is accomplished by determining the minimum reaction dose (MRD)—the smallest amount or highest dilution of the filtrate or dissolved powder that, when injected in 0.1-milliliter amounts into the skin of a hypersensitive guinea pig, results in an area of induration about 1 centimeter in diameter. The guinea pig usually is rendered hypersensitive by infection with *M. tuberculosis,* although other methods of sensitization have been advocated.

The tuberculin test can be administered by a variety of methods. The tuberculin can be rubbed into a tiny scratch on the flexor surface of the forearm. It can be added to a small patch of absorbent material (for example, filter paper) and held in place on the forearm by an adhesive band, although this method is not very sensitive. The more common testing procedure was initiated by Mantoux and involves the intradermal injection of 0.1 milliliter of the tuberculin. For mass surveys, the tuberculin may be loaded into a compressed air gun that inoculates the desired amount of tuberculin into the skin without the aid of a needle.

Different individuals vary considerably in the degree of skin hypersensitivity to tuberculin, and some highly sensitive individuals can give rather severe hemorrhagic reactions to large doses. Consequently, it is common practice to administer a high dilution (1:10,000 or 0.01 milligram) of OT tuberculin as the first dose. If the individual does not react to that dose, a second, larger dose (up to 1:100 dilution or 1 milligram) may be used. An international tuberculin unit (TU) has been established and is now available to laboratories responsible for tuberculin production and standardization. Five units of PPD is the recommended test dose.

Tuberculin hypersensitivity is classified as "delayed type" in contrast to the immediate type discussed in ruling out hypersensitivity of the diphtheria patient to animal serum antitoxin. As indicated in Chapter 4, this was the first recognized instance of cell-mediated immunity. In the positive tuberculin test no significant reaction occurs before several hours and the maximum reaction will not be seen before 24 to 36 hours. The reaction is considered positive if an area of induration 10 millimeters or more in diameter is observed. Lesser reactions may indicate a lesser degree of hypersensitivity in an early infection;

such tests should be repeated a week or two later.

LABORATORY DIAGNOSIS

The usual specimen for the diagnosis of pulmonary tuberculosis is sputum coughed up from deep inside the involved area of the lung. Only open cases will yield tubercle bacilli in the sputum. The number of tubercle bacilli in the specimen will depend upon the extent of necrosis and the number of air passages involved in the lung lesion. The technologist assigned to handle such specimens should be thoroughly trained in the techniques and dangers involved and should be provided with all necessary equipment to avoid self-infection or transmission of infection to other laboratory personnel. Accidental laboratory infections are quite common in this disease.

The first laboratory test to be performed is a Ziehl-Neelsen or equivalent acid-fast stain (see Paik and Suggs 1974) of a smear of the sputum on a clean (grease-free), new microslide. Used slides may develop microscopic etches that may retain the stain during destaining and be misinterpreted as acid-fast bacilli, thereby resulting in a false positive diagnosis. The time allotted to the microscopic examination of a stained smear before rendering a negative decision must be arbitrary and dependent upon the volume of work in the laboratory. A minimum of 10 minutes per smear would be reasonable. Workers at one TB sanitorium reported that the specimen must contain 100,000 tubercle bacilli per milliliter for reasonable certainty of obtaining a positive diagnosis by the stained smear method. Thus it is obvious that a negative stained smear result does not rule out the presence of tubercle bacilli in fewer than 100,000/milliliter numbers in the specimen. Another acid-fast staining procedure that is considered to be more sensitive than the Ziehl-Neelsen technique is the Truant et al. (1962) fluorescent staining procedure using the auramine stain. This procedure, however, requires an ultraviolet-light microscope for examining the stained specimen.

Cultivation of the specimen is essential to establish the presence of bacilli when there are too few (fewer than 10^5/milliliter) tubercle bacilli to be found in the microscopic examination of the stained smear. Cultivation of the specimen, even when the stained smear is positive, may also be desirable to determine the species of *Mycobacterium* and the drug of choice for treating the patient. Prior to inoculation of the culture media, the sputum must be treated with two objectives in mind: (1) the highly viscous, mucoid state should be digested to liquidity and (2) the non-acid-fast bacteria must be killed with minimum damage to the acid-fast bacilli present. An additional advantage to the liquefaction of the sputum is the fact that it can then be centrifuged to sediment and concentrate the tubercle bacilli present. Centrifugation should be done in a screw-capped centrifuge tube, taking precautions to prevent aerosol or other dispersion of the digested specimen. Two commonly used digestive and selective killing agents for the treatment of TB sputum are (1) 2–4 percent NaOH for 30 minutes at 37°C followed by neutralization of the NaOH with an equivalent amount of acid; and (2) the acetyl-cysteine-alkali method wherein equal amounts of sputum and digestant are placed in a sterile, screw-capped, 50-milliliter centrifuge tube, mixed for not more than 30 seconds on a vortex-type test-tube mixer, and allowed to stand for 15 minutes at room temperature before adding phosphate buffer (pH 6.8) and centrifuging. For detailed considerations of these and other methods of treating TB sputum, see Runyon et al. (1974). All inoculated media should be incubated at 37°C in an atmosphere of normal O_2 and 5 to 10 percent added CO_2, using precautions to prevent the drying of solid media.

In testing fast-growing bacteria for drug susceptibility or resistance, it is common practice to isolate the organism in pure culture and then test the isolate by exposure to the drug in broth or in or on a suitable solid medium. Since it takes 2 to 4 weeks to obtain good growth of *M. tuberculosis,* however, prior isolation and then testing the isolate for drug susceptibility would require some 4 to 8 weeks to obtain this desirable information. Consequently it is now common practice to inoculate equal amounts of the treated sputum to the surface of a vial (or quadrant of a plate) of a solid, clear-agar medium (usually 7H-10 or D-M) containing no drug and to other vials or quadrants of the same medium in each of which a test concentration of one of the therapeutic drugs has been incorporated. The originally discovered drugs for chemotherapy in tuberculosis were the antibiotic *streptomycin* and the synthetic drugs *isoniazid* (INH) and *para-aminosalicylic acid* (PAS). Long use of these drugs has resulted in many instances of the development of drug resistance by strains of *M. tuberculosis.* By incorporating test concentrations of these three and other more recent drugs in separate aliquots of the culture medium and comparing the amount (number of colonies) of mycobacterial growth resulting from equal inocula onto each drug-containing medium with that on the no-drug control medium, the susceptibility or resistance of the organism to each drug can be reported. Growth of *M. tuberculosis* on the no-drug medium, of course, yields cultural evidence of an open case of pulmonary tuberculosis. Repeat cultures at 2–4-week intervals on the no-drug medium and the drug medium (containing the drugs being used in treating the patient) can yield evidence of continuing therapeutic efficacy, or the development of resistance to the drugs by the strain of *M. tuberculosis* involved. In case of the latter, another active drug should be substituted for continuing therapy. The Texas State Department of Health (*Mycobacterium*) Laboratory routinely tests each acid-fast bacillus culture for susceptibility to each of six therapeutic drugs: streptomycin, para-aminosalicylic acid, isoniazid, ethambutol, rifampin, and ethionamide. They use the quadrant plate technique and clear 7H-10 agar medium. Microscopic colonies of mycobacteria can usually be counted on this medium after 7 to 10 days' incubation.

IMMUNITY

Koch was the first to note that infection in experimental animals, after 2 to 3 weeks, resulted in resistance to reinfection. This resistance was observed to relate to the onset of the hypersensitive state. As a consequence, many efforts to produce suitable vaccines for active immunization have been reported. Although heat-killed *M. tuberculosis* and cells of other mycobacterial species and various proteins, extractives, and emulsions of such cells have been tested (and to some extent advocated), the only immunogen widely used is a live, weakly virulent strain of *M. bovis.* This strain was obtained as a fully virulent isolate by workers at the Pasteur Institute in Paris. A. L. Calmette, the director of the institute, and his colleague Guerin spent years gradually reducing the virulence of the isolate to the point where, although it would infect and multiply to some extent in experimental animals, it would not cause progressive tubercular pathology. Oral administration or cutaneous inoculation of this isolate tended to produce tuberculin hypersensitivity in the test animals and later in humans. The relatively avirulent isolate has been designated the "bacillus of Calmette and Guerin" or BCG. It is not advocated for general immunization or for infant immunization—and certainly not for individuals who already are hypersensitive to tuberculin. In areas of high incidence of tuberculosis with poor control and treatment facilities, however, its use has been noted to be a factor in controlling the spread of the disease.

A recently (1972–1973) advocated unique use for BCG is unrelated to the disease tuberculosis. This use is based upon the fact that tubercle bacilli (dead or alive), when injected along with various antigens, exert an adjuvant effect on the associated antigens. Various workers have now experimented with the injection of BCG into a variety of animal cancers with the objective of exerting an adjuvant effect on the weak cancer antigens—and the hope that this will lead to a cancer-specific immune response and healing of the malignancy. Although some rather remarkable results in experimental animals have been reported, it is still too early to draw conclusions relative to the efficacy of this approach to cancer therapy.

Although serum antibodies can be produced by "immunization" with various mycobacterial cells or extracted antigens from such cells, these antibodies are not responsible for the tuberculin hypersensitivity or the resistance to reinfection of infected hosts. However, lymphocytes from hypersensitive experimental animals can produce hypersensitivity and resistance to infection when injected into *syngenic* animals. Although serum antibodies to tubercular antigens have no immunotherapeutic significance, they have been useful in the serotaxonomic differentiation of some mycobacterial species. For a more detailed consideration see David and Selin (1976).

CHEMOTHERAPY

Whereas the therapeutic efficacy of sulfanilamide and penicillin had been established for a variety of bacterial diseases by the early 1940s, these diseases did not include tuberculosis. Selman Waksman in 1944 reported the discovery of the antibiotic streptomycin, which became the first effective drug for therapy in this disease. Subsequently, a number of antibiotic and synthetic drugs have been advocated for tubercular therapy. Some of these, including streptomycin, give toxic reactions in some patients. Also, as indicated above, tubercle bacilli are prone to develop resistance to safe concentrations of therapeutic drugs, and the drug-resistant strains may be capable of infecting other hosts and being resistant to the drug prior to the start of therapy. For these reasons a very important function of the mycobacterium laboratory is to inform the physician of the drugs of choice for treating a given case of the disease. In this regard it is common practice to use a combination of two drugs, frequently including isoniazid, in such therapy.

Chemotherapy in tuberculosis is a slow process at best. This may be due to the frequency of quiescence of the tubercle bacilli within walled-off lesions, since some drugs are much more effective against rapidly growing organisms. It may be due also to the difficulty of therapeutic concentrations of the drug reaching the tubercle bacilli in cavitated lesions or embedded in the caseous matrix of necrotic lesions. Regardless of cause, continuous therapy for months to a year or more may be required. It has been established that rest (in bed) is an impor-

tant adjunct to healing of tubercular lung lesions. This rest function has been carried to the
extreme of temporarily collapsing (*artificial pneu-
mothorax*) a severely cavitated lung by the injection of an inert gas into the pleural cavity on that
side. By maintaining the pressure within the
pleural cavity, the lung tissue on that side is kept
at rest. After healing, the gas pressure can be
removed and the respiratory function of the
healed lung can be resumed.

CONTROL AND PREVENTION

Since there is no immunoprophylactic agent
advocated for general use, the greatest hope for
controlling the spread of tuberculosis is threefold:

1. Educate the general public regarding the
   insidious nature of the onset of symptoms
   and the contagious nature of the disease.
2. Undertake tuberculin testing to find early
   evidence of infection, followed by chest X-
   raying of tuberculin-positive individuals.
3. Initiate early chemotherapy on active cases of
   tuberculosis—both for the welfare of the
   patient and to prevent the spread of the
   disease to others.

In crowded environments where the incidence of tuberculosis is high, the tuberculin
testing might be followed by the administration
of BCG to tuberculin-negative individuals—but
not to infants.

Treatment of active cases and control of the
spread of the disease from such cases is best
accomplished in tubercular sanitoria with adequate beds, good nutrition, and trained personnel. Sputum from such cases should be collected
in cardboard or other flammable containers and
incinerated daily.

REFERENCES

David, H. L. and M. J. Selin. 1976. Immune response
    to mycobacteriae. Chapter 45 in *Manual of Clini-
    cal Immunology.*

Kilburn, J. O. and G. P. Kubica. 1968a. Reagent
    impregnated paper strips for detection of niacin.
    Am. J. Clin. Pathol. 50:530–532.

Kilburn, J. O., K. D. Stottmeier, and G. P. Kubica.
    1968b. Aspartic acid as a precursor for niacin
    synthesis by tubercle bacilli grown on 7H-10
    agar medium. *Am. J. Clin. Pathol.* 50:582–586.

Paik, G. and M. T. Suggs. 1974. Reagents, stains, and
    miscellaneous test procedures. Chapter 96 in
    Manual of Clinical Microbiology.

Philpott, J. A., A. R. Woodburne, O. S. Philpott, W. B.
    Schaefer, and C. S. Mollohan. 1963. Swimming
    pool granuloma. *Arch. Derm.* 88:158–162.

Runyon, E. H., A. G. Karlson, G. P. Kubica, and L. G.
    Wayne. 1974. Mycobacterium. Chapter 16 in
    Manual of Clinical Microbiology.

Truant, J. P., W. A. Brett, and W. Thomas, Jr. 1962.
    Fluorescence microscopy of tubercle bacilli
    stained with auramine and rhodamine. *Henry
    Ford Hosp. Med. Bull.* 10:287.

Uganda Buruli Group. 1971. Report of the epidemi-
    ology of *Mycobacterium ulceranus* infection (Buruli
    ulcer) at Kinyara, Uganda. *Trans. Roy. Soc. Trop.
    Med.* 65:763–775.

Vera, H. D. and M. Dumoff. 1974. Culture media.
    Chapter 95 in *Manual of Clinical Microbiology.*

10

Whooping Cough

Whooping cough (pertussis) was recognized as a clinical entity by Thomas Sydenham in 1670. Because of the severe coughing paroxysms, he named the disease *pertussis* from the Latin for intensive cough. Jules Bordet and O. Gengou first reported the observation of an ovoid bacillus in bronchial exudates of a child victim in 1890. They did not succeed in culturing the organism, however, until 1906. The delay was due, in part, to the fact that the organism required a higher than usual concentration (30 to 50 percent) of blood in the complex medium on which growth finally was obtained.

THE ETIOLOGICAL AGENT

The organism isolated by Bordet and Gengou was a small, gram-negative, nonmotile, ovoid rod that later was found to be encapsulated in the smooth (S) colony phase. The original Bordet-Gengou medium was composed of potato infusion, peptone, glycerol, and agar to which was added 50 percent freshly drawn blood. Because of the requirement for the high concentration of blood in the original BG medium, the organism was placed in the genus *Hemophilus* and given the species designation *pertussis*. However, Pollock (1947) and Mishulow et al. (1952) reported that activated charcoal could replace the blood in such a medium because, like the blood albumin, it functioned only to neutralize certain fatty acids in the medium that were toxic for *H. pertussis.* Therefore, since blood is not required, the organism has been removed from the genus *Hemophilus* and now is designated *Bordetella pertussis* in honor of Bordet. A related but physiologically and antigenically distinct organism, *B. parapertussis,* has been isolated from mild cases of whooping cough. Another member of the genus is *B. bronchiseptica.* All three species of the genus share at least one antigen, but each is known also to possess antigens not shared with the other two species.

Leslie and Garner in 1931 reported a significant antigenic *phase variation* phenomenon in *H. (B.) pertussis* cells. Freshly isolated, smooth (S) colony, virulent cells generally were found to be in the antigenic phase designated 1. As the cells were maintained in laboratory cultures, they tended to undergo progressive changes to antigenic phases 2, 3, and 4. Antigenic phase 4 was found to be associated with rough (R) colony, avirulent cells. Since, prior to 1931, whooping cough vaccines had been prepared from laboratory strains of *H. (B.) pertussis* without regard to their antigenic phase status, some such vaccines were found to be immunogenic whereas others were not. Since 1931, whooping cough vaccines have been prepared from S-colony antigenic phase 1 cells only.

Phase 1 *B. pertussis* cells have yielded several antigenically distinct extractable components. One of the extractable antigens is the agglutinogen; antibody specific for this antigen is responsible for the agglutination of the *B. pertussis* cells (Schuchardt et al. 1963). Two antigenic *toxins*—one heat-labile and dermonecrotic, the other a heat-stable endotoxin—have been extracted from *B. pertussis* cells. Other extractable antigens include a *hemagglutinin* that will attach to and cause agglutination of red blood corpuscles; a *histamine sensitizing factor;* a *lymphocytosis promoting factor;* and *adjuvant factors.* There have been claims for an additional antigen that functions as the protective or immunogenic antigen. The protective antigen, in contrast to the case in *S. pneumoniae,* is not the capsular antigen. Its exact nature is not clearly comprehended, however, and killed whole cells, rather than purified protective antigen, constitute the usual vaccine for whooping cough immunization (Munoz 1963a; 1963b).

PATHOGENESIS

The mechanism whereby *B. pertussis* produces pathology in the patient is not clearly comprehended. There is experimental animal evidence that the heat-labile toxin might be a factor. This seems reasonable because the organisms, although they colonize and erode the ciliated epithelium of the bronchial tree, rarely invade the bloodstream or other tissues. The

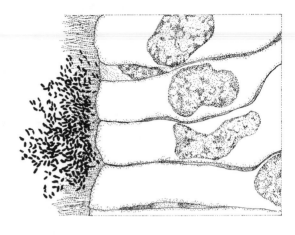

Figure 10–1. Colony of *Bordetella pertussis* among the cilia of cells lining a bronchial membrane. About 1500×. (After W. Burrows, 1973.)

systemic symptoms of the disease, therefore, would seem to result from absorbed, pharmacologically active components or products of the cells. The *B. pertussis* cells secrete a sticky substance that tends to cement them to the cilia lining the bronchial membranes. Colonies of such cells (see Figure 10-1) can interfere mechanically with the normal bronchial-clearing function of the cilia. This permits pneumococci, streptococci, and other pathogenic bacteria to complicate the *B. pertussis* infection and cause bronchial pneumonia.

Uncomplicated whooping cough is divided into three clinical stages, each lasting about 2 weeks. The *catarrhal stage* begins with symptoms indistinguishable from the common cold: nasal coryza, sneezing, and a mild progressive cough. After 10 to 14 days the *paroxysmal stage* begins— intense coughing spasms are followed by a deep inspiratory whoop as air is drawn rapidly into the depleted lungs. Sometimes multiple cough paroxysms follow each other with no intervening inspirations. This development may cause the patient to become anoxic, which may lead to severe, even fatal convulsions—particularly in infants. During the *convalescent stage* the number of coughing paroxysms gradually decreases and the patient recovers, usually with long-lasting immunity.

During the catarrhal stage *B. pertussis* cells colonize the bronchial membranes (see Figure 10-1). Since, at this stage, the disease may be considered just another cold, few if any precautions against the spread of the disease are taken. Therefore this stage, particularly by the second week, becomes the most contagious. However, because of the explosive coughing, organisms are discharged in much greater numbers during the early paroxysmal stage. Usually after 4 weeks from onset live organisms can no longer be found in respiratory discharges.

The pathogenic mechanism involved in the paroxysmal coughing is something of a mystery. Obviously the irritation due to the erosion of the bronchial membranes could be expected to trigger cough responses. Probably the mild progressive coughing during the catarrhal stage can best be explained by this irritation. The coughing of the paroxysmal stage is significantly different from that of the catarrhal stage, however, or that of coughing episodes in other diseases. It seems significant to this author that the onset of paroxysmal coughing on the tenth to fourteenth day coincides with the time that one might expect the onset of an immediate hypersensitivity response to antigenic stimulation. This, coupled with experimental animal evidence of hypersensitivity to *B. pertussis* antigens, seems to justify the conclusion that either intact cells, soluble products, or disintegration components of *B. pertussis* coming into contact with hypersensitive bronchial tissues might account for the paroxysmal coughing in this disease. The occasional coughing paroxysms continuing during the convalescent stage, after live *B. pertussis* cells can no longer be isolated, might be explained by residual dead cells or cell fragments, not coated with IgG or IgA antibody, being liberated from their attachment on the cilia and coming into contact with the hypersensitive membranes. For more details see Pittman (1970). A typical outbreak involving 31 confirmed (culture or fluorescent antibody) and 20 unconfirmed cases of whooping cough was re-ported from Knoxville, Tennessee, during the summer and early fall of 1975. Thirteen of the cases were in infants under 1 year of age (see *MMWR*, 21 May 1976).

EPIDEMIOLOGY

Whooping cough is a disease of humans only, although clinically similar infections have been produced experimentally in chimpanzees. Rabbits, rats, mice, and chick embryos have been used in experimental studies with *B. pertussis*, but the symptoms in these animals in no way resemble human whooping cough. The actual primary vehicle in the transmission of whooping cough is infected bronchial exudate—and, since this is always admixed with saliva, the mode of transmission is "traffic in saliva" as illustrated in Figure II-A. The organisms, however, are rather susceptible to external environments. Consequently, direct contact or its equivalent (respiratory droplets) is more important than secondary vehicles in whooping cough epidemiology. Carriers seem to be of no significance. As stated, the disease is highly contagious during the catarrhal and early (first week) paroxysmal stages.

LABORATORY DIAGNOSIS

The clinical laboratory is rarely called upon to aid in the diagnosis of whooping cough. If whooping cough is prevalent in a neighborhood and catarrhal symptoms are suspected of being early whooping cough, however, the laboratory can isolate and identify *B. pertussis* before the onset of the paroxysmal stage. The medium used for this isolation is some modification of that of Bordet and Gengou (BG). The modification can use either fresh blood or charcoal. The blood must be added to the sterile agar medium at a temperature of 50°C and immediately dispensed into sterile petri plates or into sterile tubes for blood-agar slants. The charcoal may be added to the medium prior to sterilization, and the melted charcoal agar can be dispensed into sterile plates or tubes at temperatures above 50°C.

Plates of BG medium may be held vertically, about 6 inches in front of the patient, during a paroxysmal cough (the cough plate method of inoculation). Droplets containing *B. pertussis* cells coughed up from the bronchial membranes will thereby seed the plate medium. During the catarrhal stage, however, a cotton swab inserted through the nares to the nasopharyngeal area is more likely to pick up *B. pertussis* cells. The swab exudate should be roll-inoculated to one edge of the BG medium and then streaked over the rest of the surface with a sterile bacteriological loop to obtain isolated colonies. Either cough plates or swab-inoculated plates should be incubated overnight at 37°C. Smears from characteristic colonies should be gram-stained; and if the colony is composed of gram-negative oval rods, it should be inoculated to a BG agar slant. After overnight incubation of the slant, the growth may be suspended in sterile saline. This bacterial suspension can be proved to be composed of *B. pertussis* cells by a serotaxonomic agglutination test using an absorbed antiserum known to contain antibodies specific for the nonshared antigens of *B. pertussis*. If fluorescent antibody specific for *B. pertussis* and an ultraviolet-light microscope are available, the organisms in a smear of the nasopharyngeal exudate may be identified as *B. pertussis* by the direct FA technique (see Donaldson and Whitaker 1960). For more detailed considerations see Pittman (1974).

Although agglutinins develop in the serum of whooping cough patients, they do not appear until late in the convalescent stage. Therefore serodiagnostic tests are of little value. There are no skin tests of practical value in whooping cough, although a susceptibility test, using the heat-labile toxin, has been described.

IMMUNITY

The fact that an attack of whooping cough confers lasting immunity is indicative of both the immunogenicity and the homogeneity of the protective antigens of *B. pertussis*. Active immunoprophylaxis consists of two or more injections of pertussis vaccine spaced 4 weeks apart.

The monovalent (P) vaccine consists of a saline suspension of killed, antigenic, phase-1 *B. pertussis* cells. As indicated in the discussion of diphtheria immunization, the *B. pertussis* cells can be suspended in diphtheria toxoid (DP) or in a mixture of diphtheria and tetanus toxoid (DPT) to give two- or threefold immune responses per injection. Moreover, the *B. pertussis* cells provide an adjuvant effect on the associated toxoid antigens. The first active immunization for whooping cough (preferably with three doses of DPT antigens) should be initiated at the age of 2 to 3 months. This immunization should be followed by a single booster injection 1 year later.

Passive immunoprophylaxis using convalescent serum antibodies has been advocated for susceptible infants exposed to known cases of whooping cough. Such serum antibodies are rarely available, however, and their prophylactic efficacy is questionable. The same holds for passive immunotherapy, which, if it has any value, must be given during the early catarrhal stage.

Whooping cough is one of the few diseases for which *active* immunotherapy (after onset of symptoms) can be advocated with reasonable justification. This justification is based upon three facts: (1) the natural clinical disease lasts a relatively long time (about 6 weeks); (2) the infection is relatively superficial and therefore results in minimal antigenic stimulation; and (3) the severe paroxysmal stage may be caused by an allergic hypersensitivity of the involved membranes. Consequently as soon as a diagnosis is made, preferably during the first week of the catarrhal stage, active immunization with monovalent (P) pertussis vaccine should be initiated. This and subsequent injections at one- to two-week intervals can supplement the immunogenic stimulation involved in the infection and, hopefully, speed up both the immune (IgG) and the desensitization (IgA) antibody responses.

CONTROL AND PREVENTION

The ideal preventive measure for whooping

cough is active immunization of all infants at age 2 to 3 months. Furthermore, active immunization should be started immediately in *nonimmune* contacts with a known case of whooping cough. This step may not prevent the development of symptoms, but it should modify such symptoms and prevent serious complications.

Chemotherapy with chloromycetin or other broad-spectrum antibiotics—but not penicillin—has been advocated for late catarrhal and early paroxysmal whooping cough.

REFERENCES

Donaldson, P. and J. A. Whitaker. 1960. Diagnosis of pertussis by fluorescent antibody staining of nasopharyngeal smears. *Amer. J. Dis. Child.* 99:423–427.

Mishulow, L., L. S. Sharpe, and L. L. Cohen. 1952. Beef-heart charcoal agar for the preparation of pertussis vaccines. *Amer. J. Pub. Health.* 43:1466–1472.

Munoz, J. 1963a. Comparison of *Bordetella pertussis* cells and Freund's adjuvant with respect to their antibody inducing and anaphylactogenic properties. *J. Immunol.* 90:132–139.

————. 1963b. Immunological and other biological activities of *Bordetella pertussis* antigens. *Bacteriol. Rev.* 27:325–340.

Pittman, B. 1974. *Bordetella.* Chapter 27 in *Manual of Clinical Microbiology.*

Pittman, M. 1970. *Bordetella pertussis*—bacterial and host factors in the pathogenesis and prevention of whooping cough. In *Infectious Agents and Host Responses,* S. Mudd (ed.). Philadelphia: Saunders.

Pollock, M. R. 1947. The growth of *Hemophilus pertussis* on media without blood. *Brit. J. Exp. Pathol.* 28:295–307.

Schuchardt, L. F., J. Munoz, W. F. Verwey, and J. F. Sagin. 1963. The relationship of agglutinogen to other antigens of *Bordetella pertussis. J. Immunol.* 91:107–111.

11

Introductory Virology

Viruses were first recognized as submicroscopic, filter-passing, infectious agents. Whereas ordinary light microscopes will resolve objects of around 0.25 micrometers (250 nanometers), viruses in general range in size from the smallest (10 to 17 nanometers) to the largest (about 250 nanometers)—all of which pass filters that restrict the passage of larger organisms. Viruses within or absorbed onto host tissue components might not pass the filters, however, and larger organisms, particularly if not rigid, might grow through or be forced through filters. Consequently filterability, although extensively used in the recognition of new viruses, is not an absolute characteristic for virus identification. Furthermore, the development of the electron microscope renders viruses no longer submicroscopic.

NATURE OF VIRUSES

All viruses are obligate parasites. This means that they have not, as yet, been cultivated in the absence of living susceptible cells. Practically all rickettsiae, some bacteria, and some protozoa also are obligate parasites. Consequently obligate parasitism is not a differential characteristic of viruses. Nevertheless, since there is no evidence of growth and binary fission during virus replication, both of which commonly occur during the replication of rickettsiae and bacteria regardless of obligate or facultative parasitism, there are obvious differences between viruses and other microorganisms. For more details see Casals (1956).

VIRUS COMPOSITION AND STRUCTURE

Two fundamental characteristics distinguish viruses from all other forms of life: (1) they possess only one nucleic acid, either DNA or RNA but not both as found in all other life forms; (2) they possess no enzymes capable of functioning in energy metabolism (that is, ATP generation). Because there is no mechanism for

123

generating ATP, viruses must depend upon the host tissues to provide both the structural components (amino acids and nucleotides) and the synthetic machinery necessary for the synthesis of viral proteins, nucleic acid, and lipids, and the assembly of these components into mature virions. When the nucleic acid of the infecting virus enters the host cell, it usurps the role of the cell genetic material and redirects the cell synthetic machinery toward the production of new virus. If enzymes not normally produced by the host cell are needed, the virus nucleic acid directs the cell to produce these enzymes.

Mature virions may be released from the infected cell by rupture of the cell, or the virion may be extruded or budded through the outer cell membrane without visible damage to the cell (see Figure 11-1). In the latter case a portion of the cell membrane may pinch off and provide an outer *lipoidal envelope* around the protein coat of the virion. In other viruses, however, there is evidence that the lipoidal envelope is synthesized independently of the outer cell membranes and such virions may be released by cell bursts. Enveloped virions, because of the lipoidal nature of the envelope, are susceptible to treatment with ether, whereas nonenveloped virions are resistant to such treatment.

Figure 11–1. A C-type RNA virus caught in the process of budding from an infected cell. 168,000×. (Courtesy of J. J. Cardamone, Jr., and J. S. Youngner.)

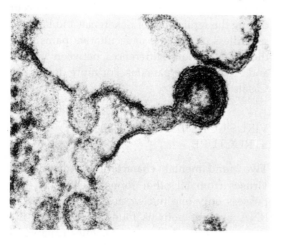

Mature virions may occur in a variety of shapes (spherical, bullet-shaped, cylindrical, cubical, polyhedral). Many bacterial viruses (bacteriophages) and possibly some animal viruses possess taillike structures. These structures may serve for attachment of the virus to specific receptors and, in the case of bacterial hosts, penetration through the cell wall. The hollow core of the tail then serves as a channel through which the nucleic acid is inoculated into the host cell (see Figure 11-2). The sites for phage attachment may be highly specific. Different phage biotypes within a bacterial species may be recognized by the susceptibility of the biotype strain to one or a few of many phages that will attack other biotype strains of that species. This use of differential bacteriophage susceptibility testing within a bacterial species is known as *phage typing* and is helpful in epidemiological studies of certain pathogenic bacterial diseases.

The shape of a given virus is determined by the arrangement of the bundles of protein molecules, designated *capsomeres*, that compose the protein coats (the *capsids*) of viruses (see Figure 11-3). The nucleic acid of the virion is housed within this protein coat, which is then designated a *nucleocapsid*. In cylindrical viruses (for example, tobacco mosaic virus) the capsomeres and the enclosed nucleic acid form a helical structure. In cubical or polyhedral nucleocapsids, the nucleic acid is randomly coiled within the nucleocapsid (see Caspar 1965). In many such virions, the nucleic acid is a single, large macromolecule. In the *Myxovirus influenzae* virion the nucleic acid is segmented into eight polynucleotide fragments. Nucleocapsids with lipoidal envelopes may develop spikes that extend beyond the surface of the envelope. Such spikes may house (1) structures that attach the virion to cells and (2) enzymes (RDE) that may destroy the receptor site. When the RDE destroys the site of attachment, the virion may detach and then attach to other intact cell receptors. The exact contribution of the RDE to the life cycle of the virus is not clearly established.

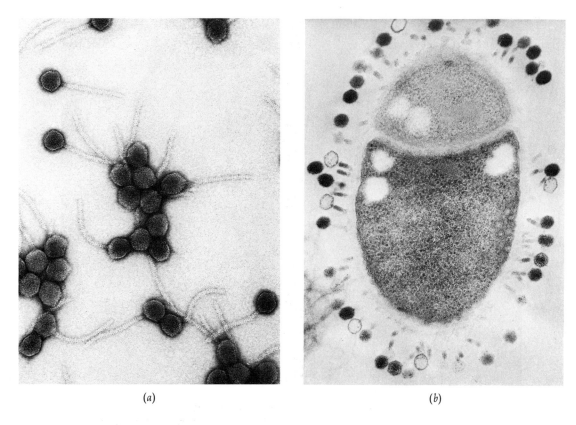

(a)   (b)

Figure 11–2. (a) Negatively-stained, purified lamda bacteriophage. Heads are about 65 nm in diameter, tails about 100 nm long. (b) ⌀CP51 bacteriophage attached to a cell of *Bacillus subtilis.* 41,400×. ((a) Courtesy of J. Griffith; (b) courtesy of S. C. Holt.)

One of the cellular manifestations of virus infection, recognized in some instances even before the virus etiology of disease was established, is the presence of inclusion bodies in the cytoplasm or nucleus of the host cell (see Figure 11-4). Since these inclusion bodies tend to stain differently from the normal cell constituents, they may serve as laboratory diagnostic signs of infection (for example, the *Negri bodies* in rabies or *Guarnieri bodies* in smallpox). The Guarnieri bodies were later demonstrated by E. Paschen to be composed of smaller bodies (*elementary bodies*) that proved to be the actual virions. Thus in this instance, at least, the inclusion body proved to be a colony of the virus particles in the cytoplasm of the infected cell.

PROPAGATION OF VIRUSES

Since all viruses are obligate parasites, they cannot be cultivated on nonliving media. In other words living, susceptible host tissue is essential for virus replication. Moreover, different viruses require different types of tissue for such replication. Obviously the virus is replicated in the natural host. When this natural host is a human being, however, practical propagation for diagnostic purposes, vaccine, or other volume production of the virus requires other types of host tissue. In some instances human viruses may infect and be replicated in adult experimental animals (such as the mouse, ferret, monkey, or chicken). In other instances

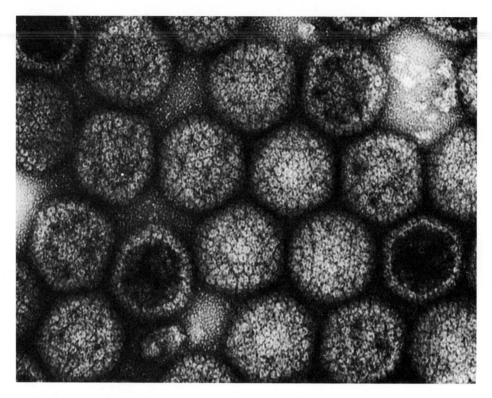

Figure 11–3. An array of negatively-stained capsids of *Herpesvirus* sp. The capsomeres composing the capsids may be seen. Capsid diameter is about 80–100 nm. (Courtesy of B. Roizman.)

the adult experimental animal may not be susceptible to infection by a given virus, whereas the infant animal of the same species is susceptible. In many instances the embryonic animal (such as the chick embryo) may be susceptible to infection and propagation of viruses that cannot be propagated in postnatal animals, either infant or adult.

Finally, with the extensive development during the 1930–1950 era of *in vitro* cultivation of animal tissues, it became apparent that such tissues could serve as hosts to certain viruses. The propagation of poliovirus in tissue cultures by John Enders and his colleagues made possible the development of the Salk and Sabin vaccines for the practical eradication of the dreaded disease paralytic poliomyelitis. Subsequently these tissue cultures have provided the means for specific diagnosis of poliomyelitis and other diseases. Tissue cultures also provide the

volume production of viruses needed for other disease vaccines. These usages of virus propagation are discussed along with other considerations of the individual viral diseases.

QUANTITATION OF VIRUSES

The virologist on frequent occasions is called upon to quantitate the amount of virus (the number of virions) in a specimen. An early, highly effective, and reproducible method of quantitation was the *plaque-forming* unit (PFU) method applied to the enumeration of bacteriophage virions. If one desired to establish the number of phage virions that would attack *Shigella paradysenteriae* in a milliliter of sewage filtrate, one could prepare dilutions of the filtrate and mix 1-milliliter amounts of each dilution with an aliquot of a young broth culture of *S. paradysenteriae.* Each mixture would then be

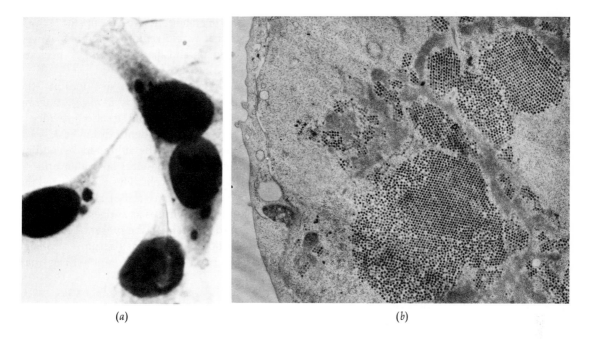

(a)   (b)

Figure 11–4. Two types of viral inclusion bodies. (a) Light micrograph of mouse fibroblast cells infected with vaccinia virus. The larger dark areas are the nuclei; the smaller dark bodies are the cytoplasmic viral inclusions. (b) Electron micrograph of crystalline aggregates of adenovirus virions in the nucleus of a HeLa cell 24 hours after inoculation. 8,870×. ((a) Courtesy of N. Sharon; (b) courtesy of S. Dales and S. L. Wilton.)

seeded to the entire surface of a suitable agar medium in a petri plate and the plates incubated overnight at 37°C. The bacterial cells would grow into a film or "lawn" on the medium. Where a phage virion was deposited, however, it would attack and lyse a bacterial cell. The liberated phage progeny from that cell would then attack and lyse neighboring cells, and this process would continue and result in a clear area of no bacterial growth (the plaque) in the bacterial lawn. By counting the number of such plaques on the plate and multiplying the count by the reciprocal of the dilution of the filtrate in that mixture, the number of phage virions in 1 milliliter of the undiluted filtrate can be established.

The PFU method of enumerating animal viruses is less readily applied to virion counts. It has, however, been used for the enumeration of viruses that attack and destroy animal tissue culture cells capable of growing as a lawn on the surface of a suitable medium.

Another method of animal virus enumeration that is less quantitative than the PFU method is the determination of the *average infectious dose* (ID/50) of a specimen containing virus. The ID/50 is the smallest amount of the specimen which will infect 50 percent or more of the experimental animals that receive the dose. If all infected animals die as a result of the infection, the dose is easily established and is reasonably reproducible. However, it is common experience to find that infecting experimental animals may require the presence of more than one virion in the dose administered and this number may vary with the type of experimental animal used.

When tissue cultures are used for the enumeration of virions, the equivalent of the ID/50 is called the *tissue cytopathogenic* or *cytopathic dose* (TCD)—the smallest amount of the virus specimen that will cause macroscopically or microscopically visible evidence of pathology (CPE) in the tissue culture cells. Usually only low power or no magnification of the infected tissue culture is required for recognizing this evidence of cytopathology. Since homologous antibody will neutralize or inhibit the capacity of a virus to infect host tissues, the ID/50 or TCD/50 technique can be used for the serotaxonomic identification of such viruses. Known antibody, for example, when added to antigenically homologous virus prior to host exposure, will inhibit infection or cytopathology. Such antibody will not inhibit antigenically heterologous viruses. Also using known antigenic viruses, a patient's serum can be tested for the presence of homologous antibody — serodiagnosis.

With some viruses (for example, parainfluenza), tissue culture cytopathology is not as readily recognized as a corollary phenomenon — *hemadsorption*. In this instance the virus infection of the tissue culture cells results in the adsorption by the infected cells of erythrocytes added to the cell environment. Noninfected cells fail to adsorb the erythrocytes.

Hirst (1941) reported a phenomenon that has been extremely valuable in demonstrating the presence of virus in a test specimen quantitating that virus, and arriving at serotaxonomic identification of the virus (or serodiagnosis of the homologous disease). This phenomenon is *viral hemagglutination* (HA) — that is, the agglutination of erythrocytes by certain viruses. Hirst first observed this phenomenon accidentally in fluids obtained from chick embryos infected with influenza virus. He noted that red blood cells, which got into the fluid as a result of the rupture of embryonic blood capillaries, were clumped (agglutinated) if the embryo was infected but not clumped in noninfected embryo fluid. He noted that by testing dilutions of the fluid from infected embryos, which received a suitable quantity of chicken red blood cells, he could establish an *HA titer* — the highest dilution of the fluid that caused agglutination of the red blood cells. He noted, also, that the HA titer correlated closely with the ID/50 of the virus in the fluid. Thus a simple *in vitro* test that can be performed in an hour or two can substitute for *in vivo* tests that would require numerous experimental animals and days or weeks to perform (Figure 11-5).

Not only will the HA test indicate the presence and quantity of a hemagglutinating virus in the specimen but it also provides a simple serotaxonomic identification test. Viral hemagglutination can be inhibited by adding specific antibody to the virus specimen prior to adding the red blood cells. This is designated the *hemagglutination inhibition* (HI or HAI) test. Also, using known HA viruses as antigens, the HI test can be used to establish the presence of homologous antibody in a patient's serum — serodiagnosis (see Hirst 1965). Different viruses may

Figure 11–5. Virus titration by hemagglutination test. Hemagglutination (a uniform mat of cells) shown from 1:10 through 1:640 dilutions of viral antigen. No hemagglutination is evident in the 1:1280 and greater dilutions — note buttons of cells in these and in control without virus.

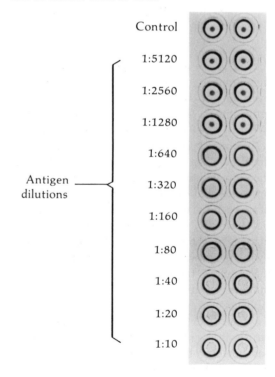

require red blood cells from different animal species for the viral HA phenomenon. Consequently, the availability of that animal species may limit the practicality of the test. Chicken, guinea pig, human, and monkey red blood cells have been the most frequently used in HA and HI testing procedures for human viral diseases. Not all viruses cause HA, however, at least not with red blood cells that have been tested to date. A modification of the HA test—the hemadsorption test—was described by Shelokov et al. (1958). For more detailed considerations, see Schmidt and Lennette (1965) and Fenner and White (1976).

TAXONOMIC CLASSIFICATION

As indicated in Chapter 3, the taxonomic classification of viruses is not yet final. The International Committee on the Taxonomy of Viruses (ICTV) has recommended new and enlightened approaches to virus taxonomy (see Fenner 1976). Taxonomists frequently have designated taxonomic groups with the names of biological scientists who have made significant contributions to the area involved. These names may do honor to those individuals, but they do nothing to indicate the nature of the organism so named. The animal virologists, in contrast, have chosen to indicate morphological or biochemical characteristics of the viruses in the names given to taxonomic groups. The names, therefore, make it possible to visualize something of the nature of the viruses included in that group. Moreover, the recommendation for ending all genus designations with the suffix -virus makes possible the use of many former common names (for example, poliovirus) as the taxonomic genus name—Poliovirus. In discussing the various viral diseases, this book gives the accepted or strongly recommended genus and species designation for each virus involved.

REFERENCES

Casals, J. 1956. Viruses: The versatile parasites. I. The arthropod-borne group of animal viruses. *Trans. New York Acad. Sci.* 19:219–235.

Caspar, D. L. D. 1965. Design principles in virus particle construction. Chapter 4 in *Viral and Rickettsial Infections of Man.*

Fenner, F. 1976. The classification and nomenclature of viruses: The current position. *Amer. Soc. Microbiol. News* 42:170–173.

Fenner, F. and D. O. White. 1976. *Medical Virology.* 2nd ed. New York: Academic Press.

Finland, M. (ed.). 1964. Current progress in virus diseases. A symposium. *Bacteriol. Rev.* 28: 367–496.

Hirst, G. K. 1941. The agglutination of red cells by allantoic fluid of chick embryos infected with influenza virus. *Science* 94:22–23.

———. 1965. Cell-virus attachment and the action of antibodies on viruses. Chapter 8 in *Viral and Rickettsial Infections of Man.*

Schmidt, N. J. and E. H. Lennette. 1965. Basic technics for virology. Appendix in *Viral and Rickettsial Infections of Man.*

Shelokov, A., J. E. Vogel, and L. Chi. 1958. Hemadsorption (adsorption-hemagglutination) test for viral agents in tissue culture with special reference to influenza. *Proc. Soc. Exper. Biol. Med.* 97:802–809.

Smith, H. 1972. Mechanisms of virus pathogenicity. *Bacteriol. Rev.* 36:291–310.

12

The Common Cold

The common cold (infectious coryza or rhinitis) is the most prevalent human infectious disease. The symptoms, with which everyone is familiar, are difficult to distinguish from noninfectious coryzas or rhinitises—the upper respiratory allergies. Moreover, the prodromal symptoms of other respiratory group diseases (sore throat, cough, coryza, conjunctivitis) frequently simulate the symptoms of the common cold. Since the common cold usually is given little serious concern, the similar onset symptoms of the more serious diseases (diphtheria, whooping cough, influenza, measles, and others) may result in epidemic spread or serious pathology before a differential diagnosis is made. The common cold also, as previously stated, can predispose the patient to the more serious complications of bronchial or lobar pneumonia. Also, because of its prevalence (estimated to average two colds per person per year) and debilitating effect, with resulting absenteeism or loss of efficiency, the common cold often is rated by industry as one of the greatest causes of economic loss.

ETIOLOGY

Many research efforts to establish an etiological agent for the common cold date back to the early twentieth century. Although a number of potentially pathogenic bacteria (such as alpha streptococci, pneumococci, staphylococci, beta streptococci, *Klebsiella pneumoniae, Neisseria catarrhalis,* and *Hemophilus influenzae*) commonly found on the normal respiratory membranes have been implicated as causing complications, none has been established as the primary cause of the common cold. W. von Kruse, in 1914, was the first to report that common cold symptoms could be transmitted to human volunteers by bacteria-free filtrates of nasal washing from cases. Between 1914 and 1960 a number of filterable viruses were demonstrated capable of causing coldlike symptoms in human volunteers and in some instances in chimpanzees and higher apes (for examples see Dochez et al. 1930 and 1938). These included certain enteroviruses, coxsackieviruses, respiratory syncytial viruses, adenoviruses, parainfluenza viruses, and influenza A viruses. None of these appeared to be *the* cause of the common cold, however.

In 1946 the British Medical Research Council set up a common cold research unit at Salisbury. Since human volunteers were required for this research and strict isolation of the volunteers was frequently essential, the director conceived the idea of housing the research in a number of well-separated housing units. These units, with all expenses paid, were offered as honeymoon cottages to war veterans and their brides. Each couple had to agree not to socialize with other cottage occupants and to remain isolated from all others except the assigned research personnel. They had to agree, moreover, to permit experiments involving transmission, immunity, and other aspects of the common cold, including etiological studies.

For 14 years this research effort, involving more than 6,000 volunteers, discovered little information about the common cold that had not previously been discovered by the Rockefeller Foundation and other research workers in the mid-1930s. Tyrrell and Parsons (1960), however, using human fetal liver tissue culture, reported the isolation of a new virus from a common cold patient. This virus they designated *Rhinovirus*. The newly isolated virus did not produce visible cytopathology in the tissue culture cells. However, the *Rhinovirus*-infected cells were found to be resistant to infection by another virus that did produce visible cytopathology in noninfected fetal tissue culture cells (the *viral interference* phenomenon). The new virus was found to grow best when the tissue cultures were continuously rotated and incubated at 33°C instead of the usual 37°C. Subsequently they found that by deleting sodium bicarbonate and maintaining the pH of the tissue culture medium between 6.8 and 7.3, microscopically visible cytopathology could be observed (see Figure 12-1).

As additional *Rhinovirus* isolates were studied, some were found capable of infecting and replicating in adult monkey kidney tissue (MKT) cultures as well as in the human embryonic tissue cultures. These were designated *Rhinovirus* M biotypes. Those that required the human tissue were designated *Rhinovirus* H biotypes. One of the M biotypes proved to be *Echovirus* 28 (enteric cytopathogenic human or-

Figure 12-1. Micrographs showing cultures of human fetal diploid lung cells. (a) Uninfected; (b) appearance of cytopathology due to infection with *Rhinovirus*. Both 160×. (Courtesy of J. H. Schieble.)

(a)

(b)

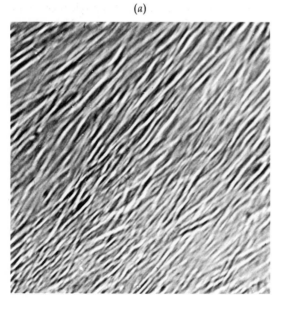
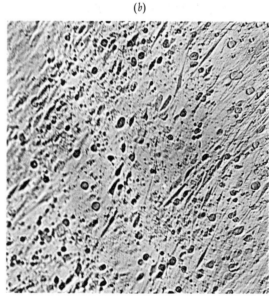

phan virus), previously isolated in a monkey kidney tissue culture. Because that MKT culture had been inoculated with fecal material from a *healthy person,* the virus isolate was designated an *orphan virus.* They soon established, moreover, that both biotypes included antigenically distinct serotypes. By 1971 this antigenic heterogeneity had reached at least 89 serotypes for the H biotype and at least 7 serotypes for the M biotype. This extent of antigenic heterogeneity of the serotypes precluded the likelihood of immunoprophylaxis as a means of controlling the common cold. For a review of the first 8 years of research on the rhinoviruses, see Hamre (1968).

LABORATORY DIAGNOSIS

Because of its complicated nature, clinical laboratory diagnosis of the common cold is never requested. Research and public health laboratories may be involved in the isolation and identification of rhinoviruses, but not for purely diagnostic purposes. Human fetal diploid cell strains constitute the tissue culture of choice for primary isolation of rhinoviruses. After isolation the rhinovirus may be adapted to growth on other human fetal tissues or on human heteroploid cell lines such as KB or HeLa. These latter cells have been in continuous culture for years and frequently yield higher rhinovirus titers and more potent antigens than the fetal diploid cells.

Reed and Hall (1973) reported that the rhinoviruses cause viral hemagglutination of sheep red blood cells, thereby permitting the simple HI test for serotype identification of new isolates. Such tests, however, require the availability of all known serotype antisera. The serotaxonomic identification of newly isolated rhinovirus serotypes generally has been accomplished by specific neutralization of tissue culture infectivity by homologous antiserum. The approximately 100 serotypes already identified, however, make any such serotaxonomy of a new isolate a burdensome chore of little practicality. For additional details of laboratory diagnosis see Schieble (1974).

CONTROL AND PREVENTION

There are no control measures of established value in either preventing or curing the common cold. In view of the antigenic heterogeneity of the many other viruses than can produce common cold symptoms and the many antigenic serotypes of the rhinoviruses, an immunological approach to control and prevention seems hopeless. A broad-spectrum antiviral protein, *interferon,* is being studied intensively as a possible prophylactic or therapeutic agent in a variety of viral diseases ranging from the common cold to cancer. Interferon was first recognized as an antiviral agent produced by cells that were infected with a virus. Subsequently a variety of inducers of interferon production, other than viral infection, have been discovered: double-stranded viral RNA; a lipid derivative of bacterial endotoxin; a soluble protein from *Escherichia coli;* old tuberculin administered to BCG-infected mice; and a synthetic polynucleotide— polyinosinic:polycytidylic acid, commonly designated poly (I):poly (C). The poly (I):poly (C) inducer and the isolated interferon have been studied extensively with some encouraging results reported in the prevention or cure of viral infections in experimental animals other than humans. The administration of isolated interferon and the induction of interferon by poly (I):poly (C) in human volunteers have both yielded promising results. Levy and Riley (1973) reported a possible mode of action of interferon. Others had reported that interferon helps cells distinguish between their own and viral messenger RNA. Levy and Riley analyzed messenger RNA from interferon-treated and from untreated cells and found the RNA of the treated cell to be slightly larger than that from the untreated cells. They noted that the RNA molecules being translated were the larger ones. They believe that the difference in size might permit the interferon-treated cells to differentiate their own RNA from that of the viruses and thereby translate only their own RNA and suppress the replication of the viruses. Much more research will be required before a final evaluation is possible.

Another future possibility for control or cure of the common cold will be the discovery of an antiviral antibiotic or chemotherapeutic agent. In spite of intensive research, none has been discovered to date (1977). Because of the extent of the market, the discoverer of such an agent will become a wealthy person almost overnight.

REFERENCES

Dochez, A. R., G. S. Shibley, and K. C. Mills. 1930. Studies on the common cold. IV. Experimental transmission of the common cold to anthropoid apes and human beings by means of a filterable agent. *J. Exper. Med.* 52:701–716.

Dochez, A. R., K. C. Mills, and Y. Kneeland. 1938. Filterable viruses in infection of the upper respiratory tract. *J. Amer. Med. Ass.* 110:177–180.

Hamre, D. 1968. Rhinoviruses. In *Monographs in Virology*, ed. J. L. Melnick. Vol. 1, pp. 1–76. Basel: Karger.

Levy, H. B. and F. L. Riley. 1973. Effect of interferon treatment on cellular messenger RNA. *Proc. Natl. Acad. Sci.* 70:3315–3319.

Reed, S. E. and T. S. Hall. 1973. HI test in *Rhinovirus* infections of volunteers. *Infect. Immunity* 8:1–13.

Schieble, J. H. 1974. Rhinoviruses. Chapter 79 in *Manual of Clinical Microbiology.*

Tyrrell, D. A. J. and R. Parsons. 1960. Some virus isolations from common colds. III. Cytopathic effects in tissue culture. *Lancet* 1:239–242.

13

Influenza

The disease influenza has been called la grippe and flu. It has also been designated in terms of the geographical area where the first case of a worldwide epidemic (pandemic) was recognized—such as Spanish, Asian, or Hong Kong influenza. This tendency of the disease to occur in pandemics, at intervals of 10 to 40 years, has been recognized since the sixteenth century but was not explained until the 1940s. The 1918–1920 pandemic of "Spanish" influenza has been classed, along with the plague of Justinian (sixth century) and the Black Death (fourteenth century), as one of the three greatest pestilences of historical times. More than 20 million deaths were estimated worldwide, over 500,000 of them in the United States. The author remembers enjoying the pandemic when schools closed and he could go fishing, but the enjoyment was short-lived. When he contracted the disease, his treatment consisted of a big dose of epsom salts daily. I am now convinced that this therapy was a carry-over of the humoral theory. I do not know whether it was yellow bile or black bile that the physician was attempting to eliminate. I only know that he eliminated everything that would come through. Fortunately for me, I survived both the treatment and the disease.

ETIOLOGY

In 1892, R. Pfeiffer isolated from a case of influenza a small gram-negative bacillus that he believed to be the cause of the disease. The isolate was designated *Hemophilus influenzae,* and many years of research were expended in attempting to prove its etiological relationship to its namesake disease. During the 1918–1920 pandemic, however, many cases of influenza failed to yield cultures of *H. influenzae* and the claim to etiology was finally disproved by the failure to meet the first postulate of Henle-Koch etiology.

Shope (1931) isolated from cases of influenza in hogs a filterable virus that appeared to be synergistically associated with *H. influenzae suis* in the virulent swine disease. No such synergistic association between human influenza virus and a bacterium has been described. However, cases of human influenza are prone to contract bacterial pneumonias that frequently are the cause of the influenza mortality.

Smith, Andrewes, and Laidlaw (1933) infected ferrets with filtered nasal washings from a human case of influenza. They noted that the only route of inoculation of the filtrate that resulted in infection was instillation into the nasal passages of the ferret. Apparently the virus has a strict portal of entry requirement involving the external surface of the nasal epithelial cells. Subcutaneous, intravenous, or other parenteral injections of the filtrate failed to cause infection.

Virus obtained from the mascerated turbinate bone epithelium of infected ferrets was first used for infectivity and immunological studies. This ferret passage virus was then adapted to mice for additional experimentation. These early studies in ferrets and mice led to the recognition of two antigenic groups—A and B. Some years later a third antigenic group C was added. Within groups A and B, antigenic subgroup serotypes were recognized; no subgroup serotype of group C virus has yet been discovered. Prior to 1975, the taxonomic designation for influenza virus was *Myxovirus influenzae* A, B, or C. During the September 1975 Congress for Virology, however, the International Committee on the Taxonomy of Viruses (ICTV) approved a change in the genus designation from *Myxovirus* to *Influenzavirus* (see Fenner 1976).

In 1940, F. M. Burnet advocated the isolation and propagation of *M. (I.) influenzae* in intact chick embryos. He and others noted that inoculation of filtered nasal washings from a human case into the amniotic cavity (see Figure 13-1) of a 9–11-day-old chick embryo resulted in a higher percentage of infections than inoculations to other sites. Following several chick

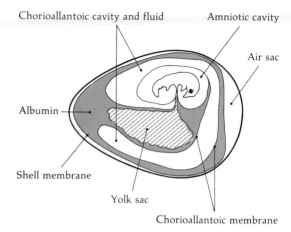

Figure 13–1.   Section of egg with a 10-day-old chick embryo.

embryo passages by the amniotic cavity route, however, the virus becomes adapted to infection of the embryo by either the amniotic or the chorioallantoic (CA) cavity routes of inoculation. After suitable incubation the virus can be found in and harvested along with the CA fluid of the infected embryo. Although tissue culture propagation of *M. (I.) influenzae* has been successful, practically all virus for diagnostic antigens and vaccine production is propagated in embryonated eggs.

STRUCTURE AND ANTIGENICITY OF *INFLUENZAVIRUS*

It was G. K. Hirst, in 1941, who reported the phenomenon of viral hemagglutination (HA) of chicken erythrocytes by influenza virus. Prior to this discovery the only way that the presence and concentration of virus in a specimen (ferret or mouse tissue or CA fluid) could be determined was by establishing the ID/50 of the specimen for a susceptible host. These were time-consuming and expensive practices. The HA titration merely requires serial dilutions of the CA fluid from the infected embryo and a suspension (0.5 percent v/v) of chicken red blood cells. The highest dilution (smallest amount) of the CA fluid that causes agglutination of red blood cells is the HA titer of the virus.

Thus within an hour or two both the presence and concentration of a hemagglutinating virus—not necessarily *M. (I.) influenzae*—can be established. Hirst noted that the infectious dose titer and the HA titer correlated closely. Moreover, the capacity of the virus to cause HA was inhibited by antibody specific for the antigenic subgroup serotype of the virus—the HI test. Thus within 2 to 4 hours after harvesting the CA fluid, the Hirst phenomenon makes possible the establishment of the presence, the concentration, and the antigenic subgroup identity of the *M. (I.) influenzae* isolated from the nasal exudate of the patient. The smallest quantity of the virus that causes HA of a standard suspension of chicken red blood cells is designated the *chicken cell agglutinating* (CCA) *unit.* Influenza vaccines must contain as much as or more than a required minimum number of CCA units of virus per milliliter.

In addition to the antigenic hemagglutinin on the virus, which attaches to the receptor sites on the chicken red blood cells, the *M. (I.) influenzae* virion possesses an enzyme (RDE) that destroys the receptor sites on the chicken erythrocytes. This enzyme is a *neuraminidase* (N) and is antigenically distinct from the hemagglutinin (H). If the virus and the red blood cells are allowed to remain suspended in buffered saline, the neuraminidase will destroy the RBC receptor site and release the virus. This procedure has been used to obtain highly purified influenza virus.

Both the hemagglutinin and the neuraminidase are components of the virion and are located on spikes that extend out from the lipoidal surface of *M. (I.) influenzae* (see Figure 13-2). The hemagglutinin constitutes the subgroup-specific viral (V) antigen found in the CA fluid. However, a significant soluble (S) antigen

Figure 13–2. (*a*) Negatively-stained virions of *Influenzavirus influenzae.* Note the spikes on the envelopes. 125,700×. (*b*) Diagrammatic illustration of the *M. (I.) influenzae* A virion. ((*a*) Courtesy of the Virus Laboratory, University of California, Berkeley.)

(*a*)

(*b*)

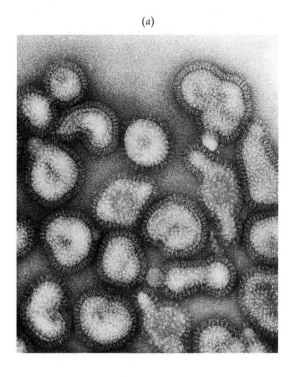

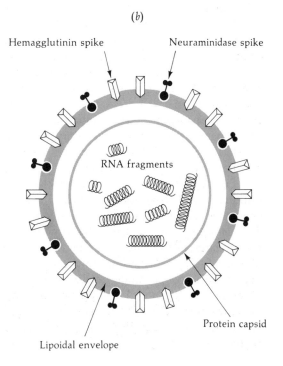

Hemagglutinin spike   Neuraminidase spike

RNA fragments

Protein capsid

Lipoidal envelope

specific for each member of the *M. (I.) influenzae* group (A, B, or C) is also present in the CA fluid of an infected chick embryo. This soluble antigen does not cause hemagglutination and has no immunological significance. But when a new antigenic mutant of *M. (I.) influenzae* is responsible for a case of the disease, the HI test will not identify the virus because no antiserum for the new mutant is available. Therefore if the HI tests with all known antisera are negative, the virus responsible for hemagglutination (1) may not be *M. (I.) influenzae* or (2) may be a new antigenic mutant of this virus for which no antiserum is available. To resolve these possibilities, the V antigen is absorbed onto chicken red blood cells, sedimented, and removed by centrifugation. This leaves only the S antigen in the supernatant CA fluid. This S antigen will be specific for *M. (I.) influenzae* A, B, or C. With antisera specific for each of these three group antigens, a positive complement fixation test, using the absorbed CA fluid (S antigen) as the unknown, can identify the virus as *M. (I.) influenzae* of the homologous A, B, or C group.

The *M. (I.) influenzae* A and B are prone to undergo antigenic mutations at frequent intervals. Some of these mutants are more or less closely related to prior antigenic strains. At intervals of about 10 to 40 years, however, a completely new antigenic mutant occurs. If no living person has had prior infection with this new mutant, there is worldwide susceptibility and a pandemic of the disease may result. The 1957–1958 pandemic (Asian influenza) was the first to be recognized as a potential pandemic at the start by the application of the virus identification procedures just summarized.

Figure 13-2*b* presents a diagrammatic illustration of the *M. (I.) influenzae* A virion. The RNA genome is segmented into eight discrete pieces. This segmentation is believed by some virologists to be responsible for the genetic plasticity of the *M. (I.) influenzae*, resulting in the high degree of antigenic mutagenicity. When two different genetic (antigenic) strains of the virus infect the host cell simultaneously (probably in swine), the segmented RNA genes can undergo segregation and random recombinations, result-

ing not only in the original genotypes but in one or more *hybrid* genotypes. These hybrids could be the completely new antigenic mutants that, transmitted to humans, constitute the initiators of a new pandemic of influenza. There are other genetic explanations (such as point mutations) for the frequent lesser antigenic changes. See Beare and Hall (1971) for another possible aspect of recombinant RNA strains of influenza virus—live virus vaccine production.

SUBGROUP SEROTYPE DESIGNATIONS

One of the first specimens of influenza virus to be isolated (into ferrets) in the western hemisphere was from a patient in Puerto Rico in August 1934. It had the same antigenicity as the strain isolated the year before by Smith and his colleagues. The isolated virus, which is still maintained in virology laboratory stocks, was designated A/PR/8/34. Subsequent isolates have been similarly designated in terms of the group antigen A, B, or C, the geographic site of isolation, and the date of isolation. Stock viruses can be kept alive indefinitely when stored in glass ampules at $-76°C$. Since the hemagglutinin (H) and neuraminidase (N) antigens have immunological and taxonomic significance, recent virus isolates have included these antigens in their subgroup classification, such as A/England/42/72(H_3N_2). The 42 in this designation indicates the forty-second A isolate of 1972. More recent A (H_3N_2) isolates that caused epidemics in New Zealand in 1973 and in Victoria, Australia, in 1975 show slight antigenic differences from A/Eng/42/72(H_3N_2), but apparently not enough to initiate a pandemic.

In February 1976 an outbreak of influenza among army recruits at Fort Dix, New Jersey, resulted in the isolation of a major new antigenic mutant designated A/New Jersey/76(Hsw_1N_1). The sw in this designation stands for swine. The New Jersey virus is closely related to the swine influenza virus isolated by R. E. Shope in 1931. Although no virus was isolated from patients during the 1918–1920 pandemic of influenza, retrospective serological studies have indicated a close relationship between the pandemic virus of 1918 and the Shope swine virus. Because the New Jersey virus represents a major antigenic mutation and owing to the fear of another pandemic as severe as the one of 1918–1920, the U.S. government funded a massive effort to immunize a major portion of the American population against this virus isolate (see Boffey 1976a and 1976b).

Subgroup serotypes of *M. (I.) influenzae* B have not been responsible for pandemics in this century. The more recent B isolates are B/Taiwan/65, B/Maryland/69, B/Massachusetts/1/71, and B/Hong Kong/5/72. As stated, there are no antigenic subgroups of *M. influenzae* C. Consequently a single HI test with an anti-C (V) antiserum, or a positive complement fixation test with anti-C(S) antiserum, will identify any antigenically homologous isolate of C group virus.

PATHOGENICITY AND CLINICAL SYMPTOMS

The mechanism whereby *M. (I.) influenzae* produces pathology is not clear. The virus attacks the nasopharyngeal mucosa and the ciliated epithelium of the respiratory tract of both experimental animals (ferrets) and humans. Following necrotic desquamation of the ciliated epithelium, inflammation, edema, congestion, and increased secretions are observed throughout the tracheobronchial tree.

The onset of symptoms usually involves a chill or chilly sensations followed by a rapid rise in temperature to 101–104°F. Headache, muscular aches, bronchitis, fatigue, weakness, or prostration are commonly observed. Although nasal congestion and sore throat may occur, these symptoms usually are not so marked as in the common cold. A watery nasal discharge associated with sneezing, or dry coughing, frequently occurs. The major symptoms that differentiate influenza from the common cold are the relative lack of coryza, the degree of fever, the severity of the muscular and other aches, and the weakness or prostration throughout and following the course of influenza.

Upper respiratory influenza is frequently followed by influenzal pneumonia. This may result from an extension of the viral bronchitis into the bronchioles, resulting in a purely viral pneumonia. Or, following the desquamation of the tracheobronchial epithelium, streptococci, staphylococci, pneumococci, or other potentially pathogenic bacteria of the upper respiratory tract may spread to the lungs, causing bacterial pneumonia. J. W. Hers and J. Mulder reported that a majority of the fatal cases of influenza they studied (during and following the 1957–1958 pandemic) had an associated coagulase-positive staphyloccal pneumonia. A study of 15,000 influenza deaths in New Guinea, in 1969, reported pneumococcal pneumonia to be the major fatal complication.

Reye et al. (1963) described an influenza B complication that has been reported to occur primarily in children 10 to 15 years of age. This complication, designated *Reye's syndrome*, involves encephalopathy and fatty degeneration of the viscera with a mortality rate of around 30 percent. Seventy cases of this complication were reported to CDC during one week in February 1974. The cases were reported from 14 different states (*MWR*, 15 February 1974).

The 1918–1920 pandemic had a much greater mortality rate than any subsequent influenza pandemic, raising the question of the relative virulence of the viruses involved in these pandemics. In 1918–1920 there were no sulfonamides or antibiotics, however, nor any other antibacterial drugs effective against bacterial pneumonias. Such drugs were available by the mid-1940s. Since a high percentage of influenzal deaths are caused by bacterial pneumonias, these therapeutic antibacterial drugs could account for the lower mortality of the more recent pandemics. This, of course, does not rule out the possibility of a more virulent strain of *M. (I.) influenzae* being involved in the 1918–1920 pandemic.

PREVALENCE AND EPIDEMIOLOGY

Localized epidemics or worldwide pandemics of influenza have occurred every year since the viral etiology was established by Smith et al. in 1933. The original A serotype (WS or PR8) was responsible for a majority of the cases through 1944. The first B serotype was isolated in 1936 and has been involved in localized outbreaks at intervals of 1 to 7 years since that time. In 1947 the first significant mutant serotype of A $(A'/FM_1/47)$ was identified and tended to replace the original A serotype between 1947 and 1957. It spread worldwide as localized epidemics, but more gradually, and was not considered a pandemic strain of the virus. The first C strain was identified in 1947. It has not been accepted as a member of the new genus *Influenzavirus*, however. In 1957 the A_2/Asian/57 pandemic strain was isolated in China and was responsible for the pandemic of 1957–1958. This strain along with B strains, and occasional C strains, accounted for the localized epidemics of influenza through 1967. In 1968 another major mutant $(A_2/HK/68)$ was first recognized in Hong Kong and spread rapidly throughout the world —accounting for the third pandemic of influenza in this century. It and minor mutants such as A_2/Eng/72(H_3N_2) and A_2/Victoria/75(H_3N_2) have accounted for most localized epidemics of A-type influenza to date (1976). A new B strain (B/HK/5/72) has caused localized outbreaks of influenza since 1973 in both the eastern and western hemispheres including Canada and the United States.

This tendency of continuous minor antigenic mutations of A and B strains of *M. (I.) influenzae*, interspersed with major (pandemic) mutations of A strains, necessitates constant surveillance by health authorities responsible for the formulation of influenza vaccines. The World Health Organization (WHO) maintains influenza typing centers worldwide. Information collected at these centers is funneled to a central office where experts determine the homology or heterogeneity of new virus isolates and whether or not a new antigenic serotype of the virus should be added to, or substituted for, a prior serotype in influenza vaccine. A good example of such studies by WHO laboratories on the B serotypes is presented in *MMWR* (19 May 1973).

The exact prevalence of influenza is impossible to assess. Difficulty of clinically differentiating febrile colds or other respiratory illness from influenza makes reporting uncertain. Rarely are laboratory diagnoses requested until an epidemic is in progress, and then the tests usually are performed by public health laboratories associated with the WHO Influenza Commission. Suffice it to say that influenza is one of the most prevalent of the human reportable diseases. In the nonpandemic year of 1970, for example, 128,394 cases of influenza were reported to the Texas State Health Department—more than any other reported disease incidence. The epidemiology of influenza involves the traffic in saliva illustrated in Figure II-A.

LABORATORY DIAGNOSIS

As stated, laboratories for diagnosing influenza and identifying the antigenic serotype of the virus have been established worldwide by WHO and other public health authorities. Such laboratories must maintain stocks of all previously identified antigenic serotypes of *M. (I.) influenzae* A, B, and C. They also must have antisera specific for each of these virus serotypes.

The laboratory specimen, for the isolation of the virus to be identified, is nasopharyngeal exudate from the patient. This can be obtained by swabbing the nasal passages and posterior nasopharynx within 48 to 72 hours after onset of symptoms. The swab should be immersed in a buffered tryptose-phosphate-gelatin solution and delivered to the laboratory within 3 hours. If delivery will require more than 3 hours, the specimen should be packed in dry (CO_2) ice.

Upon delivery to the laboratory, the specimen (thawed, if frozen) should receive suitable concentrations of a mixture of antibiotics designed to kill or suppress bacterial contaminants without affecting the virus. This is easier than filtering out the bacteria. A suitable quantity of the treated specimen is then inoculated into the amniotic cavity of two or more 9–11-day-old chick embryos. After 2 to 4 days' incubation at

32–35°C, the CA fluid of the embryo is harvested and titrated for hemagglutinating (HA) activity using a 0.5 percent suspension of chicken red blood cells. If HA occurs, it indicates the presence of a virus that might be *M. (I.) influenzae;* and the highest dilution of the CA fluid that causes HA indicates the concentration of the virus.

To identify the CA fluid virus, a suitable excess (for example, 8 CCA units) is added to each of a number of small tubes for HI tests. Each tube then receives antiserum specific for one of the possible subgroup serotypes of A and B virus or for the C group serotype. Adequate positive and negative controls are included in the HI testing procedure. Chicken red blood cells are added to all test and control preparations, which are then allowed to stand at room temperature (about 25°C) for 1–2 hours. The antiserum, which inhibits HA by the CA fluid virus, identifies that virus as *M. (I.) influenzae* of homologous antigenic serotype.

If none of the antisera inhibits HA, the virus in the CA fluid that caused HA may not be *M. (I.) influenzae,* or it may be a completely new antigenic mutant of *M. (I.) influenzae.* If the virus is *M. (I.) influenzae,* the soluble (S) antigen in the CA fluid (after removal of the V antigen by chicken RBC) can be used in three complement fixation tests with specific anti-A, anti-B, and anti-C antisera to identify the virus as a member of the homologous group. The convalescent serum of the patient from whom the virus was isolated should inhibit HA by this virus in an HI test. This virus is then recognized as a potential pandemic strain of *M. (I.) influenzae.* The new virus and antiserum specific for it are then added to the stocks of the WHO influenza virus typing centers. Biological houses that produce influenza vaccine are urged to concentrate on the production of large quantities of the new virus vaccine in the hopes of immunizing essential medical and nursing personnel and high-risk individuals ahead of the anticipated pandemic spread of the disease. This precaution—which tends to put a heavy strain on the chicken and fertile egg farmers and the vaccine producers of the world—was tried in 1976 in anticipation of

a possible human pandemic of swine flu (see Immunity).

Serodiagnosis can be performed using paired serum (acute and convalescent) specimens from the patients and the HI test procedure. The paired serum specimens are essential because most people have serum antibodies to one or more of the influenza virus serotypes at all times. Therefore only a rising antibody titer during the course of the disease has diagnostic significance. At least three titrations (serial dilutions) of both the acute and convalescent sera are prepared. Each dilution of each serum of one titration receives eight CCA units of the prevailing known *M. (I.) influenzae* A subgroup serotype stock virus. Additional serum HI titrations may be included for other A subgroup serotypes. This procedure is repeated for B subgroup serotypes and for the C serotype. Chicken red blood cells are then added to both the test and control preparations. If after 2 hours at about 25°C the patient's paired sera indicate a significantly rising HI antibody titer (threefold or more) to one of the known virus serotype antigens, this identifies the serotype of the virus that caused the influenza infection in the patient. Again, if the patient's paired sera fail to indicate a rising HI titer to any of the known virus serotypes, either the patient did not have influenza or he suffered an infection with a new antigenic mutant of *M. (I.) influenzae.* It is too late, of course, to isolate virus from this convalescent patient. If a regional epidemic is in progress, however, the causative virus should be isolated and identified by the serotaxonomic procedures described above.

IMMUNITY

Because of the antigenic mutability of *M. (I.) influenzae,* the likelihood of repeated infections in an individual is to be expected. Serological evidence of these past infections is commonly observed in HI titrations of the sera from patients or healthy individuals. The hemagglutinin and neuraminidase glycoproteins (V antigens) of the virion are the antigenic moieties by which the influenza virus is recognized by the immune mechanism in host tissues; and antibodies specific for these antigens constitute the primary response to attack by the influenza virus or to influenza vaccination.

Influenza vaccine is composed of current A and B serotype virus propagated in embryonated eggs, harvested with the CA fluid, and rendered noninfectious by treatment with formalin or ether. The former is designated *whole virus* and the latter *split virus* vaccine. New antigenic mutants usually require a prolonged period of adaptation to the chick embryo before adequate yields of virus for vaccine production are realized. In 1961 E. D. Kilbourne reported that he could hybridize the fast-growing A/PR/8/34 virus with the slow-growing recently isolated A strains of the virus and obtain virus hybrids with the fast-growing character of the PR/8 strain and the antigenic structure of the recent isolate. This process was claimed to reduce the production time for a new mutant influenza vaccine from 6 months to 4 weeks. The author is not aware of the application of this hybridization procedure to the A/New Jersey/76 virus for the swine flu vaccine production of 1976.

The 1974–1975 bivalent vaccine contained not less than 700 CCA units of A/Port Chalmers/73(H_3N_2) virus and 500 CCA units of B/HK/72 virus per immunizing dose (see *MMWR,* 13 June 1974). As a result of extensive field trials during the spring of 1976 involving the A/NJ/76 swine flu vaccine, the U.S. Public Health Service has recommended three influenza vaccine formulations for 1976–1977:

1. Monovalent A—to contain 200 CCA units of A/NJ/76 whole or split virus per dose
2. Bivalent A—to contain 200 CCA units of A/NJ/76 and 200 CCA units of A/Victoria/75(H_3N_2) whole or split virus per dose
3. Monovalent B—to contain 500 CCA units of B/HK/72 virus per dose

The Public Health Service recommends annual immunization against influenza in the high-risk population. This group includes those having such chronic conditions as heart disease; bronchopulmonary disease such as asthma, bronchitis, bronchiectasis, and emphysema; chronic renal disease; diabetes and other chronic metabolic disorders; chronic neuromuscular disorders; and malignancies. Also included are healthy individuals over 65 years of age. Usually one dose of the 1976–1977 influenza vaccines is considered adequate to provide an immune response in adults 18 or older. For the recommended immunization of high-risk individuals 3 to 18 years of age, see *MMWR* (17 September 1976). Although most of the egg protein has been removed from current influenza vaccines, they should be administered cautiously, and under close medical supervision, to individuals known to be hypersensitive to eggs.

By December 1976 a rare paralytic disease (Guillain-Barré syndrome—G-BS) of unknown etiology was reported to be occurring at a significantly greater rate in those receiving the A/NJ/76 (swine flu) vaccine than in the nonvaccinated population. During the period from 1 October through 22 December 1976, for example, a total of 172 cases of G-BS were reported to CDC. Of the 166 with known immunization status, 99 cases of G-BS and 6 deaths occurred in recipients of influenza vaccine, whereas 67 cases and 1 death occurred in nonrecipients of the vaccine. Although there has been no proof that the swine flu vaccine was the etiological agent of the Guillain-Barré syndrome, these figures, coupled with the fact that no evidence of a swine flu pandemic was developing, caused the U.S. Public Health Service to discontinue the massive effort to abort an influenza pandemic at its onset (see *MMWR,* special issue, 24 December 1976). If a causal relationship between influenza vaccine and G-BS can be ruled out, the millions of tax dollars spent on the program may pay off in terms of having established the mechanics for preventing a future pandemic.

Since the early 1960s, considerable research has been devoted to developing live, attenuated influenza vaccines. Although promising results have been reported, no such vaccine has been licensed for human use in the United States to date. Maugh (1973b) has summarized studies involving live virus vaccines. An interesting claim for some live virus vaccines is their capacity to stimulate the production of nasal secretory (IgA) antibodies at higher levels than killed virus vaccines.

CONTROL AND PREVENTION

At present the only means of preventing influenza is active immunoprophylaxis with influenza vaccine. To date this prophylaxis has been effective at a maximum of 70 to 80 percent of those exposed. Moreover, this prophylaxis is only effective in individuals exposed to the same serotypes of virus incorporated in the vaccine.

DuPont researchers have reported a chemoprophylactic agent, amantadine HCl (Symmetrel), which is effective in preventing infections caused by A serotypes of *Influenzavirus*. The drug must be given prior to infection and is not therapeutic in those already infected. This, of course, limits its usefulness markedly. See Maugh (1976) for a review of the current status of antiviral chemotherapy.

Fortunately, there are many antibacterial drugs and antibiotics that may be used to cure the complicating bacterial pneumonias responsible for many of the fatal cases of influenza. The ideal, of course, would be the discovery of a drug or antibiotic that would cure the viral disease before it reaches the pneumonic stage.

REFERENCES

Arehart-Treichel, J. 1974. Vaccines on the horizon. *Science News* 106:380–383.

Beare, A. S. and T. S. Hall. 1971. Recombinant influenza A viruses as live vaccines for man. *Lancet* 2:1271–1273.

Boffey, P. M. 1976a. Anatomy of a decision: how the nation declared war on swine flu. *Science* 192:636–641.

——. 1976b. Swine flu vaccine: a component missing. *Science* 193:1224–1225.

Fenner, F. 1976. Classification and nomenclature of viruses: the current position. *Amer. Soc. Microbiol. News* 42:170–173.

Kilbourne, E. D. (ed.) 1975. *The Influenza Viruses and Influenza*. New York: Academic Press.

Maugh, T. H. II. 1973a. Influenza: the last of the great plagues. *Science* 180:1042–1044.

——. 1973b. A persistent disease may yield to new vaccines. *Science* 180:1159–1161.

——. 1976. Chemotherapy: antiviral agents come of age. *Science* 192:128–132.

Reye, R. D. K., G. Morgan, and J. Baral. 1963. Encephalopathy and fatty degeneration of the viscera, a disease entity in childhood. *Lancet* 2:749–752.

Shope, R. E. 1931. Swine influenza. III. Filtration experiments and etiology. *J. Exper. Med.* 54:373–385.

Smith, W., C. H. Andrewes, and P. P. Laidlaw. 1933. A virus obtained from influenza patients. *Lancet* 2:66–68.

14

Measles

Rubella 145
Rubeola 146

There are two etiologically distinct types of measles: rubella (German or 3-day measles) and rubeola. Rubella is a mild disease, generally with no serious consequences to the patient. When rubella is contracted by an expectant mother during the first 3 to 6 months of pregnancy, however, the fetus can suffer serious to fatal injury.

RUBELLA

Gregg (1941) was the first to note that a high percentage of early-pregnancy rubella cases, reported in hospital records, resulted in fetal deaths, abortions, or birth of defective children (fetal teratogeny). The defects reported by Gregg and others included crippling deformities, blindness, deafness, damage to the heart or other organs, or damage to the central nervous system. Collectively these consequences of fetal infection by rubella virus during early pregnancy have been designated the *congenital rubella syndrome* (CRS), which is now a reportable disease. The rubella epidemic of 1964–1965 in the United States was estimated by the Baylor Rubella Study Group (1969) to have been responsible for 15,000 spontaneous abortions, up to 5,000 postnatal infant deaths, and between 20,000 and 30,000 birth abnormalities. These abnormalities frequently are the real tragedies of the congenital rubella syndrome.

Since the discovery of the rubella virus teratogeny, a number of other virus infections in pregnant women have been suspected of causing teratogeny (see Fuccillo and Sever 1973). Although Siegel (1973), in a carefully designed study, reported no evidence of fetal damage in mothers suffering mumps, chicken pox, rubeola, or hepatitis infections during pregnancy, certain other virus infections (cytomegalovirus and herpes simplex) have been implicated in documented teratogeny.

After Gregg, in Australia, reported rubella teratogeny in 1941, young Australian women approaching marriageable age who had not had rubella were reported to have intentionally exposed themselves to the disease in order that they might become immune and thereby eliminate any chance of rubella teratogeny in their children. Others advocated allowing young girls to associate with cases of rubella with the intent of becoming infected and immune by the natural disease process.

Rubella virus, which has been placed in the family Togaviridae, genus *Rubivirus* (see Fenner 1976), has now been propagated in tissue culture, and live-virus vaccines were licensed for human immunization in the United States in 1969. Between 1969 and November 1975, 322 proved or suspected cases of CRS were reported in the Unites States (see *MMWR,* 15 November 1975). The U.S. Public Health Service has advocated the immunization of infants with this vaccine in an effort to eliminate the disease and thereby eliminate the probability of the congenital rubella syndrome. The success or failure of this preventive approach will not be known for a good many years. In the meantime, young women who have not had rubella vaccine—and who are not yet pregnant—should consider being actively immunized with the vaccine to protect their unborn children. No one knows whether or not immunized infants will retain that immunity to young adult age. This possibility will become increasingly unlikely if the incidence of rubella is reduced to the point where repeated exposures to rubella infection might no longer serve as boosters to maintain that immunity. Under these circumstances, of course, booster injections of the vaccine could be substituted for past herd-immunization type of subclinical booster infections (see Enders 1970). For additional considerations see Rawls and Person (1974).

RUBEOLA

In contrast to rubella, rubeola is a serious disease in the infected patient, particularly in infants under 3 years of age and in debilitated older children. Moreover, rubeola virus has been removed from the group of viruses that cause fetal teratogeny (Siegel 1973).

Etiology

Although a viral etiology for rubeola was suggested as far back as 1911, the final proof was established by Enders and Peebles (1954). They succeeded in propagating the virus in primary cultures of human or simian kidney cells or human amnion cells. After serial passage in these primary cell cultures, the virus will multiply in a variety of stable cell lines (HeLa, Vero, and others) and in chick embryo tissues. It is a

large (120 to 160 nanometers in diameter), ether-sensitive, RNA virus possessing an outer envelope of lipoprotein. It produces a *syncytial* cytopathic effect (CPE) involving multinucleated giant cells in infected tissue culture cells.

Rubeola virus is antigenically homogeneous. It shares antigenicity with distemper virus of dogs and rinderpest virus of cattle, but the shared antigens do not appear to have immunogenic significance. The rubeola virus will hemagglutinate monkey or baboon red blood cells but not human. Also, sheets of rubeola-infected tissue culture cells, on glass surfaces, show the phenomenon of hemadsorption of these red blood cells. In contrast to *Influenzavirus,* however, there is no receptor-destroying enzyme (neuraminidase) on the rubeola virion and the virus does not elute from the monkey RBC. Rubeola virus has been classified by ICTV as a member of the new family Paramyxoviridae, genus *Morbilivirus* (see Fenner 1976). The species designation has not been established but might well be *rubeolae.*

Clinical Symptoms

After an incubation period averaging 9 days, rubeola commences with 4 days of prodromal symptoms that, for the first 2 days, are indistinguishable from those of the common cold: cough, coryza, and conjunctivitis. These prodromal symptoms frequently include lethargy and a gradually increasing fever. On the second day of these symptoms, the first clinically distinctive lesions occur on the inner buccal mucosa opposite the molar teeth: the *Koplik spots* or *enanthem.* These small bright red spots with bluish-white centers constitute the means for the earliest possible differential diagnosis of rubeola—a significant public health measure. If the Koplik spots are not observed, the prodromal patient may be considered to have just another febrile cold and little or no effort will be made to prevent the spread of the infection to others. Toward the end of the prodromal period the patient develops a conjunctivitis.

The conjunctivitis in rubeola tends to result in a photophobia, and the patient's eyes should be shielded from bright lights (housed in a semidarkened room). There is no convincing evidence that transient exposure to a bright light results in weakened or damaged eyesight, but the bright light can be extremely painful.

On about the fourth day after infection, the skin rash (*exanthem*) appears and a differential clinical diagnosis at this stage is grossly apparent. The rash appears as dark red macules, first on the neck or forehead and then spreading rapidly over the face, trunk, and extremities. Coincident with the rash, the fever and constitutional symptoms increase in severity. When the exanthem is in full bloom, the temperature falls by crisis or rapid lysis and the patient improves rapidly. The exanthem fades and a desquamation in the form of fine branny scales is complete in 5 to 10 days. There is no virus in these scales, which therefore are noninfectious.

Shortly after the licensing of killed-virus rubeola vaccine (see Rauh and Schmidt 1965). Fulginiti et al. (1967) reported cases of atypical measles in children who had been immunized with the killed-virus vaccine. Subsequently other such cases were reported, some in children who received live-virus vaccine within 3 months after the killed-virus immunization. A review of 177 cases of rubeola in California during 1974 and 1975 identified 56 cases of atypical measles, 47 of whom had been immunized with killed-virus rubeola vaccine. One of the 56 had been immunized with live-virus vaccine only, and in 8 the vaccination status was unknown. The average interval between killed rubeola vaccination, in this group, and the onset of atypical measles was 10.5 years; the longest interval was 12.5 years. The symptoms of atypical rubeola included high prodromal fever and no Koplik spots in at least half the cases. All had an atypical rash with raised papules, blisters, and pinpoint hemorrhages. Nausea, vomiting, pleuritic chest pains, and pneumonia were common symptoms also (see *MMWR*, 13 August 1976).

Because of its highly contagious nature and the antigenic homogeneity of the virus, rubeola is one of the classic childhood diseases. If uncomplicated, the patient recovers with long-lasting immunity. Second attacks in an individual, under current or past circumstances, have been extremely rare. Whether or not this long-lasting (lifetime) immunity will persist, after current active immunization programs have practically eliminated the chances for herd immunization by subclinical booster infections, remains to be determined. If it does not, booster vaccine immunization may be required.

Complications

The serious aspect of rubeola is the fact that it predisposes the patient to a variety of serious complications—pneumonia is the most serious and most frequent. Lack of nursing care of the patient has been reported to be a factor in this predisposition. The complicating pneumonia is particularly dangerous in infants under 3 years of age and in debilitated older children. In addition to pneumonia, ear infections (otitis media), mastoiditis, and occasionally encephalitis complicate the usual rubeola pathology.

Prevalence

Rubeola occurs worldwide, usually in localized epidemics. The peak incidence of the disease in North America usually occurs in the spring (March to June), but localized epidemics have been observed during all seasons. Butte, Montana, for example, reported an epidemic of 331 cases between 8 July and 26 November 1973. This outbreak was cited as a classic example of how not to deal with a potential rubeola epidemic. The index case on 8 July was not reported to the public health authorities, and over the next 6 weeks his five siblings contracted the disease and were not reported. The first case outside the index family occured on 1 September. On 9 September, the first case to be hospitalized occurred. Still there was no report of rubeola to the health authorities. Although no new cases developed during the following 10 days, 29 cases occurred from 28 September to 7 October, and 80 new cases occurred during each of the next three 10-day periods. The first report to the state health department of a case of rubeola in this epidemic was 16 October. Mass vaccination campaigns were carried out on preschool and elementary school children on 25 and

26 October and the epidemic ended on 26 November. If the index family cases had been reported to the health authorities and the mass vaccination campaign had been instituted in July or August, most of the 331 cases could have been prevented. Other nonspringtime epidemics include 518 cases between 1 August 1971 and 8 January 1972 in Des Moines County, Iowa, and 637 cases in Texarkana, Texas, between 28 June 1970 and 22 January 1971. An epidemic involving 1,071 cases occurred in Dallas, Texas, between 1 December 1970 and 22 May 1971; the peak incidence in this epidemic was in February and March. Additional rubeola epidemics were reported in Allegan County, Michigan, in 1975 (66 cases) and in the state of Utah (1,976 cases) between 15 May 1975 and 15 May 1976. This latter epidemic is a good example of the explosive nature of measles epidemiology, since only 15 cases had been reported in Utah during the preceding year (see *MMWR*, 13 November 1975 and 25 June 1976). The total number of cases of rubeola reported in the United States in 1964 (prior to the licensing of live rubeola vaccine) was more than 458,000. Subsequently the yearly case reports declined to a low of around 22,000 in 1968 but rose to more than 75,000 in 1971. The subsequent annual incidence through 1975 has ranged between 22,000 and 32,275 (*MMWR*, August 1976 supplement).

Epidemiology

The incubation period from the day of infection to the onset of prodromal symptoms, as indicated above, averages 9 days. The case becomes capable of transmitting the infection to others at the onset of the prodromal symptoms and remains capable of transmitting the disease for a minimum of 6 days—from 4 days before to 2 days after the development of the skin rash. However, contagiousness can persist until the cessation of abnormal mucus secretion. Knowing that a case has been contagious for only 4 days at the onset of the skin rash makes it possible to pinpoint the maximum stage of the incubation period of contacts infected by expo-

sure to this patient. This information has immunological significance that will be discussed under passive immunization.

Rubeola is one of the most highly contagious of all human diseases. It has been called the visitor's disease because even transient presence in the room of a case may result in infection. The epidemiology is the traffic in saliva type illustrated in Figure II-A.

Laboratory Diagnosis

The availability of the tissue culture means of propagating rubeola virus, and the availability of virus specific antisera, makes possible the serotaxonomic identification of cases shedding virus in upper respiratory discharges. The best procedures include (1) antibody neutralization of virus CPE in tissue cultures; (2) antibody inhibition of viral hemagglutination (HI test) of simian red blood cells; or (3) inhibition of the hemadsorption phenomenon using these RBC. Also, direct FA techniques can be used for demonstrating virus in tissue culture cells. None of these procedures, however, are used in routine clinical laboratory diagnosis. They are only occasionally used in public health laboratory confirmation of clinical diagnoses. Also, such tests may be used to establish the required concentration of viral antigen in rubeola vaccines.

Prior to the onset of the rash, rubeola-specific antibody is not present in the serum of the patient, but significant titers of such antibody develop rapidly thereafter. Therefore serodiagnosis is a distinct possibility. Using known rubeola virus as the test antigen, the patient's serum may be titrated for rubeola antibody before and after onset of the rash. A rising antibody titer will be observed if the disease is rubeola. Again, the serodiagnostic tests may be CPE neutralization, inhibition of viral hemagglutination (HI) or hemadsorption of simian red blood cells, or the indirect FA technique. In all of these serodiagnostic tests, the patient's serum is tested for the presence or absence of rubeola virus-specific antibody. For additional information see Black (1974).

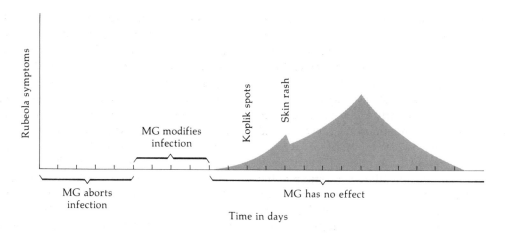

Figure 14–1. Possible effects of administration of measles globulin (MG) to *Morbilivirus*-infected individuals.

Immunity

Passive immunization using convalescent serum from rubeola patients, or measles (rubeola) globulin (MG) from pooled adult serum, has been practiced since the 1920s. It early became obvious that such immunization had no therapeutic effect once the prodromal symptoms appeared. If the MG was administered during the incubation period, however, the infection could be aborted or modified, depending upon the dosage of MG or the stage of the incubation period when the MG was administered. Figure 14-1 correlates the stages of a rubeola infection with the immunological effects of the administration of MG. If the MG is given during the first 5 days of the incubation period, the infection is aborted. Such individuals will develop no symptoms of rubeola and will be passively immune for a maximum of 10 to 12 weeks. If the MG is administered between the fifth and ninth day of the incubation period, the infection is modified to the extent that only minor symptoms of rubeola (slight fever, a few spots of rash) occur, and these possibly after an incubation period of up to 21 days. The slight symptoms, however, indicate that the rubeola virus has multiplied sufficiently, prior to MG administration, to give an adequate antigenic stimulation

for a lasting, active immune response. Prior to the development of rubeola vaccine, this was the only way, other than an unmodified case, whereby active immunity to rubeola could be acquired. At that time only high-risk contacts (under 3 years old) were given MG immediately after exposure. The administration of MG to other contacts was delayed, hopefully until the fifth to ninth day of incubation, to get the benefit of the modified-case immunity.

The availability of rubeola vaccine has eliminated the need for this delayed administration of MG. Now all susceptible contacts should receive MG immediately upon exposure to a known case of rubeola. If the contact develops mild symptoms of measles, one can conclude that the contact was infected and was between the fifth and ninth day of the incubation period. This individual should then possess long-lasting (lifetime) immunity. If the susceptible contact develops no symptoms of measles, either the exposure did not result in infection or the incubation stage of the infection was between the first and fifth day of the incubation period when the MG was administered. In either case, no long-lasting immunity will develop. Such individuals should be actively immunized with live-virus rubeola vaccine 3 months after administration of the MG.

The propagation by Enders and Peebles (1954) of the Edmonston strain of rubeola virus made possible the early development of formalin-inactivated (killed) virus vaccine. Mass tissue culture procedures were devised and the inactivated virus was tested for safety and immunogenicity. These early killed-virus vaccines proved to be weak immunogens, however, and as indicated above led to cases of atypical measles. Therefore a number of years were spent in weakening the Edmonston strain to the point where it was safe and immunogenic when administered as live-virus vaccine. Since the live-virus vaccine infects and multiplies to a limited extent in the tissues of the vaccinee, a single small dose is adequate for an immune response. The Edmonston strain of rubeola virus met the requirements for a safe and effective live-virus vaccine and in 1965 was licensed for human use in the United States. Other strains of rubeola virus have been adapted to live-virus vaccines in this and other countries.

Stokes has produced a triple live-virus vaccine composed of a mixture of weakened strains of rubeola, rubella, and mumps viruses. Such vaccines are subject to the problem of viral interference. When one serotype virus infects the host, this infection may interfere with the capacity of other serotype viruses to infect. With a triple live-virus vaccine, if all three viruses infect at once, a threefold immune response might be expected. If one or two viruses infect and interfere with infection by the others, however, repeated administration of the triple-virus vaccine may be required for a triple immune response. Live-virus rubeola vaccines, although safe, tend to produce some symptoms of rubeola such as fever and rash. Such symptoms can be ameliorated by the coincident injection of a small amount of measles globulin.

Control and Prevention

Active immunization of all infants between 3 and 6 months of age should eliminate rubeola. The use of Stokes triple vaccine would include rubella and mumps in this elimination effort. If these childhood diseases are eliminated from one, but not every, area of the world, a system of booster immunizations might be needed to maintain the immunity. In this regard, the U.S. Public Health Service in December 1975 recommended that measles vaccine boosters should be given routinely to children who were immunized prior to age 12 months—provided there is no history of an attack of measles. The booster should be administered at age 12 to 16 months or later (up to the twelfth birthday).

Immediate administration of measles globulin to known *susceptible contacts* exposed to a case of rubeola is advocated. Since MG is human serum globulin, there is no sensitization of the recipient. If these susceptible contacts develop no symptoms of rubeola within 21 days, they should be actively immunized with live-virus rubeola vaccine 3 months after the administration of the MG.

Rubeola patients should be quarantined until 4 days after the onset of the skin rash or until all abnormal discharges of mucus have ceased. Quarantine of a case should be instituted as early as possible. This necessitates early diagnosis—preferably at the onset of the prodromal symptoms. Certainly Koplik spots should be looked for by the second day of these coldlike symptoms.

Exposed susceptible children (siblings, schoolmates, and other close contacts) may be allowed freedom of movement for 7 days following the first possible exposure. This first possible exposure can be calculated as 4 days prior to the onset of the skin rash in the case that resulted in the exposure. The exposed contact should then be quarantined for the remainder of the incubation period (2–3 days). If symptoms of rubeola develop in the contact, the quarantine should be extended as indicated above for cases of the disease.

REFERENCES

Baylor Rubella Study Group. (1969). Rubella teratogeny. *Hospital Practice* 2:27–35.

Black, F. L. 1974. Measles virus. Chapter 76 in *Manual of Clinical Microbiology.*

Enders, J. F. 1970. Rubella vaccination. *New Eng. J. Med.* 283:261–263.

Enders, J. F. and T. C. Peebles. 1954. Propagation in tissue cultures of cytopathogenic agents from patients with measles. *Proc. Soc. Biol. Med.* 86: 277–286.

Fenner, F. 1976. Classification and nomenclature of viruses: the current position. *Amer. Soc. Microbiol. News* 42:170–173.

Fuccillo, D. A. and J. L. Sever. 1973. Viral teratology. *Bacteriol. Rev.* 37:19–31.

Fulginiti, V. A., J. J. Eller, A. W. Downie, and C. H. Kempe. 1967. Altered reactivity to measles virus. *J. Amer. Med. Ass.* 202:101–106.

Gregg, N. M. 1941. Congenital cataract following German measles in mother. *Trans. Opthal. Soc. Australia* 3:1126–1139.

Rauh, L. W. and R. Schmidt. 1965. Measles immunization with killed virus vaccine. *Amer. J. Dis. Child.* 108:232–237.

Rawls, W. E. and D. A. Person. 1974. Rubella virus. Chapter 77 in *Manual of Clinical Microbiology.*

Siegel, M. 1973. Congenital malformations following chickenpox, measles, mumps, and hepatitis. *J. Amer. Med. Ass.* 226:1521–1524.

15

Mumps

Mumps (*parotitis*) is a highly contagious, frequently epidemic disease that was reported in the writings of Hippocrates and other early medical practitioners. The typical clinical symptoms include swelling and tenderness of the parotid and the other salivary glands. The involvement may be unilateral, bilateral, or sequential. The involved glands usually are painful and highly sensitive to acid substances such as lemon juice or dill pickles. After viremic spread, other glands (gonads, pancreas) and the central nervous system (*meningoencephalitis*) may be involved. The disease is widespread but is rarely fatal.

ETIOLOGY

The viral etiology of mumps was established by Johnson and Goodpasture (1934) at Vanderbilt University. The virus can be isolated from patients by inoculation of salivary secretions (after treatment with antibiotics) into primary human or simian cell cultures or into the amniotic cavity or the yolk sac of the chick embryo. After adaptation to such tissues, the virus can be propagated in a variety of tissue cultures including stable cell cultures such as HeLa. In tissue culture, the mumps virus produces a syncytial type of cytopathology. Like all members of the myxovirus group (family Paramyxoviridae), the mumps virus is an RNA virus. It possesses a lipid-containing outer envelope with surface spikes (see Figure 15-1).

Like *Myxovirus (I.) influenzae,* mumps virus in infected tissues produces two types of antigens: V and S. The V antigen, located on the surface of the intact virion, is responsible for hemagglutination of chicken or human red blood cells (see Levens and Enders, 1945). It is immunogenic and antigenically homogeneous. The S (soluble) antigen is produced in the core of the virion, but excess S antigen is found in the culture fluids of infected tissue culture cells. The V and S antigens are antigenically distinct and can be separated by differential centrifugation or by the absorption of V antigen onto red blood

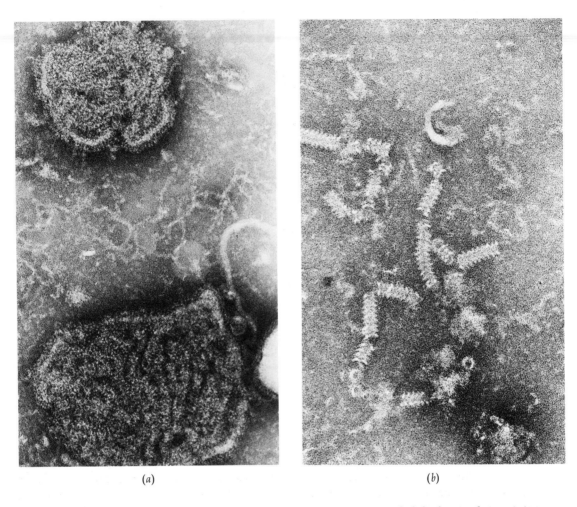

(a)   *(b)*

Figure 15–1. (*a*) These negatively-stained virions of mumps virus are slightly damaged, permitting the stain to reach the interior of the particle and stain internal components. 111,400×. (*b*) Characteristic helical nucleo-protein released from a ruptured virion of mumps virus. 162,000×. (Both courtesy of B. Wolanski, Merck Sharp and Dohme.)

cells. Both antigens may be demonstrated by complement fixation tests with specific antisera, but only the V antigen is demonstrable by the HA test or identifiable by the HI test. A suggested taxonomic designation for the mumps virus is *Paramyxovirus parotitis.*

CLINICAL DISEASE

Uncomplicated parotitis is a relatively mild disease with practically no mortality. The swollen salivary glands may or may not involve concomitant fever. The symptoms usually last for 1 to 2 weeks.

The most common complication (around 20 percent) is orchitis in the mature male. One or both testicles may be involved with painful swelling and possible atrophy. Meningoencephalitis (about 1 percent) may occur with or without salivary gland involvement. Those cases without parotitis frequently have been diagnosed as aseptic meningitis.

LABORATORY DIAGNOSIS

Clinical laboratories are rarely called upon to aid in the diagnosis of mumps. However, since live mumps virus is available in tissue culture as well as antisera specific for both the V and the S antigens, both serotaxonomic and serodiagnostic testing procedures are available to virologists. Clinical parotitis is so obvious, early in the infection, that laboratory aid in its diagnosis is not justifiable. Meningoencephalitis, or other *P. parotitis* diseases in a patient without salivary gland symptoms, however, might be diagnosed by simple serodiagnostic procedures, particularly if both V and S antigens are available. Antibody specific for the S antigen develops rapidly and may reach high titers before antibody to the V antigen reaches measurable concentrations. Antibody specific for the V antigen, however, persists much longer than that for the S antigen. Quantitative complement fixation tests on dilutions of paired sera (one collected early in the disease and a second collected 2 to 4 weeks after onset) using S antigen will yield evidence of a fourfold or greater increase in anti-S antibody titer if the patient was infected with *P. parotitis*. Comparable tests with V antigen will yield similar results, particularly if the second serum is collected at a later date. A rising HI antibody titer can be demonstrated using the patient's sera, known *P. parotitis* V antigen, and chicken or human red blood cells. For additional information see Dienhardt and Shramek (1974).

IMMUNITY

An attack of mumps confers long-lasting immunity. This is presumptive evidence for both the immunogenicity and antigenic homogeneity of the virus. Convalescent serum following a case of mumps usually contains reasonably high titers of anti– *P. parotitis* antibody. Such antisera, however, seem to yield little if any passive immunity when administered to susceptible contacts.

The isolation and propagation of mumps virus has made possible the development of both formalin-killed and live-virus vaccines for immunoprophylaxis in mumps. The killed-virus vaccines, like those for rubeola, however, are unsatisfactory in that they stimulate weak and short-lived immune responses. Passage of the virulent mumps virus in chick embryo tissues weakens the virus so that it can be used orally as a live-virus vaccine. The results of testing indicate that such live-virus vaccines are immunogenic, and they have been licensed for human immunization (see Hilleman et al. 1968). As indicated in the discussion of measles, Stokes has combined attenuated mumps, rubeola, and rubella viruses into a triple live-virus vaccine for immunization against these three diseases.

CONTROL AND PREVENTION

Since infants 3 to 6 months old certainly should be immunized against rubeola, and since the U.S. Public Health Service advocates the immunization of such infants against rubella to eliminate future cases of congenital rubella syndrome, the inclusion of immunization against mumps in this age group appears reasonable. Therefore the use of Stokes' triple virus vaccine is advocated for immunoprophylaxis in these diseases.

If the incidence of mumps falls appreciably, a system of booster immunizations should be instituted, particularly among males. Otherwise the immunity acquired in infancy may be lost at the time (young adulthood) when the serious complication of orchitis is most likely to occur.

Although the period of infectivity in a case of mumps is not clearly established, there is evidence that it might range from 6 days before to 9 days after the appearance of glandular involvement. If this is true, the initiation of quarantine measures as a means of preventing the spread of the disease will be difficult. Nevertheless, judicious quarantine of cases is advocated. For more details see Henle and Enders (1965).

POLIOMYELITIS

Poliomyelitis is a disease in which virus may be shed into the buccal cavity if the tonsils are involved in the infection. Therefore it can be transmitted by the respiratory "traffic in saliva" route. However, since all cases include infection of lymphoidal tissues (Peyer's patches) of the intestinal tract, from which virus is shed into that tract, the disease is discussed along with other intestinal group diseases in Part 3 of this book.

REFERENCES

Dienhardt, F. W. and G. J. Shramek. 1974. Mumps virus. Chapter 75 in *Manual of Clinical Microbiology.*

Henle, W. and J. F. Enders. 1965. Mumps virus. Chapter 32 in *Viral and Rickettsial Infections of Man.*

Hilleman, M. R. et al. 1968. Live attenuated mumps virus vaccine. *New Eng. J. Med.* 278:227–232.

Johnson, C. D. and E. W. Goodpasture. 1934. An investigation of the etiology of mumps. *J. Exper. Med.* 59:1–20.

Levens, J. H. and J. F. Enders. 1945. The hemagglutinative properties of amniotic fluid of embryonated eggs infected with mumps virus. *Science* 102:117–120.

16

Varicella (Chickenpox) and Variola (Smallpox)

Chickenpox and smallpox at one time were considered to be different clinical manifestations of the same disease. Now they are recognized as clinically and etiologically distinct diseases—in fact, the causative viruses are sufficiently different that they are not even included in the same taxonomic families. Both, however, are examples of dual primary vehicle diseases: The virus of each is present in and transmitted by (1) the upper respiratory discharges and (2) the exudates (including the scabs) of the skin lesions.

VARICELLA

Varicella or chickenpox is a common, highly contagious, slightly febrile disease of children. If a child escapes the disease, a clinically identical syndrome can occur in adult infections. The cutaneous lesions (exanthem) of chickenpox are characterized by successive crops of monolocular, blisterlike vesicles that may or may not become pustular prior to dehydration and crust formation. By contrast, the smallpox exanthem usually appears as a single crop of maculopapular lesions that develop multilocular vesicles on the surface of the papules. These smallpox vesicles progress to pustules prior to crust formation. The pock lesions of chickenpox, except when occasional ones are infected by staphylococci or other skin bacteria, are more superficial and much less prone to leave permanent pitted scars than are those of smallpox. The viruses of both diseases, however, are *dermotropic* and, as stated above, the pock exudates including the scabs can serve as primary vehicles of both these diseases. Chickenpox generally is a mild disease with rare mortality in children suffering no other diseases. In children or adults with leukemia or an immunodeficient disease, however, infection with chickenpox virus tends to result in an increased liability of viral pneumonia.

HERPES ZOSTER

There is convincing evidence that the same virus which causes chickenpox may cause herpes

157

zoster (shingles) in individuals who have recovered from chickenpox. Whether or not shingles results from reinfection in a partially immune (hypersensitive?) individual, or reactivation of residual latent virus in such individuals, has not been established. In contrast to the dermotropic nature of ordinary chickenpox virus, the zoster virus invades the spinal or extramedulary cranial nerve ganglia, resulting in severe and long-lasting pain, usually in the neck or trunk region. Successive crops of cutaneous vesicles, identical with those of chickenpox, tend to be distributed along one or more of the regional sensory nerves in the area of gangliar involvement.

Varicella-Zoster Etiology

The virus that causes these two clinical entities, varicella and herpes zoster, frequently is designated the V-Z virus. As indicated above, there is no generally accepted explanation for the clinical duality of the V-Z virus. Because of the relative rarity of zoster, compared to the incidence of chickenpox, there appears to be justification for concluding that zoster must involve an unknown host factor. In this respect there is evidence that leukemic and possibly other oncogenic patients, or individuals receiving bone-marrow transplants, are more prone to contract herpes zoster than the general population (see *MMWR* 18 November 1972).

The V-Z virus can be propagated in a variety of human and simian tissue cultures. In contrast to smallpox virus, however, it fails to infect chick embryo tissues. The V-Z virus is a spherical, enveloped, DNA virus. The presence and identification of the virus in tissue cultures can be established by complement fixation or by fluorescent antibody or other serotaxonomic techniques using specific anti–V-Z virus antisera. Also, rising titer serodiagnosis can be performed on acute and convalescent patients' sera by complement fixation and the indirect FA techniques using known V-Z antigens, although these tests are rarely requested of the clinical diagnostic laboratory. The recommended taxonomic designation for the V-Z virus family is Herpetoviridae and the genus is *Herpesvirus vari-*

cellae, the genus and species names indicating the clinical duality of the virus. For additional considerations see Schmidt (1974).

Control and Prevention

Since chickenpox can be transmitted by the respiratory route prior to the development of the infectious skin lesions, prevention of the epidemic spread of the disease is difficult. This is particularly true since there are no immunoprophylactic procedures available and quarantine is the only available control measure. The only preventive measure for herpes zoster is a limited supply of zoster immune globulin (ZIG) made available by the Communicable Disease Center of the U.S. Public Health Service at Atlanta. This is made available to high-risk patients who have been exposed to cases of chickenpox or zoster.

The problem of maintaining an adequate supply of ZIG is emphasized by the following request printed in *MMWR* (18 February 1977): "The increasing demand for ZIG has led to shortages, and the current stock will soon be exhausted. At the present time, CDC has no zoster immune plasma with which to begin a new lot. All those interested in supplying convalescent plasma from patients with herpes zoster should contact:

> Center for Disease Control
> Bureau of Laboratories
> Attention: Dr. Robert Ellis
>   Biological Products Division
> Atlanta, Georgia 30333
> Phone: (404) 633-3311, Ext. 3356

Plasma donations should be made between 7 and 28 days after onset of herpes zoster."

OTHER HERPESVIRUS INFECTIONS

Herpesvirus simiae (Herpesvirus B) is a monkey virus that frequently results in latent infections in these animals. Human cases have occurred mainly in individuals involved in handling monkeys, particularly those removing monkey kidneys for poliovirus vaccine production. As of 21 September 1973, there had been 24 human cases of this type of infection reported worldwide. Eighteen of these cases (75 percent) ended fatally. The significance of these latent infections in animal tissues to be used for the propagation of virus for the production of *live-virus* vaccines for human use is obvious. Stringent control measures are required to rule out the inherent dangers.

Herpesvirus simplex (H. hominis) can cause a variety of clinical symptoms in humans. The primary infection with *H. simplex* virus 1 (HSV-1) frequently results in a gingivostomatitis; primary HSV-2 infections frequently cause vaginitis or other genital pathology or dermatitis, particularly in infants. A particularly serious form of *H. hominis* infection is encephalitis. Nolan et al. (1970) treated six cases of such encephalitis with idoxuridine, four of whom showed complete recovery.

As a result of primary HSV-1 infections, the patient develops humoral antibodies and the infection becomes latent (see Docherty and Chopan 1974). The latency, however, even in the presence of persistent antibody, may be reversed by fever, emotional stress, or the common cold, resulting in recurrent "fever blister" or "cold sore" lesions. In the female, the activation of the latent virus also may result in recurrent vaginitis. Furthermore, there is growing evidence that *H. simplex* 2 might be responsible for cervical carcinoma and possibly other malignancies. For laboratory diagnosis of *Herpesvirus* infections, see Herrmann and Rawls (1974) and Taber et al. (1976).

VARIOLA

Variola or smallpox is an ancient human disease believed to have occurred in epidemic form in the early Chinese civilizations centuries prior to the birth of Christ. The disease was known to Galen in the second century A.D. and was endemic and epidemic in Asia and northern Africa thereafter. During and following the Crusades, widespread epidemics of smallpox swept over Europe and England.

Since many of the skin lesions (pocks) of smallpox almost invariably occurred on the face, and since these tended to result in permanent pitted scars in the survivors, the identity of those who had had the disease was apparent to all. This led to the recognition that those who had had smallpox did not suffer a second attack when subsequent epidemics spread through the community—they were immune. Some of the outbreaks resulted in mild cases with no mortality, moreover, whereas other outbreaks resulted in severe disease with frequently fatal results. These facts led to the recognition of different degrees of virulence in different epidemics of the disease, which in turn led to the practice of applied immunoprophylaxis (inoculation or variolation) centuries before any true knowledge of the causation of microbial diseases was established. Variolation involved obtaining matter or a scab from a pock of a mild case of smallpox and inoculating it into, or placing it on, the skin or mucus membranes of a susceptible individual. The objective of this inoculation was the production of a mild case of the disease in those who wanted to be immunized. Knowledge of this widespread practice in the Middle East was introduced by letters to western Europe (England) by Emanuel Timonius in 1713 and Lady Mary Montagu in 1718 (see Figure 16-1). The practice spread over England and to colonial America prior to the development, by Edward Jenner near the end of that century, of smallpox vaccination (see Langer 1976). Since variolation resulted in a higher percentage of mortality than vaccination, and since the practice could initiate an epidemic of smallpox, variolation was outlawed after vaccination became widespread.

Etiology

Guarnieri, in 1892, described differentially staining bodies in the cytoplasm of epithelial cells obtained from the edges of smallpox skin lesions. He believed these inclusion bodies to be protozoa. E. Paschen later described smaller bodies (elementary bodies) within and outside the Guarnieri bodies. These have been established as the etiological agent of the disease.

The elementary bodies are ovoid, spherical, or semirounded (more brick-shaped) virions (Figure 16-2). They are DNA viruses with di-

V. *An Account, or Hiſtory, of the Procuring the* S M A L L
P O X *by Inciſion, or Inoculation* ; *as it has for ſome time
been practiſed at* Conſtantinople.

Being the Extract of a Letter from Emanuel Timonius,
Oxon. & Patav. M. D. S. R. S. *dated at* Conſtantinople,
December, 1713.

Communicated to the Royal Society *by* John Woodward, M. D.
Proſeſ. Med. Greſh. *and* S. R. S.

THE Writer of this ingenious Diſcourſe obſerves, in
the firſt place, that the *Circaſſians, Georgians,* and
other *Aſiaticks,* have introduc'd this Practice of procuring
the *Small-Pox* by a ſort of Inoculation, for about the ſpace
of forty Years, among the *Turks* and others at *Conſtantinople.*

That altho' at firſt the more prudent were very cautious
in the uſe of this Practice ; yet the happy Succeſs it has
been found to have in thouſands of Subjects for theſe eight
Years paſt, has now put it out of all ſuſpicion and doubt ;
ſince the Operation having been perform'd on Perſons of all

Figure 16–1.   First account of smallpox inoculation (variolation) to appear in English. Extract from
a letter written by Emanuel Timonius at Constantinople in December 1713 and published in the
Transactions of the Royal Society of London in 1714.

mensions of 200 to 250 by 250 to 350 nanometers. Thus they represent one of the largest
viruses, and many virions can be resolved by
light microscopes. The virions are nonenveloped, are resistant to ether, glycerol, and 1
percent phenol, and are quite resistant to drying.
Living virus has been isolated from scabs kept at
room temperature for over a year and from dry
powdered exudate. Exudate dried on the bed-
clothes of a patient has been known to transmit
infection to laundry workers.

For many years variola virus has been
included in a group of similar viruses known as
the poxvirus group. This group now constitutes
the taxonomic family Poxviridae (see Fenner
1976). Variola and related viruses are placed in
the genus *Orthopoxvirus,* which includes *O.
variolae* (smallpox), *O. bovis* (cowpox), and *O.
officinalis* (vaccinia virus). These three poxviruses
are sufficiently different to justify the different
species designation, but they all share the same
immunogenic antigen. Vaccinia virus *O. officin-*

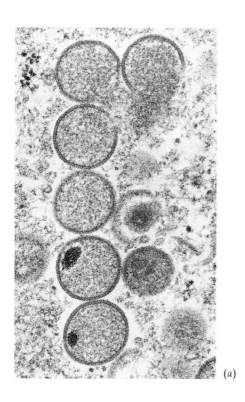

(a)

Figure 16–2. (a) Thin section of cell with immature intracellular virions of *Orthopoxvirus officinalis* (vaccinia virus); dense nucleoids are visible in several. (b) Mature negatively-stained, "brick-shaped" *O. variolae* (smallpox virus). 70,000×. ((a) Courtesy of J. J. Cardamone, Jr., and J. S. Youngner; (b) courtesy of F. A. Murphy.)

(b)

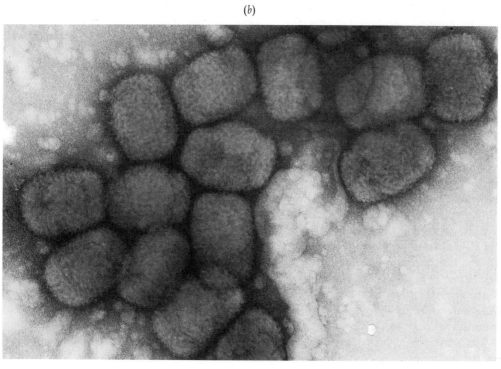

alis, although believed to have been isolated from a cowpox infection, has been artificially maintained by serial calf and rabbit passage. Over the years, it has developed taxonomic differences from the wild type *O. bovis* and *O. variolae* while retaining the immunogenic antigen. It is the official smallpox vaccine virus.

In addition to these three species of the genus *Orthopoxvirus,* other Poxviridae infect a variety of animals including mice, chickens, rabbits, and monkeys. The monkeypox virus has been reported to have caused occasional cases of human disease in South Africa (Cho and Wenner 1973). Also, monkeypox virus has been isolated from the kidneys of monkeys showing no symptoms of disease (latent infections). Although monkeypox in humans appears to be far less serious than *Herpesvirus simiae* infections, these latent infections in monkeys reemphasize the potential danger of using such animal tissue cultures for the propagation of live-virus vaccines for human immunization.

Although *O. variolae* can be propagated in a variety of tissue cultures (human or monkey), the chorioallantoic membrane (CAM) of the 11–13-day-old chick embryo is the usual experimental host for such propagation. For inoculation of the virus, the CAM is dropped to form an artificial air sac after puncturing the shell at the normal air sac. The inoculum is treated with antibiotics to suppress bacterial growth and is dropped through a pinhole onto the CAM at the artificial air sac site. After a suitable incubation period, the shell can be peeled away above the inoculum site and the infected CAM will show greyish white pock lesions. The infected CAM can be removed, emulsified, and used as a source of antigen for serotaxonomic identification. The viruses *O. bovis* and *O. officinalis* also can be propagated on the CAM of the chick embryo. The size and appearance of the pock lesions on the CAM, and the maximum temperatures at which these three poxviruses will grow, differ sufficiently to aid in their taxonomic differentiation (see Laboratory Diagnosis).

The immunobiology of *O. variolae* and *O. officinalis* has been studied much more thoroughly than other poxviruses. *Orthopoxvirus variolae* produces at least five well-recognized antigens that appear sequentially in infected cell cultures. A soluble antigen LS appears free in the cultures about 4 hours after infection. It appears to be a complex of two antigens: The L is heat-labile and the S heat-stable. Another soluble antigen, a nucleoprotein (NP), appears in the tissue culture about 5 to 6 hours after infection. A hemagglutinin (H), for selected fowl erythrocytes, appears in the cell cultures about 10 hours after infection. It is a particulate antigen about 65 nanometers in diameter. Although each of the antigenic products will stimulate animals and humans to produce homologous antibody, which may be demonstrated by appropriate GA reactions, such antibodies will not neutralize the virus and appear to have no immunological significance in smallpox. *Orthopoxvirus officinalis* produces the soluble antigens mentioned above and at least three additional ones. Antigen associated with the infectious virions (V antigen) of both *O. variolae* and *O. officinalis* appears to be responsible for the production of virus-neutralizing antibodies and the lasting immunity following smallpox infection or vaccination. In addition to *O. bovis* and *O. officinalis,* *O. variolae* shares antigenicity with the poxviruses of monkeys, rabbits, mice, and possibly others.

Pathogenic Mechanism

Although the histopathology of smallpox has been extensively described, the mechanism whereby this pathology is produced is not clear. The virus appears to invade the upper respiratory mucus membranes and, during the incubation period of 12 to 13 days, multiplies in these tissues with minimal, if any, production of infectious lesions. The virus spreads through the regional lymphatic channels and the blood (primary viremia) to visceral tissues where it multiplies extensively during the latter part of the incubation period. Onset symptoms of chills, fever, vomiting, headache, prostration, and others are associated with a secondary viremia. The virus then produces metastatic foci of infection in the buccopharyngeal mucus membranes and skin. Exudates from these lesions constitute the primary vehicle for the spread of the disease to others.

The skin lesions, as stated, appear as a single crop of maculopapular lesions that progress to a vesicular stage, followed by leucocyte infiltration of the vesicles to produce the pustular stage. Then, by fluid resorption and dehydration, the pock lesions develop the crust stage. Enormous numbers of *O. variolae* (elementary bodies) can be found in scrapings of the papular lesions, in vesicular or pustular fluid, or in the crusts of the skin lesions. After the separation of the crusts, permanent, deep-pitted scars are revealed, particularly on the face. Shortly after the onset of the skin eruption, the patient's condition improves. During pustulation there usually is a secondary rise in fever and severity of symptoms believed to be due to the absorption of toxic products of cell necrosis and bacterial complications.

The extent of pathology, the severity of symptoms, and the mortality resulting from smallpox are directly related to the number of pock lesions involved in the individual case. Exceptions to this are fulminating types of the disease wherein death may occur before the cutaneous eruption reaches recognizable proportions.

Clinical Smallpox

Detailed descriptions of clinical smallpox can be found in the text by Dixon (1962). As indicated above, the systemic symptoms of fever, prostration, various aches, and pains precede the onset of the focal eruption by several days. The focal macules appear first on the buccal and pharyngeal membranes, then on the face, forearms, and hands, and then on the trunk and elsewhere. Although the eruption does not involve all sites simultaneously, all lesions at a given site progress as a single crop all at the same stage of development. The macular rash quickly becomes maculopapular. Within 2 or 3 days the papules develop surface, multilocular vesicles, and these become pustular as leucocytes invade the area. Secondary (suppurative) fever and increased constitutional symptoms develop at this time and persist until desiccation of the pustules begins. This desiccation leads to the beginning of crust formation on the eighth to tenth day after onset of the rash, and crusting is complete in another 6 to 8 days. Most of the crusts will have separated by the twenty-first day after onset of symptoms (see Figure 16-3).

Sweitzer and Ikeda (1927) and Dixon (1962) have classified clinical smallpox as follows:

1. Variola minor (alastrim)—only a few discrete pocks; mortality nil

2. Variola major
   (a) Numerous discrete pocks; mortality about 6 percent
   (b) Confluent pocks; mortality about 45 percent
   (c) Hemorrhagic smallpox; mortality about 79–80 percent
   (d) Purpuric smallpox; mortality 100 percent

In hemorrhagic and purpuric smallpox, the typical skin pocks may not develop prior to death. One of the last cases of smallpox to be introduced into the United States was the hemorrhagic variety. This individual traveled by bus from Mexico to New York in 1947. After arrival, he became ill with symptoms of subcutaneous and buccal membrane hemorrhaging and died. His case probably would have gone undiagnosed except for the fact that a number of hospital personnel who had been in contact with the patient subsequently developed typical variola major of the pock types.

Each individual pock lesion in smallpox is about equivalent to a primary smallpox vaccination sore. With this in mind, one who has been vaccinated can visualize the discomfort, fever, and pain that many such sores scattered over the body could produce. Boils, bedsores, and skin abscesses are among the minor expected complications. Bacterial septicemia, bronchitis, bronchial pneumonia, and tetanus are more serious complications.

Prevalence

As a teenager in San Antonio, Texas, the author has two recollections that relate to the prevalence and fear of smallpox in the 1910–1920 era—a fair percentage of the people we passed

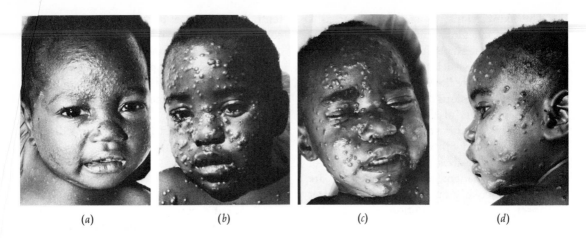

(a)   (b)   (c)   (d)

Figure 16–3.   Progression of smallpox eruption. (*a*) Papules on day 2 of eruption. (*b*) Papules on day 4 of eruption; the beginning of vesiculation may be seen on some lesions. (*c*) Pustular stage on day 6 of eruption. (*d*) Scab formation and healing on day 9 of eruption. (Courtesy of World Health Organization.)

on the streets showed the telltale pock scars on their faces; and while hunting rabbits in the mesquite brush on the west side of town, we were warned not to go near a small frame house near South Zarzamora Street. We learned later that it was the pest house where smallpox patients were housed until death or recovery. A volunteer nurse who had had smallpox was assigned to feed and care for the patients. When the house was occupied, a yellow flag was raised as a warning of danger.

As a result of extensive vaccination campaigns, smallpox had been eliminated from the western hemisphere and from Europe by 1950. Since air travel makes it possible for a person to travel to any part of the world during the incubation period, however, smallpox outbreaks in previously disease-free areas have resulted from travelers from the endemic areas of the world. By 1972 these endemic areas had been reduced to the Middle East, India, Pakistan, Bangladesh, Ethiopia, and adjacent North Africa. Smallpox was reintroduced in West Germany, for example, in January 1970. The index patient had just returned from West Pakistan and was hospitalized on the ground floor in an isolation ward. The skin rash first appeared on 13 January; during the next 3 days, after which he was removed to another hospital,

17 secondary cases were infected. The most probable explanation for at least part of the spread from the index case appeared to be airborne transmission, including ventilator shaft dissemination to the three floors of the hospital. A total of 20 cases and 4 deaths occurred in this outbreak (see *MMWR,* 20 June 1970). Another outbreak of smallpox involving 161 cases and 33 deaths occurred in Yugoslavia from 26 February to 15 April 1972 (see *MMWR,* 24 March 1972 and 8 April 1972). At the time of the index case, Yugoslavia had been free of smallpox for 42 years. The index case was believed to be a pilgrim who had traveled to Mecca and returned by bus through Baghdad, where smallpox was reported to be occurring at that time. Worldwide, a total of 132,339 cases of smallpox were reported for the year 1973.

The World Health Organization (WHO) in 1967 initiated a global eradication program against smallpox. At that time 30 countries were reporting smallpox endemicity. By the summer of 1976, WHO reported the complete eradication of this dreaded disease from the earth. As of 11 February 1977, however, WHO reported five new cases of smallpox in one family in Kenya (see *MMWR,* 11 March 1977). There has not been a case of smallpox in the United States since 1954.

Epidemiology

Although monkeys can be infected experimentally with *O. variolae*, humans appear to be the only host in which smallpox occurs in nature. Smallpox, as stated, is transmitted by dual primary vehicles: upper respiratory exudates (saliva) and cutaneous lesion exudates. The respiratory mode of transmission is that diagrammed in Figure II-A. Since the virus survives drying, however, secondary vehicles assume great significance in the epidemiology of this disease. Smallpox is probably the most highly contagious of all *serious* human diseases. Moreover, the 12-day incubation period makes possible the transportation of the virus from endemic areas to any part of the world prior to recognition of the infected status of the traveler. This characteristic necessitates constant governmental vigilance to prevent such importation. A case of the disease is infectious from just prior to the onset of the maculopapular rash to the detachment of the last cutaneous scab.

Laboratory Diagnosis

This discussion begins with a warning: Only well-trained virologists, with adequate knowledge of the dangers involved and the methods and facilities for avoiding these dangers, should undertake the laboratory diagnosis of smallpox.

Orthopoxvirus variolae or its soluble antigens can be identified in a variety of clinical specimens. Suitably stained smears of exudate or scrapings from skin pock lesions, when examined with light microscopes, will show large numbers of free elementary bodies. Epithelial cells in such smears will show Guarnieri bodies. Direct FA techniques may be used on such smears. Electron microscopic preparations of such lesion exudate will show the morphologically typical brickshape of the elementary body virions. Such microscopic demonstrations frequently take no more than a few hours but should be confirmed by more time-consuming procedures.

Primary isolation and propagation of *O. variolae* usually involves treating the clinical specimen (pock exudate or scab) with suitable combinations of antibiotics in phosphate-buffered saline (PBS) and inoculation of the mixture onto the CAM of 11–13-day chick embryos. Blood, collected aseptically, may be tested for the presence of a viremia without the addition of antibiotics. After incubation of the embryo at 36–37°C for 72 hours, the CAM is examined for characteristic pock lesions. If they are present, the infected portion of the CAM can be dissected out and ground in a sterile mortar. The soluble antigens in this emulsion can be demonstrated by complement fixation or by precipitation in agar gel (PAG) using known anti—*O. officinalis* antiserum from immunized rabbits. The latter test requires a clear agar (1 percent) gel 1 millimeter thick on a glass microslide. Four wells 4 millimeters in diameter are cut into the gel spaced at 5-millimeter centers as indicated in Figure 16-4. The wells are filled with

Figure 16–4. Agar gel precipitation (PAG) test to identify soluble smallpox antigen.

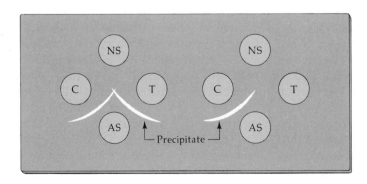

NS = normal serum
C = control (positive)
T = test extract
AS = anti-*O. officinalis* antiserum

the reagents indicated and the preparations are incubated in a moist chamber. Lines of precipitate usually appear within 2 to 3 hours. The preparation on the left illustrates a positive test result; that on the right is negative. Positive controls using known *O. officinalis* antigen (C) and negative controls using normal rabbit serum (NS) should be included in such serotaxonomic testing procedures. By judicious use of modifications of these procedures, the viruses of *O. variolae* major and minor, *O. bovis*, and *O. officinalis* (all of which will infect the CAM) and the V-Z virus of chickenpox (which will not infect the CAM) can be differentiated.

For more rapid serotaxonomic identification of *O. variolae*, the scab can be emulsified in a small amount of PBS and the supernatant fluid used as antigen in complement fixation or PAG tests. Negative results by these procedures, however, should be checked by the CAM propagation and testing procedures.

Foci of *O. variolae* infections in human (HeLa) or monkey kidney tissue cultures can be demonstrated *in situ* by hemadsorption using selected chicken erythrocytes. Prior treatment of the tissue culture with anti-*O. officinalis* antibody will block the phenomenon.

Antibodies begin to appear in the patient's serum within 5 days after the onset of the skin rash and usually reach high titers (1:320 or more) within another week. Using known *O. officinalis* antigens and the patient's serum, complement fixation, PAG, or HI serodiagnostic tests can be performed and significantly rising antibody titers established. See Nakano and Bingham (1974) for a more detailed discussion.

Immunological Measures

Although an English farmer, Benjamin Jesty in 1776, was the first to inoculate members of his family with cowpox matter with the objective of preventing smallpox, it was the medical doctor Edward Jenner who, in 1796–1798, first proved the efficacy of this procedure (vaccination) and publicly advocated its substitution for the practice of variolation. Since the early usage of this immunological procedure involved human-to-human propagation and passage of the infectious matter, other human infections could be passed at the same time. This possibility resulted in considerable opposition to the practice, so much so that new methods of propagation of the vaccine virus and new governmental safety controls were instituted.

Vaccine in use for smallpox immunization today consists of live *O. officinalis* propagated in the skin of calves (calf-lymph vaccine) or in the CAM of chick embryos inoculated with calf-lymph virus. Calf-passage virus appears to be more stable than continuous chick-embryo-passage virus. Frequent passage of the virus in rabbits prior to propagation in calves seems to enhance the production and the immunogenicity of the calf-lymph vaccine.

Biological houses licensed to produce calf-lymph vaccine must provide dust-free stalls for more than the number of calves to be used. There must be facilities for sterilizing the bedding (hay), feed, and so forth and also pens where the calves can be isolated and held for a sufficient time to establish their freedom from disease. Such calves are then washed thoroughly and moved into their assigned sterile stalls. Attendants are assigned to each calf on a 24-hour-a-day basis. When bedding is soiled, the calf is immediately moved from the stall, cleaned, and placed in a fresh sterile stall. The soiled stall is cleaned, disinfected, and made ready with fresh, sterile hay.

When all is ready, the calves are strapped down, the bellies are shaved, and multiple scratches the length of the abdomen are inoculated with the active calf-lymph seed virus. When the infections reach the confluent vesicular stage, the calves are sacrificed and bled out and the vesicular fluid (lymph) containing the virus is harvested. It is then mixed with an equal volume of glycerol that will slowly kill any bacteria present without affecting the vaccine virus. The attendants whose calves yield lymph with the least number of bacteria receive a monetary bonus for their efforts. The glycerinated calf-lymph vaccine is held and tested at intervals until demonstrated free of bacteria. It is then tested for potency (ID/50) in the skin of rabbits prior to packaging for distribution. Representative samples of the packaged product must be submitted to the National Institutes of Health for checking prior to release for human use.

E. B. M. Cook (1948) and her colleagues at the Texas Department of Health Laboratory were the first to develop and test chick-embryo, live-virus vaccine for smallpox immunization. Calf-lymph seed virus was inoculated to the CAMs of large numbers of 11–13-day-old chick embryos. After inoculation, the infected CAMs were harvested and each placed in a small, numbered petri dish. The CAM was swabbed with a sterile cotton swab and then placed in deep-freeze. The swab was inoculated to correspondingly numbered bacteriological culture media and incubated to determine the presence or absence of bacterial contamination. Any CAM showing such contamination was discarded. The uncontaminated CAMs were thawed, pooled, and emulsified, and an equal volume of glycerol was added to dilute the CAM emulsion and eliminate any bacteria that might have been missed by swabbing. The CAM method of vaccine production yields an initial bacteria-free product that is impossible to obtain with the calf-lymph method of production. Packaging and testing of chick embryo vaccine are the same as that for calf-lymph vaccine.

Smallpox vaccine is drawn aseptically into capillary tubes in 0.01-milliliter amounts. The tubes are 1.5 millimeters in diameter by 7 centimeters long and are hermetically sealed at both ends. The vaccine is packaged along with a sterile needle (sealed in another capillary tube) and a small rubber bulb that has a rigid perforation below to receive the vaccine capillary and a thin-wall perforation above to prevent pressure buildup when the capillary is inserted below. Since the vaccine is live O. officinalis, storage between 0° and −10°C is preferable to prevent death of the virus, which will occur in about 1 week at room temperature. Some authorities recommend dehydrating the virus from the frozen state (lyophilizing). This powdered virus keeps alive indefinitely at 4–6°C.

The objective of smallpox vaccination is to infect the living epithelial cells at the site of inoculation. The live O. officinalis in the vaccine may be scratched through the overlying cornefied epithelium, or it may be teased through by multiple pressures of the sterile needle supplied with the vaccine. The latter method is preferable. The site of inoculation should be cleansed—but not disinfected. One end of the capillary tube containing the vaccine should be broken off and inserted into the rubber bulb. Also, the end of the capillary tube containing the sterile needle should be broken off. Next the other end of the capillary containing the vaccine is broken off. Then, placing the finger over the upper perforation in the rubber bulb, the vaccine is deposited on the cleansed surface of the skin. The sterile needle is used to tease the virus through the cornefied and dead epithelial cells to the living cells below. This is accomplished by multiple (20–30) pressures of the point through the deposited vaccine.

Smallpox vaccination may yield four possible results:

1. *Primary (vaccinia) reaction:* This reaction consists of a papule that begins to develop on the fourth day, followed by vesiculation on the eighth day, pustulation on the tenth day, crust formation on the twelfth day, and separation of the crust on the sixteenth day after vaccination. This reaction is given by individuals with no immunity at the time of their first vaccination.

2. *Accelerated (vaccinoid) reaction:* This reaction consists of the foregoing papule, vesicle, pustule, and crust stages, all speeded up so that the crust separates on about the tenth day after vaccination. This appears to be a typical anamnestic response to infection in individuals who have been previously vaccinated. It indicates that the vaccinee had some residual immunity but not enough to prevent infection if exposed to smallpox. The case, however, probably would have been mild, even though variola major virus was involved.

3. *Immediate reaction:* This reaction consists of a papule only, which fades without vesiculation on about the sixth day after vaccination. It is believed to be a typical delayed hypersensitivity reaction to infection and probably indicates proper administration of the vac-

cine containing live *O. officinalis* virus, and immunity to smallpox. There are those who will disagree with this "probable immunity" conclusion. If so, the individual should be revaccinated with a fresh lot of vaccine.

4. *No reaction:* This lack of a reaction might be explainable on any one of three grounds — (1) it could mean immunity in a nonhypersensitive individual who was properly vaccinated with a live-virus vaccine; (2) it could have no immune significance if the live virus in the vaccine were improperly administered and did not reach the living epithelial cells; or (3) it certainly would have no immune significance if the virus in the vaccine were dead. Because of these three possibilities for explaining no reaction, such individuals should be revaccinated with a fresh lot of vaccine by someone who understands the importance of proper administration of the vaccine.

When to be vaccinated depends upon whether or not the individual resides in or plans to enter an area of smallpox endemicity or is faced with an introduced outbreak of smallpox in a previously disease-free area. Vaccination of infants when there is practically no likelihood of exposure is not warranted. In 1968, out of a total of 5,594,000 primary vaccinations and 8,574,000 revaccinations in the United States, nine deaths from vaccination complications were reported. Five deaths, per million primary infant vaccinations, were in infants under 1 year of age. The vaccination complications included encephalitis, vaccinia necrosum, eczema vaccinatum, generalized vaccinia, and accidental bacterial infections.

After smallpox vaccination was proved effective in preventing the spread of the disease, most countries passed laws making vaccination compulsory. To enforce the law, certified evidence of successful vaccination was required for entrance to public schools. During my lifetime, this requirement has resulted in a change from thousands of cases of smallpox per year in the United States in the early 1900s to no cases of smallpox in this country since 1954. When practically everyone is vaccinated at least once in their lifetime (at about 6 years of age), the immune barrier becomes sufficient to stop the epidemic spread of the disease.

The nine deaths from vaccination complications in 1968, when compared with no cases of smallpox in the United States during the past 20 years, raises the legitimate question of the justifiability of compulsory vaccination. Both the U.S. Public Health Service and state departments of health now have answered the question with an emphatic no! A certificate of recent (3 years) smallpox vaccination is no longer required for public school entrance. Such certificates, however, are required of individuals entering the United States from areas of the world where smallpox is still endemic. It is hoped that this requirement will keep the disease out of this country while the WHO smallpox eradication program eliminates the disease from the rest of the world. This elimination apparently has now been approximated.

From Jenner's time on, there have been those who fought against the practice of smallpox vaccination. The argument that the practice did not prevent smallpox was easy to refute. The argument that other diseases were transmitted with the vaccine was true when the vaccine virus was passed from human-to-human infections. It is no longer true. Of course any skin lesion can become accidentally infected with a variety of pathogenic organisms, but this is not the fault of the vaccine. The argument that compulsory vaccination constituted an infringement of personal liberty is more difficult to refute. In the past, the proponents of vaccination had to fall back on the ethics of the greatest good for the greatest number in their refutation of the infringement of personal liberty argument. Now that vaccination is no longer compulsory, the argument is moot.

Two groups who in the past have fought compulsory vaccination hardest are the Christian Scientists and the chiropractors. The irony of this opposition is the fact that both groups implicitly believe in their ability to prevent infectious disease by spiritual or manual methods. Since vaccination is merely the intentional infection of the skin with a mild disease organism, all that members of these groups have to do to prove their ability to prevent the disease (the vaccination sore) is to pray over the site of infection or manipulate the spine of the vaccinee. If by so doing they can prevent the *O. officinalis* infection in a susceptible individual, I personally will be glad to join in their beliefs and their preventive medicine procedures.

Immunotherapeutic measures (using convalescent human serum) have been reported to yield beneficial results. There has been no advocacy of the use of foreign (horse or other animal) serum antibody therapy, however.

Control and Prevention

In endemic areas, if any are discovered, children should be vaccinated at an early age and revaccinated after 3 to 4 years.

Cases of smallpox should be rigidly quarantined. All contaminated vehicles should be disinfected by burning, boiling, or autoclaving at least twice daily.

Appropriate antibiotics can be administered, particularly during the pustular stage of the cutaneous eruption, to suppress bacterial complications. The antibiotics will have no effect on the viral infection, however.

Immediate vaccination of known contacts is advocated to speed the immune response if they are infected.

The prophylactic use of N-methylisatin β-thiosemicarbazone has been advocated by Bauer et al. (1963). It is reputed to suppress the infection when given to household contacts with a case of smallpox. A new semicarbazone was being tested (1974) on rhesus monkeys by Dr. Rao in India. It has been claimed to be a good prophylactic drug and can also effect a cure if given within 72 hours of infection. For international control measures see Bennenson (1970).

REFERENCES

Bauer, D. J., L. St. Vincent, C. H. Kempe, and A. W. Downie. 1963. Prophylactic treatment of smallpox contacts with N-methylisatin β-thiosemicarbazone (Compound 33T57, Marboran). *Lancet* 2:494–496.

Bennenson, A. S. (ed.). 1970. *Control of Communicable Diseases in Man.* 11th ed. New York: American Public Health Association.

Cho, C. T. and H. A. Wenner. 1973. Monkeypox virus. *Bacteriol. Rev.* 37:1–8.

Cook, E. B. M., P. N. Crain, and J. V. Irons. 1948. A report on field use of chick membrane smallpox vaccine in Texas. *Tex. Health Bull.* 6:50–56.

Dixon, C. W. 1948. Smallpox in Tripolitania 1946: an epidemic and clinical study of 500 cases, including trials of penicillin treatment. *J. Hyg.* 46:351–377.

————. 1962. *Smallpox.* London: Churchill Publishers.

Docherty, J. J. and M. Chopan. 1974. The latent *Herpes simplex* virus. *Bacteriol. Rev.* 38:337–355.

Fenner, F. 1976. The classification and nomenclature of viruses: the current position. *Amer. Soc. Microbiol. News* 42:170–173.

Herrmann, E. C., Jr. and W. E. Rawls. 1974. *Herpes simplex* virus. Chapter 83 in *Manual of Clinical Microbiology.*

Joklik, W. K. 1966. The poxviruses. *Bacteriol. Rev.* 30:33–66.

Langer, W. L. 1976. Immunization against smallpox before Jenner. *Scientific Amer.* 234:112–117.

Nakano, J. H. and P. G. Bingham. 1974. Smallpox, vaccinia, and human infections with monkeypox viruses. Chapter 86 in *Manual of Clinical Microbiology.*

Nolan, D. C., M. M. Carruthers, and A. M. Lerner. 1970. *Herpesvirus hominis* encephalitis in Michigan. *New Eng. J. Med.* 282:10–13.

Schmidt, N. J. 1974. Varicella-Zoster virus. Chapter 85 in *Manual of Clinical Microbiology.*

Sweitzer. S. E. and K. Ikeda. 1927. Variola: a clinical study of the Minneapolis epidemic of 1924–25. *Arch. Derm. Syph.* 15:19–29.

Taber, L. H., F. Brasier, R. B. Couch, S. B. Greenberg, D. Jones, and V. Knight. 1976. Diagnosis of *Herpes simplex* virus infection by immunofluorescence. *J. Clin. Microbiol.* 3:309–312.

Subgroup B: Genital Contact

The diseases involved in this subgroup commonly are transmitted by sexual intercourse. The major primary vehicles are exudates from the infected genital tracts. The diseases frequently are classified as venereal or VD, but they may be transmitted by other modes of contact, particularly when exudates from extragenital lesions (mouth or skin) constitute the primary vehicles. Although most cases of these diseases are acquired as a result of direct physical contact, a few may be acquired from contact with freshly contaminated secondary vehicles. The causative organisms of gonorrhea and syphilis, however, die rapidly outside the tissues or body cavities of infected hosts.

17

Chancroid, Bacterial Vaginitis, Gonorrhea, and Lymphogranuloma Venereum

Three bacterial species are known to infect the urinogenital tract membranes or external genitalia: *Hemophilus ducreyi*, the cause of chancroid or Ducrey's infection; *Hemophilus vaginalis*, claimed to be the cause of a specific bacterial vaginitis; and *Neisseria gonorrhoeae*, the causative organism of gonorrhea. A rickettsia, *Chlamydia psittaci*, is the cause of lymphogranuloma venereum; *C. psittaci* also causes a variety of other diseases in birds and humans that do not involve genital contact.

CHANCROID AND BACTERIAL VAGINITIS

The causative organisms of chancroid and bacterial vaginitis are small, gram-negative rods belonging to the genus *Hemophilus*. The cause of chancroid, *H. ducreyi*, frequently tends to grow in end-to-end pairs or short chains. Chancroid *(soft chancre)* involves an ulcerated lesion of the genital membranes or skin. The ulcer enlarges in diameter as the *H. ducreyi* erode the outer walls.

The chancroid lesion is differentiated from the primary lesion of syphilis by the fact that the latter remains more circumscribed in its early crater-form status and the surrounding tissue is indurated *(hard chancre)*. Furthermore, *H. ducreyi* does not tend to penetrate the host tissues beyond the lymphatics near the lesion, whereas the causative organism of syphilis is capable of rapidly penetrating tissues throughout the body.

Chancroid is usually a disease of the tropics, although 21 cases were reported from Winnipeg, Manitoba, in December 1975 and January 1976 (see *MMWR* 14 May 1976). *Hemophilus ducreyi* may be demonstrated in gram-stained smears of scrapings from the periphery of the ulcer. Their morphology in these smears, however, may be confusing. Cultivation in high-concentration, rabbit-blood agar, or even in clotted rabbit blood, has been described. Sheep blood, however, inhibits growth of the organism. Chancroid may be cured by topical disinfection or by a single dose of suitable antibiotics. Syphilis cannot be so easily cured.

The specific vaginitis caused by *H. vaginalis* was first discovered by H. L. Gardner and C. D. Dukes in 1955 when they were studying cases of "nonspecific" (viral?) vaginitis in women. The causative organism was studied by Redmond and Kotcher in 1963, but it is still too early to assess the etiological relationship and the epidemiology of the vaginitis caused by *H. vaginalis*. It may be a venereal disease, particularly if a specific urethritis or latent infection or carrier state could be established in the male. The relative rarity of reported cases of the disease indicates the unlikelihood of the male being a factor in the spread of the disease, however. See Hobson and Holmes (1977) for other nongonococcal urethritis and related infections.

GONORRHEA

Gonorrhea (specific urethritis or clap) is a disease that, in adults, practically always involves the mucus membranes of the urethra. This involvement is pyogenic and results in a copious discharge of pus that is more obvious in the male than the female. The designation gonorrhea was used in the writings of Galen during the second century A.D.; its usage then implied a "flow of seed." Thereafter, for many years, gonorrhea and syphilis were confused. Paracelsus, in 1530, taught that gonorrhea was an early symptom of syphilis. Petritius, in 1591, was the first to state that the gonorrheal discharge consisted mainly of pus. The two diseases, at that time, frequently were present together in infected patients. The confusion was heightened by the classic error reported by the eminent English physician John Hunter in 1767. Hunter intentionally inoculated himself with pus from a patient supposedly infected with gonorrhea only. When he reported early symptoms of gonorrhea followed by symptoms of syphilis, the case for gonorrhea being an early symptom of syphilis seemed to be proved. It took almost another 200 years to finally delineate gonorrhea and syphilis as two distinct diseases.

Etiology

The causative organism of gonorrhea is designated *Neisseria gonorrhoeae* or commonly the gonococcus. It was first described by A. Neisser, in 1879, in the pus discharges of a case. It was first cultivated from such exudates by Bumm in 1885. Its etiological relationship to the disease was later established by using human volunteers to fulfill the experimental animal requirement of the Henle-Koch etiology postulates.

The organism is a gram-negative, coffee-bean-shaped diplococcus indistinguishable by these criteria from *N. meningitidis*. It frequently is found intracellularly in the polymorphonuclear leucocytes of the pus exudate. The gonococcus appears to be slightly less susceptible to temperature changes than the meningococcus, but it is equally susceptible to drying, ultraviolet light, and other external environments.

A variable percentage of the gonococcal strains are more fastidious in their cultural requirements than other *Neisseria* (see Lankford and Snell 1943; Lankford and Skaggs 1946). Hemoglobin, yeast extract, glutamine, cocarboxylase, and possibly other supplements added to special peptone (Proteose no. 3, Difco) media have been advocated for maximum chance of isolating all strains of the gonococcus. Proteose no. 3 (Difco) peptone contains hypoxanthine, which stimulates the growth of *N. gonorrhoeae*. Thayer and Martin (1964) described a selective agar plating medium (T-M) that meets the cultural requirements of most *N. gonorrhoeae*. Also, it is designed to suppress the growth of saprophytic *Neisseria* species, *Mima polymorpha*, *Proteus* species, and other bacteria that might complicate the isolation of gonococci. After the hemoglobin is added, the T-M medium is heated at 75°C, which causes it to turn chocolate brown in color and improves its nutritional qualities. Gonococcal cultures should be incubated at 35–36°C in an atmosphere of 3 to 10 percent added CO_2. A candle jar may be used to provide the minimal CO_2 requirement. Another commonly used culture medium (Transgrow) is a modified T-M agar medium, usually dispensed into flat-sided, screw-capped bottles containing the added CO_2. This is used to transport clinical specimens by mail to distant diagnostic laboratories (see Laboratory Diagnosis). Commercial lots of these culture media (usually in the dehydrated form) should be checked carefully for promotion of gonococcal growth, and for suppression of contaminant growth, prior to use in diagnostic laboratory work.

Kellogg et al. (1963, 1968) described four distinct biotypes of *N. gonorrhoeae* based on the appearance of the colonies and the presence or absence of pili on the cells (see Figure 17-1). Type 1 colonies predominate in primary isolation from purulent exudate from acute gonorrhea. The cells of colony types 1 and 2 possess pili. The other colony biotypes appear rapidly during culture passage until all colonies have the appearance of old laboratory strains (type 4), the cells of which lack pili and are avirulent when tested on human volunteers. Type 1 colony cells are virulent and produce urethritis when inoculated to such volunteers. Only firsthand experience in observing gonococcal colonies will make the characteristics of these biotypes apparent to the technical worker.

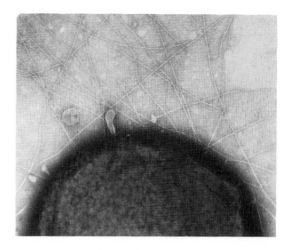

Figure 17–1. Pili on the surface of a negatively-stained cell of *N. gonorrhoeae* (T2 colony type). About 44,880×. (Courtesy of J. L. Swanson.)

Neisseria gonorrhoeae has long been known to be antigenically heterogeneous. Repeat gonorrheal infections are quite common, probably as a result of this heterogeneity. Since humans are the only hosts and only experimental animal, there have been few, if any, significant immunological studies with *N. gonorrhoeae*. Even serotaxonomic studies using agglutination and complement fixation tests have yielded little of generally accepted practical value. Deacon (1961) reported a "K-type" antigen present in virulent gonococci found in urethral exudate or in very young primary cultures. He noted that this surface antigen disappears rapidly in cultured cells and is no longer present in cultures more than 30 hours old. He advocated demonstrating the K-type antigen by means of specific fluorescent anti-K antibody. He also claimed that the antigen was highly specific for *N. gonorrhoeae*. Other experts in the field are prone to disagree with Deacon's conclusions. However, Thayer in 1970 advocated the serotaxonomic use of a direct FA test using gonococcal antiserum that had been absorbed with *N. meningitidis* type B cells to make it more specific for the gonococcal antigens.

Quinn and Lowry of Vanderbilt University reported studies in which they prepared extracts of their gonococcal isolates and used these in precipitin tests comparable to the Lancefield streptococcal grouping technique. When the extracts were tested against homologous and heterologous antisera, Quinn and Lowry were able to distinguish nine antigenic groups of the gonococci. They observed that isolates from a localized gonorrheal outbreak tended to yield extracts characteristic of a single group. Although it is too early to assess the immunological or serotaxonomic significance of these reports, they do extend another approach for future studies in these areas.

Clinical Symptoms

Uncomplicated gonorrhea in the adult male, after an incubation period of 2–8 days, consists of an inflammatory and pyogenic involvement of the lining membranes of the anterior urethra (a specific urethritis). The involvement commonly extends to the posterior urethra; in the female the cervix of the uterus also may be involved. In the male, the inflammatory involvement results in intense burning and pain upon urination, and variable constitutional symptoms may result. Disease symptoms in the female are much less obvious, and estimates of asymptomatic infections in females have ranged as high as 90 percent. The pyogenic discharge from the male varies from a scant mucoid exudate in the early disease to a copious flow of yellow to greenish pus during the acute phase. The gonococci may invade the prostate, cervical, or other glands along the urinogenital tract and establish chronic infections with little or no pus exudate. The chronic and asymptomatic cases are common sources of infection in sexual partners.

In adult gonorrhea the primary infections may be complicated by extension along the genital tract channels. In addition to the prostatitis mentioned above, the infection in the male may extend to the testicles and result in a gonococcal *orchitis*. In the female the cervical involvement may extend through the uterus to the fallopian tubes resulting in a salpingitis; to the ovaries resulting in an ovaritis; or to the peritoneum resulting in an inflammatory peritonitis. The involvement of the testicles, fallo-

pian tubes, or ovaries may result in sterility. Arthritis is a common sequel following chronic gonorrhea.

In female infants and young children, a nonvenereal gonorrheal vulvovaginitis may occur. Outbreaks of this type of involvement have been reported in pediatric wards in hospitals and in other concentrations of female children.

In addition to the urinogenital membranes, the epithelial cells of the eyes are highly susceptible to gonococcal infection. Since the gonococcus does not invade through tissues, congenital transmission from the infected mother to the child *in utero* does not occur. At the birth of such a child, however, the eyes are invariably exposed to infection by gonococci in the urinogenital exudates of the infected mother. Gonococcal infection of the corneal epithelium of the newborn (opthalmia neonatorium) can lead to blindness. Such gonorrheal ophthalmia was quite common (estimated to be the cause of 12 percent of all cases of blindness) prior to the widespread practice of disinfecting the eyes of *all* newborn infants—usually by using a drop of 1 percent silver nitrate ($AgNO_3$) in each eye. Some authorities advocate a prophylactic injection of penicillin or other chemoprophylaxis along with or substituted for the $AgNO_3$ prophylaxis.

Epidemiology

Gonorrhea in the adult is almost invariably transmitted by sexual intercourse. This is even more true for gonorrhea than for syphilis. In the latter disease, infectious lesions frequently occur in the mouth or other extragenital sites. Such extragenital lesions are extremely rare in gonorrhea. During the 1970s, however, an increasing number of nasopharyngeal isolates of *N. gonorrhoeae* have been reported. An occasional case of adult gonorrhea has been attributed to contact with freshly soiled secondary vehicles. Also, cases of infant or young female vulvovaginitis usually are acquired by extragenital contact with an infected adult or with other infected children or with freshly contaminated secondary vehicles.

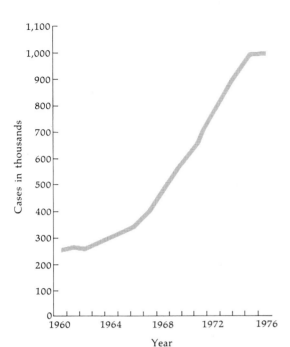

Figure 17–2. Gonorrhea, United States, 1960–1976. (From *MMWR* 14 January 1977.)

ent recovery, and can be shed intermittently into the lumen, repeated testing is necessary to prove recovery and noninfectivity. Repeatedly culturing on suitable media (see Laboratory Diagnosis) is the best available means of ruling out persistent infectivity; and this requires *multiple negative* test results to be significant.

Laboratory Diagnosis

Diagnosis of acute gonorrhea in the male usually can be accomplished with a single gram-stained smear of the pus discharged from the orifice of the urethra. Finding large numbers of intracellular or extracellular, gram-negative, coffee-bean-shaped diplococci in the pus is generally considered diagnostic (see Figure E2 on the back cover).

Laboratory diagnosis of gonorrhea in the female is a more complex problem and frequently requires cultural procedures for success. The exudate for such a diagnosis usually is collected on a cotton swab with the aid of a vaginal speculum. The swab should be inserted into the orifice of the urethra where it empties into the vaginal cavity. Also, the opening of the cervix uteri and possibly the posterior nasopharynx should be swabbed. The exudate on the swab should be roll-inoculated immediately to a

The incidence of gonorrhea is directly proportional to the sexual promiscuity of the population. Since both the male and the female can develop infections with no overt symptoms, such promiscuous individuals can serve as the source of infection for multiple sexual partners. This promiscuity during the 1960s and continuing into the 1970s has resulted in a continuously increasing incidence of gonorrhea that is reaching epidemic status both in the United States and elsewhere in the world (see Figure 17-2). As indicated in Table 17-1, the Venereal Disease Control Division of CDC reported an increase of newly reported civilian cases of gonorrhea from 351,735 in 1966 to 1,001,994 in 1976 (see *MMWR* supplement, August 1976, and VD Branch CDC report, March 1977).

An infected individual can transmit the gonorrheal infection from shortly before the pyogenic stage until all *N. gonorrhoeae* have been eliminated. Since live organisms can persist within or between cells of the urinogenital membranes or glands after treatment or appar-

Table 17-1. New civilian cases of gonorrhea and syphilis reported to CDC: 1966–1976.

Year	Gonorrhea	Syphilis
1966	351,735	105,159
1967	404,836	102,581
1968	464,563	96,271
1969	534,872	92,162
1970	600,072	91,383
1971	670,268	95,997
1972	767,215	91,149
1973	842,621	87,469
1974	898,943	83,771
1975	999,937	80,356
1976	1,001,994	71,761

plate of T-M medium and streaked for isolated colony production using a sterile bacteriological loop. The plate should be incubated overnight at 35–36°C in an atmosphere of 3–10 percent added CO_2. If typical colonies develop, well-isolated ones may be numbered on the bottom of the plate and transplanted to a fresh plate of T-M medium by touching each colony with a sterile, straight bacteriological needle. The transplant plate should be incubated as described above. After each such transfer, the residual cells on the needle may be smeared in a tiny drop of water on a microslide for staining by the gram method. The original plate may then be sprayed or flooded with an oxidase test solution consisting of 0.5 to 1.0 percent tetramethyl-p-phenylenediamine dihydrochloride. Gonococcal colonies on the plate will rapidly turn pink, then red, and finally dark purple to black. Since colonies of other *Neisseria* and some other bacterial species will give a positive oxidase reaction, a positive test result is not proof of identity. Nevertheless, if the plating medium is T-M selective agar, the growth of most non-gonococcal species will be suppressed. If further taxonomic testing on live cells is needed, it may be performed on the transplant growth from the oxidase-positive colonies.

If the specimen for cultural isolation of *N. gonorrhoeae* must be sent to a laboratory at some distance, it should be roll-inoculated and streaked to the surface of the agar medium in a Transgrow bottle. Since the bottle contains not only a nutrient medium but also the necessary CO_2, the screw cap should be tightened immediately and the culture sent to the laboratory for incubation and study. Positive isolations of *N. gonorrhoeae* have been obtained in Transgrow cultures inoculated from 1 to 5 days prior to delivery and incubation in the laboratory. Obviously, the sooner the cultures are incubated and studied, the better.

In diagnosing chronic gonorrhea, or in establishing cure after treatment of either male or female cases, repeated negative cultures comparable to those described above may be required. In diagnosing gonorrheal vulvovaginitis in children, the exudate should be collected on a swab inserted well into the vagina. The use of an ear speculum may be helpful in collecting this specimen. In diagnosing gonorrheal ophthalmia, pus from the conjunctival sac should be collected on a sterile swab. Such swab specimens should be roll-inoculated to plates of T-M agar and streaked for isolated colony cultivation as described above.

J. D. Thayer in 1970 advocated the use of FA anti–*N. gonorrhoeae* that has been absorbed with *N. meningitidis* (group B) cells for the final taxonomic test for the identification of *N. gonorrhoeae* isolates. This direct FA test also may be used on smears of exudates if there are sufficient numbers of the diplococci to be found in microscopic examinations. If an ultraviolet-light microscope is not available, the absorbed anti–*N. gonorrhoeae* antiserum may be used in a complement fixation test with a suspension of the cultured diplococci serving as the test antigen. Biochemical differentiation of *Neisseria* species has been advocated, but frequently equivocal results are obtained.

Control and Prevention

Immunological procedures have never proved successful either in preventing or in curing gonorrhea. Finding and treating (disinfecting) cases and carriers, and avoiding sexual promiscuity, are the only successful means of preventing infection. Disinfecting the eyes of *all* newborn infants will prevent gonorrheal ophthalmia.

Practically all gonococci developed resistance to sulfonamides by the late 1940s. Fortunately the penicillin family of drugs then proved effective in gonorrhea therapy. During the Korean War some cases of penicillin-resistant gonorrhea were reported. The gonococci isolated from these cases were, however, susceptible to penicillin. Further study indicated the presence of penicillinase-producing avirulent staphylococci on the genital membranes of the gonorrheal patients. The staphylococci were destroying the penicillin, thereby permitting the gonococci to resist the penicillin therapy!

In February and April of 1976, however, the first known penicillinase-producing *N. gonor-*

rhoeae (PPNG), one from Maryland and one from California, were identified by CDC (see *MMWR,* 27 August 1976). Consequently, a search for additional cases was instituted. By 21 January 1977, 94 PPNG isolates were confirmed by CDC from 16 states in the United States. Thirty-nine of the 94 cases yielding PPNG were linked with military personnel or others returning from the Far East. One PPNG isolate also proved resistant to spectinomycin but was susceptible to tetracycline (see *MMWR,* 4 February 1977). Forty cases of such gonorrhea have been reported from Liverpool, England, and one case from London. Eleven of the Liverpool cases have been linked epidemiologically with individuals who recently traveled from the Far East.

The treatment recommended by CDC for uncomplicated gonorrhea remains one of the penicillins or tetracycline. However, patients with a positive follow-up culture 7 to 10 days after initial treatment—with the recommended doses of penicillin, ampicillin, or tetracycline— should receive 2 grams of spectinomycin intramuscularly. If the patient's infection is related to the Far East, the follow-up cultures should be performed 3 to 7 days after initial treatment (see *MMWR,* 1 October 1976).

LYMPHOGRANULOMA VENEREUM

Etiology

Lymphogranuloma venereum (LGV; LG inguinale) also has been designated tropical or climatic bubo because of its major incidence in tropical regions and because of the frequent involvement of the inguinal lymph nodes resulting in groin swellings similar to those of bubonic plague. The tropical distribution of the disease probably is due to the frequency of the depressed socioeconomic status of such populations, with associated ignorance and lack of adequate medical facilities. In the early part of this century, LGV, psittacosis, and diseases caused by taxonomically related organisms were believed to be due to filterable viruses (see Bedson and Bland 1932; Bedson 1936). Subsequently the etiological agents of these diseases were found to possess both DNA and RNA, thereby removing them from the taxonomic category of viruses.

Since these organisms were observed to multiply by binary fission and possessed bacteria-like cell walls, but were obligate parasites and possessed other characteristics of rickettsiae, they have been classified as members of the taxonomic order Rickettsiales and family Chlamydiaceae. Some authorities advocate *Bedsonia* for the genus designation; others prefer *Chlamydia;* we will use the latter. One species of the genus *Chlamydia* is designated *C. psittaci.* Different strains of this species share antigens, but each is believed to possess an additional strain-specific antigen as well as strain-specific pathogenicity. One strain of *C. psittaci* is responsible for psittacosis in the parrot family of birds; ornithosis in turkeys and other nonpsittacine birds; and psittacosis (ornithosis) in humans, the latter only as a result of contact with infected birds. Another strain of *C. psittaci* has been established as the cause of lymphogranuloma venereum, which usually is transmitted from human to human by genital contact. This strain appears to be the only member of the genus *Chlamydia* that is classified as the etiological agent of a human venereal disease.

Chlamydia psittaci and other chlamydiae share a unique developmental sequence in infected tissue cells. The infection is initiated by a small (perhaps 300 nanometers) spherical elementary body with a central dense nucleoid. The elementary body gains entrance into a vacuole in the cytoplasm of a mononuclear cell by phagocytosis. Inside this vacuole the elementary body enlarges to 500 to 1,000 nanometers. It then undergoes repeated division by binary fission, filling the vacuole and forming a characteristic inclusion body within the cytoplasm of the cell. The elementary-body progeny of this binary fission can then be liberated to infect adjacent cells or other individuals.

The elementary bodies of *C. psittaci* stain purple with Giemsa stain, as do the inclusion bodies, which are tightly packed colonies of the elementary bodies. Other polychrome stains, but not the gram stain, may be used for demonstrating the elementary and inclusion body stages of *C. psittaci.*

Clinical Symptoms

Usually, after an incubation period of a few days, the initial vesicular lesion develops on the head or skin of the penis in the male, or on the labia, vaginal walls, cervix, or anal region in the female. The vesicle may be painless and easily overlooked. It may burst and leave a shallow lymphogranulomatous chancre that may heal, and the infection may be terminated at this stage. Chlamydiae infections have been observed to persist for long periods of time in latent or subclinical status, however, and overt disease in the natural host is more the exception than the rule.

If the infection is not terminated, the second stage of LGV involves the regional lymph nodes, usually in the groin. Mild fever, muscle pains, pain in the groin, and malaise are common early constitutional symptoms. Anorectal involvement usually results in perianal and deep pelvic lymph node involvement, particularly in the female. The lymphadenitis may be unilateral or bilateral. The adenitis may heal spontaneously, or the nodes may suppurate. As the lymphadenitis and more generalized involvement increases, the fever, prostration, and other constitutional symptoms increase in severity. In severe cases, the infection may progress to pneumonitis or meningoencephalitis. Elephantiasis of genital tract tissues may develop late in the infection.

Diagnosis

An intradermal diagnostic test was reported by Frei (1925), who used exudate from human lesions diluted 1:5 in saline and heated at 60°C for 3 hours to kill the then unknown causative organism. After intracutaneous injection of 0.1 milliliter, the results were read at 48 and 96 hours. A raised papule at the test site significantly larger than that at the control site was considered positive and had diagnostic significance comparable to that of a positive tuberculin test in the diagnosis of tuberculosis. After *C.*

psittaci was found capable of infecting mice, chick embryo yolk sac, and other animals and tissue cultures, the Frei test antigen was derived from these sources. The control consists of a comparable preparation from noninfected tissues. A commercial Frei test antigen (Lygranum) is available for diagnostic use. Furthermore, *C. psittaci* antigen for serodiagnostic tests (complement fixation) is derived from infected animal hosts or tissue cultures. Some authorities consider a rising titer serodiagnostic test as more sensitive and more diagnostically significant than the Frei test.

Control and Prevention

There are no immunological measures available for the prevention or cure of LGV. Since the World Health Organization is involved in a worldwide effort to find and treat syphilis using serological testing for locating cases, the logical approach to the control of LGV is the use of these same sera for the serodiagnosis of the latter as well as the former disease. Of course, finding cases of such communicable diseases has no value unless adequate facilities for treatment are available. Fortunately LGV can be cured by treatment with sulfonamides or antibiotics.

REFERENCES

Bedson, S. P. 1936. Observations bearing on the antigenic composition of psittacosis virus. *Brit. J. Exp. Pathol.* 17:109–121.

Bedson, S. P. and J. O. W. Bland. 1932. A morphological study of psittacosis virus, with the description of a developmental cycle. *Brit. J. Exp. Pathol.* 13:461–466.

Deacon, W. E. 1961. Fluorescent antibody methods for *Neisseria gonorrhoeae* identification. *Bull. World Health Org.* 24:349–455.

Frei, W. 1925. Eine neue Hautreaktion bei "Lymphogranuloma inguinale." *Klin. Wschr.* 4:2148–2149.

Hobson, D., and K. K. Holmes (eds.). 1977. *Nongonococcal Urethritis and Related Oculogenital Infections.* Washington: American Society for Microbiology.

Kellogg, D. S., Jr., I. R. Cohen, L. C. Norins, A. L. Schroeter, and G. Reising. 1968. *Neisseria gonorrhoeae. J. Bacteriol.* 96:596–605.

Kellogg, D. S., Jr., W. L. Peacock, Jr., W. E. Deacon, L. Brown, and C. I. Pirkle. 1963. *Neisseria gonorrhoeae.* I. Virulence genetically linked to clonal variation. *J. Bacteriol.* 85:1275–1279.

Lankford, C. E. and E. E. Snell. 1943. Glutamine as a growth factor for certain strains of *Neisseria gonorrhoeae. J. Bacteriol.* 45:410–411.

Lankford, C. E. and P. K. Skaggs. 1946. Cocarboxylase as a growth factor for certain strains of *Neisseria gonorrhoeae. Arch. Biochem.* 9:265–283.

Thayer, J. D. and J. E. Martin, Jr. 1964. A selective medium for the cultivation of *N. gonorrhoeae* and *N. meningitidis. Pub. Health Rep.* 79:49–58.

18

Syphilis

Syphilis (lues, great pox) is a human disease with conflicting evidence relative to its geographical origin. There is histological evidence (mummies) that the disease occurred in ancient civilizations in Africa and Asia. There are, moreover, mild, nonvenereal forms of syphilis (bejel) in the Middle East and parts of Africa that might have resulted from evolutionary host-parasite adaptations requiring thousands of years. By contrast it is a well-authenticated historical fact that a highly virulent form of the disease spread over Europe after the return of Columbus. The early clinical aspects of the disease at that time were much more severe than those of the current disease. The skin rash of the fifteenth and early sixteenth-century syphilis, in Europe, frequently included large ulcerative lesions that were designated "great pox" to distinguish the affliction from the disease smallpox. Much of the medical reputation of Paracelsus (around 1530) was based on his discovery that mercury would heal these skin ulcers.

Assuming that there had been no syphilis in Europe prior to 1492, the introduction of a new disease organism for which there was no population immunity might account for the high virulence of the disease at that time regardless of the geographical source. Again, the lesser virulence of the current disease as contrasted to the 1492 form in Europe could be the result of host-parasite evolution over the past 450 years. Whether the new, virulent strain of the spirochete was introduced into Europe from the West Indies by Columbus' sailors or from some African or Asian source by the mass movement of crusaders will, of course, never be established. Regardless of the source, the 1492 causative agent must have had different virulence and probably different antigenic characteristics from any prior disease organism experienced in epidemic form by the Europeans of that day.

ETIOLOGY

Determination of the etiology of syphilis took about 20 years from the time of Koch's establishment of the germ theory of disease and the etiology of anthrax in 1876. This was not due to

181

lack of effort—Lassar, in 1905, stated that "125 causes of syphilis have been established in the past 25 years." That same year two protozoologists, Shaudinn and Hoffman (1905), described the organism that has come to be regarded as the true cause of syphilis, even though it cannot be cultivated in its virulent form in nonliving media.

Because of the difficulty of seeing the organism with ordinary light microscopy, it was designated the pale spirochete and given the name *Spirochaeta pallida* or *Sp. pallidum.* Later it was placed in the genus *Treponema* with retention of the species designation *T. pallidum.*

Treponema pallidum is a tightly coiled, corkscrew-shaped organism ranging from 4 to 14 microns in length and possessing 6 to 15 coils (see Figure 18-1). The genus *Treponema* contains at least three other species pathogenic for humans or animals, and several saprophytic species, but *T. pallidum* is the only member of the genus commonly transmitted by genital contact and, therefore, considered to be the cause of a venereal disease. Due to its corkscrew shape and

Figure 18–1. Treponema pallidum. (a) FA stain. *(b)* Darkfield micrograph. (Courtesy of the Center for Disease Control, Atlanta, GA.)

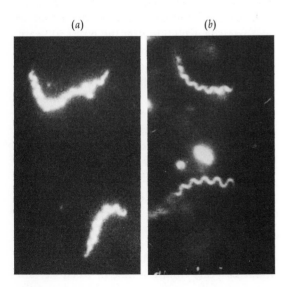

(*a*)   (*b*)

motility, *T. pallidum* has the capacity to penetrate thin, moist tissue membranes and travel into and out of lymph and blood channels.

Treponema pallidum, as stated, is difficult to see under ordinary light microscopy. Therefore, for demonstrating live motile treponemes, the use of dark-field microscopy is required. Moreover, the organisms are very difficult to stain with the ordinary bacterial stains. Negative staining has been advocated for demonstrating *T. pallidum* in smears on microslides. Zeigler et al. (1976) demonstrated capsular, envelope, or slime layer material on unwashed virulent *T. pallidum* but not on washed cells and not on avirulent strains.

In spite of claims to the contrary, virulent *T. pallidum* has never been cultivated on nonliving media. Culture strains, originally believed to be *T. pallidum* (for example, *T. reiteri*) either are not *T. pallidum* or, in adapting to growth on artificial media, have lost virulence for experimental animals and humans. Although all mammals tested appear to be at least partially susceptible to experimental infection (including latent infections) with *T. pallidum*, human beings are the only known host to be naturally infected. The rabbit is the experimental animal host usually used for the propagation of virulent *T. pallidum* for research or serodiagnosis.

Treponema pallidum is very susceptible to external environments. Heat (above 41°C), drying, ultraviolet light, and various chemicals, including ordinary soap, are treponemacidal. However, the spirochetes will survive and retain motility for some hours in fluid exudate from skin or mucus membrane lesions when collected and sealed in a capillary tube—a common means for delivering such specimens to the laboratory for taxonomic testing. Nelson (1948) formulated a sustaining medium that will maintain survival of *T. pallidum* for 4 to 7 days at room temperature (about 25°C). There is no evidence, however, that the spirochetes multiply during this survival period.

Treponema pallidum possesses a variety of antigens, some of which are shared by other treponemes, both saprophytic and pathogenic.

Although the location of a unique antigen on the spirochete has not been established, infection by *T. pallidum* results in the production of antibody that will react with alcoholic extracts of beef heart and certain other normal animal tissues. This Wasserman type antigen was one of the first recognized examples of the biological species (spirochete and bovine) heterogeneity of antigen distribution. Since *T. pallidum* could not be cultivated, the Wasserman type antigen was adapted to the serodiagnosis of syphilis. Subsequently, many other examples of heterophile species distribution of antigens have been discovered. One of these involves the alcohol-soluble Forssman's antigen, which is shared by certain pathogenic and nonpathogenic organisms, and certain normal animal tissues (guinea pig kidney and sheep red blood cells). Fortunately, beef heart tissue does not possess Forssman antigen—fortunate because normal human sera frequently possess Forssman antibody. Consequently, many false positive reactions could be expected if the serodiagnostic test antigen for syphilis also contained Forssman-type antigen. Even so, the anti–sheep-RBC Forssman antibody in the patient's serum may have to be absorbed onto sheep red blood cells and removed by centrifugation prior to performing a complement fixation test on the serum.

In addition to the heterophile antigen, *T. pallidum* possesses at least one antigen that is highly (but not absolutely) specific for virulent *T. pallidum*. Consequently, when a Wassermann-type antigen serodiagnostic test (for example, VDRL) is suspected of being falsely positive, it is common practice to test the individual's serum for the presence of the highly specific virulence antibody using virulent *T. pallidum* as the test antigen. Some means of absorbing or blocking the test serum antibodies to the cross-reacting antigens on the spirochetes is used to increase the specificity of the test (see Laboratory Diagnosis). For additional details, see Kelly (1974).

As indicated above, practically all body tissues, including placental, can be invaded by *T. pallidum*. Since there is little, if any, evidence of toxin production by the organism, the mechanism whereby the tissue damage (pathology) is accomplished is not comprehended.

CLINICAL SYMPTOMS

Regardless of the mechanism of pathogenicity by *T. pallidum*, the fact that practically any body tissue can be damaged results in clinical symptoms that vary from case to case. Sir William Osler called syphilis the great imitator, because in different cases it could imitate the symptoms of any other disease that might tend to damage the same tissues. One authority, during the era of Edgar Bergen, the ventriloquist, and Charlie McCarthy, his dummy, called syphilis the great ventriloquist among diseases because, in its final stages, it may speak out from any organ or tissue of the body. It should be noted, moreover, that periods of latency, or asymptomatic infections in syphilis, are quite common.

Clinical syphilis commonly is divided into three stages, although some authorities prefer two: early and late. We will discuss the three-stage category: primary, secondary, and tertiary syphilis.

Primary Syphilis

Primary syphilis usually is characterized, within 10 to 40 days after exposure, by an ulcer at the site of invasion by *T. pallidum*. The edges and base of this ulcer are indurated (the hard or Hunterian chancre). This primary chancre may occur on the skin of the genitalia in both male and female patients or on the vaginal membranes of the female where it can easily be missed. Since infectious lesions of secondary syphilis frequently occur in the mouth, the disease also may be transmitted by kissing. In such transmission, the primary chancre may occur on the lips, the cheeks, or the buccal membranes. This primary chancre is relatively painless and does not tend to expand laterally as does the soft chancre of Ducrey's infection. There are few, if any, constitutional symptoms at this stage. However, large numbers of *T. pallidum* are found in the walls and exudate within the primary chancre, making this a highly infectious stage of the disease. Also, spirochetes rapidly migrate away from the chancre through the underlying lymphatics. This results in a significant enlargement of the regional lymph node draining the area of the primary chancre. Therefore, although topical disinfection of the ulcer (as practiced by Paracelsus) may kill the local spirochetes and heal the chancre, it will not cure the disease. If the primary chancre does not occur, or if it is missed or ignored and the patient is not treated, there is a gradual change during the primary stage from seronegative to seropositive as syphilitic antibody is produced in response to the antigenic stimulation provided by the infection. Exudate from the primary chancre provides the earliest possible specimen for the diagnosis of a case of syphilis (see Laboratory Diagnosis).

Secondary Syphilis

The symptoms of secondary syphilis may onset from 2 weeks to 3 or more months after termination of the primary stage. Inadequate treatment during the primary stage may delay this onset even longer. The infectious lesions of secondary syphilis may involve the skin or the mucus membranes of the urinogenital tract, the mouth, and the eyes. Other secondary lesions containing spirochetes are found in various visceral organs, bone, blood, and other tissues. A common manifestation of secondary syphilis is a cutaneous rash. The rash may be papular, acneiform, erythematous, or pustular. The rash may be quite extensive or it may be so scanty and transient that it can easily be missed. The secondary lesions of the mucus membranes (mucus patches) contain large numbers of *T. pallidum,* and those in the urinogenital tract and the mouth are common sources of infection. Again, the lesions of secondary syphilis generally are relatively painless and the patient usually remains ambulatory. During secondary syphilis, serodiagnostic tests become increasingly positive, approaching 95 to 100 percent in

middle or late secondary stages. There are reported estimates that 20 to 25 percent of untreated cases either undergo spontaneous healing or prolonged latency following the secondary stage of the disease.

Tertiary Syphilis

The symptoms of tertiary syphilis may follow shortly after the secondary stage, or they may be delayed for months or occasionally years of latency. Nodular or ulcerative cutaneous lesions may occur. Subcutaneous or visceral gummatous (nodular) lesions up to the size of a hen's egg may develop. These may rupture with the discharge of a bloody, viscous fluid leading to deep and persistent ulceration. The accumulation of these ulcerative and necrotic tissue products may finally overwhelm the patient, thereby resulting in death. Live *T. pallidum* are difficult to find in the tertiary lesions, but their presence may be established by animal inoculation. The cardiovascular system may be damaged, weakening the arterial walls and resulting in aortic aneurisms and possible rupture. Neurosyphilis usually is a late development of the tertiary stage. Tabes dorsalis is a crippling form of neurosyphilis leading to locomotor ataxia or loss of coordination (the shuffling gait) due to degeneration of the dorsal columns of the spinal cord. General paresis is another form of neurosyphilis leading to progressive loss of mental faculties. This form is frequently associated with delusions of grandeur. One case in the Texas State Hospital at Austin enjoyed counting the cars on Guadalupe Street, because in his delusions he was the inventor of the automobile and was drawing a royalty on each one built. Unfortunately for him, general paresis usually terminates in more severe dementia and death in a few months to 5 years.

Along with decrease of the numbers of viable spirochetes in tertiary syphilis, the positivity of serodiagnostic tests decreases to approximately 75 percent. Also, transmissibility of the disease decreases during the tertiary stage.

As stated, *T. pallidum* in an infected mother can penetrate through the placenta to the fetus *in utero,* giving rise to congenitally acquired syphilis. About 40 percent of untreated cases of congenital syphilis lead to death and abortion of the fetus. Of the remaining congenital cases in which a live child is born, the child may show secondary or tertiary symptoms at birth. These usually result in death shortly after birth. Others may show no symptoms at birth but develop secondary or tertiary symptoms any time from the first to the tenth year after birth or occasionally later. Hutchinson reported a triad of symptoms, one or more of which commonly occur in congenital syphilitics who survive the infection:

1. Hutchinson teeth—in which the central permanent incisors (usually upper) are peg-shaped and possess a crescentic notch in the cutting edge (see Figure 18-2)
2. Interstitial keratitis—resulting in inflammation and cloudiness of the cornea leading to blindness
3. Deafness

Since fetal damage may occur early in the pregnancy of an infected mother, early diagnosis and treatment of the disease in the mother must be performed to prevent congenital syphilis. Obstetric care, therefore, should include a serodiagnostic test for syphilis early in pregnancy. If there is evidence of syphilitic infection, the

Figure 18–2. Hutchinson teeth of congenital syphilis (lower jaw). Note notches in incisors. (Courtesy of the Center for Disease Control, Atlanta, GA.)

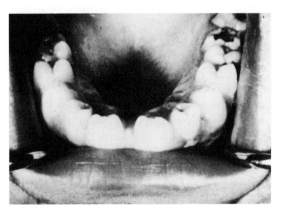

mother should be treated adequately to prevent congenital syphilis in her child.

PREVALENCE AND EPIDEMIOLOGY

Syphilis occurs worldwide and, like gonorrhea, the incidence is directly proportional to the sexual promiscuity and medical ignorance of the populace in the area under study. The incidence of syphilis, however, does not approach that of gonorrhea. The annual number of new civilian cases of syphilis reported in the United States climbed during the early 1960s to peak at 114,314 in 1964. Since that time there has been a continuous, gradual decrease in the United States to 80,356 in 1975 (see Table 17-1). This decreased incidence is the result of a nationwide program of syphilis eradication instituted by WHO and other public health authorities during the 1960s.

The major mode of transmission of syphilis, as stated, is by sexual intercourse. The primary vehicle for this genital contact transmission is exudate from infectious lesions, mainly chancres or mucus patches in or on the genitalia. Since, however, these infectious lesions can also occur at extragenital sites (skin, lips, buccal membranes), the exudate from such lesions can serve as a second or as the only primary vehicle. These extragenital contact infections are fairly frequent worldwide, and in the nonvenereal form of syphilis in the Middle East and Africa (bejel) such extragenital infections are the common mode of transmission. Blood on freshly contaminated razors and hypodermic needles (drug addicts) can serve as a primary vehicle also. Moreover, transfused infected blood can infect the recipient. Consequently blood donors must be screened to make sure they are free of this and other blood-borne diseases.

Freshly contaminated secondary vehicles have been claimed to be responsible for the transmission of syphilis. Possibly this is true in highly unsanitary environments, but the spirochetes of syphilis are very susceptible to conditions outside the body. Consequently noncontact (secondary vehicle) transmission of the disease, if it occurs, is extremely rare.

The incubation period of syphilis (from exposure to onset of primary chancre) is usually about 3 weeks (range 10 days to 6 weeks). If the primary chancre does not develop or if it is missed, the onset of recognizable secondary symptoms may be delayed for months. The patient becomes infectious to others with the development of the primary chancre and remains infectious as long as open lesions on skin or mucus membranes persist. In untreated syphilis, the infectious stage averages about 2 years. However, chemotherapy (penicillin) can render a patient noninfectious to others (including the fetus *in utero*) even though the therapy is inadequate to cure the patient permanently.

LABORATORY DIAGNOSIS

Serotaxonomy

The earliest possible means of diagnosing a case of syphilis is the demonstration of virulent *T. pallidum* in exudate from a primary chancre. The specimen for such a diagnosis is serous fluid from the untreated chancre. Before the specimen is collected, the chancre should be cleansed with cotton moistened with sterile saline—avoid using disinfectants on the chancre. After cleansing, the walls of the chancre should be pressed slightly to accumulate serous fluid (not blood) in the crater of the ulcer. A capillary tube inserted into this chancre fluid will accumulate around 0.05 milliliter of the specimen. If there is to be any delay in the microscopic examination of this specimen, it should be sealed in the tube by jabbing both ends into a semisolid beeswax-Vaseline mixture.

For preliminary examination, a small amount (about 0.01 milliliter) of the specimen should be mounted under a coverslip on a microslide and be examined by dark-field microscopy. The presence of morphologically typical, highly motile spirochetes in the specimen would be presumptive, but not definitive, evi-

dence of the presence of *T. pallidum* in the lesion. The spirochetes could be saprophytic treponemes or possibly other saprophytic or pathogenic genera of spirochetes, which might not be recognized as such by an inexperienced technologist.

If the laboratory is equipped for ultraviolet-light microscopy, the surest way to identify the spirochetes in the chancre fluid as *T. pallidum* is the direct FA technique. For this test, antiserum from an animal that has been immunized with virulent *T. pallidum* is needed. This antiserum must be absorbed with cultured *T. reiteri* to remove cross-reacting antibodies. The IgG from this absorbed anti–*T. pallidum* is then tagged with fluorescein isothiocyanate and may be kept in the refrigerator for subsequent use. Also, fluorescent (F) anti–*T. pallidum* can be purchased commercially. To perform the test, a smear of the chancre fluid containing the unknown spirochetes is fixed on a microslide. The smear is covered with the F anti–*T. pallidum* and allowed to react for 30 minutes at 37°C in a moist chamber. The antiserum is then washed off and the preparation is dried and examined with the ultraviolet-light microscope. If the spirochetes fluoresce, they are identified as *T. pallidum* or a treponeme with comparable antigenic identity (see Figure 18-1).

During secondary syphilis, the specimen for the serotaxonomic identification of *T. pallidum* may be (1) exudate from mucus patches, (2) scrapings from skin rashes, or (3) aspirated fluid from enlarged lymph nodes. Mucus patches are most likely to yield a sufficient number of treponemes to be found in microscopic examinations.

Serodiagnosis

As stated above, the first serodiagnostic test for syphilis was reported by August von Wassermann. He adapted the complement fixation test procedures developed by Bordet and Gengou in 1901 to the diagnosis of syphilis. For his test antigen, Wassermann used an emulsion of the liver of a stillborn fetus from a syphilitic mother.

This emulsion contained large numbers of *T. pallidum,* which Wassermann considered essential for a diagnostic test antigen. However, when controls using liver emulsion from a nonsyphilitic fetus also yielded positive test results with syphilitic sera and negative results with nonsyphilitic sera, the concept of a heterophile diagnostic antigen was first visualized. A variety of animal tissues were tested, and beef heart proved to be the choice for such a test antigen. The beef heart tissue was extracted with a variety of solvents, and an alcohol-soluble lipid proved to be the best test antigen for the routine serodiagnosis of syphilis. This alcoholic extract of beef heart tissue is frequently referred to as Wassermann-type antigen, and the complement fixation test for syphilis using this antigen is commonly known as the Wassermann test. Michaelis (1907) was the first to report that the Wassermann-type antigen could be used in a precipitation test as well as in a complement fixation test for the serodiagnosis of syphilis. The globulin in the patient's serum, with which the Wassermann-type antigen reacts, has been called *reagin.* Since the term *reagin* has been used in another antibody context, this author prefers to designate this reactive globulin as Wassermann-type antibody.

Over the years, the tests devised by Wassermann and by Michaelis have been modified extensively by various other serologists, each of whom gave their own name to the modified test—Kolmer, Eagle, Kahn, Kline, and others. A recent modification involved extensive purification of the beef heart extract by the personnel of the Venereal Disease Research Laboratory (VDRL) on Long Island, New York. They purified the alcoholic extract of beef heart to the extent of obtaining a reproducible product they designated cardiolipin. This cardiolipin, however, was so pure that it would not react with syphilitic antibody unless it was supplemented with lecithin. The earlier, crude alcoholic extracts of beef heart contained variable amounts of lecithin. The cardiolipin, however, can be supplemented with a known optimum amount of lecithin obtained in purified form from sources other than beef heart tissue. Also, the cardiolipin is supplemented with a sensitizing agent (cholesterol) that has been used since 1909 in Wassermann test antigens. The cholesterol does not react with Wassermann-type antibody, but it makes possible a positive reaction with smaller amounts of antibody (a more sensitive test) than is the case with the noncholesterolized antigen.

The VDRL cardiolipin-lecithin-cholesterol (CLC) antigen has been adapted to use in both complement fixation and precipitation tests for the routine serodiagnosis of syphilis. One of these, the VDRL precipitation test, is the most widely used test in the United States. It is a slide test in which a measured amount of the heat-inactivated (56°C for 30 minutes) test serum is mixed with a pretitrated amount (in one drop) of the antigen. The mixture, in a circumscribed ring on the slide, is rotated for a specified time on a mechanical rotator and then examined under low-power microscopic magnification. The size of the aggregates in the test preparation correlates the degree of reactivity of the serum (1+ to 4+). Positive and negative controls are always included in the testing procedure. As in other serodiagnostic tests, a quantitative VDRL test can be performed by using serial dilutions of the test serum in the foregoing procedure.

In serodiagnostic tests in which the Wassermann-type test antigen (beef heart, CLC) is so far removed taxonomically from the causative organism of the disease (*T. pallidum*), one might expect that diseases other than syphilis would give positive test results. Although this does occur, it is remarkably rare except in other treponemal human diseases such as yaws and pinta. Some, but not all, cases of leprosy and malaria and some smallpox vaccinees give false positive results with the CLC antigen serodiagnosis of syphilis. Very occasionally, the serum of an individual with no evidence of disease will give a false positive. Some authors call these "biological false positive" reactions. Since both true and false positive reactions are biological phenomena, the term in either context seems superfluous. However, no false positive laboratory diagnostic test is potentially more emotionally disconcerting than a false positive test for syphilis.

Consequently, much effort has been expended in attempts to design tests that would distinguish between true and false positive serodiagnostic results. These tests have tended to substitute treponemal antigen for the Wassermann-type (CLC and other) test antigen. One of these is the *T. pallidum* immobilization (TPI) test. In this test, live, virulent *T. pallidum* from infected rabbits are mixed with the patient's heat-inactivated serum and added guinea pig serum complement. This spirocheticidal test is examined with a dark-field microscope to determine whether or not the *T. pallidum* are immobilized (killed) as a result of anti–*T. pallidum* in the patient's serum. As perfomed, the TPI test does not distinguish satisfactorily between true and false positive results; nor does the *T. pallidum* complement fixation (TPCF) test or the *T. reiteri* complement fixation (TRCF) test, in which the respective killed treponemes serve as the test antigen.

An indirect FA test—designated the FTA-ABS test—has been designed, using a smear of virulent *T. pallidum* on a microslide, as the test antigen. The killed *T. pallidum* can be purchased in lyophilized form, thereby making the testing procedure more available to qualified laboratories (see Hunter et al. 1964). In addition to the smear of virulent *T. pallidum*, the test requires the following reagents and major equipment:

1. The patient's serum
2. Sorbent—an extract containing *T. reiteri* antigens
3. Fluorescent (F) anti–human IgG antibody
4. An ultraviolet-light source
5. An ultraviolet-light microscope

The test is performed by diluting the patient's serum 1:5 in sorbent. This blocks or absorbs cross-reacting antibodies in the patient's serum that are not specific for the *T. pallidum* virulence antigen. The *T. pallidum* smear on the microslide is covered with the sorbent-treated patient's serum. The slide is placed in a moist chamber at 37°C for 30 minutes to allow specific antibody in the patient's serum, if any, to react with the virulent *T. pallidum* antigen. If the patient's serum possesses unblocked antibody specific for virulent *T. pallidum,* that antibody globulin will be attached to the *T. pallidum* on the slide, but it cannot be seen. The excess serum is washed off the slide. The smear is then covered with F anti–human IgG and replaced in the moist chamber for 30 minutes at 37°C. This allows the F anti–human IgG to react with the human IgG, if any, on the surface of the *T. pallidum* cells. The excess F anti–human IgG is washed off and the slide is prepared for examination with the ultraviolet-light microscope. If the spirochetes on the slide fluoresce, it indicates that the patient's serum had antibody specific for the virulent *T. pallidum*. If they fail to fluoresce, the FA test is negative.

As a general rule, a false positive VDRL (or other Wassermann-type antigen test) is indicated by a negative FTA-ABS test. In 1970, however, a young woman was given a routine VDRL test as a prerequisite to being granted a marriage license. When the test was positive, the young woman was most upset. She denied having had sexual intercourse or any symptoms that might have been syphilis. Upon physical examination her hymen was found to be intact. Her fiancee also had no evidence of syphilis, past or present. An FTA-ABS test was performed on the young woman's serum and it, too, was positive. A quantitative VDRL test was positive at a 1:8 serum dilution. The patient had received a smallpox vaccination a month earlier. Since smallpox vaccination is known to cause occasional false positive reactions, and since there was no clinical or epidemiological evidence of syphilis, the marriage license was granted. Two weeks later, the two serodiagnostic tests were repeated and the VDRL titer had decreased to 1:2 and the FTA-ABS test was negative. When the patient was retested 3 months later, after marriage, both tests were negative. This decrease in antibody titer would not have occurred if the individual had been and continued to be infected with *T. pallidum*. Thus it is obvious that even the FTA-ABS test is not absolute in its ability to distinguish between true and false positive Wassermann-type antigen serodiagnostic results. Nevertheless, the FTA-ABS test, combined with the follow-up quantitative serodiagnostic tests to note a falling antibody titer, is the best means available for establishing the absence of syphilis in an individual giving a false positive serodiagnosis. For additional considerations see Wood (1974).

IMMUNOLOGY

As indicated above, a variety of antibodies, including treponemacidal antibodies, result from *T. pallidum* infections. Although some cases of syphilis undergo spontaneous cure, there is no conclusive evidence that these cures are a consequence of the presence of humoral antibody. Moreover, there appears to be an infection-associated immunity in that syphilitics rarely develop a second primary chancre when reexposed during the course of their infection. Jones et al. (1976) reported results of studies of syphilis vaccines in rabbits. Using *T. pallidum* with intact capsules as killed vaccines, they reported encouraging results. They also studied the effects of a variety of adjuvants on the immunogenicity of their vaccine. However, there are no immunoprophylactic or immunotherapeutic procedures available for human use.

CONTROL AND PREVENTION

The surest individual means of preventing syphilis is the avoidance of sexual promiscuity. Prostitutes, both male and female, and other promiscuous individuals, heterosexual or otherwise, constitute the major sources of infection. Disinfection of external genitalia or the use of vaginal douches after exposure may or may not prevent infection. Treponemacidal drugs can be used both prophylactically or therapeutically. After Paul Ehrlich reported the therapeutic efficacy of his six hundred and sixth chemical compound tested (arsphenamine), this drug and later modifications became the drugs of choice for the treatment of syphilis and other spiro-

chetoses. Because of the toxicity of the arsenicals, however, massive doses could not be used and prolonged weekly administration (for about 18 months) was required for reasonable certainty of cure. It soon became clear, however, that even though a few doses of the arsenicals would not cure the patient, they would prevent the transmission of the disease to others, including transmission to the fetus *in utero*. Thus early diagnosis and treatment of the pregnant mother became routine obstetric practice to prevent congenital syphilis.

With the discovery that the relatively nontoxic penicillin was effective in both the prophylactic and therapeutic aspects of syphilis, this drug has replaced the arsenicals and related compounds for these purposes. Both the prevention of congenital syphilis and the cure of the pregnant patient can now be accomplished by a few weeks of treatment with massive doses of penicillin. The earlier a diagnosis is made (primary chancre preferably), the greater the chances of cure. If the patient is hypersensitive to penicillin, then tetracycline or other broad-spectrum antibiotics can be substituted. For treatment schedules recommended by the CDC, see *MMWR* (9 April 1976).

Public health procedures for the prevention of syphilis include (1) providing laboratory facilities for finding cases, including the "sero-diagnostic dragnet" in high-incidence environments; (2) clinical (VD) facilities for treating and thereby disinfecting cases; (3) epidemiological services to trace known contacts and thereby enable early diagnosis and treatment of these potential new sources of infection. For a detailed discussion of national and international (WHO) control measures, see Bennenson (1970).

REFERENCES

Bennenson, A. S. (ed.). 1970. *Control of Communicable Diseases in Man.* 11th ed. New York: American Public Health Association.

Hunter, E. F., W. E. Deacon, and P. E. Meyer. 1964. An improved test for syphilis—the absorption procedure (FTA-ABS). *Pub. Health Rep.* 79: 410–412.

Jones, A. M., J. A. Zeigler, and R. H. Jones. 1976. Experimental syphilis vaccines in rabbits. I. Differential protection with an adjuvant spectrum. *Brit. J. Vener. Dis.* 52:9–17.

Kelly, R. T. 1974. *Treponema*. Chapter 36 in *Manual of Clinical Microbiology*.

Michaelis, L. 1907. Precipitinreaktion bei Syphilis. *Klin. Wschr.* 44:1477.

Nelson, R. A. 1948. Factors affecting the survival of *Treponema pallidum* in vitro. *Amer. J. Hyg.* 48: 120–132.

Schaudinn, F. and E. Hoffmann. 1905. Ueber Spirochatenbefunde in Lymphdrusensaft Syphilitischer. *Deutsch. med. Wschr.* 31:711.

Wood, R. W. 1974. Tests for syphilis. Chapter 51 in *Manual of Clinical Microbiology*.

Ziegler, J. A., A. M. Jones, R. H. Jones, and K. M. Kubica. 1976. Demonstration of extracellular material at the surface of pathogenic *T. pallidum* cells. *Brit. J. Vener. Dis.* 52:1–8.

19

Unusual or Exotic Contact Diseases

The miscellaneous contact subgroup diseases include those transmitted from animals to humans as a result of occupational or recreational contacts among other modes of transmission—such as tularemia (discussed in Chapter 22). Also included is contact with contaminated surfaces such as shower stalls, swimming pool facilities, and other moist environments involved in many of the fungal diseases discussed in Chapter 21. This subgroup may be further extended to the staphylococcal and the nosocomial (hospital-acquired) diseases discussed in Chapter 20. Thus Chapter 19 serves as a sort of catch-all chapter for diseases that involve unknown or unusual types of contact in their transmission or are rare or absent in America although they may be prevalent and even epidemic in other parts of the world. Such diseases as anthrax, leprosy, yaws, ornithosis (psittacosis), Q fever, aseptic pneumonitis, infectious mononucleosis, Lassa fever, and Marburg fever are considered briefly here.

ANTHRAX

Etiology

As indicated in Chapter 2, the animal disease anthrax (charbon) occupied a prominent historical niche in pathogenic microbiology. Davaine demonstrated the presence of anthrax bacilli in the blood of all diseased sheep examined and the capacity to transmit the disease by the inoculation of blood from infected sheep to healthy animals. Thereby he fulfilled two of the etiological requirements postulated by Professor

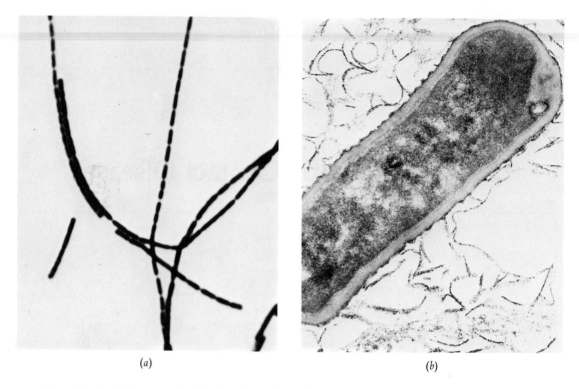

(a)   (b)

Figure 19–1. (a) Gram-stained chains of *Bacillus anthracis* cells from a patient's lesion after culture on artificial media. (b) Electron micrograph of a cell of *B. anthracis;* note the gram-positive cell wall morphology. 26,420×. ((a) Courtesy of P. S. Brachman; (b) courtesy of S. C. Holt.)

Henle at Göttingen. It remained for Robert Koch, in 1876, to isolate the anthrax bacilli in pure culture and to use these in the transmission of the disease. Also he proceeded to reisolate the same bacilli from the experimentally infected animals. Pasteur then spectacularly demonstrated the efficacy of his weakened anthrax bacillus vaccine to immunize sheep against exposure to virulent anthrax bacilli.

The anthrax bacillus is a nonmotile, gram-positive, aerobic, spore-forming rod with flattened ends (Figure 19-1) and a tendency to grow in chains. The taxonomic designation is *Bacillus anthracis.* It can be cultivated on simple peptone, beef-extract nutrient agar, although the addition of 5 percent sheep blood to such agar media frequently is preferred. Capsules develop when sodium bicarbonate is added to the medium and incubation is in an increased CO_2 atmosphere. Spores generally are not demonstrable in blood

or exudate from infected animals. *Bacillus anthracis* colonies do not hemolyze the blood in the agar medium as do most common *Bacillus* species that might be mistaken for *B. anthracis* — such as *B. cereus.* (However, rare nonhemolytic strains of *B. cereus* have been reported.)

Epidemiology and Clinical Symptoms

Anthrax is primarily a disease of herbivorous animals — cattle, horses, sheep, goats, camels, deer, and others. Two north Texas counties reported the deaths of 160 cattle and horses from confirmed or presumptive anthrax during July to September 1976 (see *MMWR,* 24 September 1976). Because of the spores, which develop after the death of the infected animal, *B. anthracis* can live almost indefinitely in contaminated soil or on animal products such as the hides or hair from infected animals (see Figure 19-2). Anthrax

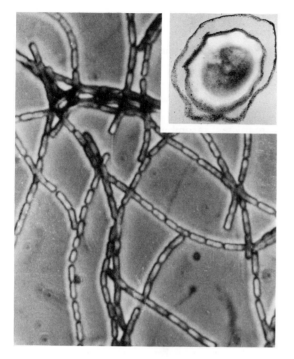

Figure 19–2. Chains of *B. anthracis* cells showing spores; the material from a patient's lesion has been incubated for more than 24 hours on artificial media. About 5250×. Inset: Electron micrograph of a thin section through a free-spore. 26,600×. (Courtesy of P. S. Brachman; inset courtesy of S. C. Holt.)

bacilli or their spores can infect human beings through scratches or abrasions in the skin, where they cause a characteristic cutaneous lesion with a black center surrounded by blisterlike vesicles (see Figure 19-3). The anthrax spores can also infect human beings by the respiratory route, resulting in pneumonic symptoms; in Pasteur's time this respiratory anthrax was designated woolsorter's disease. If untreated, anthrax infections may result in a massive, highly fatal septicemia. Imported goatskin bongo drums, rugs, pack saddle pads, and other goatskin items from the West Indies have been incriminated in the transportation of anthrax spores into the United States. Twenty-three of 42 such items (55 percent) imported from Haiti and tested by CDC in 1976–1977 yielded anthrax spores. Unfortunately there is no practical means of disinfecting such items

(see *MMWR*, 4 February 1977). In January 1976, mixed goat and camel hair yarn imported from Pakistan was found to be heavily contaminated with anthrax spores after it caused the death of a California male. Sixty-two pounds of this yarn were collected locally by the Houston Health Department and destroyed (personal communication from R. A. MacLean, M.D.). Nevertheless, even including these cases, only 13 cases of human anthrax were reported in the United States during the 5-year period from 1971 through 1975. For more details see Wright (1965).

Laboratory Diagnosis

The specimens for the laboratory diagnosis of human anthrax are (1) scrapings from the vesiculated periphery of skin lesions, (2) exudate coughed up from pulmonary anthrax, or (3) blood from septicemic anthrax. Smears of the specimen should be gram-stained and examined for morphologically typical organisms. If ultraviolet microscopy is available, a fluorescent antibody stained smear should be examined. The specimens should be streak-inoculated to blood agar with and without added sodium bicarbonate and should be incubated aerobically at 35°C for 18 to 24 hours in an atmosphere of 5

Figure 19–3. Cutaneous anthrax on arm of a woman who had been a carder in a wool factory. (Courtesy of the Center for Disease Control, Atlanta, GA.)

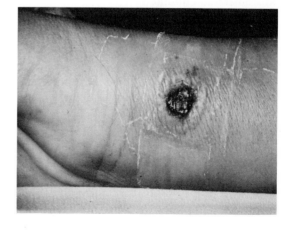

percent added CO_2. The diagnosis of anthrax in animals usually is performed by veterinary medical laboratories (see Stein 1944). For differential characteristics of *B. anthracis* and the common soil saprophyte *B. cereus* and for other laboratory diagnostic considerations, see Feeley and Brachman (1974).

Control and Prevention

The major measures for control of anthrax are directed against the disease in domestic animals. These are enforced by the Bureau of Animal Industry (BAI) and include (1) prompt vaccination of the healthy animals, on infected premises, with the Sterne modification of the Pasteur vaccine; (2) quarantine against the shipment of animals from the infected area; (3) burning or burying (in lime) of dead animals; and (4) a vigilant search for new cases. Anthrax should be suspected whenever an herbivorous animal has died suddenly; and an ear or other specimens should be submitted to a veterinary laboratory for confirmatory diagnosis.

Immunity and Chemotherapy

Animals recovering from an attack of anthrax are immune to subsequent exposure. As previously indicated, Pasteur used weakly virulent anthrax bacilli as a vaccine to protect animals against the disease. M. Sterne, in 1939, devised a safer and more stable modification of the Pasteur vaccine that is approved by the BAI for use in animal immunization.

Although no widely used anthrax vaccine for the protection of high-risk humans is available, sulfonamides, penicillin, and broad-spectrum antibiotics have been proved effective as chemotherapeutic agents. Early diagnosis and treatment will cure most cases of anthrax.

LEPROSY

Etiology

Leprosy, a disease of great antiquity, dates back to the early Chinese civilizations and was well recognized in early biblical times (see Skinsnes 1964; Skinsnes and Elvove 1970). In those times the leper was required to go about crying "unclean" in order to prevent contact transmission to others.

Hansen was the first to report the presence of acid-fast bacilli in leprosy lesions. These organisms resemble tubercle bacilli both in morphology and staining characteristics but have never been grown on nonliving media. Therefore, although they have been found in every case of leprosy examined, their claim to etiology has not been proved by the Henle-Koch postulate requiring isolation in pure culture. The organisms are straight or slightly curved, slender, nonmotile, acid-fast rods found in packets or bundles in the cytoplasm of infected cells.

For years no experimental animal was available for research on leprosy until C. C. Shepard, in 1963, reported the experimental infection of mice by means of inoculation of human leprous material into the mouse footpads. Since the common cutaneous and nasal mucosa lesions of leprosy in humans are areas of low body temperature, the infection of mice in the low temperature footpad provides an interesting man/mouse temperature correlation. Eleanor Storrs of the Gulf South Research Institute of Louisiana, in 1971, reported experimental infection of the armadillo with leprosy bacilli from human lesion material. This again provides a low-temperature correlation because the whole body temperature of the armadillo ranges between 87 and 92°F. The Storrs group later reported finding seven armadillos from widely scattered areas of Louisiana to be naturally infected with leprosy bacilli. This finding suggests a possible animal reservoir for this disease. Although the Henle-Koch etiology postulates for leprosy have not yet been fulfilled, the taxonomic designation for the accepted etiological agent is *Mycobacterium leprae.*

Epidemiology and Clinical Symptoms

Human leprosy occurs as cutaneous nodular lesions, as neural anesthetic lesions, or as a combination of both. The disease has been classified as *lepromatous* or *tuberculoid*. In the lepromatous type, the lesions contain many bacilli, the lepromin skin test (comparable to the tuberculin test in TB) is negative, and the prognosis is poor. In the tuberculoid type, the lesions contain few bacilli, the lepromin skin test is positive, and the prognosis is good.

In nodular leprosy, the raised skin nodules usually occur on exposed surfaces such as the face, arms, or legs. The nodules frequently ulcerate and the exudate contains large numbers of *M. leprae.* In neural leprosy the peripheral nerves, especially the sensory nerves, are attacked, producing anesthesia in the area of involvement. The cartilage of the nose is often destroyed, moreover, and many other organs or tissues, with the exception of voluntary muscles, may be attacked. Fingers or toes may atrophy and drop off. One cured leper at the medical school in Galveston formerly took especial delight in displaying a mummified finger he carried in his coat pocket. During the decade 1966 through 1976, some 1,227 cases of leprosy were reported in the United States. The annual incidence ranged from a low of 81 cases in 1967 to a high of 162 cases in 1975—with an average of 122.7 cases per year. In 1975, the Pacific states of California (78), Hawaii (30), and Oregon (4) accounted for 112 of the 162 reported cases (see *MMWR* supplement, August 1976).

Although contact transmission involving exudate from open lesions is the obvious mode of infection, the factors involved are not clear. Seemingly, prolonged close association with a leper is essential for transmission of the infection.

Laboratory Diagnosis

In nodular or lepromatous leprosy, large numbers of acid-fast bacilli can be demonstrated in specimens from the lesions. A superficial incision of the skin covering a leprosy nodule is used to prepare multiple impression smears on a microslide. These smears are fixed and stained for acid fastness by techniques described for *Mycobacterium tuberculosis* (see Chap-

ter 9). Smears of exudate from any suspected leprosy lesions should be comparably stained and examined for acid-fast bacilli, with the expectation that few organisms will be found in lesions of tuberculoid leprosy. For extensive considerations of the laboratory diagnosis of *Mycobacterium* species see Runyon et al. (1974).

Control and Prevention

For years the only means of controlling the spread of leprosy was lifelong commitment to a leprosarium with no expectation of cure. The leprosarium for the continental United States is located at Carville, Louisiana. Following the discovery of the sulfonamides, however, a related drug (a sulfone) was proved to be effective in leprosy therapy. Consequently commitment to a leprosarium no longer involves the hopelessness of the former patient. Many cures have been reported, and now, with mice and the armadillo as experimental animals, new therapeutic drugs for leprosy can be anticipated.

YAWS

Etiology

Yaws (frambesia) is a human disease virtually restricted to the tropical areas of the world and is most prevalent in socioeconomically depressed populations living under poor hygienic conditions. The causative organism is *Treponema pertenue,* which in motility, morphology, staining, and certain other characteristics is indistinguishable from *T. pallidum* (the causative agent of syphilis). A third human treponematosis (pinta) is caused by *Treponemea carateum* with characteristics similar to the human treponemes described above. Furthermore a fourth (nonhuman) treponeme, *T. cuniculi,* is a common rabbit pathogen that shares certain antigens and other characteristics with the human pathogens. Since rabbits are used as experimental animals for treponemal research and for the production of test antigens (virulent *T. pallidum*) and antisera for the diagnosis of syphilis, natural *T. cuniculi* infections in these animals must be ruled out.

Epidemiology and Clinical Symptoms

The initial lesion in yaws appears, after an incubation period of 3 to 4 weeks, as a painless florid papule surrounded by an area of inflammation. The papule gradually increases in size, erodes, and ulcerates. The exudate dries to form a dark crust. From 6 weeks to 3 months later, either before or after the "mother yaw" has healed, generalized secondary lesions of the mother yaw type occur. Successive crops of such lesions may appear over a period of months to years. When the papules develop on the soles of the feet, a hyperkeratosis develops, leading to "crab yaws"—one of the most common and incapacitating lesions. Late symptoms may include deep ulcerative skin lesions, rhinopharyngeal lesions, and crippling bone and joint lesions. The mode of transmission of yaws involves contact with exudate from open lesions. Although *T. pertenue* will not penetrate unbroken skin, even microscopic abrasions may serve as the portal of entry.

Laboratory Diagnosis

Generally the characteristics of the mother yaw are sufficient to warrant a clinical diagnosis. In any case, highly motile *T. pertenue* can be demonstrated in the lesion exudate by dark-field microscopy. Moreover, infection with *T. pertenue* (as well as *T. carateum*) tends to stimulate the production of Wassermann-type antibody in the patient, which can be demonstrated by the VDRL or other Wassermann-type antigen serodiagnostic tests.

Control and Prevention

As indicated in Chapter 18, WHO has been involved for a decade or more in a "find and treat" campaign to eradicate syphilis, and the same serological test procedures have uncovered many cases of yaws. The latter disease has proved to be even more amenable to treatment with penicillin than is syphilis. Consequently the incidence of yaws has been reduced spectacularly wherever these diagnostic and treatment procedures have been applied.

PSITTACOSIS (ORNITHOSIS)

A mild human disease contracted by contact with members of the parrot family of birds (psittacine birds) was recognized in Switzerland in 1880 and designated *psittacosis* (parrot fever). In the 1930s, however, a number of severe to fatal cases of psittacosis were recognized in various parts of the world including the United States. The American cases were traced to recently imported parrots or parakeets from South America. Subsequently the disease organisms were found in wild psittacine birds living in the bush country of Australia. The infection was also established in parakeets bred and raised in the United States and Germany. Later, the disease was traced to petrels, sea gulls, pigeons, chickens, ducks, turkeys, and other nonpsittacine birds. Since ornithology includes both psittacine and nonpsittacine birds, the more inclusive designation *ornithosis* has been accepted as a proper name for the human disease regardless of the source of infection.

Etiology

The causative agent of psittacosis was first considered to be a virus, but extensive studies of different strains of the agent isolated from cases of psittacosis-ornithosis, from lymphogranuloma venereum (see Chapter 17), and from birds and mammals have ruled against the viral nature of the agent. It still is a mystery how such a variety of clinical entities can be caused by different strains of the same genus and species *Chlamydia psittaci*. As indicated in Chapter 17, *C. psittaci* possesses both DNA and RNA, has cell-wall material characteristic of bacteria, and is an obligate intracellular parasite. As a consequence of these and other characteristics, it is now classified as a member of the order Rickettsiales. See Meyer (1965) for a more comprehensive discussion.

Epidemiology and Clinical Symptoms

Human ornithosis infections can range from asymptomatic to mild, to severe, to fatal. The disease in the natural hosts frequently is asymptomatic (latent), even though the *C. psittaci* may be shed in respiratory and fecal discharges. Fatal epizootics, however, have been reported in birds in captivity (aviaries). The human disease usually involves a pneumonitis. After an incubation period of 1 to 2 weeks, the onset symptoms include chills and fever, sore throat, nausea, and vomiting. A persistent dry cough may be the main symptom of pneumonic involvement. This pneumonitis is best demonstrated by chest X-ray examination, but it is very apparent at autopsy of fatal cases. A septicemia can be demonstrated during the first week of symptoms. Neurological symptoms may indicate central nervous system involvement. Necropsy evidence of focal necrotic lesions in the liver, spleen, kidneys, heart, and other organs indicates the possible generalized nature of pathological involvement.

Prior to the recognition of the extent of asymptomatic and mild cases, the mortality rate in human psittacosis was reported to be 20 to 30 percent. This was later reduced to about 10 percent; and, with the advent of effective antibiotic (tetracycline and others) therapy, the mortality of early diagnosed cases is nil.

As indicated above, *C. psittaci* is shed in the respiratory secretions and fecal discharges of infected birds. Early cases of psittacosis were attributed to respiratory infection due to contact exposure to parakeets (love birds). It was later established that *C. psittaci* could remain viable for a year or more in dried fecal droppings from infected birds, and airborne infection by this vehicle appeared to be a major mode of transmission. Several outbreaks of human ornithosis have occurred in workers involved in processing turkeys for the market. One such outbreak in June 1976 occurred in a Nebraska poultry processing plant—it involved 28 of the plant's 98 employees, who at the time were processing turkeys raised in Texas (see *MMWR*, 1 October 1976). Efforts to establish the presence of infection in turkey flocks by using the direct complement fixation test failed, however. Turkey antiornithosis antibody, even though it reacts with and blocks ornithosis antigen determinant sites, fails to fix complement—it is an incomplete antibody. Consequently an indirect complement fixation test had to be devised. This involved the use of rabbit, human, or other animal antiornithosis antiserum that *will* fix complement when it reacts with ornithosis antigen. When a turkey serum test is negative, it could mean either the presence of no antiornithosis antibody or incomplete antiornithosis antibody in the serum. To resolve these possibilities, a duplicate of the negative turkey serum test receives rabbit antiornithosis antiserum, following incubation with the turkey serum, before adding the indicator system. If this test continues to be negative, whereas a control with only rabbit antiornithosis antibody is positive, it proves the presence of incomplete antibody in the turkey serum that had reacted with and blocked the ornithosis antigen as indicated by the continued negativity of the indirect complement fixation test. This procedure makes possible the certification of ornithosis-free turkey flocks by complement fixation testing. Ornithosis also can be passed from human to human by the respiratory mode of transmission.

Laboratory Diagnosis

Warning: Accidental infections among clinical laboratory personnel are quite common, especially when experimental animal inoculations are involved in the diagnostic procedures. The laboratory diagnosis of ornithosis should thus be performed by adequately trained personnel in laboratories properly equipped for rickettsial and viral diagnostic procedures. Preferably the laboratory specimens (blood, sputum, or autopsy material) should be submitted to a state or national public health laboratory that is equipped and specializes in these diagnoses. For details of laboratory diagnosis of *C. psittaci* infections see Hanna et al. (1974).

Control and Prevention

There are no immunological measures applicable to the control or prevention of ornithosis. As indicated above, human *C. psittaci* infections can be cured by treatment with the tetracyclines. Therefore early diagnosis and adequate tetracycline therapy are the best control measures for human ornithosis. From the public health point of view, constant vigilance against the importation of psittacine birds from known endemic areas of the world is justified. The certification of ornithosis-free aviaries and turkey flocks has been a widely practiced control measure in the past.

Q FEVER

Etiology

Q fever is a rickettsial disease that was first recognized as a new human clinical entity by E. H. Derrick in a study of nine cases of a febrile illness among abattoir workers in Australia in 1935. Derrick questioned the nature of the disease and, therefore, designated it Q (query) fever. Because F. M. Burnet identified the causative agent as a rickettsia, it was named *Rickettsia burneti*. Davis and Cox (1938) identified a filterable (Berkefeld W) agent from a tick (*Dermacentor andersoni*) in Montana as a rickettsia and designated their isolate *R. diaporica*. Subsequent studies by R. E. Dyer indicated that *R. burneti* and *R. diaporica* were identical. Cox et al. (1947) reported an outbreak of Q fever among slaughterhouse workers in the United States. Because of marked differences between the rickettsiae of Q fever and those of other members of the genus *Rickettsia*, the Q fever etiological agent has been designated *Coxiella burneti*. It and the disease Q fever have been found to occur practically worldwide (see Ormsbee 1965).

Several characteristics differentiate *C. burneti* from members of the genus *Rickettsia*: its tendency to include a filterable stage in its life cycle; its greater resistance to drying; its failure to form a toxin; its failure to cause skin rashes; its independence of an arthropod vector in its transmission; and its antigenic distinction from other rickettsiae. Like other rickettsiae, however, *C. burneti* is an obligate intracellular parasite; it infects and grows extensively in the yolk sac membranes of embryonated eggs; it can be transmitted from animal to animal by arthropods (ticks); and it causes febrile infections in guinea pigs.

Epidemiology and Clinical Symptoms

Although fatal cases of Q fever do occur, they are much less common than those caused by spotted fever of the Rocky Mountain type, epidemic typhus fever, and other diseases involving rickettsiae of the genus *Rickettsia* (see Chapters 31 and 32). Animal host infections frequently are asymptomatic, and human infections range from mild to severe but are rarely fatal. After an incubation period of 2 to 4 weeks (average 20 days), the onset of symptoms is sudden: chilly sensations or frank chills followed by fever and persistent severe headache, general malaise, myalgia, and frequent chest pains in some outbreaks. Although the disease usually involves a primary atypical pneumonia, the extent of pulmonary involvement may vary considerably. It is best demonstrated by chest X ray. Loss of appetite is common and in combination with nausea and vomiting may contribute to marked weight loss.

When Q fever was first diagnosed among abattoir workers, it was assumed that contact with the carcasses of infected cattle was the mode of transmission. Further study indicated that workers in the pens were more prone to contract the disease than those in the butchering area, however. Moreover, human cases were traced to dusty sheep pens on California ranches. The fact that *C. burneti* are shed in large numbers in the feces of infected ticks and in the milk and urine of infected animals, and survive for months in the dried state in these vehicles, tends to implicate dust aerosols as the probable mode of transmission to humans. Person-to-person transmission of Q fever, although reported, is believed to be rare. Yet it is difficult otherwise to explain some of the extensive epidemics that have been reported, particularly those in the Mediterranean area during World War II. For more extensive considerations, see Ormsbee (1965).

Laboratory Diagnosis

Clinically, the early stages of Q fever can simulate the onset of a variety of other infectious diseases—typhoid and other salmonelloses, brucellosis, hepatitis, and leptospirosis (see Part III) and dengue fever and other rickettsioses (see Part IV). Even the symptoms of atypical pneumonia are the same as those caused by a number of viruses. Consequently, laboratory aid is essential to clinch a specific diagnosis of Q fever. If the patient gives a history of direct or indirect contact with cattle or sheep, Q fever should be suspected. The laboratory specimens from early cases include blood, urine, and sputum. Although guinea pigs and hamsters are highly susceptible to *C. burneti*, inoculation of these animals poses a hazard to laboratory and other personnel in the building. Blood specimens may be inoculated into the yolk sac of 5–6-day-old chick embryos that are incubated at 36.5°C. Prior to animal or yolk sac inoculation, urine or sputum should be treated with bactericidal antibiotics (penicillin, streptomycin, erythromycin) that do not affect the growth of *C. burneti*. The yolk sac can be harvested 7 to 11 days after

Figure 19–4. FA stain of *Coxiella burneti* in yolk sac smear of experimentally infected chick embryo. 1080×. (Courtesy of W. Burgdorfer.)

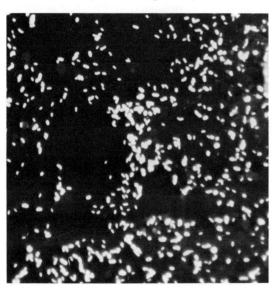

inoculation or on the death of the embryo. A smear of the infected yolk sac membrane may be stained with Giemsa or other polychromatic stains and will reveal large numbers of coccus, coccobacillary, or bacillary forms. If fluorescent anti–*C. burneti* antibody is available, this may be used to identify *C. burneti* in the yolk sac smear (see Figure 19-4). The serotaxonomic complement fixation test can be used to identify the *C. burneti* in the yolk sac membrane. Tissue cultures can also be used to propagate *C. burneti*.

In serodiagnostic studies, an antigenic phase variation phenomenon was reported by Berge and Lennette and was explained by Stoker and Fiset (1956). Upon isolation from patients or animals, *C. burneti* is in antigenic phase 1, which is characterized by reacting only with late (convalescent) serum antibody. After 8 to 20 passages in chick embryo yolk sac the *C. burneti* isolate converts to antigenic phase 2, which will react with antibody produced much earlier in the infection. Obviously phase 2 *C. burneti* is the serodiagnostic antigen of choice. A single passage of phase 2 *C. burneti* through a guinea pig, however, will cause a reversion to phase 1. The quantitative complement fixation test is performed on paired sera (early and late) to establish a rising titer to *C. burneti* phase 2 antigen. A single high titer to antigenic phase 1 *C. burneti* has been interpreted as evidence of a persistent or chronic infection. For a comprehensive discussion of the laboratory diagnosis of rickettsial diseases in general, including Q fever, see Ormsbee (1974).

Control and Prevention

Killed *C. burneti* vaccines have been used to immunize persons in high-risk jobs, but the severe nodular and frequent persistent abscess reactions at the site of vaccine injection have tended to restrict their usage. Live, attenuated *C. burneti* have been experimented with as vaccines; but to this author's knowledge, such vaccines are not commercially available for preventive purposes.

For chemotherapeutic purposes, the tetracyclines appear to be the drug of choice, although they have not always proved effective. Penicillin, erythromycin, and streptomycin, as indicated above, are *not* effective in Q fever therapy.

VIRAL DISEASES

A number of viral diseases including viral pneumonia might be included in the miscellaneous contact subgroup. Most cases of aseptic pneumonia (viral pneumonitis) probably are better included in the respiratory contact subgroup, however. Usually their diagnosis is idiopathic—based on not finding a bacterial or other nonviral cause for the pneumonic pathology. Another viral disease, infectious mononucleosis (IM), is better included in the respiratory contact subgroup. In fact, it might be considered a prototype of this group: Such close contact is required for transmission that it has been designated the "kissing disease." The diagnosis of IM is aided by the fact that the leucocytosis that develops during the course of the disease consists of a relatively high percentage of mononuclear leucocytes (monocytes) and a relatively low percentage of polymorphonuclear leucocytes. Furthermore, the IM patient develops a high titer of heterophile antibody demonstrable by the agglutination of sheep erythrocytes. Two viral diseases that definitely belong in the miscellaneous contact subgroup are Lassa fever and Marburg fever.

LASSA FEVER

Etiology

The first three cases of a new and highly virulent disease were reported by Frame and Troup (1970). The first case involved a missionary nurse in the village of Lassa on the Jos plateau in Nigeria who became ill on 12 January 1969. The source of her infection was unknown. After being moved to a hospital in Jos, she died on 26 January 1969. The second case, who nursed case 1 after her arrival at Jos, became ill on 3 February and died on 13 February 1969. The third case nursed the first two cases and became ill on 20 February 1969. She was flown to New York via Lagos, Nigeria, and arrived at the Presbyterian hospital on 4 March 1969. After a prolonged critical illness, she gradually improved and was completely recovered by 29 May 1969. A cytopathic agent was grown in tissue culture inoculated with a serum specimen from case 3. It was Frame et al. who suggested the name of Lassa fever for this disease.

Leifer et al. (1970) reported two laboratory-acquired cases of Lassa fever, one fatal. The other was treated with 500 milliliters of plasma from the recently recovered case 3 and survived. The patients yielded positive cytopathic agents in tissue cultures inoculated with blood serum, throat washings, and urine. The convalescent plasma seemingly aborted the course of the disease and the surviving patient recovered without complications.

Buckley and Casals (1970) recovered 14 cytopathic isolates from tissue cultures inoculated with serum, throat washings, pleural fluid, or urine from four Lassa fever patients. They noted that the viremia lasted for 1 to 2 weeks after the onset of illness. The virus infected mice and Vero cell (African green monkey kidney) tissue cultures but failed to infect cultures from two species of *Aedes* mosquitoes tested. One-day-old mice, inoculated intracerebrally, failed to develop symptoms, although complement fixation antibodies developed in the mice and Lassa virus was isolated from the urine as late as 83 days after inoculation. Comparably inoculated adult mice became ill and died.

The Lassa virus isolates appeared to be spherical RNA viruses with lipid-containing envelopes and surface projections (see Figure 19-5). Lassa virus proved to be antigenically distinct from the arboviruses (see Chapter 34) tested. It showed a low degree of antigenic cross-reactivity with lymphocytic choriomeningitis (LCM) virus.

Epidemiology and Clinical Symptoms

The onset of Lassa fever symptoms was reported to be gradual, with fever, weakness, muscle aches, and mouth or pharyngeal ulceration being prominent. In the severe cases these symptoms progressed to pneumonitis, fre-

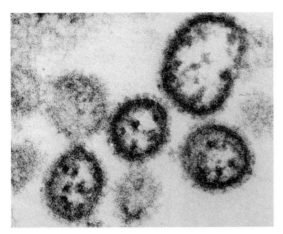

Figure 19–5. Lassa virus in Vero (green monkey) cell culture after isolation from a patient in Sierra Leone. Note the well-resolved envelopes and surface projections. 121,000×. (Courtesy of F. A. Murphy.)

quently with pleurisy, myocarditis, and nephritis. Cases also developed encephalopathy and intestinal bleeding. In the Jos plateau outbreak of 1969–1970 there were 26 cases and 10 deaths at the Jos hospital. At a nearby hospital six cases were reported. One of the six died of "nephritis" after apparent recovery from the Lassa fever symptoms. This and subsequent epidemics have involved a total of more than 100 cases of Lassa fever (Jawetz et al. 1976). Serological evidence from household contacts of five Lassa fever patients indicates the possibility of mild or even asymptomatic infections among human beings (see Troup et al. 1970).

Since Lassa virus was isolated from both throat washings and urine of infected patients, transmission of the disease from human to human could involve either respiratory or urinary modes. Considering the tendency toward intestinal bleeding, this mode of transmission would also seem to be possible. Naturally infected African house rats have been reported, and urinary transmission from these animals could initiate human disease outbreaks.

Laboratory Diagnosis

Warning: Because of the virulence of Lassa virus and the history of accidental infections among diagnostic and research laboratory personnel, diagnosis should be undertaken only by highly trained technologists in adequately equipped laboratories. Since the Lassa virus can be propagated in Vero cell tissue cultures, vaccines for the prophylactic immunization of laboratory and other high-risk (medical and paramedical) personnel should be made available in known endemic areas of the world.

Laboratory specimens for the isolation of Lassa virus include blood serum (during the first 2 weeks of illness), nasopharyngeal swabs or throat washings, and urine. The specimens may be inoculated to mice—which is dangerous—or to Vero cell tissue cultures. If cytopathic effect (CPE) develops in the Vero cells, the presence of Lassa virus can be established by serotaxonomic complement fixation or direct FA tests using known positive Lassa virus antiserum.

Serodiagnostic complement fixation tests using paired sera (early and late) from the patient and known Lassa virus antigen can be used to establish a rising Lassa virus antibody titer. In such serological testing, care must be exercised to avoid problems arising from the shared antigens of other arenaviruses.

Control and Prevention

Rodent control, such as that practiced in bubonic plague (see Chapter 29) and in Bolivian hemorrhagic fever (Chapter 34) may prove to be the most effective means of controlling rat-to-human transmission of Lassa fever. Awareness of the danger of human-to-human transmission and, hopefully, prophylactic immunization of high-risk personnel will prevent future outbreaks of the disease.

The only known treatment for Lassa fever is convalescent serum from recovered patients. A limited supply of such serum is available at CDC and other WHO-associated laboratories.

MARBURG FEVER

Etiology

An outbreak of severe febrile disease occurred in 1967 in a group of laboratory workers in Marburg, Germany who were involved in the

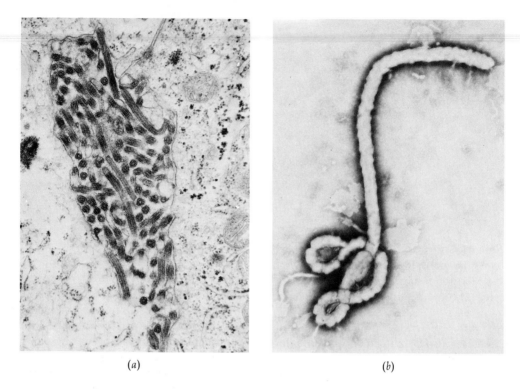

(a)   (b)

Figure 19–6.   (*a*) An ultra-thin section of Marburg virus particles in a Vero cell from a culture inoculated with a liver specimen from the fatal case in South Africa. The long filamentous structures are
unlike any other known type of virus. 30,000×. (*b*) Negatively-stained electron micrograph of the
"Marburg-like" (now named Ebola) virus from a cell culture inoculated with serum from a patient
in Zaire. The virus is morphologically indistinguishable from Marburg virus but appears to be
serologically unrelated. 45,580×. (Both courtesy of Viral Pathology Branch and Special Pathogens
Branch, Center for Disease Control, Atlanta.)

removal of kidneys from African green (vervet) monkeys to be used in monkey kidney tissue cultures for polio and other virus propagation. A total of 31 workers in the Marburg and neighboring laboratories became infected either from contact with the monkey viscera or from exposure to ill patients. Seven of the cases proved fatal. The infectious agent proved to be a morphologically unique virus and was designated Marburg virus. See Figure 19-6*a*.

Epidemiology and Clinical Symptoms

No field infections with Marburg virus were reported prior to 1975. Then, on 15 February 1975, a 20-year-old man was admitted to a hospital in Johannesburg, South Africa, complaining of muscle pains, headache, nausea, and chills. His clinical condition worsened rapidly, with continued high fever and slow pulse. Two days after admission a hemorrhagic syndrome appeared with "coffee-ground" vomitus, diarrhea, and intestinal and other mucus membrane bleeding. The patient died on 18 February.

This man and a woman companion had been hitchhiking around southern Africa for several months, visiting Rhodesia during the 10 days prior to returning to South Africa. His companion was admitted to the same hospital on 22 February with high fever. Because Lassa fever was suspected, a unit of Lassa fever convalescent serum was administered on 24 February. The patient thereafter showed gradual signs of improvement and eventually recovered. An attending nurse reported muscle pains and high fever on 28 February but began to improve and recovered thereafter (see *MMWR*, 8 March 1975).

An epidemic hemorrhagic fever caused by a "Marburg-like" virus (see Figure 19-6b) had resulted in at least 325 deaths in the Zaire-Sudan area of Africa by 3 December 1976 (see *MMWR*, 29 October, 5 November, 3 December 1976). Although numerous bites by hemophagus arthropods have been reported in some cases, no vector has been incriminated and the initiation of infection of human cases remains a mystery. Contact with the viscera of asymptomatic monkeys is the only proved means of acquiring Marburg fever. Human-to-human transmission, by respiratory or other direct contact, appears to be almost a certainty, however.

Laboratory Diagnosis

The Marburg virus has been propagated from autopsy liver specimens in Vero cell tissue culture. Laboratory aid in diagnosis of suspected Marburg fever should be left to CDC or other WHO-associated laboratories that have the personnel and equipment necessary to deal with this and other dangerous exotic viral diseases.

REFERENCES

Buckley, S. M. and J. Casals. 1970. Lassa fever, a new virus disease of man from West Africa. III. Isolation and characterization of the virus. *Amer. J. Trop. Med. Hyg.* 19:680–691.

Cox, H. R., W. C. Tesar, and J. V. Irons. 1947. Q fever in the United States. IV. Isolation and identification of rickettsiae in an outbreak among stock handlers and slaughterhouse workers. *J. Amer. Med. Ass.* 133:820–821.

Davis, G. E. and H. R. Cox. 1938. A filter passing agent isolated from ticks. I. Isolation from *Dermacentor andersoni*, reactions in animals, and filtration experiments. *Pub. Health Rep.* 53:2259–2267.

Feeley, J. C. and P. S. Brachman. 1974. *Bacillus anthracis*. Chapter 15 in *Manual of Clinical Microbiology*.

Frame, J. D. and J. M. Troup. 1970. Lassa fever, a new virus disease of man from West Africa. I. Clinical description and pathological findings. *Amer. J. Trop. Med. Hyg.* 19:670–676.

Hanna, L., J. Schachter, and E. Jawetz. 1974. Chlamydiae (psittacosis-lymphogranuloma venereum-trachoma group). Chapter 87 in *Manual of Clinical Microbiology*.

Jawetz, E., J. L. Melnick, and E. A. Adelberg. 1976. *Review of Medical Microbiology*. 12th ed. Los Altos, Calif.: Lange.

Leifer, E., D. J. Gocke, and H. Bourne. 1970. Lassa fever, a new virus disease of man from West Africa. II. Report of a laboratory acquired infection treated with plasma from a person recently recovered from the disease. *Amer. J. Trop. Med. Hyg.* 19:677–679.

Meyer, K. F. 1965. Psittacosis-lymphogranuloma venereum agents. Chapter 47 in *Viral and Rickettsial Infections of Man*, ed. F. L. Horsfall and Igor Tamm. Philadelphia: Lippincott.

Ormsbee, R. A. 1965. Q fever rickettsia. Chapter 52 in *Viral and Rickettsial Infections of Man*.

———. 1974. Rickettsiae. Chapter 88 in *Manual of Clinical Microbiology*.

Runyon, E. H., A. G. Karlson, G. P. Kubica, and L. G. Wayne. 1974. *Mycobacterium*. Chapter 16 in *Manual of Clinical Microbiology*.

Skinsnes, O. K. 1964. Leprosy in society. II. The pattern of concept and reaction to leprosy in Oriental antiquity. *Leprosy Res.* 35:106–122.

Skinsnes, O. K. and R. M. Elvove. 1970. Leprosy in society. V. Leprosy in occidental literature. *Int. J. Leprosy* 38:294–307.

Speir, R. W., O. Wood, H. Liebhaber, and S. M. Buckley. 1970. Lassa fever, a new virus disease of man from West Africa. IV. Electron microscopy of Vero cell cultures infected with Lassa virus. *Amer. J. Trop. Med. Hyg.* 19:692–694.

Stein, C. D. 1944. Differentiation of *Bacillus anthracis* from nonpathogenic aerobic spore-forming bacilli. *Amer. J. Vet. Res.* 5:38–54.

Stoker, M. C. and P. Fiset. 1956. Phase variation of the Nine Mile and other strains of *Rickettsia burneti*. *Canad. J. Microbiol.* 2:310–321.

Troup, J. M., H. A. White, A. Tom, and D. E. Corely. 1970. An outbreak of Lassa fever on the Jos Plateau, Nigeria in January-February 1970. A preliminary report. *Amer. J. Trop. Med. Hyg.* 19:695–696.

Wright, G. C. 1965. The anthrax bacillus. Chapter 22 in *Bacterial and Mycotic Infections of Man,* ed. R. J. Dubos and J. G. Hirsch. Philadelphia: Lippincott.

20

Staphylococcal and Nosocomial Diseases

By Thomas W. Huber

Staphylococcal and nosocomial (hospital-acquired) infections have been transmitted in a variety of ways—respiratory, direct contact, airborne infection, contaminated secondary vehicles, wound inoculation, and bite inoculation. Transmission by catheters (urinary and intravenous), by contaminated sutures and other items used in surgery, and by respiratory assist apparatus has been documented. Yet-to-be-discovered life-support and diagnostic apparatus probably will be added to the long list of mechanisms that have been incriminated as inanimate vehicles of these diseases. Awareness of the problem of nosocomial infections has led the Joint Commission on Accreditation of Hospitals to require hospital personnel to become active in internal epidemiology. Hospital infection control efforts are usually the responsibility of an infection control committee or an infection control officer or both. Microbiologists, nurses, pharmacists, physicians, and administrators should be representatives on such committees. Infection control officers, in most instances, have been nurses, but it is becoming apparent that microbiologists and physicians also have training that is valuable in controlling hospital infec-

tions. Hospital epidemiology is developing rapidly, and it is likely that in the future infection control officers will have specialized advanced training in that field.

Staphylococcal disease has been a perennial problem for hospital epidemiologists. During the 1950s and early 1960s, staphylococcal infection was synonymous with nosocomial infection. Staphylococcal diseases commonly occur in nonhospitalized individuals also, but the mechanisms of transmission are similar if not identical. Gram-negative bacilli (such as *Escherichia coli*, *Salmonella*, and *Shigella* species and others) have now replaced the staphylococci as the most frequent causes of nosocomial infections, even though staphylococci have remained a problem.

STAPHYLOCOCCAL DISEASES

Staphylococci are gram-positive spherical organisms that occur in microscopic clusters resembling bunches of grapes (see Figure C on the back cover). A. Ogston in 1881 reported staphylococci in smears of exudates from chronic and acute abscesses. Rosenbach (1884) grew the organisms in pure culture and reported that many abscesses were caused by staphylococci. Bacteriological cultures of the nose and skin of normal individuals also commonly yielded staphylococci. Rosenbach described two pigmented colony types of staphylococci and proposed appropriate species nomenclature: *Staphylococcus aureus* (golden) and *Staphylococcus albus* (white). Culture of disease lesions such as boils or other abscesses usually resulted in the growth of *S. aureus.* The golden pigment was believed to be correlated with the virulence of the staphylococci, and early bacteriologists used pigment production as a key differential. It was soon recognized, however, that there was a disturbing lack of correlation between virulence and pigment production, and other virulence or correlative factors were sought. For a technical discussion of the classification of staphylococci see Baird-Parker (1965).

A great variety of enzymes, hemolysins, and toxins are produced by pathogenic staphylococci. With its discovery, each extracellular product was proposed to be the long-awaited absolute indicator of virulence. The following are some of the staphylococcal products or characteristics proposed at one time or another to be of virulence or other taxonomic significance:

1. Alpha hemolysin—a hemolytic factor that lyses rabbit erythrocytes and involves a toxin that kills leucocytes and is lethal for mice and rabbits.

2. Beta hemolysin—lyses sheep erythrocytes and the lytic activity is potentiated by chilling after 37°C incubation (hot-cold lysis).

3. Delta hemolysin—lyses human and horse erythrocytes and exhibits toxic factors for leucocytes.

4. Leucocidins—kill polymorphonuclear leucocytes.

5. Deoxyribonuclease (DNAase)—an enzyme that hydrolyzes DNA to nitrogen-base components.

6. Fibrinolysin—an enzyme that causes the dissolution of fibrin clots.

7. Coagulase—an enzyme that catalyzes the conversion of fibrinogen to a fibrin coagulum in the absence of calcium ions.

8. Ability to ferment mannitol.

9. Lysed by lysostaphin—a staphylolytic enzyme discovered by C. A. Schindler and V. T. Schuhardt (1964–1965) that exhibits specificity for organisms with pentaglycine linkages in their cell wall. All strains of *S. aureus,* a few coagulase-negative staphylococci, but no other known bacteria, possess these pentaglycine linkages.

10. Protein A—a surface protein of many strains of *S. aureus* that adsorbs gamma globulin due to an attraction for the Fc portion of the molecule.

Over the years, proposals and counterproposals were made concerning the relation of each of these characteristics to staphylococcal virulence. In 1965, the Subcommittee for Taxonomy and Nomenclature of Micrococcaceae agreed to select a single characteristic of overriding taxonomic significance, since the issue of the virulence of staphylococci could not be resolved. The committee selected the capacity of the isolate to produce coagulase. Therefore coagulase-positive staphylococci are now classified as virulent *S. aureus* and coagulase-negative as "avirulent" *S. epidermidis* (see Buchanan and Gibbons 1974). Hereafter the term *Staphylococcus* or staphylococci will refer to *S. aureus; S. epidermidis* will be designated by name when it is discussed. For an excellent and comprehensive discussion of staphylococci, the reader is referred to Cohen (1972).

Pathogenesis

The mechanism by which *S. aureus* produces disease is unknown. Many of the factors mentioned in the introduction conceivably could play a role. Hemolysis of erythrocytes evokes a toxic reaction and eventually results in anemia. Leucocidins kill leucocytes and could thereby protect the phagocytized staphylococci. Fibrinolysin could digest fibrin, deposited as a response to injury, allowing "walled-off" staphylococcal infection to spread. Coagulase could deposit fibrin around staphylococcal cells and protect them from phagocytosis. Staphylococcal isolates from significant disease usually produce all of these potential virulence factors, and perhaps some combination if not all contribute to virulence. Unknown host factors may be even more important than staphylococcal virulence factors. Staphylococci are ubiquitous and are present in the anterior nares, other mucus membranes, skin, or hair of almost every human. Indeed, pure cultures of supposedly virulent staphylococci have been spread on the skin of human volunteers without pathological effect. The minimal pus-forming dose (MPFD) was determined for human volunteers using freshly isolated staphylococci and intradermal injections. The MPFD proved to be 2.8×10^6 organisms in 0.1 milliliter. The same number of organisms was required to cause infection when inoculation was subcutaneous or into incisions through the skin. The MPFD did not seem to vary whether the source of isolation was from human lesions or normal nose or skin. The insertion of a suture in the skin resulted in a 10,000-fold reduction of the MPFD.

Elek and Conen (1957) concluded that the foregoing studies showed the importance of host defense mechanisms in the establishment of infection, since natural infection is unlikely if 10^6 organisms are required. Staphylococcal virulence is not demonstrated in mouse challenge studies. Smith (1963) challenged mice with up to 5×10^8 organisms by intravenous injection. With 58 strains isolated from human disease, mouse mortality ranged from 7 to 70 percent but was low with most isolates. Animal models analogous to human infection are not readily available, even though an encapsulated isolate, designated the Smith strain (Sv) of *S. aureus,* is lethal to the mouse when injected by the intraperitoneal route.

Clinical Disease

Human staphylococcal infections occur frequently but generally are localized at the portal of entry by normal host defenses. The portal may be a hair follicle but usually is a break in the skin. The break may be minute or it may be a traumatic or surgical wound. Foreign bodies, including sutures, provide a favorable habitat for staphylococci and make infection difficult to eradicate. Another portal by which staphylococci may enter is the respiratory tract. Respiratory infection resulting in pneumonia frequently is a complication of influenza but can result from metastasis. The localized host response to staphylococci is one of inflammation characterized by an elevated temperature at the site, swelling, the accumulation of pus, and necrosis of tissue. Around the inflamed area, body defenses develop a wall consisting of fibrin and migratory tissue cells. This results in the formation of an abscess filled with bacteria, dead and dying leucocytes, and other necrotic tissue. Skin and subcutaneous tissue infections—impetigo, pyoderma, boils, furuncles, carbuncles—are commonly caused by staphylococci. Localized infection of the bone is called osteomyelitis, and *S. aureus* is the most common cause. Serious consequences of staphylococcal infection frequently occur when organisms invade the bloodstream. The resulting staphylococcal septicemia may be rapidly fulminant; or a bacteremia may result in seeding internal abscesses, boils and other skin and subcutaneous tissue lesions, lungs, kidneys, heart, skeletal muscle, or the meninges.

Epidemiology

The epidemiological aspects of hospital and community staphylococcal disease are challenging because of several unique features. The physiology of *S. aureus* enables it to survive under suboptimal conditions. It is resistant to bile, sodium chloride, and potassium tellurite, characteristics that are used in designing selective media for staphylococci. The reservoir of asymptomatic carriers and subclinical cases is immense. Staphylococci can be transmitted in a variety of ways, and the response of the infected host can be extremely variable, ranging from no symptoms to severe disease. Special typing techniques are required to differentiate epidemic strains from endemic *S. aureus*. Each of the unique features merits further discussion.

Staphylococci resist drying and with low relative humidity can survive for extended periods in a state of "suspended animation." Because of this resistance, the inanimate environment serves as an additional reservoir of staphylococci. Staphylococci have been recovered from blankets, sheets, curtains, baths, floor dust, and all common fomites (substances that can absorb and transport germs). Cultures of air often yield *S. aureus*. The degree of air contamination is probably directly proportional to the proximity and activity of people near the air sampler. Humans represent perhaps the largest and most important reservoir. Williams et al. (1966) reported that during epidemics some 70 percent of hospital patients and personnel become colonized with *S. aureus* and that normally 35 to 50 percent of adults are nasal carriers. An additional 5 to 10 percent harbor staphylococci on their skin. Newborn infants soon become colonized with staphylococci, but the carrier rate normally drops to 10–20 percent by the age of 1 year and by the age of 10 approximates that of adults. The high incidence of staphylococcus carriers plus its ubiquity in the environment make the potential mechanisms of transmission almost limitless.

The widespread natural distribution of *S. aureus* complicates the tracing of epidemic strains since one must be able to distinguish the epidemic from the normal flora. The pattern of antibiotic resistance (antibiogram) of the staphylococcal isolates may differentiate the organisms into broad groups. Isolates with unusual antibiograms have more chance of being related to epidemics than those with common antibiotic susceptibility patterns. A system for serotyping strains of *S. aureus* has been described. This serotyping was used as an adjunct to a phage typing scheme during the 1950s and 1960s when large hospital outbreaks were prevalent. Individual strains were detected by agglutination patterns in carefully cross-adsorbed specific antistaphylococcal antisera.

Individual strains of staphylococci can be distinguished by the pattern of their susceptibility to lysis by a set of staphylococcal bacteriophages. The phages have been derived from lysogenic strains of *S. aureus* and are able to lyse most but not all isolates. Using a set of phages with different *S. aureus* specificities, similarity of staphylococcal strains can be determined by their susceptibility patterns. Each phage selected for incorporation into the typing set is first standardized by determining its host range against *S. aureus* strains of known phage type. The lytic activity of each phage suspension is titrated by testing dilutions of the suspension on known susceptible strains called propagating strains. Figure 20-1 shows the appearance of a plate used to determine the routine test dilution (RTD) of a phage suspension. In this illustration, spot 5 shows a pattern of incomplete lysis. Many strains of *S. aureus* show less than complete lysis with one or more of the typing phages. The following scheme for recording reactions has

Figure 20–1. Plate illustrating RTD of a staphylococcal phage suspension. The 10^{-4} dilution, being the highest dilution showing complete lysis, represents the RTD for this phage suspension. (Courtesy of P. B. Smith.)

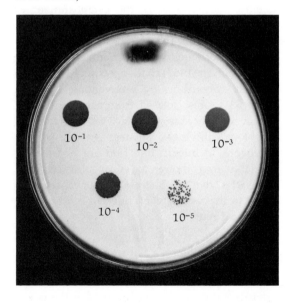

29	52	52A	79	
80	3A	3C	55	71
6	42E	47	53	54
75	77	83A	84	85
	81	94	95	96

Figure 20–2. Template with phage type numbers.

been advocated: fewer than 20 isolated plaques, ±; 20–50 plaques, +; not confluent but more than 50 plaques, + +; confluent lysis, + + +.

Phages are designated by numerals. The phages most commonly used in the typing set are shown in a template used for applying phages and reading the lytic reactions (see Figure 20-2). The phage type of an isolate of *S. aureus* is reported as the type number(s) of the phages giving major (+ + or greater lysis) reactions. For example, a strain lysed + + or greater by one RTD of phage type numbers 6, 47, and 53 would be reported as phage type 6/47/53. Minor reactions may be disregarded or listed in parentheses following major reactions. In recent years, many strains have begun to show resistance to lysis by the phages in the typing sets, resulting in up to 50 percent of all *S. aureus* isolates being nontypable. Increasing the concentration of the applied phages to 100 RTD allows lysis and therefore differentiation of many otherwise nontypable strains. The phage type of strains lysed by only the 100 RTD concentrations are reported with the type numbers enclosed in brackets or designated in some other manner as being the result of testing

with an increased phage concentration. The typing set currently (1976) used is this: group I phages—29, 52, 52A, 79, and 80; group II phages—3A, 3C, 55, and 71; group III phages—6, 42E, 47, 53, 54, 75, 77, 83A, 84, and 85; unassigned phages—81, 94, 95, and 96. For a complete discussion of phage typing, the reader is referred to Cohen (1972: chap. 18).

The correlation of phage type with the virulence or epidemic-producing potential of *S. aureus* is controversial. To be sure, infections due mainly to staphylococci of phage types 80/81 reached pandemic proportions from the mid-1950s to the early 1960s. Staphylococcal infection was said to be one of the most important public health problems during that period. Up to 30 percent of hospital personnel carried strains 80/81 in their anterior nares and many developed staphylococcal lesions. Almost all infants in hospital newborn nurseries became colonized with these staphylococci; many developed skin lesions and others more serious disease such as staphylococcal sepsis. Twenty percent or more of some hospitalized patients developed staphylococcal infections of strains 80/81. Dismissed patients and hospital personnel spread the 80/81 strains to their families and to other members of the community. Outbreaks occurred in institutions other than hospitals and in groups working in close contact (for example, football teams). The 80/81 strains were estimated to be involved in 1 to 2 percent of all hospital deaths. These statistics indicate the possibility of increased virulence of the 80/81 strains. The danger inherent in placing emphasis on 80/81 strains, however, is the tendency to assume that other strains of *S. aureus* are less significant in epidemic infections. Williams et al. (1966) found that many phage types and even nontypable staphylococci have caused epidemic outbreaks in surgical and maternity units. Furthermore, despite the disappearance of 80/81 strains in the mid-1960s, *S. aureus* was second only to *Escherichia coli* as a cause of hospital-acquired infection in 1970, a trend that has continued (see Bennett et al. 1971). The most appropriate usage of phage typing of *S. aureus* is as an epidemiological tool to trace the origins of staphylococcal infections. If an inordinate amount of staphylococcal infection is detected, phage typing should be applied to isolates from patients and from suspected carriers or other probable sources of infection. The isolation of a common phage type *S. aureus* from these sources indicates a common source outbreak, whereas a variety of phage types would implicate multiple sources of infection. In the latter cases endogenous infection from the patient's own flora must be considered.

Laboratory Diagnosis

The laboratory diagnosis of staphylococcal disease is based upon the isolation and identification of *S. aureus* from lesion exudate. Observation of clusters of gram-positive cocci in smears is helpful, but staphylococci cannot be differentiated microscopically from other aerobic and anaerobic cocci. Staphylococci grow readily on sheep blood agar plates and normally produce a zone or multiple zones of hemolysis surrounding a large, flat, opaque, frequently golden colony. Aerobic incubation is preferred. Staphylococci can be reliably distinguished from streptococci by transferring a bit of the colony, with a bacteriological loop, to a drop of 3 percent hydrogen peroxide on a glass microslide. The violent formation of bubbles indicates that the organism produces catalase, an enzyme that destroys hydrogen peroxide with concomitant release of gaseous oxygen. Streptococci do not produce catalase. Staphylococci are differentiated from the other catalase-positive, gram-positive cocci (*Micrococcus*) by differential carbohydrate fermentation tests or by lysostaphin susceptibility tests (see Schuhardt 1965; Klesius and Schuhardt 1968).

The clinically significant *S. aureus* is differentiated from the usually saprophytic *S. epidermidis* by the coagulase test. The organism to be tested is inoculated into a tube containing citrated rabbit plasma. After 3–18 hours' incubation in a water bath at 37°C, the tube is examined for the presence of a fibrin clot. A slide test for coagulase production has been described. Rabbit plasma is stirred into a heavy

suspension of staphylococci in a drop of saline. A rapid (within 10 seconds) clumping of the organisms is seen in a positive slide coagulase test. Some *S. aureus* strains that are coagulase-positive in the tube test, however, fail to clump in the slide test. Therefore all slide-test-negative organisms should be retested by the tube technique. A staphylococcal isolate giving a negative coagulase test by the tube technique is identified as *S. epidermidis*. The isolation of *S. epidermidis* has little clinical significance, except from urine when present in large numbers (10^5/milliliter) or from blood after open-heart surgery. Rare cases of bacterial endocarditis due to *S. epidermidis* have, however, been reported.

Therapy

The institution of proper and effective treatment is dependent upon the site of the infection, the susceptibility of the isolate to the antibiotic, whether or not foreign bodies are involved, and the allergies of the patient. As previously indicated, foreign bodies lower the host's resistance to staphylococcal infection and make eradication of the organism difficult. Infected foreign bodies such as sutures and drainage tubes should be removed if possible. The site of the infection is important in that closed abscesses or body cavities that fill with pus in response to staphylococcal infection must be surgically drained. The presence of even sterile pus prevents normal healing and can be responsible for persistent fever. Infected pus is dangerous in that organisms continue to multiply and the lesion will ultimately rupture and drain. Lesions near body surfaces frequently drain through sinus tracts formed through the skin. Spontaneous healing can occur after suitable drainage. In other instances, abscesses rupture into body cavities containing vital organs or gain access to the blood by erosion of adjacent capillaries. Furthermore, antibiotic therapy may not be effective for organisms in an abscess since by definition an abscess is a focal area that has lost blood circulation. Drainage of pus from closed abscesses is as important as the administration of antibiotics.

Penicillin was used widely in staphylococcal disease following the drug's commercial availability in the 1940s, and soon thereafter penicillin-resistant strains of *S. aureus* became common. In present-day hospitals, up to 90 percent of *S. aureus* isolates are resistant to penicillin. In almost all instances *S. aureus* resistance is due to the production of a penicillin-destroying enzyme—penicillinase. Now the choice of antibiotics for the treatment of staphylococcal disease has been simplified by the availability of semisynthetic, penicillinase-resistant penicillin compounds such as methicillin and nafcillin. Prior to the early 1960s, staphylococci were frequently resistant to all available antibiotics. Methicillin is a penicillin molecule chemically altered to resist the action of penicillinase; before it and its analogs became available penicillin-resistant staphylococcal infections were treated with tetracycline or erythromycin. Widespread usage of these antibiotics resulted in the selection of strains of staphylococci also resistant to these drugs, especially in hospitals. The cessation of the use of tetracycline and erythromycin in the early 1960s has resulted in the reemergence of strains of *S. aureus* susceptible to tetracycline and erythromycin. A propensity for developing resistance to methicillin has not been shown despite many reports of the isolation of methicillin-resistant *S. aureus.* Susceptibility testing of isolates should be done in all *S. aureus* infections. Penicillin is the treatment of choice in penicillin-sensitive strains of *S. aureus* because it is cheaper than its semisynthetic analogs and the development of penicillin resistance during the course of therapy of an individual patient has never been observed. Methicillin or a related analog is the drug of choice for penicillin-resistant strains, but an allergy to penicillin also precludes the use of the penicillin analogs. Potentially effective alternative drugs for *S. aureus* disease are the cephalosporins and vancomycin.

The results of treatment of *S. aureus* disease and the eradication of staphylococci from carriers have proved to be quite different. During appropriate treatment of the disease staphylococci are suppressed so that cultures usually become and remain negative. Staphylococci, however, rapidly reemerge or recolonize treated carriers. Often the same phage type recurs, suggesting mere suppression of the staphylococcal flora rather than sterilization and reseeding. Furthermore, it is believed that the action of antibiotics destroys normal nasal flora facilitating the reseeding or reemergence of antibiotic-resistant strains of *S. aureus.* Parenteral as well as topical application of lysostaphin in carriers appeared to give more promising results (Martin and White 1967). The specificity of lysostaphin for *S. aureus* left the normal flora unaffected, and the reacquisition rate was considerably slower than with other forms of treatment. The unique attack by lysostaphin on the *S. aureus* cell wall has been described by Schuhardt et al. (1969) and is illustrated by Figure 20-3.

The parenteral use of lysostaphin has been thwarted by the fact that, as a large protein molecule (molecular weight 30,000), it is antigenic and can induce hypersensitivity. Although lysostaphin is not as large as or more antigenic than the horse serum antitoxin molecule used in diphtheria and other therapy, the therapeutic use of lysostaphin probably could only be justified, at this time, to treat life-threatening infections due to staphylococci that are highly resistant to other potential therapeutic agents. For a comprehensive review of the literature on lysostaphin see Zygmunt and Tavormina (1972).

Control and Prevention

The hospital strains of staphylococci (phage type 80/81) caused epidemics of surgical, maternity, and neonatal infections during the 1950s and early 1960s. By mid-1960 the prevalence of the 80/81 strains, and concomitantly widespread hospital staphylococcal infections, diminished. The reason for this abatement of staphylococcal infections is unknown. Some speculate that hospital strains became lysogenized with phages 80 and 81 and in the process lost virulence. Another conjecture is that the effective treatment offered by the discovery of penicillinase-resistant penicillins controlled in-

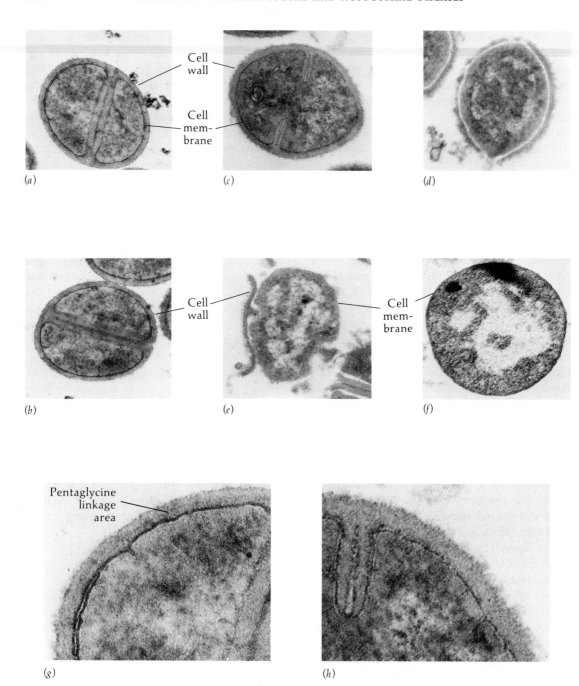

Figure 20–3. Electron micrographs of ultra-thin sections of lysostaphin-treated *Staphylococcus aureus* cells in 24% NaCl solution. Parts *a* and *b* are 2 and 10 minute controls (no lysostaphin) respectively; *c, d, e,* and *f* are 2, 5, 10, and 30 minute test preparations (5 units of lysostaphin per ml); *g* and *h* are enlargements of portions of *a* and *c* respectively. Figures *a* through *f* are 63,840×; *g* and *h* are 167,200×. Variations in size here are explained partly by the locations of the sections through the cells. (Photography courtesy of L. M. Pope.)

fections. Still others believe that the institution of hospital control measures was responsible.

In order to be of value, control measures must be directed at preventing the most probable means of transmission—which are quite diverse due to the high carrier rates and the survival of staphylococci on inanimate objects as well as in the animate environment. One important difference should be noted: Usually no multiplication occurs in the inanimate environment other than culture media. Though their survival in the environment is superior to that of most other infectious organisms. Staphylococci will eventually die without proper nutrients. It is logical, then, that animate hosts are more important reservoirs than the inanimate environment since the environment only becomes contaminated by the shedding of organisms from staphylococcal carriers and cases.

Control and prevention measures that have been instituted to protect against staphylococcal spread are as varied as the potential routes of transmission. Laminar airflow apparatus has been installed to provide sterile air in the operating theater but with very little reduction in surgical infection rates. Staphylococci have been isolated from every inanimate object tested in a hospital, and disinfection procedures have been instituted with some success to control such sources of infection. Attempts to identify carriers have resulted in specimens from innumerable noses and other body areas having been cultured and the isolates phage-typed and correlated with dissemination of epidemic staphylococci. To incriminate a carrier as the source of an outbreak, it must be established by epidemiological investigations that the suspect was the only plausible source of dissemination. It must be remembered that hospital personnel can become carriers following contact with an infected patient. A person identified as causing infections should be treated, removed from the vicinity of highly susceptible patients, and retrained in hygienic practices. Personnel should be examined for the presence of skin lesions and transferred to noncritical areas until such lesions are healed and culture-negative. Isolation of infected patients is good practice and provides

effective control. Proper hand washing is the most obvious and effective means of curbing the spread of staphylococcal as well as other infectious disease. Unfortunately, hands are probably the most common means of transmission of hospital epidemics because busy hospital personnel (including nurses and physicians) are apt to omit proper hand washing before and after handling each patient.

NOSOCOMIAL DISEASES

Hospital epidemics of staphylococcal disease were responsible for an awareness that disease could be transmitted from patient to patient or from personnel to patient within the confines of the health care facility. *Nosocomial* (which means hospital-acquired) infections are caused by many organisms. The gram-negative bacilli (see Figure C on the back cover) have surpassed the staphylococci in frequency as the etiology of nosocomial infections. *Escherichia coli*, *Proteus*, *Pseudomonas*, and *Klebsiella-Enterobacter* species cause almost half the reported nosocomial infections. A survey of United States hospitals revealed that 2 to 15 percent of patients admitted acquired an infection during their hospital stay (Bennett et al. 1971). A working definition of nosocomial infection is an infection that occurs more than 48 hours after admission. Not all nosocomial infections are preventable, since many result from traumatic wounds or from dirty surgery made necessary by life-threatening crises. Constant surveillance of charts of hospital patients to document infections and monitoring bacteriology laboratory results provide data pertinent to preventable (cross-infection) and nonpreventable (self or endogenous) infections. Cross-infections are those with common etiology and therefore presumably are due to a common source of contamination or transmission. Cabrera and Davis (1961) reported 14 cases of meningitis that occurred in a neonatal nursery. The etiology was unusual in that the causative organism was identified as *Flavobacterium meningiosepticum* and suggested a common source of the outbreak. Environmental sampling revealed the organisms to be present in a faulty sink trap. It was postulated that babies were infected by aerosolization of the organisms from the trap during bathing. Repairing the trap eliminated the organisms and terminated the epidemic.

Documented Outbreaks

A few examples of other nosocomial disease outbreaks resulting from cross-infections merit discussion here. An outbreak of *Salmonella enteritidis*, serotype *typhimurium* (see Chapter 24), was documented by the isolation of the organism from 12 infants in a diarrhea ward. The organisms were recovered from fecal specimens obtained more than 2 days after admission, whereas admission cultures were uniformly negative. Epidemiological investigation revealed an index case of *S. enteritidis ser-typhimurium* admitted to the ward a month prior to the outbreak. Cultures of the environment (air, bassinets) and the feces of hospital personnel were negative for the causative organism. However, the to-do made about culturing the hospital personnel brought the problem to their attention. Awareness of the problem plus a renewed vigor in insisting upon proper hand washing brought about the termination of the outbreak. The exact mechanism of transmission will never be known, but the usual means is via unwashed or improperly washed hands.

In one hospital in Utah six cases of *Streptococcus pyogenes* wound infection occurred in a 45-day period (see *MMWR*, 14 May 1976). All infections occurred within 48 hours after surgery. In fact, major surgery was the only experience shared by all. An investigation of the medical records of these and other patients undergoing surgery during the same period revealed that exposure to one anesthesiologist and one surgeon was unique to the infected cases. Cultures of the throat and anus of the two doctors showed that the anesthesiologist was an anal carrier of the same M-type *S. pyogenes* isolated from the infected patients. The anesthesiologist withdrew from surgery and underwent a course of penicillin therapy that eliminated the organism. No further infections occurred.

In the early 1970s many hospitals across the United States practicing active infection surveillance reported an increased incidence of sepsis due to an organism related to *Erwinia* (a plant pathogen), now known to be *Enterobacter agglomerans*. All patients who developed sepsis had received intravenous fluid prepared commercially by a large company with nationwide distribution. Quality control records and initial cultures indicated that the fluid was sterile. Subsequently, it was discovered that contamination was present between the seal and the closure lid. Organisms leaked into the bottles only if the lids were sufficiently jarred as they frequently are during preparation for use. A different closure provided the necessary control for this nationwide epidemic. The discovery and prevention of this epidemic depended on hospital surveillance and cooperative reporting to the National Nosocomial Infections Study program of the Center for Disease Control.

Control Measures

The cross-infections discussed in the preceding paragraphs are examples of established common-source transmission of nosocomial diseases. The source and mode of transmission often are not discovered, however. Surveillance may indicate the presence of a problem, general control measures are instituted, the problem disappears, and the causative agent and the source are undetermined. One can only presume that the source of infection subsided circumstantially or that the rededication of personnel to proper hygienic procedures resulted in the termination. The prompt disappearance of cross-infections soon after hospital personnel became aware of them testifies to the importance of an infection control officer and a surveillance program that promptly detects the onset of infections.

The occurrence of unusual organisms such as *E. agglomerans* or *F. meningiosepticum* or organisms of known pathological significance, such as *Salmonella* or *Streptococcus pyogenes*, usually indicates cross-infection rather than endogenous infection. Cross-infections can result from the spread of common organisms that constitute the normal flora indigenous to humans. Unfortunately, these organisms are also the most common cause of endogenous infection. To distinguish cross- from self-infections, the infection control officer needs to document the expected (baseline) incidence of infection for common organisms in the institution. An increased incidence of infections due to a common organism (such as E. coli) is evidence that hospital transmission may be occurring. Elaborate typing schemes are available to differentiate individual strains of common organisms. Some of the typing schemata available are:

1. For *Escherichia coli*—serological typing based upon somatic (O), flagellar (H), and envelope (K) antigens

2. For *Salmonella*—serological grouping based upon O antigens and typing based upon H antigens; also phage typing in some instances (see Chapter 24)

3. For *Shigella*—serological grouping based upon major O antigens and typing based upon minor O antigens (see Chapter 23)

4. For *Klebsiella*—serological typing based on capsular antigens

5. For *Pseudomonas aeruginosa*—pyocyanin typing, phage typing, and serological typing

6. For *Proteus, Serratia,* and *Enterobacter*—bacteriocin typing based upon the pattern of inhibition of members of a set of indicator bacteria

Reagents for these schemata are available at reference control centers, but most tests are not performed in clinical or hospital laboratories. The delay between collection of specimens and the return of a typing report makes it important that hospital epidemiologists learn to use other keys to strain individuality. Foremost is the antibiogram of the suspected epidemic strains. The antibiogram is the microbial susceptibility pattern of the isolate, which usually can be established within 48 hours after the collection of the specimen. Most isolates of E. coli are sensitive to all antibiotics normally tested. If E.

coli is suspected of causing a nosocomial outbreak and every isolate exhibits the same *unusual* pattern of resistance to one or more antibiotics, presumptive evidence is gained for a cross-infection. Another guide that can be used before special typing results are available is to compare biotypes of the isolates. The biotype of an organism is its pattern of carbohydrate fermentation and other biochemical reactions. Examples of the expected biotype for gram-negative bacilli of the gastrointestinal tract are given in Table III-A in the introduction to the intestinal group diseases. The isolation of organisms with identical but unusual biotypes (such as lactose-negative E. coli) indicates relatedness. The hospital epidemiologist should use this data base to estimate the expected number of infections with each organism, compare antibiograms and biotypes, and develop the expertise to decide whether or not cross-infection is occurring with the frequently isolated organisms. If preliminary indicators point to cross-infection, the isolates should be referred to state or national health laboratories for special typing procedures.

Thus far we have not discussed the control and prevention of endogenous infections that arise from infection with an organism from the patient's own flora. Although these cannot be suppressed to the extent that cross-infections can, one should not assume that nothing can be done. Endogenous infections can be reduced by observing the best possible surgical techniques, by proper care and changing of indwelling urinary and intravenous catheters, by proper care and cleansing of respiratory assist equipment, and by good housekeeping practices. The reduction of endogenous infections offers a stiff challenge to everyone involved in the operation of hospitals—only through a combined effort to change human habits will progress be made.

REFERENCES

Baird-Parker, A. C. 1965. Staphylococci and their classification. *Ann. New York Acad. Sci.* 128:4–25.

Bennett, J. V., W. E. Scheckler, D. G. Maki, and P. S. Brachman. 1971. *Current national patterns in the United States.* Proceedings of international conference on nosocomial infections. American Hospital Association. Baltimore: Waverly Press.

Buchanan, R. E. and N. E. Gibbons (eds.). 1974. *Bergey's Manual of Determinative Bacteriology.* 8th ed. Baltimore: Williams & Wilkins.

Cabrera, H. A. and G. H. Davis. 1961. Epidemic meningitis of the newborn caused by flavobacteria. *Amer. J. Dis. Child.* 101:289–296.

Cohen, J. O. (ed.). 1972. *The Staphylococci.* New York: Wiley.

Elek, S. D. and P. E. Conen. 1957. The virulence of *Staphylococcus pyogenes* for man. A study of the problems of wound infection. *Brit. J. Exp. Pathol.* 38:573–586.

Ivler, D. 1974. *Staphylococcus.* Chapter 7 in *Manual of Clinical Microbiology.*

Klesius, P. H. and V. T. Schuhardt. 1968. Use of lysostaphin in the isolation of highly polymerized deoxyribonucleic acid and in the taxonomy of aerobic Micrococcaceae. *J. Bacteriol.* 95:739–743.

Martin, R. R. and A. White. 1967. The selectivity of lysostaphin in vivo. *J. Lab. Clin. Med.* 70:1–8.

Rosenbach, F. J. 1884. *Mikroorganismen bei den Wund-Infections-Krankheiten des Menschen.* Weisbaden: J. F. Bergmann.

Schindler, C. A. and V. T. Schuhardt. 1964. Lysostaphin: a new bacteriolytic agent for the *Staphylococcus. Proc. Nat. Acad. Science* 51:414–421.

————. 1965. Purification and properties of lysostaphin—a lytic agent for *Staphylococcus aureus. Biochim. Biophys. Acta.* 97:242–250.

Schuhardt, V. T. 1965. See discussion following Baird-Parker (1965), listed above.

Schuhardt, V. T., T. W. Huber, and L. M. Pope. 1969. Electron microscopy and viability of lysostaphin-induced staphylococcal spheroplasts, protoplast-like bodies, and protoplasts. *J. Bacteriol.* 97:396–401.

Smith, D. D. 1963. Mouse virulence and coagulase production in *Staphylococcus aureus. J. Path. Bacteriol.* 86:231–236.

Williams, R. E. O., R. Blowers, L. R. Garrod, and R. A. Shooter. 1966. *Hospital Infection: Causes and Prevention.* Chicago: Yearbook Medical Publishers.

Zygmunt, W. A. and P. A. Tavormina. 1972. Lysostaphin: model for a specific enzyme approach to infectious disease. *Progress in Drug Research.* Vol. 16, pp. 310–331. Basel: Birkhauser Verlag.

21

Fungal Diseases

By Thomas W. Huber

Fungal diseases can result from inhalation, from contact with contaminated moist surfaces such as shower stalls, or from inoculation of infectious particles that occur in nature (exogenous infection). Fungal disease also can result from organisms present within the body as normal flora (endogenous infection). In general, the potential to produce disease is unrelated to the ability of the fungus to survive and even multiply outside host tissues. Most fungi have established an ecological niche in nature and the infection of humans and animals is not essential to their survival. These incidental infections, however, can be quite frequent if highly endemic areas are inhabited by human or other animal hosts. The recognition that many fungal diseases previously considered to be rare and fatal are common and usually mild emphasizes the need to understand the basic principles of mycology. Descriptive and taxonomic terms in mycology texts may appear formidable but are useful and will not be avoided here. See Webster (1970), Emmons et al. (1970), and Conant et al. (1971) for more details.

THE ACTINOMYCETALES

Although pathogenic genera of the order Actinomycetales *(Actinomyces, Nocardia,* and *Streptomyces)* are taxonomically considered to be bacteria (see Table 1-1), they share certain characteristics, including epidemiology, with the fungi. Moreover, as indicated in the textbook references of Chapter 1, the diseases caused by these organisms frequently are included in medical mycology. Characteristics of Actinomycetales shared with bacteria are size (1 micron or less in diameter), cell-wall composition, and sensitivity to antibacterial agents (Figure 21–1a). Members of Actinomycetales, however, also share taxonomic characteristics with the true fungi (Eumycetes)—namely, filamentous growth with true branching, slow growth, and the ability to grow on the usual fungal culture media.

Briefly the major actinomycetes of pathogenic significance for humans are:

1. *Actinomyces israelii,* an anaerobic organism indigenous to the upper respiratory tract of humans. Infections usually involve the mouth or lower respiratory tract following trauma or aspiration of saliva into the lungs.

2. *Nocardia asteroides,* a partially acid-fast aerobic environmental organism. Infections usually are acquired by inhalation of airborne organisms into the lungs. Pulmonary infections are most common, but systemic and wound infections may occur.

3. *Nocardia brasiliensis, N. caviae, Streptomyces,* and *Actinomadureae* species are aerobic, environmental organisms. Characteristically, infections with these organisms occur on the extremities following traumatic injury. The ensuing localized disease of subcutaneous tissue with suppuration (pus formation) and drainage is called *mycetoma.* Mycetomas (*myce*—fungal; *toma*—tumor) caused by members of Actinomycetales are referred to as actinomycotic mycetomas.

Actinomycosis

Actinomycosis formerly was a fairly common disease of cattle designated *lumpy jaw.* The etiological agent of the cattle disease was an actinomycete named *Actinomyces bovis.* A related species, *A. israelii,* is found as a normal inhabitant of the human mouth. Human infections have resulted from trauma as a consequence of tooth extraction or dental surgery or other causes. The actinomycotic lesions are suppurative, and the pus frequently contains macroscopically visible yellow granules—"sulfur granules." When examined microscopically these granules are found to be colonies of club-shaped bacteria arranged radially around the periphery of the granule (see Figure 21–1b). Coccoid cells also are found within the granule.

The *Actinomyces* are anaerobic species that can be cultivated on brain-heart infusion agar or similar media, although some authorities prefer to supplement the media with blood. The cultures must be incubated anaerobically at 30–37°C. The club-shaped organisms in the sulfur granules can be stained with eosin for better resolution. The coccoid or branching filaments are gram-positive cells.

Some antigenic serotype heterogeneity among *A. israelii* strains has been reported, but apparently they have no immunobiological significance. The *Actinomyces* are susceptible to sulfonamides, penicillins, tetracycline, and other antibiotics. Therefore early diagnosis and treatment is the best means of controlling the disease.

Nocardiosis

Nocardiosis in humans usually is caused by two of the many species of the genus *Nocardia: N. asteroides* or *N. brasiliensis.* The latter species is not so geographically restricted as the name would imply—it is found in South and Central America and in Mexico and the United States. The *Nocardia* cells tend to be acid-fast in their staining characteristics, but not as uniformly so as the tubercle bacilli. These and other aerobic actinomycetes are common saprophytic soil organisms. Usually, but not always, *Nocardia* infections are opportunistic, tending to occur in debilitated patients, especially those on immunosuppressive or steroid medication. The primary infection in human nocardiosis usually is pulmonary and can range from a single suppurative lesion to scattered lesions to lobar consolidation. Following any degree of pulmonary involvement, the *Nocardia* may invade the bloodstream and metastasize to various body organs including the liver, spleen, kidneys, and brain, thereby causing a variety of organ-related pathological symptoms.

V. T. Schuhardt once was present at an autopsy performed on an elderly person who

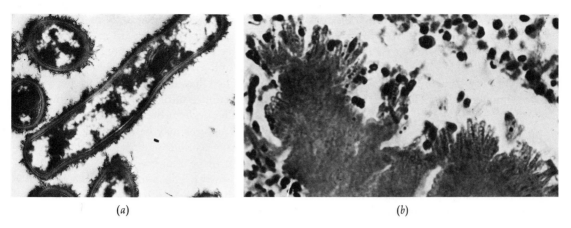

(a)   (b)

Figure 21–1. (a) Electron micrograph of a thin section through cells of *Actinomyces israelii;* procaryotic features, including a gram-positive cell wall, are demonstrated. (b) Hematoxylin and eosin (H and E) stain of a section through a sulfur granule showing peripheral clubs. About 2815×. (Both courtesy of M. A. Gerencser and J. M. Slack.)

had been diagnosed as tubercular. The few observed acid-fast bacilli found in his sputum had been atypical, however, and tubercle bacilli had not been isolated. When the bone saw used to open the chest cavity cut through a portion of the attached diaphragm, a spray of pus was dispersed widely in the autopsy room. Upon physical examination a walled-off abscess several inches in diameter was found attached to the diaphragm, the peritoneal wall, and the liver. *Nocardia asteroides* was isolated from the pus in the abscess. Those in the room at the time of autopsy spent several anxious weeks wondering whether or not they had inhaled enough of the aerosol to result in infection.

The Nocardia species grow well, but slowly, on most laboratory media incubated aerobically at 25 to 37°C. The colonies on agar media may be glabrous (skinlike consistency), wrinkled, and bright orange in color; or they may be butyrous (butter consistency), smooth, glistening, and ranging in color from white to pink, salmon, or brown. Dry powdery colonies with moldlike aerial mycelia have occasionally been reported. Sulfadiazine and nalidixic acid appear to be the drugs of choice for the treatment of nocardiosis. For more detailed information concerning the pathogenic Actinomycetaceae see Gordon (1974) and Dowell and Sonnenwirth (1974).

TRUE FUNGI (EUMYCETES)

Eumycetes are characterized by a simple plant body (thallus) that lacks chlorophyll and is not differentiated into roots, stems, or leaves. The thallus of fungi may exhibit three forms: bacterialike, yeastlike, or moldlike. The moldlike thallus is composed of branching intertwined filaments (hyphae) producing a dense mat of growth (mycelium). The mycelium produces various types of reproductive bodies (spores). The form and manner in which spores are produced, together with the appearance of the hyphae and mycelium, provide the major characteristics used to classify filamentous fungi. Eumycetes formerly were divided into four classes: Phycomycetes, Ascomycetes, Basidiomycetes, and Deuteromycetes, the latter being composed of imperfect (asexual spores) fungi. Now, however, the class Phycomycetes has been subdivided into six classes yielding a current total of nine classes of Eumycetes (see Webster 1970; Baker 1971). Spores may be produced as sexual spores (the result of nuclear fusion and recombination) or asexual spores, which are produced in, on, or by the mycelium without nuclear fusion. The majority of pathogenic fungi are found in the class Deuteromycetes. These *fungi imperfecti* either do not possess sexual forms or the sexual sporulation forms have yet to be discovered. A brief description of asexual spores is in order since their appearance is of great taxonomic value (see Figure 21-2).

Thallospores are produced by changes in the mycelium or thallus. There are three types of thallospores:

1. Blastospores—spores produced by budding (yeasts); see Figure 21-2a

2. Chlamydospores—spores produced by hyphal cells changing into thick-walled resistant structures; see Figure 21-2b

3. Arthrospores—spores produced by hyphal fragmentation; see Figure 21-2c

The more specialized types of asexual spores are conidia and sporangiospores. True conidia are produced by a structure called a *conidiophore*. The conidia are free (not in a sac) and are produced mainly by the Ascomycetes (see Figure 21-2d). Sporangiospores are produced inside a sac called a *sporangium* that develops on the end of a sporangiophore (see Figure 21-2e).

With the exception of bacterialike (Actinomycetales) and yeastlike fungi (*Cryptococcus* and *Candida* species), the fungi cannot be identified by bacteriological techniques. They are identified primarily by morphological criteria. Since the identification of filamentous fungi depends upon their microscopic appearance, preparations must be made that will allow the observation of undisturbed fungal elements. Preliminary examination of the growth may be made with low-magnification microscopy or the use of a dissecting microscope. "Teased preparations" may be made by teasing some of the mycelium with bacteriological needles in a drop of lactophenol—cotton blue on a microslide (see Paik and Suggs 1974). Placing a coverslip on the preparation readies it for microscopic observation.

Often it is impossible to disperse the mycelium without destroying important identifying characteristics, making it necessary to prepare a slide culture. This culture allows observation without disturbing fungal growth. One method of preparing such a culture is to place a block of Sabouraud's or other appropriate agar on a sterile glass microscope slide. The sides of the block are inoculated with the fungus and a sterile coverslip is placed on the block. Then the slide culture is placed in a sterile moist chamber until typical fungal growth appears. The undisturbed arrangement of sporulation structures may be observed in this manner. (*Caution:* Slide cultures should never be prepared using fungi with white, cottony mycelial growth. The genera *Coccidioides, Histoplasma,* and *Blastomyces* have that appearance and are highly infectious by the airborne respiratory route. These agents should only be handled by skilled laboratory workers who have access to specialized safety equipment.) The agents of systemic mycoses exhibit dimorphism; that is, they exist as filamentous fungi in nature but change into another morphological structure (usually yeast) in the tissues of an infected host. Demonstration of dimorphism in a fungus is of taxonomic value.

DERMATOPHYTOSES

Etiology and Epidemiology

The dermatophytoses certainly belong in the miscellaneous contact subgroup of diseases since they may be acquired from contact with infected humans, animals, or contaminated moist environments. Dermatophytoses are fungal infections of the skin commonly known as ringworm, athlete's foot, or "jock itch." The term *ringworm* developed from a period in the history of infectious disease when only macroscopically visible parasites were known. The disease was believed to be the result of a worm (*Tinea*) in the skin. Current medical terminology reflects this notion by referring to ringworm of the scalp as "tinea capitis," athlete's foot as "tinea pedis," and jock itch as "tinea cruris."

Several species of fungi are etiological agents of dermatophytoses, but they all are classified within three genera: *Trichophyton, Microsporum,* and *Epidermidophyton. Epidermidophyton* and certain species of *Trichophyton* and *Microsporum* are *anthropophilic*—that is, they cause

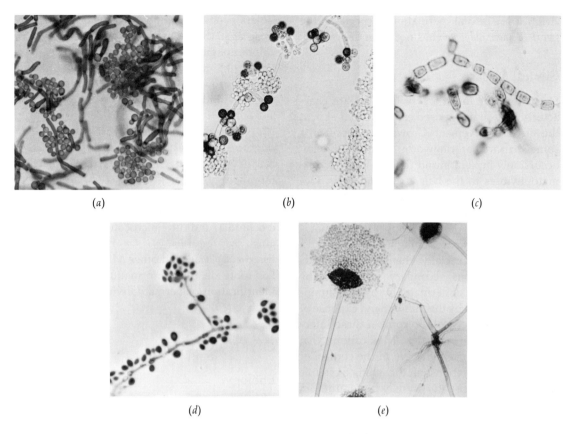

Figure 21–2. (a) Clusters of blastospores of *Pityrosporum furfur* among hyphae or pseudohyphae.
(b) Spherical chlamydospores of *Candida albicans* among pseudohyphae and clusters of smaller blastospores. (c) Arthrospores of *Coccidioides immitis*. (d) Conidia of *Sporothrix schenckii* around tip and on sides of conidiophore and along hypha. (e) Sporangia of *Rhizopus arrhizus*; one has been ruptured, releasing sporangiospores. ((a) Courtesy of J. T. Sinski; (b) through (e) courtesy of the Center for Disease Control, Atlanta, GA.)

disease only in humans and are isolated only from humans. Transmission of anthropophilic fungi is through contact with infected peeled skin or with secondary vehicles such as moist environments previously contaminated by an infected individual (for example, swimming pool walkways or shower stalls). Other members of *Trichophyton* and *Microsporum* are said to be zoophilic, which indicates a predilection for animals. Humans become infected with zoophilic fungi by contact with infected animals or animal hair. Other agents, *Microsporum gypseum* in particular, are *geophilic*. Humans acquire geophilic fungi through contact with contaminated soil or plant matter.

Sexual forms of some dermatophytic species have now been discovered—a development that necessitates reclassification with a concomitant change in nomenclature. Such taxonomic changes, resulting in the alteration of long-accepted names, are always confusing. For the purpose of completeness, the following nomenclature changes are mentioned: (1) *Microsporum* species with sexual sporulation now belong in the genus *Nannizzia*; (2) such species of the genus *Trichophyton* now belong to the genus

Arthroderma. Sexual sporulation in species of the genus *Epidermidophyton* has not been discovered.

Clinical Disease

Dermatophytic infections of the skin are characterized by slightly raised erythematous skin at the site of involvement. Growth may occur in a somewhat circular (ringworm) fashion. Infection occurs only in keratinized tissues, limiting dermatophytoses to the hair, skin, and nails. Despite this limitation, extensive skin, hair, or nail involvement with resulting inflammation can occur, but the major problems with dermatophytoses are cosmetic. Itching in the lesions can be bothersome, especially when scratching leads to a more serious secondary infection. The economic impact of dermatophytoses is significant when judged by the number and expense of antifungal products sold to combat these infections in the United States. Medications that contain tolnaftate are effective in the control of some fungal infections of the skin. Systemic treatment with griseofulvin may be required in particularly severe or refractory infections.

Most of the dermatophytes can cause any of the types of infections mentioned above. Some host specificity occurs, in that *Microsporum* infection usually causes tinea capitis in prepubescent individuals.

Laboratory Diagnosis

The diagnosis of dermatophytosis can usually be established by the classic symptoms supported by microscopic examination of scrapings of infected tissue. The tissue is first cleared with 10 percent potassium hydroxide (KOH) and gentle heat. Potassium hydroxide clears the tissue but leaves the mycelial elements unaffected, permitting visualization. Or cultures of the fungus can be stained by treatment with lactophenol–cotton blue. The appearance of the hyphae in the tissue is similar regardless of the dermatophyte etiology. To establish the specific etiology of the infection, the affected tissues must be cultured. The medium of choice for the isolation of dermatophytes is Sabouraud dextrose agar (SDA) modified by the addition of chloramphenicol (0.05 mg/ml) and cycloheximide (0.5 mg/ml). Chloramphenicol inhibits the overgrowth of bacterial contaminants while cycloheximide inhibits saprophytic fungi such as *Penicillium* and *Aspergillus.*

Generic and species identification of *Microsporum, Trichophyton,* and *Epidermidophyton* is based upon subtle differences in microscopic morphology, pigment production, and growth requirements. Figure H on the back cover presents the features—thick-walled echinulate macroconidia and no microconidia—that distinguish *Microsporum gypseum* from *Trichophyton, Epidermidophyton,* and other *Microsporum* species. For more detailed information concerning the identification of dermatophytes, see Ajello and Padhye (1974).

CRYPTOCOCCOSIS

Etiology

Cryptococcosis is a disease of the pulmonary system acquired by the inhalation of the infectious agent. Suppurative infections of the skin have been reported but are rare. Dissemination of the infection can result in cryptococcal meningitis.

Cryptococcosis is caused by a yeastlike fungus known as *Cryptococcus neoformans.* Perfect stages of the cryptococci may subdivide the genus *Cryptococcus* into several genera in the class Basidiomycetes, such as *Leucosporidium, Filobasidiella,* and perhaps others depending upon the morphological features of the isolates showing sexual sporulation. Regardless of the newer taxonomic trends, medical literature continues to refer to the disease as cryptococcosis.

Clinical Disease and Epidemiology

The portal of entry of the cryptococci usually is the upper respiratory tract. The primary focus of infection is the lungs, where the infection may remain localized or disseminate. Dissemination may occur with very little lung involvement or following apparent resolution of the lung lesions. Skin lesions may occur as a result of dissemination via the bloodstream or by direct inoculation.

Pulmonary cryptococcosis is probably a common disease that heals after minimal discomfort or symptomatology in the host. Fulminant cases of pulmonary disease are rare but do occur. Lesions may occur in any part of the lung with more extensive involvement and fever in severe cases. Lesions may be small and go unnoticed. Unlike lung lesions of tuberculosis and other systemic fungal diseases, cryptococcal lesions may heal without causing permanent evidence of infection. The severity of disease seems to depend upon the size of the infectious dose and the host's state of health. Regardless of the extent of multiplication of cryptococci, little tissue reaction is apparent, as evidenced by the rare occurrence of cavities, calcification, or caseation necrosis comparable to that described in tuberculosis (Chapter 9). Changes in normal tissue in many cases may be due mainly to the growth of yeast cells that physically displace tissue. Exact pathogenic mechanisms are not known.

Dissemination may occur at any state of lung involvement. The fact that the most frequently diagnosed form of cryptococcosis is meningeal is evidence that dissemination usually occurs with a minimum of pathology at the primary focus of infection. The reason for the predilection of Cryptococcus for nervous tissue can only be speculated upon. Perhaps the reputed inhibitory factors of serum are not present in the central nervous system, or the presence of nutritional factors such as creatinine or amino acids may provide selective advantages for central nervous system disease. The onset of cryptococcal meningitis is gradual; a common complaint is headache of increasing severity. Fever is present, and with progressing disease other signs of meningitis such as nuchal rigidity and positive Kernig's and Brudzinski's signs develop. The clinical course of untreated cryptococcal CNS disease extends from several months to several years, but the eventual outcome is almost always death.

Cryptococcus neoformans is closely associated in nature with pigeon nests. The organisms can be recovered in large numbers (up to 10^7 per gram) in debris from pigeon roosts. Dry material from the roost contains nutrients that appear to provide a selective advantage for cryptococci—in fact, the cryptococci may predominate over all other microorganisms in this environment. Pigeons were commonly raised on farms prior to 1940; since that time the number of rural pigeons has declined, but the number of urban pigeons is ever-increasing.

Cryptococcosis is worldwide in distribution and occurs more commonly in males than females, perhaps because outdoor occupations make significant exposure more likely in males. In the environment, cells of cryptococci usually possess little capsular material. Thoroughly dried, naturally occurring cryptococci are smaller in size than cultural or *in vivo* forms. The small size allows the organisms to become airborne more easily and elude the protective action of the ciliated epithelium of the respiratory bronchi.

Disease is more severe and systemic dissemination more likely in persons with an underlying debilitating disease. Compromise of the immune system of individuals by cancer or immunosuppressive drugs can reactivate old, inactive, walled-off lesions, resulting in a delayed onset of dissemination and cryptococcal meningitis. Although exposure to infectious cryptococci must be common, large outbreaks of cryptococcosis are unknown, indicating that the infected individual's state of health is the most important factor in determining the development of severe disease.

Laboratory Diagnosis

Since the symptoms of cryptococcal disease, even in the disseminated forms, are idiopathic in nature, laboratory demonstration of the causative yeast is the only way to establish a specific diagnosis. In a case of pulmonary disease, the laboratory specimen would be sputum; in CNS disease, spinal fluid. The *C. neoformans* are fragile and distort during drying or fixation for staining. Cells stain irregularly or not at all and are impossible to distinguish as cryptococci in dried, stained preparations. The observation of *C. neoformans* in clinical specimens is best accomplished by a negative contrast stain, which is efficacious because of the presence of a wide capsule in most clinically significant isolates.

Spinal fluid should be centrifuged and the sediment used to prepare negatively stained smears. Sputum can be used directly or after N-acetyl-cysteine digestion and centrifugal concentration. A negatively stained smear can be prepared by placing a drop of India ink and a loop of the specimen on a microslide and placing a coverslip on the mixture. Figure 21-3 shows the appearance of *C. neoformans* in such a preparation. The distinctive capsule appears as a clear area, since it is unpenetrated by India ink particles. Inside the capsule, budding double-walled yeast cells are seen. Yeast cells from

Figure 21–3. India ink preparation of spinal fluid showing yeasts of *Cryptococcus neoformans;* note the capsule around each. The considerably smaller, irregular cells in the field are white blood cells.

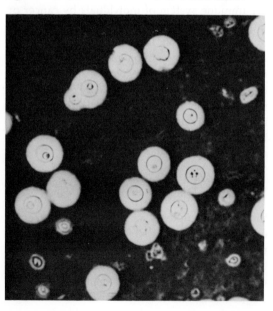

clinical material are round to ovoid and may range in size from 4 to 8 microns. The microscopic observation of typical yeast cells suggests the diagnosis of cryptococcosis.

Clinical specimens should be cultured regardless of the outcome of direct examination. The appearance of artifacts (such as powder from surgical gloves and leucocytes) that may be present in the specimen can be confusing. Isolates of *C. neoformans* vary in the size of their capsules, although some degree of encapsulation is required for virulence. Specimens containing too few organisms to visualize microscopically may yield a diagnosis through culture.

The medium of choice for the isolation of *C. neoformans* is SDA. Cycloheximide should not be incorporated into the medium since it inhibits many strains. Antibacterial inhibitors such as chloramphenicol may be used to advantage. Colonies of cryptococci may develop as early as 24 to 96 hours of incubation but may be delayed; cultures should be incubated 4 to 6 weeks before discarding them as negative. Generic features of significance are production of urease, lack of mycelia on cornmeal-Tween agar, and the presence of a capsule. A number of saprophytic *Cryptococcus* species exist that may require additional tests to differentiate.

The taxonomic characteristics of greatest significance in the identification of *C. neoformans* are culture growth at 37°C and pathogenicity for mice when injected intravenously or intracerebrally. Tests to determine the pattern of sugar and nitrate assimilation are useful in the speciation of the genus *Cryptococcus.*

Serological tests are especially useful in the diagnosis of cryptococcosis. Cases of CNS involvement may have focal lesions in the brain without contaminating the spinal fluid with yeasts. Culture of the spinal fluid from such patients would be misleadingly negative. Serodiagnostic tests may aid in the diagnosis of culturally unprovable pulmonary cases. During the acute stages of the cryptococcosis, an antigenemia occurs. It appears that the system is overburdened with excessive amounts of capsular polysaccharide to the extent that as the disease progresses, capsular antigen excess appears in the serum, urine, or spinal fluid. The serological tests of most value, therefore, are designed to detect the cryptococcal antigen in body fluids of the patient. A latex flocculation test was designed by Bloomfield et al. (1961) to detect circulating cryptococcal antigen. Latex particles are sensitized with anticryptococcal globulin. In the presence of cryptococcal antigen, the latex particles will flocculate as the specific GA reaction occurs. A positive latex test indicates cryptococcal disease. As a patient overcomes the disease, the antigenemia disappears and cryptococcal antibodies appear in the serum. Thereafter a latex test, using latex particles sensitized with antigen, will give a GA reaction that has prognostic value and can monitor the efficacy of therapy.

Therapy

The discovery of the antifungal drug amphotericin B has decreased the mortality of all systemic fungal infections. As mentioned in the section on clinical disease, CNS cryptococcosis was almost uniformly fatal in the past. Now, with amphotericin B therapy, the mortality is less than 10 percent, but retreatment is often necessary because of a tendency to relapse after treatment.

HISTOPLASMOSIS

Etiology

Histoplasmosis is a disease of the pulmonary system acquired by inhalation of spores produced by a free living fungus. The disease is worldwide in distribution but occurs more frequently in areas inhabited by large numbers of birds, particularly starlings. In the United States the area of highest incidence is the Mississippi-Ohio River Valley. In highly endemic areas, the total human population can experience histoplasmosis. Most infections are asymptomatic, but severe disease occurs in about 5 percent of those infected. Severe forms can range in degree from moderately severe pulmonary disease to disseminated and possibly fatal cases involving

the bone marrow, liver, spleen, and other reticuloendothelial tissues.

Histoplasma capsulatum was first described by Darling (1906) in tissue sections from a fulminant infection that he decided was a protozoal disease. Subsequent study has shown the agent to be a fungus exhibiting dimorphism— that is, a morphological form in tissue different from that in *in vitro* culture. Discovery of a sexual sporulation state of *H. capsulatum* resulted in the addition of the name *Emmonsiella capsulata* to the taxonomic literature dealing with this organism.

Of all the systemic fungi, *H. capsulatum* is possibly the most nutritionally fastidious. Growth will occur on SDA, but enhanced growth and increased isolation rates result from the use of a richer medium. Brain-heart infusion (BHI) blood agar, or a mixture containing both BHI and SDA called SaBHI, are proposed by leading mycologists. Regardless of the medium chosen, the use of one richer than SDA is advantageous. The addition of cycloheximide and chloramphenicol is recommended by some workers. *Histoplasma capsulatum* will exhibit two cultural forms *in vitro,* one of which corresponds to the yeast phase found in infected tissue and the other to the mold phase that occurs in soil. Media and conditions of incubation influence culture forms—yeast forms develop at 37°C on rich medium (blood agar), whereas mold forms develop at 25°C on less nutritious media such as SDA.

Clinical Disease and Epidemiology

Microconidia—asexual reproductive spores produced by the mold form—are the infectious agents of histoplasmosis. The portal of entry of these airborne spores is the respiratory tract. In the lungs the spores convert to budding yeast cells that multiply and metastasize to the liver, spleen, and bone marrow. Metastasis occurs via blood, and the yeast cells probably are transported in macrophages. In most cases the infection abates at this point and the only residual indication of histoplasmosis is calcified lesions in the lung. Histoplasmosis may be completely asymptomatic, or symptoms may range from a mild influenzalike illness to a more severe disease characterized by fever, night sweats, weight loss, and occasional productive cough with *hemoptysis* (coughed-up blood that occurs when an infectious process erodes into contiguous pulmonary vasculature). The prognosis for these forms of acute pulmonary histoplasmosis is good, the disease resolving in 1 to 2 weeks with few residual effects except for pulmonary calcifications and hypersensitivity to the histoplasmin skin test comparable to the tuberculin test. This hypersensitivity usually persists for a lifetime. Reactivation of histoplasmosis can occur with the onset of a debilitating disease or immunosuppressive therapy. Reactivated histoplasmosis is more serious than the original disease and more closely resembles disseminated or chronic histoplasmosis. Mortality is uncommon in primary histoplasmosis.

Disseminated histoplasmosis may ensue closely after the primary infection or may develop slowly during chronic histoplasmosis. Fever, anemia, leucopenia, cough, adrenal involvement, and enlargement of the liver and spleen occur as the infection disseminates. False negative skin tests are frequent in the disseminated disease. The mortality of this form of the disease, if untreated, is at least 80 percent.

Chronic histoplasmosis may closely follow the primary disease or may develop after a period of latency. Chronic disease is characterized by a low-grade fever, productive cough, and pulmonary cavitations typical of those seen in tuberculosis and other chronic lung infections. Chronic disease rarely resolves and usually progresses into disseminated histoplasmosis. Mortality in chronic disease is 30 percent unless the disease is interrupted by treatment.

The pathogenesis of histoplasmosis is similar to that of tuberculosis (see Chapter 9) in that systemic hypersensitivity plays a pathological role. Once infected, a person is refractory to reinfection, indicating an immunizing effect. The allergic reaction that occurs in the lungs following reexposure to the sensitizing allergens may partially account for the severity of chronic, reactivated, and disseminated histoplasmosis.

Histoplasmosis is worldwide in distribution and may occur as sporadic individual cases or as large epidemics. Though the disease is wide in distribution, a number of conditions are necessary for histoplasmosis to become endemic in an area. The role of climatic conditions has been studied extensively, but the most important correlation seems to be a large bird or bat population. High concentrations of starlings in the wooded areas of Ohio, Kentucky, Tennessee, and other Ohio-Mississippi River Valley states are characteristic of areas of high endemicity. *Histoplasma capsulatum* often has been isolated from air and soil. Soil with a high content of composting bat guano or bird droppings has been found to be the richest source of natural infection. Nitrogenous compounds of bird manure enhance the growth of *H. capsulatum* in culture. Seeding of dropping-laden soil is probably accomplished by the fecal droppings from infected birds, aided to some degree by transportation on bird feathers. Guano in caves is probably seeded by droppings from intestinally infected bats.

Infections are more common in adult males than females, but no sex selectivity is apparent in children. Occupation and recreation involving outdoor activities do not fully explain the higher incidence in males. In highly endemic areas almost all individuals give positive skin tests by the age of 20, indicating that infection is almost universal.

Epidemics of histoplasmosis are frequent. In fact, public health and medical school epidemiologists often present histoplasmosis outbreaks as models. One such outbreak occurred among children in a school in Ohio who decided to commemorate Earth Day, 1970, by cleaning the school ground. Dust created by the vigorous cleaning activities in the school ground contained *H. capsulatum* spores. Air conditioning intake ducts sucked in and disseminated the dust and spores, resulting in the infection of many of the school's students and thereby increasing their ecological awareness.

Histoplasmin

The skin test material used to detect delayed hypersensitivity to infection by *H. capsulatum* is called *histoplasmin*. Histoplasmin is a filtrate of a

2–4 month culture of the mycelial phase growth in nonallergenic broth. The filtrate is diluted to give appropriate reactivity and is administered intradermally. A 5-millimeter-diameter area of induration (turgid swelling) at 48 hours is a positive test. Histoplasmin hypersensitivity has no diagnostic value unless the patient with symptoms compatible with histoplasmosis was a documented nonreactor just prior to the onset of symptoms. This set of circumstances is rare and impractical, thereby relegating the use of histoplasmin to surveillance studies. Such surveys were essential in establishing that histoplasmosis is a common mild disease with rare complications rather than a rare but uniformly fatal disease.

Laboratory Diagnosis

The diagnosis of histoplasmosis can be established by microscopic observation of the etiological agent in tissues or exudates, growth of the agent from specimens, or the serodiagnostic reactivity of the patient's serum. Direct examination of clinical specimens reveals fewer positives than other methods but, because of its rapidity, should always be attempted in suspect cases. Clinical material should be smeared on a glass microslide, dried, fixed, and stained with Giemsa or a special fungal stain such as the periodic-acid Schiff (PAS) or Grocott-Gomorimethenamine silver (GMS) stains. The observation of yeast cells 2 to 5 microns in diameter occurring intracellularly in macrophages or histiocytes will confirm a diagnosis of histoplasmosis (see Figure 21-4).

For culture the specimen should be inoculated to medium suitable for the growth of both phases of the dimorphic fungus. Some mycologists believe that isolation of the yeast phase is less likely because of bacterial overgrowth and that only attempts to isolate the mold phase are practical. The growth of both forms from a normally sterile clinical specimen, however, results in a more rapid diagnosis. The yeast phase of H. capsulatum is tough and glabrous (skinlike) to smooth and yeastlike. A wet mount of the growth will reveal oval, budding yeast cells 2 to 5 microns in size. Upon inoculation to SDA and

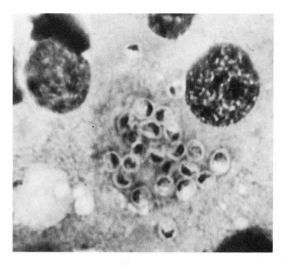

Figure 21–4. Giemsa-stained smear of liver tissue showing intracellular yeasts of *Histoplasma capsulatum*. (Courtesy of the Center for Disease Control, Atlanta, GA.)

incubation at 25°C, the yeast phase will convert to mycelial growth. The mycelial or mold phase produces a white to buff-brown fluffy colony. Since the mycelial growth is highly infectious, extreme care must be exercised in handling such cultures. Microscopic examination of a teased preparation of the colony will reveal delicate septate hyphae bearing two types of sporulation (see Figure 21-5). Large (8–16 microns) tuberculate (rough-walled) macroaleuriospores and small (2–5 microns) microconidia are produced. The microscopic appearance of the mold phase of *H. capsulatum* is mimicked by two saprophytic genera, *Sepedonium* and *Chrysosporium*. Conversion of mold to yeast phase is necessary to confirm the isolates as *H. capsulatum*, since the saprophytic genera produce only the mold phase. Conversion to the yeast phase is often fraught with problems, and it may be necessary to inoculate mice to effect the conversion. It is necessary to incubate primary cultures for a minimum of 6 weeks to be able to report a negative culture with certainty. *Histoplasma capsulatum* is slow-growing and may take 4 weeks or more for macroscopically visible growth to occur.

Serological techniques are a valuable adjunct to culture. Cultures can be overgrown with

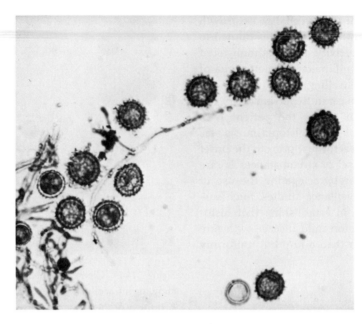

Figure 21–5. Wet mount of mycelial phase of *Histoplasma capsulatum* showing tuberculate macro-aleuriospores. About 1540×. (Courtesy of J. E. Steadham.)

contaminants or be negative because the organisms are in "closed" lesions. The serological test of most significance is a complement fixation test using both yeast and mold phase (histoplasmin) antigens. This test provides both diagnostic and prognostic information. Diagnostically significant titers are usually present 2 to 4 weeks after infection. A rising titer in subsequent serum specimens indicates progressing disease; a falling titer indicates successful therapy or recovery from the disease. Occasionally false positive reactions occur in the serum of patients with other systemic mycoses (coccidioidomycosis and blastomycosis). For this reason, the complement fixation test should be performed using not only histoplasmal antigens but also antigens from *Coccidioides immitis* and *Blastomyces dermatitidis.* Reactions tend to occur at higher titer in the homologous system, facilitating the interpretation of the test results. Other serological tests such as a latex flocculation and an immunodiffusion test have been advocated for the serodiagnosis of histoplasmosis, but the complement fixation test is the most widely used. For additional information concerning the

serodiagnosis of systemic fungal infections, see Kaufman (1974).

Therapy, Control, and Prevention

Treatment of clinically significant cases of histoplasmosis is the same as for other systemic fungal diseases—basically the use of amphotericin B. Control and prevention of histoplasmosis can be practiced only on a limited scale relative to its widely distributed natural occurrence. A localized area, known to be highly contaminated as a result of case exposure or culture, can be disinfected by spraying the ground with 3 percent formalin. This measure is limited but has been useful in curbing epidemics such as the Earth Day outbreak described above. Control of starling populations is desirable for many reasons, some unrelated to disease, but effective methods are not known. A mask could be worn or the ground wetted to control dust when cleaning out old chicken coops containing composted chicken or other bird droppings. Avoiding woods where birds roost or caves with infected bats would seem to be indicated. Persons living in highly endemic areas can probably do little to prevent infection, however, since winds can carry infectious particles for miles.

COCCIDIOIDOMYCOSIS

Etiology

Coccidioidomycosis is a pulmonary disease of the semidesert areas of the southwestern United States and South America. The disease is acquired by inhaling arthrospores of the fungus. As with histoplasmosis, almost all the individuals living in highly endemic areas become infected. The majority remain asymptomatic, but severe pulmonary disease can occur. Dissemination to multiple organs, skin, and the central nervous system occurs in a small percentage of cases and is often fatal.

Coccidioides immitis was originally reported in tissues obtained at autopsy from an Argentine soldier in 1891. It was first believed to be related to protozoa similar to those causing coccidiosis in chickens (hence the name Coccidioides). The true nature of the etiological agent was revealed when bacteriological cultures from lesions were consistently "contaminated" with a mold. Coccidioides immitis is considered to be a dimorphic fungus, even though the tissue phase is not demonstrable by ordinary in vitro culture techniques. The perfect stage of C. immitis, if any, is unknown.

Clinical Disease and Epidemiology

Clinical coccidioidomycosis exhibits a spectrum of disease pathology, ranging from asymptomatic pulmonary to fatal meningeal infections. The range of pulmonary disease is similar to that discussed in the section on histoplasmosis. The most common form is asymptomatic pulmonary disease; the second most common is symptomatic pneumonitis. Dissemination to the meninges, skin, and bone is rare but results in serious disease. Meningitis is the most common cause of death due to coccidioidomycosis. Fortunately, serious life-threatening disease is rare, occurring in less than 1 percent of the infections.

In the body, the arthrospores of C. immitis convert to tissue forms called spherules (see Figure 21-6). Specialized structures (endospores) form within the developing spherules. Mature spherules rupture, releasing a multitude of endospores, each with the ability to form spherules and repeat the cycle. Irritation of pulmonary tissues by arthrospores and spherules evokes a pyogenic response. The disease may be arrested at this stage with little residual evidence of lung pathology; or the lesions may progress by varying degrees. In all cases a delayed type of hypersensitivity develops by the second week. This is shown by conversion to a positive skin test reaction to the injection of coccidioidin. In mild forms of the pneumonitis, microabscesses and tubercles form. In disease of increased severity necrosis, caseation, and granuloma formation are correspondingly more extensive.

Figure 21-6. Endospore-containing spherules of Coccidioides immitis in a tissue section from a case of coccidioidomycosis. (Courtesy of the Center for Disease Control, Atlanta, CA.)

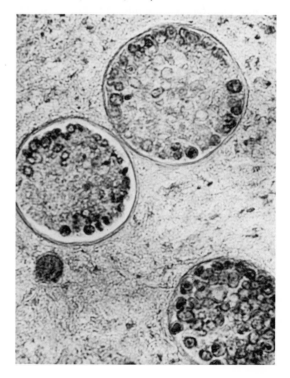

The organisms may disseminate after either extensive or little lung pathology. Metastasis to bone results in coccidioidal osteomyelitis, to skin in cutaneous coccidioidomycosis, and to the brain in coccidioidal meningitis. The infection also can become generalized, involving any of the tissues of the body. The meningeal form may have an acute or a protracted onset. Typical symptoms of meningeal irritation occur—headache, nuchal ridigity, positive Kernig's and Brudzinski's signs, and a pleocytosis in the spinal fluid. Untreated meningitis is almost always fatal. Treatment provides an ameliorative effect but often does not prevent the ultimate fatality of the disease. The pathogenic mechanism of C. immitis is not known, but a deleterious hypersensitivity reaction similar to that seen in tuberculosis and histoplasmosis is believed to play an important role.

Coccidioidomycosis is predominantly a New World disease. The proper natural conditions to support the endemicity of C. immitis occur in the ecological region classified as the Lower Sonoran Life Zone. Representative flora indigenous to the zone are yuccas, cacti, mesquites, and the creosote bush; the fauna include kangaroo rats, desert fox, and a variety of desert bats and birds. The zone is semiarid, averaging 10 inches of rainfall per year. Probably C. immitis grows around animal burrows where droppings provide organic material for rapid mycelial growth following desert showers. Mycelial elements develop resistant arthrospores that tend to survive dry spells. Winds pick up the arthrospores and disseminate them to other ecologically attractive sites or to the lungs of a person or animal unfortunate enough to be caught in a desert dust storm.

The disease shows no sex preference until after puberty. Adult males are more likely to have disseminated cases than are women. Dark-skinned races are more susceptible to systemic dissemination of coccidioidomycosis, the rate being up to 10 times that of light-skinned races. The size of the infectious dose seems to influence the severity of disease in any race. Occupational groups at risk are agricultural, construction, and other outdoor workers. Those who enjoy frequent outdoor recreation are also more prone to infection. Coccidioidomycosis is ordinarily an endemic disease with cases occurring sporadically. Epidemics have occurred in groups of susceptible individuals who spend time or dig in areas infected with C. immitis arthrospores. Epidemics among students on biology field trips and archaeology digs and soldiers on maneuver have been reported.

Coccidioidin

As mentioned in the preceding section, a person becomes hypersensitive to mycelial antigens by the second week of the disease. This hypersensitivity lasts for life unless systemic disseminated disease occurs or extremis (near death) develops. These conditions result in *anergy* (loss of responsiveness to any antigenic stimulation). Hypersensitivity is determined by a skin test using intradermally injected coccidioidin. (Coccidioidin is the filtrate of broth cultures of the C. immitis mold phase growth. The filtrates are standardized for reactivity.) The delayed hypersensitivity skin reaction is read at 48 to 72 hours after injection, and an induration of 5 millimeters is the minimum reaction considered positive.

The coccidioidin test is useful in determining the incidence or endemicity of coccidioidomycosis in an area. The test has no diagnostic value and, in fact, is contraindicated. Hypersensitive individuals can have a severe reaction resulting in necrosis and sloughing of a large portion of the dermis of the arm. In addition the antigenic stimulation of the skin-test material often results in an anamnestic response of serodiagnostic complement-fixing antibodies. Hence skin testing an individual can cause a false positive serological diagnosis in hypersensitive individuals. For additional details of this and other systemic mycoses see Larsh and Goodman (1974).

Laboratory Diagnosis

As in histoplasmosis, the diagnosis of coccidioidomycosis may be made in three ways: direct

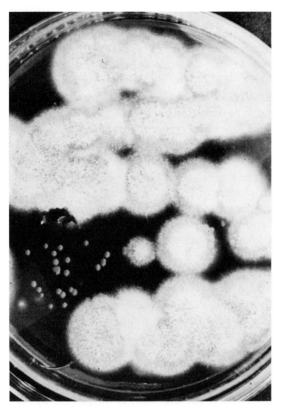

Figure 21–7. Colonies of *Coccidioides immitis* on Sabouraud's dextrose agar at room temperature. (Courtesy of J. E. Steadham.)

observation of spherules in exudate or tissue; recovery of *C. immitis* from cultures of exudate or tissue; demonstration of a high or rising antibody titer to *C. immitis* antigens.

The direct observation of spherules is facilitated by their large size (10–80 microns), thick walls, and endospores as seen in Figure 21-6. Staining of exudates is usually not helpful. The spherules may be visualized readily by clearing the specimen with 10 percent KOH. Observing the cleared specimen between a microslide and coverslip with subdued light can provide a rapid diagnosis. Tissues should be histologically sectioned with a microtome and stained to allow the observation of spherules. Usual histological stains such as hematoxylin and eosin are adequate, but the spherules also stain with special fungal stains.

Coccidioides immitis is readily cultured on simple SDA with or without inhibitors such as cycloheximide and chloramphenicol, which are recommended for contaminated specimens. Fluffy white, cottony mycelial growth (see Figure 21-7) may appear after several days' incubation; but, as with other fungi, negative cultures must be held 4 to 6 weeks before discarding. Slide preparations of the growth may be made only if a biological safety cabinet is available in which to work. Microscopic observation of slide preparations of teased mycelial growth will reveal typical delicate branched hyaline hyphae, which produce characteristic barrel-shaped arthrospores in alternating cells (see Figure 21-2*c*). Confirmation of the isolate as *C. immitis* can be done by animal inoculation. A carefully prepared suspension of the mycelial growth is injected into the testis of a guinea pig. The animal is sacrificed subsequent to the development of orchitis (inflammation of the testicle). Microscopic examination of tissue fluids from infected testes will reveal numerous spherules containing endospores.

Coccidioidomycosis, as stated above, can also be diagnosed serologically. Precipitin, immunodiffusion, latex particle agglutination, and complement fixation tests have been described. The most widely used of these is complement fixation. The antigen is prepared similarly to coccidioidin but cannot be autoclaved. Complement-fixing antibodies are slow to appear, sometimes requiring more than a month. Reactivity correlates well with disease. Rarely are symptomatic patients nonreactive. An increasing titer indicates a bad prognosis, whereas a falling titer indicates recovery or efficacious therapy. A single titer of 1:32 or greater signifies disease. Because of potential cross-reactions, a battery of fungal antigens is employed. The best practice is to include histoplasma yeast and mycelial phase antigens, *C. immitis,* and *B. dermatitidis* antigens.

Therapy, Control, and Prevention

Amphotericin B is currently the only efficacious therapeutic agent for serious fungal infections.

Nephrotoxicity of this drug is a serious side effect that is spurring the search for newer and safer drugs. Treatment of disseminated cases other than meningitis is usually successful. The development of meningitis is a bad prognostic sign. The control of a disease caused by organisms that thrive in vast natural habitats and whose survival does not depend upon causing infection is difficult, if not impossible. In geographically limited areas, dust control procedures have decreased infections. Limiting oneself to indoor or urban activities should diminish chances for infection. On the other hand, more than 95 percent of infections are mild or asymptomatic and have an immunizing effect. Consequently, extreme inconvenience to avoid natural coccidioidomycosis seems unwarranted. The disease is particularly severe in immunologically depressed individuals who, therefore, should avoid dusty conditions in endemic areas.

BLASTOMYCOSIS

Two forms of blastomycosis exist in two geographically distinct areas—North and South America. North American blastomycosis is caused by *Blastomyces dermatitidis* (the perfect stage of which is *Ajellomyces dermatitidis*). The natural habitat of *B. dermatitidis* is believed to be soil, but isolation from soil is rarely possible. Although the major portal of entry is the respiratory tract, some cases appear to result from traumatic inoculation. The clinical forms of blastomycosis are so similar to those of coccidioidomycosis and histoplasmosis that the reader is referred to those sections. Blastomycosis is rare, but sporadic cases occur over a wide geographical area. A skin test material, blastomycin, was once available but was found to have little usefulness because of nonspecific reactivity. The serodiagnosis of blastomycosis is complicated by cross-reactivity with other systemic mycoses, as discussed in the laboratory diagnosis of histoplasmosis. The surest laboratory diagnosis is the observation or isolation and identification of *B. dermatitidis* in exudate or tissue. The clearing of exudates with potassium hydroxide will reveal the characteristic yeast forms (see Figure 21-8). The tissue forms of this dimorphic fungus are spherical, thick-walled, and 8 to 15 microns in diameter with broad-based buds. The buds cause yeast pairs to appear like the figure 8. In cultures, the organism exhibits dimorphism: yeast on a rich medium at 37°C, mold on a poor medium at 25°C. Microscopic examination of the mold phase reveals only delicate, septate hyphae with microconidia borne singly (see Figure 21-9). Treatment is with amphotericin B.

South American blastomycosis is more properly called paracoccidioidomycosis since its etiology is *Paracoccidioides brasiliensis*. The routes of infection and disease caused by *P. brasiliensis* are similar to those of the other systemic fungi except that (1) a predilection for cartilage and mucocutaneous tissue exists and (2) the distribution is limited to Central and South America. Diagnostic methods are microscopic observation and culture. The appearance of *P. brasiliensis* in tissue differs from that of *B. dermatitidis* in that multiple buds occur from a central large yeast cell. Laboratory isolation is confirmed by the demonstration of dimorphism—the mycelial phase is indistinguishable from that of *B. dermatitidis* (shown in Figure 21-9).

Figure 21–8. Budding yeast forms of *Blastomyces dermatitidis*. About 4890×. (Courtesy of the Center for Disease Control, Atlanta, GA.)

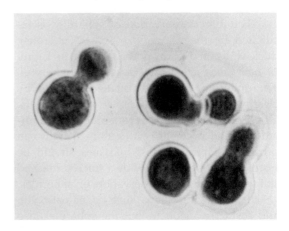

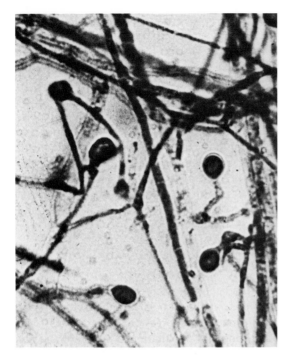

Figure 21–9. Mold phase of *Blastomyces dermatitidis* showing hyphae and microconidia. About 1720×. (Courtesy of J. E. Steadham.)

OPPORTUNISTIC FUNGAL INFECTIONS

The term *opportunistic* is applied to organisms that have little primary disease potential but can cause disease in a host with altered or compromised defense mechanisms. Organisms that usually cause opportunistic infections are common environmental organisms or constitute a portion of the "normal" human flora. Opportunistic infection can follow a drastic alteration of the normal flora through extensive antimicrobial therapy. The selection for resistant normal flora sometimes provides the stimulus for infection when normal flora alone would have maintained a healthy status quo. For example, the treatment of cancer with radiation, nucleic acid base analogs, or cytotoxic drugs results in impairment of the immune system, as does steroid therapy. In the sections on cryptococco-

sis, histoplasmosis, and coccidioidomycosis it was pointed out that immunosuppression could reactivate old chronic lesions from past disease. Impairment of resistance mechanisms also predisposes individuals to many other infectious problems, bacterial and viral as well as mycotic. *Candida, Aspergillus,* and *Rhizopus* species are common fungi that are opportunistic in their pathogenicity.

Candidiasis

Not all *Candida* infections are opportunistic, since some primary, apparently unprovoked, cases of candidiasis do occur: oral mucocutaneous candidiasis (thrush), vaginitis, onychomycosis (infection of the nails), and dermatitis (such as diaper rash). These appear to be primary infections or at least the triggering mechanism is unknown. *Candida* are common flora of the upper respiratory, alimentary, and urogenital tracts. Ordinarily, little disease potential is exhibited by these ubiquitous organisms. Antibiotic therapy (*Candida* are resistant), diabetes, leukemia, and cytotoxic drugs can convert them into pathogens causing systemic or locally severe disease. Candidiasis can affect any or all tissues of the body with pathological symptoms commensurate with the organ involved. For an example of the pathogenic potential of *Candida,* see Figure 21-10.

Candidiasis may be caused by a number of *Candida* species, but by far the most common agent is *Candida albicans.* A few of the other species that may be isolated are *C. parapsilosis, C. stellatoidea, C. guilliermondi, C. pseudotropicalis,* and *C. krusei. Candida* are oval, nonencapsulated, fermentative yeasts that produce pseudomycelia in cornmeal-Tween agar (CTA) inoculated by cut streak (needle cutting into the agar). *Candida albicans* is identified by the ability to produce terminal chlamydospores in CTA (see Figure 21-11). The speciation of other *Candida* is based upon sugar fermentation and assimilation patterns (see Silva-Hutner and Cooper 1974). The discovery of perfect stages of some species of *Candida* introduces the new generic designations

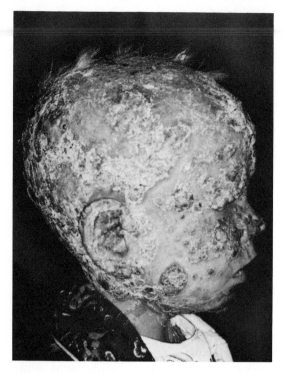

Figure 21–10. A severe case of candidiasis in an immune-deficient patient at age five years. (Courtesy of R. J. Schlegel.)

of *Pichia, Lodderomyces,* and *Kluyveromyces* in the class Ascomycetes, and several others appear to be lower Basidiomycetes. The isolation of *Candida* from clinical material is best accomplished on blood agar at 37°C or 25°C. Colonies are often apparent after overnight incubation.

The mechanism by which *Candida* causes disease is unclear. Colonizing organisms grow as yeasts on skin or mucocutaneous body surfaces. Filamentous forms similar to the pseudohyphae in CTA are seen when tissue invasion occurs. The direct observation of exudates or tissues the moment they are obtained is of utmost importance, since the morphological characteristics of the fungus can indicate more about the disease state than can the culture results. Infection can spread hematogenously or by contiguous extension.

The control of opportunistic infection depends upon how essential the predisposing factor is to the life of the patient. Where possible, cessation of antibiotic therapy or the discriminate use of antibiotics will control or prevent *Candida* infections. The periodic relocation of indwelling intravenous catheters will prevent catheter colonization and subsequent candidemia. Removal of indwelling urinary catheters will control or prevent bladder and higher urinary tract infections by *Candida*. Treatment of candidiasis depends upon the location of the infection. Nystatin is effective in bladder irrigation or topical ointments, whereas systemic infections require amphotericin B or 5-fluorocytosine therapy.

Aspergillosis

The predisposing factors of aspergillosis are leukemia, organ transplantation with subsequent immunosuppression, tuberculosis, and other causes of debilitation. Although there are over 200 species of *Aspergillus,* it is *A. fumigatus* that causes most cases of aspergillosis. The

Figure 21–11. Chlamydospores and pseudohyphae of *Candida albicans* grown on cornmeal agar. (Courtesy of the Center for Disease Control, Atlanta, GA.)

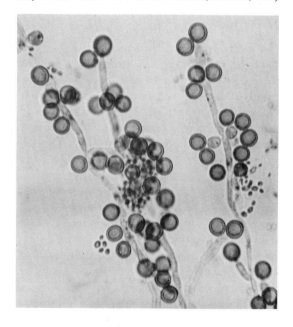

portal of entry is the respiratory tract. The pulmonary disease results in necrosis that spreads by extension. Dissemination to other organs can occur but is rare (see Campbell and Clayton 1964). *Aspergillus fumigatus* can grow in old tubercular or in systemic fungal cavities, resulting in a radiological picture known as "fluff" or "fungus ball." Fungus balls were once thought to be innocuous but can provide the nidus (point of origin) for invasive aspergillosis. Invasive aspergillosis is a life-threatening disease that is slowed but often not resolved by treatment with amphotericin B.

Aspergillus fumigatus grows well on SDA. Morphological features of the asexual conidiophores and conidia are used in identification. Serological techniques are available to identify *A. fumigatus* colony growth and serodiagnostic antibodies (see Warnock 1974). However, the serodiagnostic tests generally do not detect evidence of invasive aspergillosis.

Mucormycosis

Metabolic acidosis is the most important predisposing factor of rhinocerebral disease, the most severe mucormycotic infection. The term *mucormycosis* is used to describe disease produced by species of the genera *Rhizopus, Absidia,* and *Mucor,* all of which belong to the order Mucorales (bread molds). Diseases are similar, so the causative agent must be isolated and identified to establish the specific etiology. Metabolic acidosis usually is a result of uncontrolled diabetes, but other causes are known. The mechanism whereby an increased tissue concentration of acids, ketones, or glucose allows these ubiquitous saprophytic fungi to proliferate is unclear. The portal of entry is respiratory; the primary focus of infection is the paranasal sinuses. The fungi proliferate rapidly and spread by extension to the nose, eye, and brain. A predilection is shown for arterial vessels, and as the vessels are invaded emboli (blockages) occur. Infected emboli occlude vessels, and infarction (tissue death) and necrosis of dependent tissue ensue. The rhinocerebral form of mucormycosis is acutely fulminant; death can occur within 2 days after infection.

Reversing the acidotic condition of the patient causes remission, but the infection only becomes quiescent. Further invasion can occur if acidosis recurs. Prompt treatment with amphotericin B is recommended.

The survival of the patient is dependent upon rapid diagnosis. Direct examination of scrapings of infected tissues will show broad, aseptate ribbonlike hyphae coursing through the tissues. Clearing the tissues with potassium hydroxide aids the observation. A considerable amount of clinical judgment is required, since hyphae are scarce or absent in most obtainable tissue. Scrapings or aspirated sinus material should be cultured. It is difficult to interpret the clinical significance of the laboratory isolation of *Rhizopus, Mucor,* or *Absidia* species as they are frequent contaminants. Nevertheless, the isolation of these Mucorales should always be reported. The fungi grow abundantly on simple SDA at 37°C, often filling the tube in 1 or 2 days with fluffy white growth interspersed with black dots. Microscopic characteristics of the hyphae allow the generic identification of isolates. The species identifications are more difficult and require expert analysis.

The control of mucormycosis induced by diabetes lies in efficient public health programs involving the identification and control of diabetes. Prompt diagnosis and treatment of cases reduces the mortality significantly. Control of the etiological agents is impractical because of the ubiquity of these bread mold fungi as well as their usual harmlessness.

WOUND INOCULATION FUNGI

Mycetomas

The wound inoculation group of fungal diseases includes the mycetomas and sporotrichosis. Mycetomas have multiple etiology and may be a result of actinomycotic infection (see the section on the Actinomycetales in this chapter) or eumycotic infection. Eumycotic mycetoma results from traumatic inoculation of a naturally occur-ring fungus into the skin of an extremity. The disease involves chronic, slowly progressing nodular or suppurative lesions of the skin and subcutaneous tissue with little propensity for systemic dissemination. Local involvement can become quite extensive, however, and may ex-tend to underlying bones or joints. Joint in-volvement over many years leads to difficulty in normal joint movement. Subcutaneous and other tissue distension causes the severe dis-figuration pictured in most mycology texts. The most frequent cause of mycetoma in the United States is *Allescheria boydii* (the imperfect stage of which is *Monosporium apiospermium*).

Other etiological agents of mycetomas are *Madurella mycetomae, Phialophora jeanselmei* and *P. verrucosa, Fonsecaea pedrosoi* and *F. compacta,* and *Cladosporium carrionii.* The latter four fungi occur within the tissues as dark brown septate bodies (see Figure 21-12) rather than as grains in draining sinuses as in other mycetomas. The observation of these bodies in tissue provides the diagnosis of chromomycosis. Mycetomas are rare and may be treated by early surgical exci-sion of the infectious particles. Sporotrichosis also is transmitted by wound inoculation and is more common, so it merits consideration in more detail.

Sporotrichosis

Sporotrichosis is acquired by traumatic inocula-tion with an object contaminated with spores of *Sporothrix schenckii.* The disease is common among gardeners and is known as "rose fever" because of its frequent association with the prick of rose thorns. A rarer pulmonary form of the disease results from the inhalation of *S. schenckii* spores.

The spores of *S. schenckii* gain entrance into the skin and subcutaneous tissues by traumatic inoculation. There they convert to pleomorphic yeast cells, which multiply and form a subcu-taneous nodule at the site of the inoculation. The incubation period ranges from a week to

Figure 21–12. Septate, pigmented (sclerotic) bodies of chromomycosis in a tissue preparation cleared with KOH. About 2230×. (Courtesy of J. E. Steadham.)

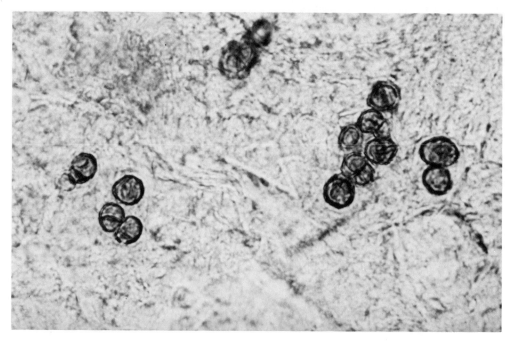

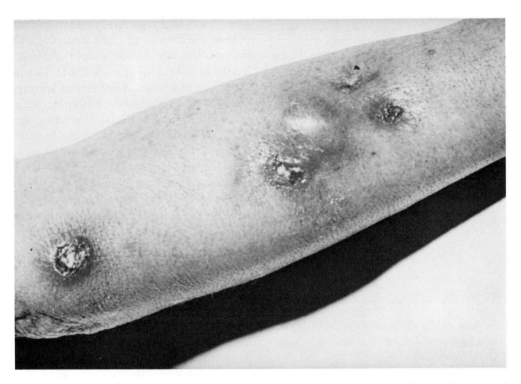

Figure 21–13. Lymphatic-associated skin lesions of sporotrichosis on a patient's arm. (Courtesy of the American Society of Clinical Pathologists.)

months, so that the insignificant wound may not be remembered by the patient. The nodule enlarges into a bubo, but little reaction occurs in the surrounding tissue. With time the skin covering the bubo becomes necrotic and drains. The lesions may heal with no other complications, or the yeasts may metastasize along lymph channels to the next lymph node. Here the process repeats itself. At one time a patient may have small, intermediate, and large closed nodules and necrotic draining lesions (see Figure 21-13). Lymphatic spread usually continues until a large regional lymph node is reached. Here the infection usually stops, but if dissemination to internal organs is to occur, it occurs as a result of the regional lymph node being unable to limit the infection. Metastasis to bones, liver, spleen, and lungs is found in the disseminated disease. The mode of pathogenesis is unknown, but observation of tissue reveals necrosis and caseating granulomas.

The natural habitat of *S. schenckii* is soil and plant matter. Isolation has been reported from tree bark, timbers, grass clippings, tree moss, and sphagnum (peat) moss. Epidemics of sporotrichosis have been traced to each of the sources mentioned. One unusual epidemic occurred in tennis players who, in their zest to volley, fell into piles of composting clippings from the grass tennis courts. Luckily the disease was mild in most of the well-nourished and physically fit individuals. An epidemic of sporotrichosis involving 13 Mississippi Forestry Commission workers and 4 pine seedling planters was described in detail in *MMWR* (23 July 1976).

The laboratory diagnosis of sporotrichosis is made by microscopically or culturally demonstrating the presence of *S. schenckii*. Aspiration of material from closed nodules provides the best specimen. Smears of the material can be dried, fixed, and stained with special fungal stains or a specific fluorescent antibody conju-

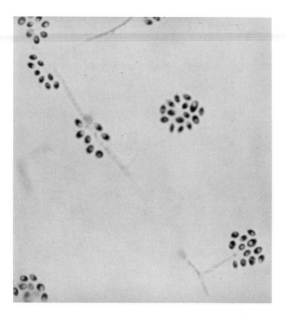

Figure 21–14. Conidia of *Sporothrix schenckii* borne singly along hyphae and in terminal clusters. (Courtesy of G. D. Roberts.)

Figure 21–15. yeast phase of *Sporothrix schenckii* illustrating pleomorphism. About 1960×. (Courtesy of J. E. Steadham.)

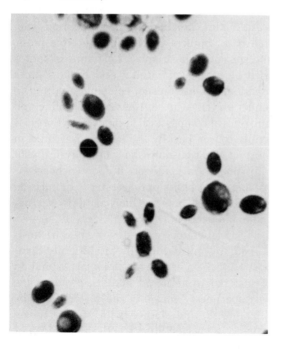

gate. Yeasts are frequently sparse and difficult to observe microscopically. The medium (SDA) for the isolation of *S. schenckii* should contain cycloheximide and chloramphenicol, and the cultures should be incubated at both room temperature and at 37°C. The fungus is dimorphic and grows as a yeast on rich media (such as blood agar) at 37°C. The mycelial phase of the fungus may appear in 3 to 5 days as off-white moldlike growth that develops tan to brownish-black coloration with time. A slide culture is usually necessary to demonstrate the delicate clusters and singly borne microconidia characteristic of *Sporothrix* (see Figure 21-14). The conversion of the mold phase to yeast phase (see Figure 21-15) is necessary to identify the isolate as *S. schenckii,* since some saprophytic fungi exhibit similar mycelial morphology.

Sporotrichosis is treated by the intravenous infusion of potassium iodide or amphotericin B. The control of sporotrichosis is compounded by its worldwide distribution, the necessity or desire to work with plants or to be outdoors, and the relative rarity of the disease. Control measures are best directed to areas or product lots that have proved to be infectious. Recall or warning of potentially hazardous material probably would occur too late to be of value because of the prolonged incubation periods. Attention to cleaning and topical disinfection of wounds, however minor, in individuals exposed to plant products is indicated.

REFERENCES

Ajello, L. and A. A. Padhye. 1974. Dermatophytes and the agents of superficial mycoses. Chapter 54 in *Manual of Clinical Microbiology.*

Baker, R. D. 1971. *Human Infection with Fungi, Actinomycetes, and Algae.* New York: Springer-Verlag.

Bloomfield, N., M. A. Gordon, and D. F. Elmendorf, Jr. 1961. Detection of *Cryptococcus neoformans* antigen in body fluids by latex particle agglutination. *Proc. Soc. Exper. Biol. Med.* 114:64–67.

Campbell, N. J. and Y. M. Clayton. 1964. Bronchopulmonary aspergillosis. *Am. Rev. Resp. Dis.* 89: 186–196.

Conant, N. F. 1965. Medical mycology. Chapter 37 in *Bacterial and Mycotic Infections of Man,* eds. R. J. Dubos and J. G. Hirsch. Philadelphia: Lippincott.

Conant, N. F., D. T. Smith, R. D. Baker, J. L. Callaway, and D. S. Martin. 1971. *Manual of Clinical Mycology.* 3rd. Philadelphia: Saunders.

Darling, S. T. A. 1906. A protozoan general infection producing pseudotubercles in the lungs and focal necrosis in the liver, spleen, and lymph nodes. *J. Amer. Med. Ass.* 46:1283–1285.

Dowell, V. R., Jr. and A. C. Sonnenwirth. 1974. Gram-positive, nonsporeforming, anaerobic bacilli. Chapter 42 in *Manual of Clinical Microbiology.*

Emmons, C. W., C. H. Binford, and J. P. Utz. 1970. *Medical Mycology.* 2nd ed. Philadelphia: Lea & Febiger.

Gordon, M. A. 1974. Aerobic pathogenic Actinomycetaceae. Chapter 17 in *Manual of Clinical Microbiology.*

Kaufman, L. 1974. Serodiagnosis of fungal diseases. Chapter 62 in *Manual of Clinical Microbiology.*

Larsh, H. W. and N. L. Goodman. 1974. Fungi of systemic mycoses. Chapter 57 in *Manual of Clinical Microbiology.*

Larone, D. H. 1976. *Medically Important Fungi.* Hagerstown, Md.: Harper and Row.

Paik, G. and M. T. Suggs. 1974. Reagents, stains, and miscellaneous test procedures. Chapter 95 in *Manual of Clinical Microbiology.*

Silva-Hutner, M. and B. H. Cooper. 1974. Medically important yeasts. Chapter 56 in *Manual of Clinical Microbiology.*

Slack, J. M. and M. A. Gerencser. 1975. *Actinomyces, Filamentous Bacteria: Biology and Pathogenicity.* Minneapolis: Burgess.

Warnock, D. W. 1974. Indirect immunofluorescence test for the detection of *Aspergillus fumigatus* antibodies. *J. Clin. Pathol.* 27:911–912.

Webster, J. 1970. *Introduction to Fungi.* New York: Cambridge University Press.

22
Tularemia

The animal disease tularemia was discovered (in ground squirrels) by G. W. McCoy in 1910 while searching for evidence of bubonic plague in rodents in Tulare County, California. The visceral lesions in trapped ground squirrels resembled those of the plague bacillus, but the causative organism could not be cultivated on media commonly used in the isolation of plague bacilli. This organism was finally isolated from the ground squirrel lesions by McCoy and Chapin in 1911 on egg-yolk agar medium. Subsequently they found that the essential growth constituent of this medium was cystine. Since this discovery, the organism has been cultivated on beef-infusion blood agar supplemented with cystine, thiamin, and glucose.

ETIOLOGY

McCoy and Chapin designated their ground squirrel isolate *Bacterium tularense*. Subsequently it was placed in the genus *Pasteurella*, which at that time included the species *P. pestis*, the causative organism of bubonic plague. Since

Pasteur was not involved in research on either organism, however, recent bacterial taxonomists have placed *P. pestis* in the genus *Yersinia* and have converted *P. tularense* to *Francisella tularensis*. The first human case of tularemia was reported by Wherry and Lamb in 1914.

Francisella tularensis is a tiny, coccoidal to rod-shaped, nonmotile bacillus. Capsules are not produced in cultures but have been reported in lesion exudates. The organisms stain gramnegative, but much better staining is obtained with dilute carbol fuchsin or polychromatic eosin–methylene-blue stains. In such environments as water, moist soil, hides, and infected carcasses, *F. tularensis* shows remarkable survival capacity.

Francisella tularensis can be cultivated on 5 percent rabbit-blood agar supplemented with glucose, cystine, and thiamin. Broth cultures are rarely used and require either a decreased oxygen tension or large inocula to initiate growth. Although the pathogenic mechanism of *F. tularensis* is generally believed to be endotoxic, a Russian worker, Khatenever, has published claims that the organism produces an exotoxin in semisolid, colloidal media. *Francisella tularensis* appears to be antigenically homogeneous. Although it shares antigenicity with *Brucella* and *Pseudomonas* species, it can be identified by agglutination or by the direct FA test using specific (absorbed) anti–*F. tularensis* antiserum.

EPIDEMIOLOGY

Humans can be infected with *F. tularensis* by a variety of modes of transmission. Edward Francis, in 1937, stated that there are 20 known methods whereby human beings can be infected. As stated, the most common mode of transmission is physical contact while skinning or dressing infected animals. This is justification for placing tularemia in the miscellaneous contact subgroup of the contact group diseases. Tularemia can also be contracted by eating inadequately cooked meat from infected animals. Moreover, an outbreak in Russia was traced to drinking or bathing in river water below an infected water-rat colony. These types of transmission justify including tularemia in a subgroup of the intestinal group of diseases. Various hemophagus arthropods (ticks, flies, mosquitoes) have also been incriminated in the transmission of tularemia to humans, as have the bites of infected vertebrate animals. These modes of transmission justify inclusion of tularemia in the inoculation group of diseases. It should be noted that a number of species of ticks have been incriminated in the transmission of *F. tularensis*. These include several species of the genera *Dermacentor* and *Haemaphysalis* and at least one species of the genus *Ixodes*. Probably the *Dermacentor* (wood ticks) are mainly involved in transmitting the disease among animal hosts. As in all tick-transmitted diseases, *F. tularensis* can be passed from infected female ticks transovarially to the next generation of larval, nymphal, and adult ticks with no intervening infectious blood meal. This transovarial transmission generally is not true in the case of hemophagus insects (flies, fleas, mosquitoes).

Cooney and Burgdorfer (1974) and Burgdorfer et al. (1974) reported the results of several years of studying the potential for animal-to-human transmission of tularemia and Rocky Mountain spotted fever in a large recreational area in the Tennessee Valley. They found serological evidence suggesting the wide distribution of both pathogenic agents in a variety of medium-sized mammals collected in the area. They isolated *Francisella tularensis* from 7 and *Rickettsia rickettsi* from 51 *Dermacentor variabilis* ticks collected. For additional epidemiological studies of tularemia see Boyce (1975).

Finally, *F. tularensis* frequently invades the lungs, resulting in tularemic pneumonia, which in the preantibiotic days had a high mortality rate. This is the only form of tularemia considered to be transmissible from human to human. It justifies inclusion of tularemia in the respiratory subgroup of the contact group diseases. Table 22-1 summarizes the vehicles involved in the various epidemiological groups in which tularemia might be included. For more details see McCrumb (1961) and Meyer (1965).

In 1968 and 1969, epizootics of tularemia occurred in muskrat colonies in upper New York state and Vermont. At least 76 cases of tularemia were reported among trappers in these areas during the epizootic. Two cases of pneumonic tularemia, one fatal, were reported from Indiana in 1969. The two patients, while on a picnic, had shot and extensively handled a squirrel. Again, in 1969, a case of tularemia was contracted in Washington state while skinning a bobcat. In all, more than 48 different species of animals, including beaver, sheep, grouse, and even a bull snake, are reported to have been naturally infected with *F. tularensis*.

In spite of the number and variety of naturally infected hosts and the many methods whereby humans can be infected, tularemia is not one of the major human diseases. During the 10-year period from 1966 through 1975 only 1,682 cases of tularemia were reported in the United States (see *MMWR* supplement, August 1976). Generally, although Texas leads the nation, fewer than 20 cases of tularemia are reported annually there. If one enjoys hunting, the chances of a fatal hunting accident greatly outweigh the chances of contracting fatal tularemia.

Table 22-1.   Epidemiology of tularemia.

Disease Group	Vehicles	
	Primary	*Secondary*
Miscellaneous contact	Infected animal tissues	None
Intestinal	Undercooked meat	None
	Water-rat carcasses	Water
Inoculation		
Arthropod	Infected animal blood	Vectors
Vertebrate	Buccal exudate	None
Respiratory contact	Human lung exudate	None
Laboratory infection	Animal tissues	Cultures, aerosols

Nevertheless, precautions should be taken while hunting, camping, and picnicking in known epizootic areas, and dead or sickly animals should not be handled. If a hunter or camper develops febrile illness within 7 to 10 days after handling a dead animal or being bitten by ticks, the clinician should be alerted to the possibility of tularemia. This is particularly important because tularemia therapy differs from that of most other febrile diseases.

CLINICAL SYMPTOMS

The clinical symptoms of tularemia vary considerably and depend upon the method of infection. If the organisms invade through the skin as a result of handling an infected animal or by arthropod bite, an inflamed papule develops in a variable percentage of cases. This papule usually ulcerates, and the organisms tend to travel the lymph channels to the regional lymph node in the armpit or groin. The lymph nodes tend to become indurated and quite painful—resembling, to some extent, the buboes of bubonic plague. A high and sustained fever accompanies these physical symptoms.

If the organisms are transmitted from contaminated fingers to the eye, severe inflammation and swelling of the eyelids may be the first evidence of infection. Again the organisms may penetrate the associated lymph channels and result in regional lymphadenitis (indurated lymph glands) and fever.

If the organisms are transmitted from contaminated fingers to the mouth, or if inadequately cooked meat from an infected animal is eaten, the organisms may penetrate the gastrointestinal mucosa and no visible papule or ulcer results. In such infections the symptoms may simulate typhoid fever. While working for the Texas State Department of Health Laboratory, the author noted a number of instances wherein a serodiagnostic test for typhoid fever was requested by the clinician. Although the agglutination tests for typhoid proved negative, tests for tularemia in these cases yielded significant agglutination titers for the latter disease.

By any route of infection, the *F. tularensis* organisms may invade the bloodstream and become septicemic from early in the infection. Such infections may be fulminating and result in death within a few days. Or bloodstream invasion may result in transient bacteremias followed by necrotic foci in the liver or other viscera. If the lungs are invaded, a tularemic pneumonia with necrotic lesions results. Since the discovery of streptomycin and its proof of efficacy in tularemia therapy, even the formerly highly fatal tularemic pneumonia can be cured if therapy is begun early. The penicillins have no therapeutic value in tularemia. Although chloramphenicol and tetracycline have been reported to have therapeutic efficacy, streptomycin is certainly the drug of choice for treating tularemia. Therefore a differential diagnosis of a febrile disease, which might be tularemia, should be made as early as possible.

LABORATORY DIAGNOSIS

Tularemia is a disease in which the prior 2-week case history may be more important than any laboratory test in arriving at an early diagnosis. If the patient gives a history of having skinned or handled a dead rabbit or other potential animal host or having been bitten by ticks or other hemophagus arthropods during the 2 weeks prior to onset of febrile symptoms, tularemia should be suspected. If there is a visible papular swelling, which tends to ulcerate, on a finger or at the site of the arthropod bite, the clinical diagnosis of tularemia is indicated. If there is inflamed swelling of the conjunctiva following contact with a dead rabbit or other potential animal host, tularemia should again be suspected. If none of these visible local lesions develops, the laboratory becomes essential to a differential diagnosis between tularemia, typhoid and other enteric fevers, typhus fever, and acute brucellosis, all of which may share the same early symptoms.

Since a blood culture is the test of choice for typhoid and other *Salmonella* enteric fevers during the first week of symptoms, such a culture certainly should be performed. The typhoid bacillus and other *Salmonella* will grow in relatively simple broth media, but not *F. tularensis* and rarely *Brucella* species and never the *Rickettsia* of typhus fever. Since the diagnosis of the latter three diseases may depend upon demonstrating a rising antibody titer, enough blood should be drawn as early as possible for both the blood culture in an ordinary nutrient-broth medium and for the determination of acute-phase serodiagnostic (agglutinin) titers to antigens of each of these suspect diseases.

If a blood culture to isolate *F. tularensis* is requested, an additional 5 milliliters of blood should be drawn. Since this organism requires special media supplemented with glucose, blood, cystine, and thiamin and grows best on

agar media, such a medium minus the blood should be prepared and dispensed in 20-milliliter amounts in large sterile test tubes. The medium should be melted and held at 50°C in a water bath. One milliliter of the patient's blood should be added to the 20 milliliters of agar medium, mixed by rotation, and poured into a sterile petri plate. This process should be repeated for each of the four other tubes of medium. The plates should be incubated and examined for colonies at 24 and 48 hours. As indicated, this early blood culture for tularemia is not as likely to be positive as is the early blood culture for typhoid. However, isolation and identification of any one of the bacterial species responsible for the suspect diseases will give the earliest possible laboratory diagnosis.

If the first blood culture is negative, a second blood specimen should be submitted to the laboratory 7 to 10 days after the first. If tularemia is suspected, secondary blood cultures may be performed by the procedure indicated above. In any case, the serum from the second blood specimen should be tested for antibody titers to the same antigens used in the first serodiagnostic tests. If there is a significant (threefold or more) rising antibody titer indicated by the two blood specimens for only one of the test antigens, the homologous disease is indicated. This frequently is the only means whereby a laboratory diagnosis of tularemia, typhus fever, or brucellosis can be accomplished. If the patient has an ulcerated skin lesion or inflamed and swollen conjunctiva or buccal membranes, exudate from these sites may be collected on a swab and inoculated to cystine—blood-agar plates. Also, fluid may be aspirated from enlarged lymph nodes and inoculated to such plates. The medium in plates that are inoculated with swab exudate should contain penicillin and other antibiotics that suppress bacterial contaminants while having no adverse effect on the growth of *F. tularensis*.

If suspicious *F. tularensis* colonies develop on any of the cystine—blood-agar plates, they may be fished to other plates or tubes of the same medium to obtain enough growth for a serotaxonomic agglutination test. This test requires a high-titer anti—*F. tularensis* antiserum from an actively immunized rabbit or fowl. To make the antiserum more specific for *F. tularensis*, it can be absorbed with killed *Brucella abortus* and *Pseudomonas* cells. Agglutination of the cells from the isolated colony to the titer of the specific antiserum or a positive FA test on a smear of the cells is accepted as identification of the isolate as *F. tularensis*.

Guinea pigs or other rodents can be infected by the inoculation of material containing *F. tularensis*. Although cultural isolation of the organism is reported to be easier from such animals than directly from humans, the increased hazard of infection to laboratory personnel hardly justifies the use of such means of laboratory diagnosis. In fact, only well-trained technologists should be allowed to undertake the isolation and identification of *F. tularensis*. For additional details see Eigelsbach (1974).

Two types of skin tests have been advocated by Foshay (1950) and others for aid in the diagnosis of tularemia. Both are claimed to be positive during the first week of the disease. One, a tuberculin-type hypersensitivity test, requires 48 hours for the development of the reaction. *Caution:* Reactions can be severe in hypersensitive individuals. The other test involves the intradermal injection of a small amount of goat anti—*F. tularensis* antiserum. It is based on the assumption that soluble antigens of *F. tularensis* circulating in the bloodstream will react with the injected antiserum in the skin and cause the immediate allergic reaction. Obviously an equal amount of normal goat serum would have to be injected into the other arm as a control. Although the rationale for this test appears logical, either the results are unreliable or the demand for the test materials has not justified commercial production. In other words, if you wanted to use the test you would have to produce your own test materials.

IMMUNITY

The relative rarity of tularemia makes the accumulation of statistics on immunity difficult to obtain. The antigenic homogeneity of *F. tularensis* would indicate that an attack of the disease should confer lasting immunity and that

an effective vaccine might be produced. A number of vaccines have been proposed, but their efficacy in humans has been difficult to prove. Russian workers produced a live, weakly virulent *F. tularensis*—strain vaccine, designated LVS, which they claimed to be highly immunogenic. However, there are reports of laboratory workers contracting one or two infections with *F. tularensis* after immunization with live hypovirulent vaccines. Moreover, animals immunized with *F. tularensis* vaccines have not always proved resistant to challenge with virulent strains of the organism. For the results of more recent experimental studies on immunity in tularemia, see Andron and Eigelsbach (1975) and Eigelsbach et al. (1975).

CONTROL AND PREVENTION

Eradication of tularemia from the rodent and other wild animal populations appears to be impossible at the present time. The wearing of rubber gloves and face masks, which should be required of laboratory personnel, is hardly practical for hunters or trappers. Fortunately streptomycin, chloramphenicol, and tetracyclines are effective therapeutic drugs when administered early in the disease. Therefore the most practical control measure at present is early diagnosis and treatment.

REFERENCES

Andron, L. A. II and H. T. Eigelsbach. 1975. Biochemical and immunological properties of ribonucleic acid-rich extracts from *Francisella tularensis*. *Infect. Immunity* 12:137–142.

Boyce, J. M. 1975. Recent trends in the epidemiology of tularemia in the United States. *J. Infect. Dis.* 131:197–199.

Burgdorfer, W., J. C. Cooney, and L. A. Thomas. 1974. Zoonotic potential (Rocky Mountain spotted fever and tularemia) in the Tennessee Valley region. II. Prevalence of *Rickettsia ricketisi* and *Francisella tularensis* in mammals and ticks from Land Between the Lakes. *Amer. J. Trop. Med. Hyg.* 23:109–117.

Cooney, J. C. and W. Burgdorfer. 1974. Zoonotic potential (Rocky Mountain spotted fever and tularemia) in the Tennessee Valley region. I. Ecologic studies of ticks infesting mammals in Land Between the Lakes. *Amer. J. Trop. Med. Hyg.* 23:99–108.

Eigelsbach, H. T. 1974. *Francisella tularensis.* Chapter 28 in *Manual of Clinical Microbiology.*

Eigelsbach, H. T., D. H. Hunter, W. A Janssen, H. G. Dangerfield, and S. G. Rabinowitz. 1975. Murine model for study of cell-mediated immunity: protection against death from fully virulent *Francisella tularensis* infection. *Infect. Immunity* 12:999–1005.

Foshay, L. 1950. Tularemia. *Ann. Rev. Microbiol.* 4:313–330.

McCrumb, F. R., Jr. 1961. Aerosol infection of man with *Pasteurella tularensis. Bact. Rev.* 25:262–267.

Meyer, K. F. 1965. *Pasteurella* and *Francisella.* Chapter 27 in *Bacterial and Mycotic Infections of Man,* eds. R. J. Dubos and J. G. Hirsch. Philadelphia: Lippincott.

PART THREE

Intestinal Group Diseases

Subgroup A: Excreta-Borne Diseases

The causative organisms of most if not all of the intestinal group diseases included in this text utilize the mouth as the portal of entry. An obvious primary vehicle of intestinal diseases is infected human fecal excreta. Infected animal and human urine also may serve as a primary vehicle. Figure III-A illustrates the major epidemiology of subgroup A of the intestinal group diseases. The segregation of oysters from other foods in this epidemiology is based upon three facts: (1) oyster beds frequently are found in shallow bays subject to heavy sewage contamination; (2) oysters tend to pass large quantities of water (around 18 gallons) through the gills daily, from which they filter out microscopic organisms as a source of food; and (3)—of most importance—oysters are the only worldwide seafood frequently consumed in the raw state.

When fecal or urinary excreta from infected animals constitute the primary vehicle, the epidemiology of the subgroup A diseases lacks only such secondary vehicles as bedding, bedpans, and fingers; and the paws of the animals may serve as a substitute for the human fingers.

The more important causative organisms of the human intestinal group diseases are found in five taxonomic genera, three of which are bacteria and two are viruses. The common pathogenic genera of bacteria are *Vibrio, Salmonella,* and *Shigella.* Occasionally one species of the genus *Yersinia* is included in the group. The *Vibrio* are slightly curved (comma-shaped) gram-negative rods. In addition to the type species, *Vibrio cholerae,* there are other vibrios pathogenic for humans or animals and numerous saprophytic vibrios. Some of the latter are found in the intestinal tract; others are found in water, moist soil, and other external environments. The genus *Vibrio* is included in the taxonomic family Vibrionaceae, which includes several other genera.

The two other bacterial genera, *Salmonella* and *Shigella,* are composed of short gram-negative, non-spore-forming (*asporogenous*) rods.

PRIMARY
VEHICLE   SECONDARY VEHICLES   PORTAL
                                                                                                OF ENTRY

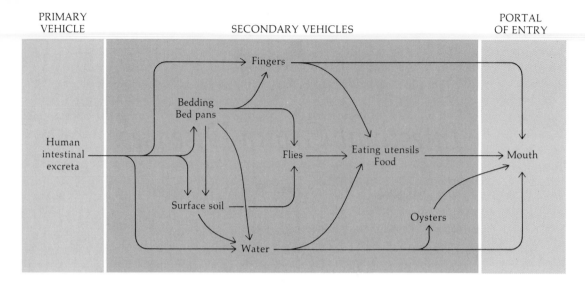

Figure III–A.   The major modes of transmission of intestinal group diseases of human origin.

Both genera contain multiple species or sero-types, all of which are actually or potentially pathogenic for human beings or other animals. The *Salmonella* and *Shigella* are grouped, along with a number of usually saprophytic genera of gram-negative bacilli, in the taxonomic family Enterobacteriaceae. This family also includes the genus *Yersinia.* Many of the saprophytic Enterobacteriaceae may occasionally become pathogenic (see Chapter 20). All these bacteria can be grown on relatively simple culture media, and differentiation of the pathogenic and the saprophytic members of the family is a frequent responsibility of the clinical laboratory bac-teriologist. Table III-A illustrates the biotype taxonomy of a few of these ubiquitous bacteria. For a comprehensive discussion of the taxonomy of the Enterobacteriaceae see Cowan (1974).

The two major excreta-borne virus diseases of humans are poliomyelitis, caused by three serotypes of *Poliovirus hominis,* and hepatitis, caused by two distinct antigenic types of *Hepatitis* virus. Since *P. hominis* and other enteroviruses (*Coxsackievirus* and *Echovirus*) can be propagated in and are cytopathogenic for monkey kidney tissue cultures, the virologist frequently is con-fronted with the problem of differentiating the

multiple serotypes of these three genera of enteroviruses.

In addition to the human diseases trans-mitted by intestinal excreta, the mouth serves as the portal of entry for subgroup B diseases of the intestinal group, in which the primary vehicle may be secretions (milk) or tissues (meat) from infected animals. As indicated in the preceding chapter on miscellaneous contact subgroup dis-eases, tularemia, when contracted by eating inadequately cooked meat from an infected animal, would be an example of this aspect of the intestinal group disease transmission. How-ever, this mode of transmission is relatively rare in tularemia compared to physical contact with infected animals. By contrast, brucellosis, which has a miscellaneous contact transmission aspect (veterinarians and abattoir workers) in its epi-demiology, was discovered as a consequence of the ingestion of milk or milk products from infected goats or cows. Moreover, brucellosis can be contracted by eating inadequately cooked pork or pork sausage from infected hogs. Brucellosis, therefore, will be considered as a member of subgroup B of the intestinal group diseases.

It should be obvious that food is an important vehicle of all intestinal group diseases. The major difference between the excreta-borne (subgroup A) and the infected animal milk- or meat-borne (subgroup B) diseases of this group is the fact that food is the *primary vehicle* in the latter diseases and there are no secondary vehicles of epidemiological significance. In the diseases of subgroup A, food is a secondary vehicle subject to contamination by the modes outlined in Figure III-A. However, disinfection (cooking or pasteurization) of the food prior to ingestion will prevent human infection by either vehicular mode of transmission.

The diseases of subgroup C of the intestinal group are not infectious. They are caused by the ingestion of preformed bacterial toxins (*enterotoxins*) in contaminated foods.

REFERENCES

Cowan, S. T. 1974. Enterobacteriaceae. Part 8 of *Bergey's Manual of Determinative Bacteriology.*

Table III-A. Taxonomic characteristics of selected saprophytic and pathogenic gram-negative bacilli of the intestinal tract.

Taxonomic Characteristics	*Escherichia coli*	*Citrobacter fruendii*	*Enterobacter aerogenes*	*Proteus vulgaris*	*Klebsiella pneumoniae*	*Vibrio cholerae*	*Salmonella typhi*	*Salmonella enteritidis*	*Salmonella choleraesuis*	*Shigella dysenteriae*	*Shigella flexneri*	*Shigella boydii*	*Shigella sonnei*	*Yersinia enterocolitica*
Motility	+	+	+	(+)	−	+	+	+	+	−	−	−	−	+*
Fermentation tests														
Glucose	G	G	G	(G)	(G)	A	A	G	G	A	A	A	A	−
Lactose	G	(G)	G	−	(G)	(A)	−	−	−	−	−	−	(A)	−
Arabinose	G	G	G	−	G	−	A	G	−	nt	nt	nt	−	(A)
Mannitol	G	G	G	(G)	G	A	A	G	G	−	A	A	A	A
Dulcitol	(G)	(G)	−	−	(G)	−	−	G	(G)	(A)	−	(A)	−	−
Sucrose	(G)	(G)	A	(G)	G	A	−	−	−	−	−	−	(A)	+
Citrate utilization	−	+	+	nt	(+)	(+)	−	−	−	−	−	−	−	−
H₂S from TSI	−	(+)	−	(+)	−	−	+	+	(+)	−	−	−	−	−
Lysine decarboxylation	+	−	(+)	(−)	(−)	+	+	+	+	−	−	−	−	−
No. of serotypes	~	?	?	?	?	3	1	†	†	10	6–8	15	1	17

*Motile at temperatures below 30°C, not at 37°C.

†Multiple serotypes.

() = Late or variable. A = acid. G = acid and gas. nt = not tested.

TSI = Triple sugar in iron agar (see Figure B on front cover).

~ = Infinite number of serotype combinations of 150 somatic O, 90 capsular K, and 50 flagellar H antigens.

23

Cholera and Dysentery

Cholera and bacterial dysentery are diseases in which the causative organisms tend to be restricted to the lumen or lining of the intestinal tract. Both may involve severe to massive diarrhea.

CHOLERA*

Cholera (frequently designated Asiatic cholera) has been endemic in parts of India (especially the Ganges delta) for centuries. It is a disease commonly associated with unsanitary excreta disposal and inadequate water purification—conditions frequently found in overcrowded and economically depressed areas of the world. Prior to 1873 a number of cholera epidemics spread worldwide (pandemics), invading even the western hemisphere. The United States has not been involved in a cholera epidemic since 1873, but a single case of cholera was reported in Port Lavaca, Texas, in the summer of 1974. This case

may in some as yet unknown manner be related to the most recent pandemic of cholera, although no additional cases have been reported in the United States.

The most recent pandemic (El Tor cholera, named after the Tor quarantine station in the Sinai) started as a localized epidemic in the Celebes in 1937 and remained localized to the East Indies for a considerable period of time. It broke out in epidemic form in Indonesia and Hong Kong in 1961. It then spread eastward to the Philippines and New Guinea and north to Korea and probably to China. By 1966 it had spread from Thailand westward through Singapore, India, Pakistan, Iran, and Iraq. By 1970 it had spread south to Africa and north and west to Russia, Syria, and other Middle Eastern countries. By 1970–1971 it had reached the west central and northern coasts of Africa and westernmost Europe (Spain and Portugal), where cases were still being reported in 1974. Also in 1974, six cases of El Tor cholera in Guam occurred in a group of 13 construction workers who dined together. The source of infection in this group appeared to be a fish caught in a local

---

*For a comprehensive review of the literature on cholera see Finkelstein (1973).

bay (Agana) and salted and preserved in brine. Subsequently, El Tor vibrios were isolated from the bay waters and more recently from storm sewers in Guam (*MMWR*, 31 August 1974). As implied above, the source of the single case of El Tor cholera in Texas in 1974 has not been determined.

The pandemics of cholera contrast with the pandemics of influenza, described in Chapter 13, in their selectivity for individuals living in excreta-contaminated environments and in their rate of spread throughout the world. Influenza pandemics usually spread worldwide with minor concern for sanitation and are practically over, except for localized outbreaks, within a period of 1 to 2 years. These time relationships indicate the greater contagiousness of respiratory group diseases compared to those of the intestinal group.

Etiology

Pacini in 1854 described the organism that was rediscovered by Robert Koch in 1884. Koch reported long spiral organisms in the watery stools of cholera patients. When grown in culture, however, the organisms became short comma-shaped bacilli (see Figure 23-1). They were motile as a result of a single polar flagellum. The organisms stain gram-negative, although they stain better with dilute carbol fuchsin. Even though Koch's organism was found in all cases of cholera and readily isolated in pure culture, proof of etiology was difficult because of the absence of a suitable experimental animal. Even human volunteers were not always infected. The Koch isolate commonly is designated *Vibrio cholerae*, although the 1957 edition of Bergey's taxonomic manual listed the organism as *Vibrio comma*. In addition to the enteropathogenic *V. cholerae*, a number of noncholeragenic vibrios (NCV) have been isolated from the human enteric tract and other sources. Although *V. cholerae* is accepted as the etiological agent of cholera, there still is considerable mystery as to how and why some persons contract the disease whereas others, equally exposed, fail to develop illness.

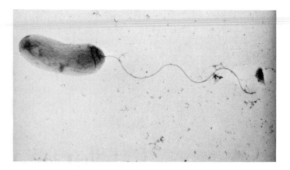

Figure 23–1. Negatively-stained electron micrograph of *Vibrio cholerae* showing comma shape and single polar flagellum. 13,015×. (Courtesy of L. M. Pope.)

As indicated above, *V. cholerae* is a slightly curved bacillus. In stained smears, however, only about half the cells assume the comma shape. The others, because of their orientation at the time of fixation on the microslide, appear as straight rods.

Vibrio cholerae and other vibrios (NCV) will grow in simple meat extract–peptone broth or agar media. They are aerobes and usually are cultured at 37°C in alkaline media (pH 7.8–9.0). They are highly susceptible to acid (pH 6.0), and acid in the stomach may be a factor in the variable infectivity of the organism for exposed human beings. Selective media for *V. cholerae* have been formulated using tellurium salts, bile salts, or bismuth sulfite as inhibitory agents for the saprophytic Enterobacteriaceae and gram-positive bacteria of the intestinal tract. *Vibrio cholerae* is not inhibited by the concentrations of these inhibitors used in the selective media. Factors affecting the virulence of cultured *V. cholerae* have been reviewed by Lankford (1960). Guentzel and Berry (1975) cited evidence incriminating motility as a contributing factor in the virulence of the three biotypes of *V. cholerae*.

The most distinctive biotype of *V. cholerae*, in terms of differing from the classic vibrio isolated by Koch, was isolated in 1906 from individuals passing through the Tor quarantine station. These were designated El Tor vibrios and differed from the classic *V. cholerae* in their production of a soluble hemolysin (not hemodigestion) for sheep erythrocytes when grown in broth culture. For some time the El Tor vibrios were thought to be noncholeragenic; however, as stated above, they not only are choleragenic but are responsible for the 1937–1974 pandemic of cholera.

Two serotypes of *V. cholerae*—Ogawa and Inaba—have long been recognized. These share a common, heat-stable, somatic antigen A. Ogawa possesses an additional somatic antigen B (AB), whereas Inaba has an additional somatic antigen C (AC). Burrows et al. (1946) reported a third serotype—Hikojima—with somatic antigens A, B, and C. Thus it would appear that, by using three monospecific antisera for the somatic antigens (anti-A, anti-B, and anti-C), a *V. cholerae* isolate might be identified as to serotype by three simple agglutination tests. Occasional vibrios may possess only the somatic antigen A, however, and instances of both *in vitro* and *in vivo* serotype variation have been reported. Moreover, vibrios have been isolated from the human enteric tract that do not agglutinate in any of these antisera. If one of the vibrio serotypes produces a soluble hemolysin for sheep erythrocytes, it is designated a homologous serotype El Tor *V. cholerae* (such as *V. cholerae* El Tor Ogawa or Inaba).

The hemolysin produced by the El Tor vibrios does not appear to have pathogenic significance in the human host. All choleragenic strains of *V. cholerae* produce a soluble vascular-permeability factor (PF). This PF, found both in culture filtrates and in the watery stools of cholera patients, produces a characteristic skin reaction when injected intracutaneously. This factor seems to be identical with a heat-labile enterotoxin produced by *V. cholerae*. The enterotoxin (designated *choleragen* by Finkelstein) is distinct from the endotoxin found in the cell walls of *V. cholerae*. The enterotoxin is a secretory protein of the *V. cholerae* and has the typical exotoxin characteristics of antitoxinogenicity in animals and being neutralized in multiple proportions by this antitoxin. The enterotoxin adsorbs to gangliosides on the surface membranes of the microvilli of the small intestine. It is not absorbed through these membranes, however.

As a result of the attachment of the choleragen, the inactive tissue enzyme, *adenyl cyclase,* is activated and this leads to increased levels of adenosine-3'-5'-cyclic monophosphate (cAMP) in the intestinal epithelial cells. The increased cAMP induces a net secretion of chloride and bicarbonate ions and water from each cell, leading to the massive diarrhea of cholera. For additional details see Pierce et al. (1971) and Carpenter (1972).

The choleragen is produced in association with an antigenically homologous, nontoxic toxoid (*choleragenoid*). The choleragen and choleragenoid are sufficiently different in size and charge, however, that they can be separated by gel chromatography. Antitoxin specific for choleragenoid will neutralize both the PF activity and the enterotoxicity of choleragen (Finkelstein and LoSpalluto 1970). However, efforts to convert choleragen to a practical toxoid for human immunization, by treatment of the toxin with formaldehyde, have failed because of the tendency of the formol toxoid to revert to toxicity. Although choleragenoid also adsorbs to the intestinal receptor sites for the enterotoxin, it does not activate adenyl cyclase and does not result in cholera. In fact choleragenoid can block the receptor sites and prevent the adsorption of the subsequently administered enterotoxin.

Clinical Symptoms

Classic cholera, following a short (1–4-day) incubation period, has a sudden onset of massive diarrhea. This appears to result from the adenyl cyclase activation by the enterotoxin. The patient may lose gallons of protein-free fluid and associated electrolytes, bicarbonates, and other ions within a day or two. This loss leads to dehydration, anuria, acidosis, and shock. The watery stools, which have practically none of the usual fecal odors, are cream-colored, contain enormous numbers of vibrios, and are speckled with flakes of mucus and epithelial cells ("rice-water stools"). The loss of potassium ions may result in cardiac complications and circulatory failure. Untreated cholera frequently results in high (50 to 60 percent) mortality rates.

In spite of the massive diarrhea, there rarely is hemorrhaging or necrotic damage to the lining membranes of the intestine. The symptoms described here are those of the average acute case. Many cases with less severe symptoms are common during epidemics. Finkelstein et al. (1976) described a case of clinical cholera caused by enterotoxigenic *Escherichia coli.*

Treatment of cholera involves the rapid intravenous replacement of the lost fluid and ions. Following this replacement, administration of isotonic maintenance solution should continue until the diarrhea ceases. If glucose is added to the maintenance fluid it may be administered orally, thereby eliminating the need for sterility and intravenous administration. By this simple treatment regimen, patients at the brink of death have been cured miraculously. Tetracycline therapy has been reported to decrease the amount and duration of maintenance fluid required for such cures. Sulfonamides, penicillin, and streptomycin have *no value* in cholera therapy.

Laboratory Diagnosis

Since cholera is a disease associated with unsanitary, excreta-contaminated environments, diarrheas of miscellaneous etiology might be expected to occur. Consequently laboratory demonstration of the etiological agent of the diarrhea is essential to make a specific diagnosis. This is particularly true in sporadic cases or early cases of an epidemic of cholera. A number of agar media have been formulated for the isolation of *V. cholerae* from the stool specimen. These media usually contain selective bile or tellurium salts or thiosulfite to suppress the growth of the common saprophytic Enterobacteriaceae of the intestinal tract (see Feeley and Balows 1974).

After streaking the stool specimen to such an agar plate medium (at pH 8.2 to 9.0), the plate is incubated overnight at 37°C. The selection of *V. cholerae* colonies on such agar plates is facilitated by examination with a broad-field microscope using oblique lighting of the agar surface (see Henry 1933). Typical colonies may be subcultured to indicator agar slants for over-

night incubation. Both the colony growth (if adequate) and growth on the agar slants can be tested by slide agglutination using monospecific *V. cholerae* anti-A, anti-B, and anti-C antisera. Positive agglutination will identify the isolate as *V. cholerae* of homologous serotype. If the isolate is suspected of being the El Tor biotype, this identification can be accomplished by one or more of several tests: (1) demonstration of the production of a true soluble hemolysin for sheep or goat erythrocytes; (2) a positive hemagglutination test using chicken red blood cells; (3) relative resistance to polymyxin B; and (4) susceptibility to specific bacteriophage—ϕH 74/76 (Basu and Mukerjee 1969).

The paucity of suitable experimental animals has complicated cholera research. Injection of *V. cholerae* parenterally into animals usually results in fatal bacteremias that in no way resemble the natural disease in humans. The infant rabbit and mouse and some adult dogs (about 50 percent) appear to be the only animals capable of being infected by oral administration of live *V. cholerae* cells. Cholera symptoms also can be produced in these animals by the oral administration of cholera enterotoxin. Infant animals, however, are not suitable for immunological studies. Much research in the past has been accomplished by injecting the *V. cholerae* cells or the choleragen into the lumen of ligated intestinal loops of adult rabbits. Both the infection or the intoxication result in a copious discharge of fluid into the ligated loop (see Figure 23-2). Measurement of the volume of this fluid permits some quantitation of the experimental results.

During the 1970s some interesting observations have been reported on the effect of cholera enterotoxin on tissue culture and isolated cells. Greenough et al. (1970) reported that cholera toxin stimulated isolated fat cells from rats to produce lipolytic activity in the suspending medium. The lipolytic activity was toxin-dose-dependent and quantitation of the activity could be established by measuring the quantity of glycerol liberated. Cuatrecasas (1973) used isolated fat cells from young rats to study the mechanism of activation of the lipolytic response to cholera enterotoxin.

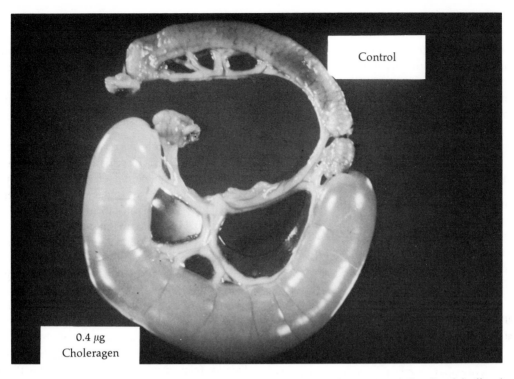

0.4 µg
Choleragen

Control

Figure 23–2.   Ligated ileal loop of rabbit intestine. Control (upper ligation) inoculated with buffered saline solution. Lower ligation inoculated with cholera enterotoxin (choleragen). (Courtesy of R. A. Finkelstein.)

Guerrant et al. (1974) reported a morphological alteration of cultured Chinese hamster ovary (CHO) cells after treatment with cholera enterotoxin. These workers correlated the morphological changes in the CHO cells with increases of cAMP in the cells. The changes were blocked by the presence of cholera antitoxin. Identical results were reported for *Escherichia coli* enterotoxin, including the neutralization of the latter by the cholera antitoxin. They advocated the CHO cell-alteration test as a rapid means of assaying both enterotoxins.

Immunity

Recovery from a case of cholera appears to confer a short-term (about 6 months) immunity to reinfection. Workers at the Haffkine Institute in India long ago developed vaccines consisting of suspensions of killed *V. cholerae* cells. Current vaccines usually include equal numbers of the two serotypes—Ogawa and Inaba (4 to 5 $\times$ 10^9 cells of each type per milliliter of vaccine). Field tests of such vaccines have yielded evidence of limited protection ranging from 50 to 75 percent of those vaccinated.

Eubanks et al. (1977) compared a number of surface components of *Vibrio cholerae* with commercial vaccine as immunogens in mice. They reported that a crude mixture of flagella and vesicular material provided fifty- to a hundredfold greater protection than the commercial vaccine. These and fluorescent antibody studies by Guentzel et al. (1977) tend to support the conclusion by Guentzel and Berry (1975) regarding the relationship between the motility and virulence of *V. cholerae.*

There are current efforts to develop live avirulent *V. cholerae* vaccines. As indicated above, efforts to produce a practical cholera toxoid (comparable to diphtheria toxoid) by the treatment of cholera enterotoxin with formaldehyde have failed—the detoxified enterotoxin reverts to toxicity *in vivo*. Finkelstein has suggested that the natural choleragenoid might be immunogenic for humans if it could be produced in adequate quantities free from the enterotoxin (see Mekalanos et al. 1977). The possibility of the selection of a mutant *V. cholerae* that produced only choleragenoid is also being investigated.

Control and Prevention

Under conditions that exist in most areas of endemic or epidemic cholera in the world, control of the disease is practically impossible. The limited efficacy of active immunoprophylaxis contributes to this pessimistic outlook. For more details see Barua et al. (1970).

Other Vibrios

A number of noncholeragenic vibrios (NCV) have been described. The most important human pathogenic NCV is *Vibrio parahaemolyticus*. This organism is a *halophile*, growing well in media containing 7 percent sodium chloride. It appears to be distributed worldwide, but human infections are concentrated in populations (Oriental) where raw fish and shellfish are a common food item. Occasional infections with *V. parahaemolyticus* in North America have been associated with the consumption of inadequately cooked shrimp and crabs (see Davidson et al. 1973). The clinical syndrome resulting from this food-borne disease is a gastroenteritis of variable severity. For additional details see Feeley and Balows (1974).

BACILLARY DYSENTERY (SHIGELLOSIS)

Dysentery is an idiopathic designation for a clinical entity involving gastrointestinal distress and diarrhea of variable severity. Such symptoms may be caused by infectious agents ranging from viruses to bacteria, to protozoa, to helminths. Such symptoms may be caused also by the ingestion of preformed bacterial enterotoxins in contaminated food. The designation

bacillary dysentery, however, usually is restricted to the dysenteric symptoms caused by infection with small, gram-negative, nonmotile, asporogenous bacilli belonging to the taxonomic genus *Shigella*. Since there are a number of species and antigenic serotypes within this genus, dysentery caused by any one of these is designated a *shigellosis*.

The Japanese bacteriologist K. Shiga in 1896 isolated and described the first dysentery bacilli from the stools of patients in Japan. Although epidemic dysentery was recognized as far back as Hippocrates, Shiga's discovery was the first time that a distinction was made between the bacillary and the amebic (*Endamoeba histolytica*) etiology of the disease syndrome. The Shiga isolate is now designated *Shigella dysenteriae* and fails to ferment both lactose and mannitol among other biochemical characteristics (see Table III-A).

Simon Flexner at the turn of this century isolated a mannitol-fermenting (acid but no gas) *Shigella* from dysentery patients in the Philippines. This isolate is now designated *Shigella flexneri*. Other biochemically and antigenically distinct, mannitol-fermenting shigellae were isolated by Carl Sonne (*Shigella sonnei*) and by J. S. K. Boyd (*Shigella boydii*). *Shigella sonnei* is the only member of the *Shigella* genus that ferments lactose. This fermentation is slow, however, taking 2 days to a week or more. The lactose fermentation and certain cross-breeding characteristics tend to relate these shigellae to some members of the genus *Escherichia*. Practically all members of the latter genus are motile bacilli, however, whereas the shigellae are nonmotile. *Shigella sonnei* is an antigenically homogeneous species, whereas the other three species of the genus are composed of a number of antigenic serotypes each (see Table III-A). The serotypes of the genus *Shigella*, however, have little practical value except for taxonomic identification and epidemiological studies.

Clinical Dysentery

Although both bacillary dysentery and cholera cause severe diarrheas, that of dysentery is not likely to be as overwhelming as that of a severe case of cholera. There is, however, a greater tendency toward ulceration and hemorrhaging in shigellosis than in cholera. Moreover, the stools of shigelloses are more likely to yield foul odors than are those of cholera.

The shigellae invade the epithelial cells of the intestinal walls (particularly the colon) apparently by pinocytosis—invaginations of surface membranes. They tend to multiply in the deeper layers of the intestinal wall and cause ulceration by endotoxins produced *in situ*. However, at least one serotype of *S. dysenteriae* produces a typical exotoxin—a neurotoxin that affects the central nervous system. Except for this neurotoxicity, the shigella exotoxin is similar in many ways to that of *C. diphtheriae*. Further, some *S. dysenteriae* have been reported to produce an enterotoxin of the *V. cholerae* or *Escherichia coli* type. These two shigella exotoxins, however, have not been sufficiently purified to establish their independent identities.

Bacillary dysentery frequently is an epidemic disease associated with crowding and unsanitary environments, especially in the tropics and hot summer months in temperate zones. In the past it frequently has been a scourge of armed forces during warfare, sometimes determining the outcome of such operations. For example, dysentery was claimed to be the cause of the failure of the Japanese to take Port Moresby in New Guinea during World War II. In recent years there has been a trend toward infant and childhood dysentery. Eichner et al. (1968) reported that between 65 and 70 percent of 9,142 cases reported to United States public health authorities were in children 1 to 9 years of age. A water-borne outbreak of *S. sonnei* shigellosis involving 1,200 cases was reported from Richmond Heights, Florida, in 1974. An outbreak of *S. sonnei* gastroenteritis at a girl's camp in Pennsylvania (see Figure 23-3) illustrates the explosive nature of shigellosis epidemiology (*MMWR*, 20 September 1975)

The natural disease appears to be restricted to humans, although epizootics have been reported in certain other primates in captivity. Mortality rates in the human disease have

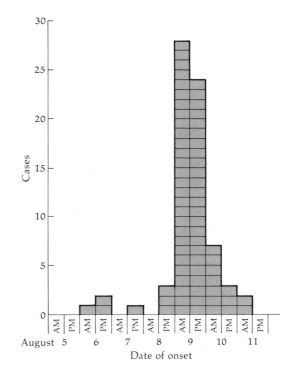

Figure 23–3. Gastroenteritis cases in 71 interviewed campers by date of onset—Wayne County, Pennsylvania, August 1974.

ranged from less than 2 percent to as high as 20 percent. The higher mortality usually has been associated with *S. dysenteriae* infection—particularly in the tropics. Shigelloses generally are characterized as ulcerative colitis; the causative organisms rarely penetrate body tissues beyond the intestinal tract membranes.

Etiology

There are four species of the genus *Shigella*, all but one of which (*S. sonnei*) involve multiple serotypes. In addition to all being gram-negative, asporogenous bacilli, some of the other differential taxonomic characteristics of the four species are listed in Table III-A. A key differential is the failure of *S. dysenteriae* to ferment mannitol. Also, *S. sonnei* can be identified by its late fermentation of lactose and its antigenic homogeneity. Other biotype and serotype characteristics are needed to distinguish *S. flex-neri* and *S. boydii.* If a shigella suspected of belonging to either of these two species is isolated in the average clinical laboratory, the technologist should report the presence of a *Shigella* (either *S. flexneri* or *S. boydii*) and submit the culture to a public health laboratory with adequate facilities for species and serotype identification. The only practical value to such identification is their epidemiological significance. It is questionable whether or not the patient should be required to pay for such differential diagnoses. However, since antibiotic and sulfonamide-resistant strains of *S. dysenteriae* and *S. flexneri* have been reported, the isolates should be tested for susceptibility to chemotherapeutic agents (see *MMWR,* 30 November 1974).

Laboratory Diagnosis

Two facts should be kept in mind when the laboratory is called upon to aid in the diagnosis of dysentery: (1) diarrheas in shigelloses may range from mild to severe; (2) such symptoms also may be caused by other gram-negative bacilli of the intestinal tract such as *Salmonella* and *Escherichia coli* serotypes. Consequently techniques and choice of media for isolation and identification of the causative organism should be chosen with these facts in mind.

Usually a fecal specimen is submitted for such diagnosis. The specimen should be inoculated to plating media as soon as possible after collection. Some authorities advocate selenite F or tetrathionate broth as enrichment media for use prior to the inoculation of plating media, especially for carriers. If delivery time to the laboratory and time of plate inoculation is to be delayed more than a few hours, suspending a portion of the specimen in an enrichment broth and submitting it along with the fecal specimen might increase the chances of isolating the causative organism. These enrichment media are more likely to be effective in the isolation of *Salmonella* (Chapter 24) than *Shigella* species.

There are a number of plating media available—many of them can be purchased in dehy-drated form. The plating media generally are characterized as nonselective or selective indicator media. Plain meat-infusion–peptone agar and Eosin methylene blue (EMB) agar are nonselective media; EMB and MacConkey's agar are differential media. For example, *Shigella, Salmonella,* and other non-lactose-fermenting colonies can be distinguished from *Escherichia* and other lactose-fermenting colonies after 18 to 24 hours' incubation on these differential media. The addition of lactose and a pH indicator, such as bromthymol blue or phenol red, to infusion agar makes it a nonselective, differential medium. MacConkey's agar is somewhat selective in that gram-negative organisms are selected for by the presence of bile salts and gram-positive organisms are suppressed by the presence of crystal violet. More selective media are brilliant green (BG) agar, bismuth sulfite (BS) agar, and *Salmonella-Shigella* (SS) agar. The latter two media contain both bismuth sulfite and brilliant green as selective agents active against *Escherichia* and other lactose-fermenting Enterobacteriaceae. For maximum chance of isolating a *Shigella* species, the fecal specimen should be streaked to three plates: infusion indicator agar, MacConkey agar, and SS agar. Both BG agar and BS agar suppress the growth of some or all strains of *Shigella.* In infantile diarrhea, where the etiological agent may be either *Shigella, E. coli,* streptococci, or other more fastidious bacteria, blood agar may be added to these three plating media.

If typical colonies develop on one or all of the inoculated plates, two or more representative colonies should be circled on the bottom of the plate and numbered. Since organisms other than the predominant type may be present in the colony on selective media and since the suppressed contaminants usually are located beneath the colony at the surface of the agar, the selected colony should be very carefully fished by barely touching the surface with a *straight* bacteriological needle. The organisms on the needle should be stab-inoculated to the base of a triple sugar iron (TSI) agar slant and then streaked on the entire surface of that slant. Repeat this inoculation procedure for one or more additional colonies and incubate the TSI cultures overnight at 37°C.

If the isolate is a *Shigella* colony, the TSI agar slant will be neutral or slightly alkaline, the butt will be acid, and there will be no evidence of gas or hydrogen sulfide (H_2S) production. Any H_2S production is indicated by brownish discoloration along the stab (see Figure B-4 on the front cover). The surface growth on the TSI slant can be inoculated to fermentation tubes of mannitol and lactose indicator broth and incubated overnight. If neither carbohydrate is fermented and the isolate is a gram-negative, nonmotile bacillus, it can be tentatively identified as *S. dysenteriae*. If the mannitol is fermented with acid but no gas and the lactose is not fermented within 24 hours, the isolate can be any one of the other three *Shigella* species. If the lactose is fermented with acid but no gas after 24 to 48 hours, it probably is *S. sonnei*.

If the laboratory has polyvalent antisera for each of the three multiserotype *Shigella* species and monovalent antiserum for *S. sonnei*, the species identification of the isolate can be established with practical certainty by four serotaxonomic agglutination tests. If the individual serotype identity of the isolate is desired, the culture should be submitted to a reference laboratory that specializes in such identification. Probably of greater significance than species identification is the determination of the susceptibility or resistance of the isolate to potential chemotherapeutic agents (see *MMWR*, 30 November 1974).

Although serum antibodies are produced as a result of *Shigella* infections, serodiagnosis has little or no practical value. One reason for this is the frequency of finding shigella antibodies in normal human sera.

Immunity

Although there is evidence of herd immunity in endemic areas of shigellosis, there are no immunological measures of practical value.

Control and Prevention

Sanitary disposal of human excreta is the best means of preventing shigelloses. Temporary or prolonged carriers are frequently the source of infection, and food contaminated by a carrier or case is a common secondary vehicle in shigellosis.

Chemotherapy and prophylaxis using soluble sulfonamides have proved effective in shigellosis. Streptomycin and broad-spectrum antibiotics also are effective. Chemoprophylaxis is best applied to persons proved to be carriers by the bacteriological diagnostic procedures described above. *Shigella* isolates, as indicated, should be tested for susceptibility to prospective chemotherapeutic agents.

REFERENCES

Barua, O., W. Burrows, and J. Gallut. 1970. Cholera control: a concise review and guide to practical measures. Supplement to *Principles and Practice of Cholera Control*. Pub. Hlth. Paper 40, WHO, Geneva.

Basu, S., and S. Mukerjee. 1969. A specific phage for pathogenic *Vibrio cholerae* biotype El Tor (ΦH 74/64.). *Bull. Wld. Hlth. Org.* 43:509–512.

Burrows, W., A. N. Mather, V. G. McGann, and S. M. Wagner. 1946. Studies on immunity to Asiatic Cholera. II. The O and H antigenic structure of the cholera and related vibrios. *J. Infect. Dis.* 79:168–197.

Carpenter, C. C. J. 1972. Cholera and other enterotoxin-related diarrheal diseases. *J. Infect. Dis.* 126:551–564.

Cowan, S. T. 1974. Enterobacteriaceae. Part 8 of *Bergey's Manual of Determinative Bacteriology*.

Cuatrecasas, P. 1973. Cholera toxin-fat cell interaction and the mechanism of activation of lipolytic response. *Biochem.* 12:3567–3576.

Davidson, T. A., Jr., R. Nelson, J. R. Molenda, and H. J. Garber. 1973. *Vibrio parahaemolyticus* gastroenteritis in Maryland. *Amer. J. Epidemiol.* 96:414–426.

Eichner, E. R., E. J. Gangarosa, and J. B. Goldsby. 1968. Current status of shigellosis in the United States. *Amer. J. Pub. Health* 58:753–763.

Eubanks, E. R., M. N. Guentzel, and L. J. Berry. 1977. Evaluation of surface components of *Vibrio cholerae* as protective immunogens. *Infect. Immunity* 15:533–538.

Feeley, J. C., and A. Balows. 1974. Vibrio. Chapter 21 in *Manual of Clinical Microbiology*.

Finkelstein, R. A. 1973. Cholera. *Critical Rev. in Microbiol.* 2:553–623.

Finkelstein, R. A., and J. J. LoSpalluto. 1970. Production, purification, and assay of cholera toxin. Production of highly purified choleragen and choleragenoid. *J. Infect. Dis.* 121(Supplement): S63–S72.

Finkelstein, R. A., M. L. Vasil, J. R. Jones, R. A. Anderson, and T. Barnard. 1976. Clinical cholera caused by enterotoxigenic *Escherichia coli. J. Clin. Microbiol.* 3:382–384.

Greenough, W. B., III, N. F. Pierce, and M. Vaughn. 1970. Titration of cholera enterotoxin and antitoxin in isolated fat cells. *J. Infect. Dis.* 121(Supplement):S111–S114.

Guentzel, M. N., and L. J. Berry. 1975. Motility as a virulence factor for *Vibrio cholerae. Infect. Immunity* 11:890–897.

Guentzel, M. N., L. H. Field, E. R. Eubanks, and L. J. Berry. 1977. Use of fluorescent antibody in studies of immunity to cholera in infant mice. *Infect. Immunity* 15:539–548.

Guerrant, R. L., L. L. Brunton, T. C. Schnaitman, L. J. Rebhun, and A. G. Gilman. 1974. Cyclic adenosine monophosphate and alteration of Chinese hamster ovary cell morphology: a rapid, sensitive in vitro assay for the enterotoxins of *Vibrio cholerae* and *Escherichia coli. Infect. Immunity* 10:320–327.

Henry, B. S. 1933. Dissociation in the genus *Brucella. J. Infect. Dis.* 52:374–402.

Lankford, C. E. 1960. Factors of virulence of *Vibrio cholerae. Ann. N.Y. Acad. Sci.* 88:1203–1212.

Mekalanos, J. J., R. J. Collier, and W. R. Romig. 1977. Simple method for purifying choleragenoid, the natural toxoid of *Vibrio cholerae. Infect. Immunity* 16:789–795.

Pierce, N. F., W. B. Greenough, and C. C. J. Carpenter. 1971. *Vibrio cholerae* enterotoxin and its mode of action. *Bacteriol. Rev.* 35:1–13.

24

Salmonelloses

The genus *Salmonella*, like other members of the family Enterobacteriaceae (see Table III-A), is composed of small, gram-negative, asporogenous rods. They generally are motile by means of peritrichous flagella (see Figure 24-1)—*S. gallinarum (pullorum)* being the only constant nonmotile exception. Most strains grow on simple or even chemically defined culture media without enrichment or special growth factors. Most strains are aerogenic and ferment glucose with the production of both acid and gas. *Salmonella typhi* is an important exception, however, never producing gas in its carbohydrate metabolism. Other anaerogenic variants of normally gas-producing strains may occur naturally—for example, *S. dublin.* Table 24-1 lists additional activities that have been advocated for the biotype identification of most Enterobacteriaceae isolates as probable members of the genus *Salmonella.* A simple test for the presumptive identification of members of the genus *Salmonella* is susceptibility to the bacteriophage 01 discov-

ered by Felix and Callow in 1943. This phage has been reported to lyse 99.5 percent of *Salmonella* strains tested and only 0.3 percent of other Enterobacteriaceae (see Thal and Kallings 1955). Other bacteriophages are specific for certain species or serotypes within the genus *Salmonella.* There are, for example, a number of biotypes of *S. typhi* Vi that can be differentiated by typing with phages specific for each type. This phage typing of *S. typhi* and other *Salmonella* is mainly significant in epidemiological studies designed to determine the source of infection, such as a carrier or another case, in an outbreak of salmonellosis.

THE KAUFFMANN-WHITE SCHEME

More than 1,400 serotypes have been identified within the genus *Salmonella.* This serotype identification, initiated by F. Kauffmann in Denmark and P. B. White in England, is commonly referred to as the Kauffmann-White classification

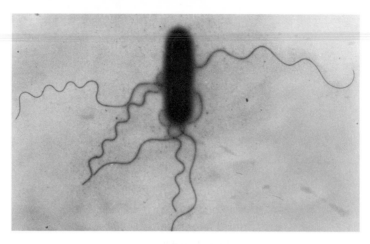

Figure 24–1. A negatively-stained cell of *Salmonella* sp. showing peritrichous flagellation. (Courtesy of W. L. Dentler.)

scheme. It involves the identification of the surface antigens on the body (somatic or O antigens) and on the flagella (flagellar or H antigens) by simple agglutination tests using the intact cells and known *monospecific* antisera. For example, *S. paratyphi* was found to possess two O antigens originally designated with roman numerals I and II and one flagellar antigen designated with the letter a. Later a third O antigen, XII, was discovered. Thus the serotype formula for *S. paratyphi* originally was established as I,II,XII:a. An isolate that possessed this antigenic formula could be identified as *S. paratyphi* by noting that it agglutinated in each of the mono-specific antisera: anti-I, anti-II, anti-XII, and anti-a. When comparable studies were performed on *S. schottmuelleri (paratyphi B)*, the O antigens were established as I,IV,V,XII. Some strains possessed an H antigen that was designated b, whereas other strains possessed two different H antigens. When it was established that the different H antigens were different antigenic phases of the same flagella, the phase 1 antigen was designated b whereas the phase 2 antigens were designated by the arabic numerals 1 and 2. Thus the original antigenic formula of *S. schottmuelleri* in phase 1 was was I,IV,V,XII:b, whereas that of phase 2 was I,IV,V,XII:1,2. Therefore a laboratory would

need seven monospecific antisera to be sure of identifying an isolate as *S. schottmuelleri* in one or the other of the two H antigen phases. *Salmonella schottmuelleri*, therefore, was found to have di-phasic H antigenicity (b⇋1,2), whereas *S. para-typhi* has monophasic H antigenicity (a).

Table 24-1. Characteristics of the four biotype subgroups of the genus *Salmonella* (Cowan et al. 1974).

Differential Characteristics	Biotypes			
	I	II	III	IV
Dulcitol	+	+	−	−
Lactose	−	−	+ or (±)	−
β-Galactosidase	−	(±)	+	−
d-Tartrate	+	−	−	−
Mucate	+	+	d	−
Malonate	−	+	+	−
Gelatin	−	(+)	(+)	(+)
KCN	−	−	−	+

(±) = Late or irregularly positive.
(+) = Late, but always positive.
 d = Different reactions by different strains.

As additional *Salmonella* somatic antigens were discovered (65 by 1974), the use of roman numerals for designation became too clumsy. Now, for example, the *S. paratyphi* serotype formula is written 1,2,12:a and that for *S. schottmuelleri* is 1,4,5,12:b:1,2. As additional *Salmonella* H antigens were discovered, the new phase 1 antigens exceeded the alphabet and subsequent discoveries were designated z_2, z_3, . . . , z_{59}. Ironically the new phase 2 numbered antigens have not exceeded 7. In retrospect the phase 1 antigens should have been number-designated and the phase 2 antigens letter-designated, but no one could foresee this in the beginning. Moreover, as new phase 2 antigens were discovered some turned out to be previously discovered phase 1 antigens of other *Salmonella*. For example, the diphasic formula for *S. loma-linda* was found to be 9,12:a:e,n,x. Table 24-2 lists a few examples of the Kauffmann-White serotypes. The groups are established on the basis of sharing certain somatic (O) antigens. Group D *Salmonella* all share O antigen 9, for example.

The Kauffmann-White scheme for the identification of serotypes of the genus *Salmonella* is a legitimate serotaxonomic procedure, and *Salmonella* typing centers have been established worldwide. They maintain stocks of monospecific antisera for all previously discovered *Salmonella* O and H antigens, and they add to these stocks with each newly discovered *Salmonella* antigen. Anyone isolating a biotypical *Salmonella* may submit the isolate to a *Salmonella* typing center for serotype identification. Unfortunately, since the first identified serotypes of the genus had previously been given medically significant species designations—*S. paratyphi* and *S. typhi* for example—*Salmonella* serotaxonomists started giving comparable (species) designations to each newly discovered serotype. As the number of new species grew they started naming the serotypes after the town or area of isolation. This led to a ridiculous number (more than 1,200) of species within the genus. For an example of illegitimate species designations see group E of Table 24-2, where differences in a single phase 1 H antigen result in two distinct species designations. This situation contrasts sharply with that of the *Streptococcus (Diplococcus) pneumoniae* (Chapter 7) serotaxonomy—there 82 (far more significant) serotypes are all included in the single species *S. pneumoniae*. Efforts to rectify this taxonomic megalomania in the genus *Salmonella* are under consideration (see Ewing and Martin 1974); but as indicated in the eighth edition of *Bergey's Manual of Determinative Bacteriology* (Buchanan and Gibbons 1974), none of the present methods of nomenclature of *Salmonella* species is entirely satisfactory.

The taxonomy of the genus *Salmonella* is further complicated by the fact that both genetic variations—including mutations and sexual (plasmid) recombinations—and phenotypic variations may occur. These include: (1) the aerogenic → anaerogenic variations mentioned above; (2) changes in serotype antigenicity in-

Table 24-2. Examples of *Salmonella* serotypes (see *Bergey's Manual* for complete listing).

Species Designation	O Antigens	H Antigens Phase 1	H Antigens Phase 2
Group A			
S. paratyphi	1,2,12	a	—
Group B			
S. schottmuelleri	1,4,5,12	b	1,2
S. typhimurium	1,4,5,12	i	1,2
Group C			
S. hirschfeldii	6,7,(Vi)	c	1,5
S. belfast	6,8	c	1,7
Group D			
S. typhi	9,12,Vi	d	—
S. dublin	1,9,12,(Vi)	g,p	—
S. loma-linda	9,12	a	e,n,x
*S. gallinarum**	1,9,12	—	—
Group E			
S. weybridge	3,10	d	z_6
S. stockholm	3,10	y	z_6

*Nonmotile.

( ) = May be absent.

duced by phage transduction-lysogeny and by plasmid gene transfer; (3) the alterations in antigenicity of the H antigens in phase 1 $\leftrightharpoons$ phase 2 variations; or (4) loss variations such as loss of the virulence (Vi) antigen (OHVi → OH) or loss of the flagellar antigens (OH → O). The latter may be induced phenotypically by growth of the organisms in certain environments (such as phenol agar) or it may occur as a permanent genetic mutation (S. typhi H901 → S. typhi O901). There also may be variations in colony characteristics such as the smooth (S) → rough (R) colony strains. The S → R variation includes changes in antigenicity and in virulence. In spite of all the taxonomic complexities, isolation and identification of Salmonella is a common requirement of the clinical, veterinary, or public health laboratory.

PATHOGENIC MECHANISM

During the past several years enterotoxic proteins have been extracted from at least two serotypes of Salmonella—S. enteritidis and S. typhimurium (see Koupal and Deibel 1975; Sandifur and Peterson 1976). These enterotoxic proteins share certain characteristics with those of Vibrio cholerae and Escherichia coli and probably participate in Salmonella gastroenteritis-type pathology. Whether or not they are involved in other aspects of Salmonella virulence and pathology remains to be determined.

Prior to the discovery of the enterotoxic proteins, the pathogenic mechanism for all Salmonella serotypes had been presumed to be endotoxic. The endotoxins appear to be present in the cell walls and can be extracted from the cells by a variety of solvents. The purified endotoxins are lipopolysaccharide complexes. They are antigenic with specificity associated with the polysaccharide moiety. Antibodies produced by immunization with endotoxins show high agglutination and precipitation titers, but they are characteristically weak in toxin neutralizing activity. The pathogenic manifestations of the endotoxins include fever, changes in vascular permeability, hemorrhage, and shock.

CLINICAL MANIFESTATIONS

Human salmonelloses commonly are divisible into two clinical types: (1) gastroenteritis, occasionally complicated by Salmonella septicemia, and (2) enteric fever of the typhoid or paratyphoid type. Although some Salmonella serotypes are more prone to cause one or the other of these two clinical syndromes, every serotype is potentially capable of causing both. Gastroenteritis frequently is contracted by the ingestion of food heavily contaminated with Salmonella. The food may be inadequately cooked meat from infected animals, such as chickens and turkeys, or food contaminated by the excreta of infected animals or humans. The gastroenteritis results in cramping and diarrhea of variable severity and frequently is confused with food poisonings of the staphylococcal enterotoxin type (see Chapter 28). The Salmonella gastroenteritis, however, is a true infection that may lead to more serious complications. The uncomplicated disease is rarely fatal.

Typhoid and other Salmonella enteric fevers and septicemias are serious diseases that in preantibiotic days resulted in 5 to 10 percent mortality. After an incubation period averaging 2 weeks, typhoid and other Salmonella enteric fevers usually commence with prodromal symptoms of chills, vomiting, malaise, and a dull headache. These signs are followed by a stepwise rise in temperature to approximately 104°F. Untreated, the temperature continues spiking at this high level for about 3 weeks followed by gradual defervescence. During the second week of fever the patient frequently is acutely ill with great prostration, mental dullness, or delirium. Intestinal hemorrhaging or perforation may occur during this stage, leading to a poor prognosis. Prior to antibiotic therapy, this stage was frequently fatal. Although this is the average symptomatology, typhoid and other Salmonella enteric fever cases may range in severity from almost asymptomatic (slight fever and malaise, so-called walking typhoid) with no mortality to fulminating fatal pathology. An S. typhi bacteremia occurs during the first week of fever after which the organisms may no longer be found in the bloodstream. They invade lymphoid tissue including *Peyer's patches* from which they are shed into the lumen of the intestine. The bacteremias and *Salmonella* septicemias can be demonstrated only by positive blood cultures. After the blood becomes negative, the organisms may continue to be isolated from the fecal excreta of patients and recovered carriers. Carriers usually harbor the *S. typhi* in the gall bladder.

Salmonella serotypes are isolated from both human and nonhuman sources. Although the serotype incidence varies from year to year, the following figures are representative for at least one year in the past decade—1969—during which 21,413 *Salmonella* were isolated in the United States. The most frequently isolated serotype from humans was *S. typhimurium* (5,733 or 27 percent); *S. typhimurium* also was the most frequently isolated serotype from nonhuman sources. The other nine most frequent human isolates in order of frequency during that year (see *MMWR* Supplement, 1970) were: *S. enteritidis* (9.3 percent), *S. newport* (7.5 percent), *S. heidelberg* (6.7 percent), *S. infantis* (5.1 percent), *S. thompson* (4.9 percent), *S. saint-paul* (4.6 percent), *S. typhi* (2.6 percent), *S. blockley* (2.4 percent), and *S. javiana* (2.2 percent).

EPIDEMIOLOGY

In Europe and at least one North African country, a heretofore rare serotype—*Salmonella wein*—has become the predominant cause of human salmonellosis. This serotype is resistant to ampicillin, chloramphenicol, tetracycline, streptomycin, kanamycin, and sulfonamides. It is sensitive to gentamicin, colistin, and cephalosporin (see *MMWR*, 4 January 1975). This serotype has now invaded the United States.

During 1972–1974 Mexico reported more than 6,500 cases of typhoid fever caused by a chloramphenicol-resistant strain of *S. typhi*. One hospital in Mexico City reported 2,548 cases and 73 deaths from typhoid during the 1972–1974 epidemic (see *MMWR*, 26 April 1975).

Outbreaks of gastroenteritis due to *Salmonella newport* were reported from Colorado and Maryland during 1975. The source of the infections was traced to raw ground beef. Whether the beef was the primary vehicle or a contaminated secondary vehicle was not reported. The isolated *S. newport* cells were found to be resistant to tetracycline and to sulfonamides. These mutations of *Salmonella* to drug resistance indicate the importance of testing such isolates for drug susceptibility as an aid to both epidemiological studies and to therapy in salmonelloses.

Several hundred cases of typhoid fever occurred in the area of Port-au-Prince, Haiti, during October and November 1974. At least 11 cases of the disease, in New York City, acquired their infections in Haiti. The *S. typhi* isolated from the Haitian source were susceptible to all antibiotics and sulfonamides usually considered for therapy in typhoid fever (see *MMWR*, 21 December 1974 and 12 July 1975). Another outbreak of 12 culture-proven cases of typhoid was traced to a restaurant in New York City in 1975. The 12 cases were reported from four different states, but all had eaten dinner at the New York restaurant on the evening of 13 December 1975 (see *MMWR*, 17 January 1976). At the last report, which included five of the cases not previously reported, the search for the carrier of the infection had not been successful.

An interesting case of *Salmonella* gastroenteritis was reported from Oregon in 1974. This involved a 6-year-old girl whose stool culture yielded both *S. typhimurium* and an *Arizona* sp. (now designated a *Salmonella arizonae* serotype). The same two *Salmonella* serotypes were isolated from her pet turtle and from other turtles at the pet store where it was purchased. The turtles were shipped from Louisiana to California, and a portion of the same lot was sent to the pet shop in Oregon. Other turtles from this lot were shipped to Texas and these and the California turtles were found to be infected. The original turtles in this lot were certified as free from *Salmonella* and *Arizona* sp. prior to shipment from Louisiana (see *MMWR*, 28 December 1974). In addition to pet turtles, infected mice, rats, dogs, chickens, turkeys, and other animals have been incriminated as nonhuman sources of human salmonellosis. Certain *Salmonella* serotypes such as *S. typhi* and *S. paratyphi*, however, occur naturally only in human infections.

LABORATORY DIAGNOSIS

The only sure way of diagnosing a salmonellosis is the isolation and identification of the causative organism. For a comprehensive coverage of the laboratory procedures involved in the diagnosis of salmonelloses and other infections caused by members of the family Enterobacteriaceae, see Edwards and Ewing (1972) and Ewing and Martin (1974).

Specimens submitted for the cultural isolation of bacteria should be collected prior to the initiation of antimicrobial therapy. If the clinical symptoms are those of uncomplicated gastroenteritis, a freshly passed stool is the specimen of choice. If the symptoms are those of enteric fever or if high fever develops in the case of gastroenteritis, one or several blood specimens

should be cultured. If the primary cultures are negative, they should be repeated.

In typhoid fever and other enteric fever salmonelloses, a blood culture is most likely to be positive during the first week of fever whereas the fecal cultures will become increasingly positive during the second week of fever. For blood culture, 5 milliliters of the blood should be inoculated aseptically into 50–100 milliliters of broth. The culture medium may be a good beef-infusion–peptone broth or fluid thioglycolate medium or preferably both. Since a number of other infections yield first-week symptoms simulating typhoid or other *Salmonella* enteric fevers, inoculation of some of the blood specimens to enriched infusion broth or agar media designed for the cultivation of more fastidious organisms, such as streptococci, *Brucella* sp., *F. tularensis,* and others, might aid in the diagnosis of the unknown fever. Enough blood should be collected at the time of blood culture to allow for the establishment of onset agglutinin titers for the diagnostic antigens of typhoid and other symptomatically similar diseases. The

Figure 24–2. Laboratory diagnosis of *Salmonella* enteric fever (typhoid) and clinically similar diseases.

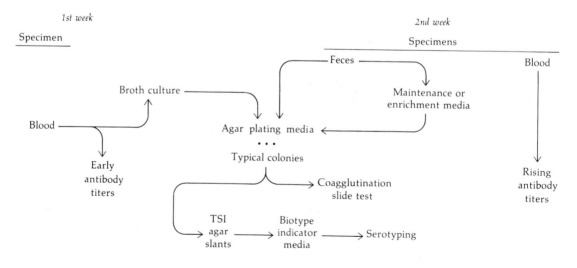

TSI = Triple sugar iron. (See Figure B on front cover.)

blood cultures should be incubated for 18 to 24 hours at 35–37°C. If there is no evidence of bacterial growth, the incubation and examinations should be continued up to 2 weeks or more. With or without visible evidence of bacterial growth, the broth should be streaked to agar plating media designed for colony isolation.

Fecal specimens may be streaked directly to agar plating media. If there is to be a delay in transporting the fecal specimen to the laboratory, however, it is desirable to inoculate some of the specimen to a fluid maintenance medium designed to keep the bacterial flora of the specimen unchanged until it can be streaked onto plating agar. If the specimen is from a suspected carrier, or if there is other reason to suspect the presence of relatively few *Salmonella* organisms, a portion of the fecal specimen may be inoculated to an enrichment broth medium designed to favor the growth of *Salmonella* while suppressing the growth of nonpathogens.

Figure 24-2 gives a simple diagrammatic illustration of the sequence of procedures involved in the culture and serodiagnosis of typhoid or other enteric salmonelloses and clinically related diseases. The fecal culture diagnostic procedures are the same as those advocated for the laboratory diagnosis of shigelloses and gastroenteritis caused by other Enterobacteriaceae (Chapter 23).

After typical colonies appear on the agar plating media, growth from the surfaces of the selected colonies should be carefully fished and inoculated (stab base and streak surface) to triple-sugar-iron (TSI) or a comparable tubed agar-slant medium. However, Edwards and Hilderbrand (1976) have advocated the use of a rapid coagglutination test (see Chapter 8) to tentatively identify the colony as a *Salmonella* prior to the inoculation of the TSI agar slant. The slide coagglutination test (see Kronvall 1973) requires the availability of a saline suspension of protein-A–containing *Staphylococcus aureus* Cowan with adsorbed antibody specific for the *Salmonella* serogroup antigens. When a bacteriological loop is touched to the surface of a suspected colony and then mixed with a drop of the staphylococcal-antisalmonella reagent, the staphylococci and the test cells will coagglutinate within 15 seconds to 2 minutes if the colony is a *Salmonella* serotype (see Figure 24-3). After inoculation the TSI agar culture should be incubated at 37°C overnight to give preliminary taxonomic evidence of the carbohydrate metabolism and H_2S production by the isolate (see Figures B-2 and B-3 on the front cover). Also the TSI agar slant provides sufficient growth for the inoculation of other media (see Tables III-A and 24-1) for additional taxonomic identification of the biotype. If the biotype evidence indicates a *Salmonella* other than *S. typhi*, this should be reported to the clinician who submitted the specimen. If there is reason to identify the serotype or phage type, the isolated culture should be submitted to a laboratory that specializes in these procedures. The clinical laboratory, however, should determine the drug susceptibility or resistance (antibiogram) of the isolate to aid the clinician in choosing the appropriate drug therapy. The antibiogram may also aid the epidemiologist in relating sources of infection in new or multiple cases of the disease. The chloramphenicol-resistant strain of *S. typhi* that caused the 1972–1974 epidemic of typhoid fever in Mexico was indicated by its antibiogram to be the source of a number of cases of typhoid in the United States involving tourists who had returned from Mexico.

As in all cases of serodiagnosis a rising antibody titer during the course of the disease is more significant than a stationary or falling antibody titer. The serodiagnostic test commonly employed in typhoid and other salmonelloses is agglutination of a killed suspension of *S. typhi* or other *Salmonella* serotypes by dilutions of the patient's serum. Consequently when a blood specimen is collected early in the disease for blood culture, an additional 3 to 5 milliliters of blood should be submitted to establish early antibody titers. These antibodies, if present, have no relationship to the current infection. The early serum antibodies have resulted from prior antigenic stimuli as a consequence of prior infections or prior active immunizations. These early serodiagnostic titrations should include diagnostic antigens for

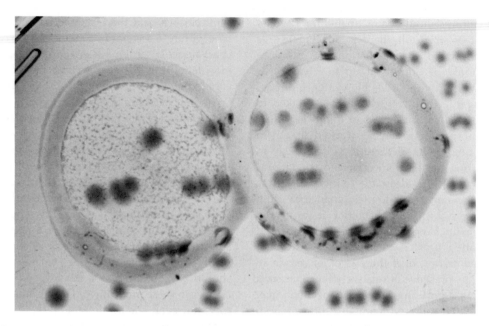

Figure 24–3.   Left: enlargement of a typical coagglutination reaction which occurred when *Salmonella typhi* was added to a polyvalent *Salmonella* antiserum-sensitized staph reagent; note mottled appearance. Right: absence of a coagglutination reaction when a nonsensitized staph reagent is used. (Courtesy of E. A. Edwards.)

other diseases that *always* (typhus fever; see Chapter 32) or *may* show early clinical symptoms indistinguishable from those of typhoid, such as tularemia and acute brucellosis. If a cultural diagnosis has not been established during the first week of the fever, a second blood specimen should be submitted 7 to 10 days later for a repetition of the serodiagnostic titrations using all the antigens used in the early titrations. If the antibody titer to one of these antigens shows a fourfold rise between the first and second week, this indicates that the antibodies were produced as a consequence of the current antigenic stimulation.

The rising-titer serodiagnosis is particularly valuable in identifying cases of typhus, tularemia, and brucellosis wherein cross-sharing of antigens by the etiological agents is rarely significant. Moreover, the culture media used for the diagnosis of salmonelloses never yield growth of the obligately parasitic *Rickettsia* of typhus fever and rarely yield growth of *F. tularensis* or *Brucella* sp. Therefore rising-titer serodiagnosis is the usual means of differentiat-

ing the diseases caused by these organisms from typhoid and other salmonelloses.

Rising-titer serodiagnostic differentiation of typhoid fever from other salmonelloses is complicated by the fact that there is extensive sharing of antigens by different *Salmonella* serotypes. At least 290 serotypes share one or more of the three antigens (9,12:d) of *S. typhi*; 69 serotypes share O antigens 9 and 12; and at least six serotypes share all three antigens. Consequently infections with any one of the *Salmonella* serotypes that share antigens with *S. typhi* could be expected to show a rising antibody titer for *S. typhi* as well as for their own serotype cells and for cells of other serotypes that share these antigens. Fortunately, because of the ease of cultural isolation of *S. typhi* and other *Salmonella* serotypes, dependence upon serodiagnosis is rarely essential in these diseases.

IMMUNITY

During the Boer War the British Army in South Africa (1899–1902) immunized the armed forces with a saline suspension of killed *S. typhi.* The results were reported as a significant lowering of both morbidity and mortality from typhoid in the immunized personnel. Many subsequent studies in animals and humans have established the efficacy of prophylactic immunization with typhoid "vaccine." The United States armed forces have required typhoid immunization since 1911.

Felix and Pitt (1934) discovered the Vi antigen of *S. typhi* and indicated it to be a surface masking antigen of freshly isolated *virulent* organisms. This antigen tends to disappear from most isolates after a few transplants on culture media. In at least one strain (*S. typhi* Vi Panama) the Vi antigen is stable. Since this discovery, *S. typhi* cells to be used in the preparation of typhoid vaccine are tested to ensure the presence of the Vi antigen. The vaccine is prepared by suspending the killed *S. typhi* Vi cells to a concentration of 10^9 per milliliter in sterile isotonic saline. If it is desirable to immunize against other *Salmonella* serotypes, killed cells of these serotypes may be incorporated in divalent or trivalent vaccines to a maximum combined concentration of 2.5×10^9 cells per milliliter. The usual subcutaneous prophylactic adult doses of these vaccines are 0.5, 1.0, and 1.0 milliliter at weekly intervals. Young children may receive smaller doses. Unfortunately there is no satisfactory method, comparable to the Schick test in diphtheria, for proving the immunogenic efficacy of this regimen on an individual basis.

The efficacy of typhoid vaccination is attested to by the fact that typhoid fever has been practically eliminated from the armed forces. Moreover, typhoid fever has been practically eliminated from all areas where good sanitary practices are enforced, irrespective of prophylactic immunization. At least one situation occurred in the South Pacific during World War II that differentiates the value of prophylactic immunization and sanitation in suppressing typhoid. During the Spanish-American War (1898) with troops engaged in the South Pacific area, one study involving approximately 10,000 men indicated a typhoid morbidity rate of more than 41 percent (more than 4,400 cases) with a

mortality rate of 5.65 percent. During World War II, with operations involving far greater numbers of men in the same Pacific area, but with all men immunized against typhoid, there was no mortality and practically no morbidity due to this disease. That sanitation was not the factor in this decreased incidence of typhoid fever is indicated by the fact that dysentery, for which there is no satisfactory vaccine, was rampant among the troops of both antagonists.

Passive immunization has never been proved to have either prophylactic or therapeutic value in typhoid or other salmonelloses. This probably is related to the endotoxic pathogenicity of these organisms.

CONTROL AND PREVENTION

Chloramphenicol has long been the drug of choice for the treatment of typhoid fever and possibly other salmonelloses. With the widespread prevalence of the chloramphenicol-resistant strain of *S. typhi* in the western hemisphere, however, other drugs will have to be substituted. Furthermore, the multiresistant antibiogram of *S. wein* in Europe and elsewhere, including the recent (1973) introduction into the United States, emphasizes the need for establishing the efficacy of other drugs for the treatment of salmonelloses. As indicated above, *S. wein* has been found to be susceptible only to gentamicin, colistin, and cephalosporin out of the nine drugs tested.

Sanitation is a major control measure in all intestinal group diseases involving fecal excreta as the primary vehicle. Sanitation in clinical cases of such diseases is the responsibility of the clinical and nursing personnel associated with the case. Disinfection of excreta, bedpans, bed linens, hands of attendants, and other secondary vehicles should be performed routinely. Flies should be excluded from these vehicles and from the environment of the patient. Eating utensils and food used by the patient should be disinfected. A cheap and excellent disinfectant is boiling water or, in the case of disposable vehicles, incineration.

Community sanitation is the combined responsibility of the citizens and the public health personnel. Community sewage (excreta) disposal should involve treatment that, under all weather conditions, results in a treatment plant effluent which is bacteriologically more pure than the community water source. This can be a big and expensive engineering problem in large urban communities.

Water purification is also a community problem in urban areas. Whereas usually only a gallon or less of water per day is ingested, the per capita use of water for all purposes can reach several hundred gallons per day. This necessitates the purification of 10^6 gallons or more of water every day for every 10,000 people in the community. Enforcement of food and milk sanitation ordinances is a community public health responsibility also.

Prophylactic immunization is an effective control measure in typhoid fever and possibly a few other salmonelloses. This immunization is not required in most sanitary environments. It is, however, recommended for those who travel to areas where the sanitary quality is either unknown or known to be bad.

Since most recent outbreaks of typhoid fever have been traced to carriers working in kitchens or other food-handling jobs, the problem of detection of typhoid carriers is a major one. Repeated fecal cultures frequently are required to determine the intermittent shedding of S. typhi by the carrier. Considering the number of food handlers in a community or state, this carrier detection can become a time-consuming and expensive public health undertaking. Felix and others (see Schubert et al. 1959) have claimed that typhoid carriers possess serum agglutinins specific for the Vi antigen of S. typhi. They contend that a Vi agglutination test should be performed on the food handlers and only those showing positive test results should be subjected to the repeated fecal cultures necessary to rule out the S. typhi carrier status of the individual. Even after the carrier state is established, the problem of what to do with the carrier remains. Since the S. typhi in most typhoid carriers persist in the gall bladder, the surgical removal of this nonessential organ has been advocated to cure the carrier state.

For a more comprehensive coverage of the *Salmonella* and other Enterobacteriaceae, see Edwards and Ewing (1972) and the microbiology textbooks and taxonomic and laboratory manuals listed among the general references of Chapter 1.

REFERENCES

Buchanan, R. E., and N. E. Gibbons. 1974. *Bergey's Manual of Determinative Bacteriology.* 8th ed. Baltimore: Williams & Wilkins.

Cowan, S. T., L. Le Minor, and R. Rohde. 1974. Enterobacteriaceae, Genus IV *Salmonella.* In Part 8 of *Bergey's Manual of Determinative Bacteriology.*

Edwards, E. A., and R. L. Hildebrand. 1976. Method for identifying *Salmonella* and *Shigella* directly from the primary isolation plate by coagglutination of protein A-containing staphylococci sensitized with specific antibody. *J. Clin. Microbiol.* 3:339–343.

Edwards, P. R., and W. H. Ewing. 1972. *Identification of Enterobacteriaceae.* 3rd ed. Minneapolis: Burgess.

Ewing, W. H., and W. J. Martin. 1974. Enterobacteriaceae. Chapter 18 in *Manual of Clinical Microbiology.*

Felix, A., and R. M. Pitt. 1934. A new antigen of *B. typhosa.* Its relation to virulence and to active and passive immunization. *Lancet* 2:186–191.

Koupal, L. R., and R. H. Deibel. 1975. Assay, characterization, and localization of an enterotoxin produced by *Salmonella. Infect. Immunity* 11:14–22.

Kronvall, G. 1973. A rapid slide agglutination method for typing pneumococci by means of specific antibody absorbed to protein A-containing staphylococci. *J. Med. Microbiol.* 6:187–190.

Sandifur, P. D., and J. W. Peterson. 1976. Isolation of skin permeability factors from culture filtrates of *Salmonella typhimurium. Infect. Immunity* 14:671–679.

Schubert, J. H., P. R. Edwards, and C. H. Ramsey. 1959. Detection of typhoid carriers by agglutination tests. *J. Bacteriol.* 77:648–654.

Thal, E., and L. O. Kallings. 1955. Zur Bestimmung des Genus *Salmonella* mit Hilfe eines Bakteriophagen. *Nord. Vet. Med.* 7:1063–1071.

25

Hepatitis

The term *hepatitis* is the idiopathic designation for diseases that damage the liver, frequently resulting in jaundice *(icterus).* Although a number of disease organisms might cause such pathology (including yellow fever virus—see Chapter 34), only a few belong to the intestinal group of diseases. These include: (1) hepatitis A virus (HAV), which generally is transmitted by human intestinal excreta; (2) hepatitis B virus (HBV), which generally is transmitted by parenteral injection (blood transfusion or blood-contaminated hypodermic needle inoculation) but can be transmitted by intestinal-group routes; and (3) *Leptospira* serotypes, which cause leptospirosis. The *Leptospira* commonly are parasites of rats or other animals and are frequently transmitted by urinary excreta.

A third hepatitis virus (HCV) has been identified as possibly the most common cause of blood transfusion hepatitis (see *MMWR*, 7 January 1977). The hepatitis viruses have failed to grow in tissue cultures, and natural infections are restricted to human hosts. Recently, however, chimpanzees and some species of marmo-

sets have been experimentally infected with hepatitis viruses.

VIRAL HEPATITIS

HAV Hepatitis—Etiology and Epidemiology

The hepatitis A virus possesses cubic symmetry and ranges in size from 25 to 28 nanometers (see Figure 25-1.) This virus is shed into the human intestinal tract, and the epidemiology, involving infected fecal excreta, is typical of the intestinal subgroup A epidemiology illustrated in Figure III-A.

An increasing number of epidemics of hepatitis A have been recognized since 1950. Statistical evidence indicates that young children frequently develop mild or subclinical infections, whereas older children and adults are more prone to develop severe illness. In grossly unsanitary community environments, therefore, a high incidence of hepatitis A infections might be expected to occur in infants and young

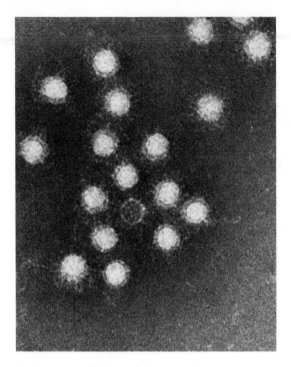

Figure 25–1. Virions of hepatitis A virus concentrated from the stool of an infected chimpanzee. 256,300×. (Courtesy of E. H. Cook, Jr., and C. R. Gravelle.)

(anicteric) cases were diagnosed in this outbreak. Epidemiological studies traced the infections to a food handler (salad preparer) who worked in the dining hall where the infected recruits ate their meals.

Raw oysters and clams, grown in sewage-contaminated water, also have been incriminated in the epidemiology of hepatitis A. Oyster-borne outbreaks were reported in Georgia and in Texas in 1973 (*MMWR*, 3 November 1973). Fourteen cases were reported from Calhoun, Georgia, and 65 cases from Houston, Texas. The latter cases were traced to a single restaurant and involved a number of out-of-state employees of Houston-based industries. The oysters responsible for both outbreaks originated from a single supplier in Louisiana. Since the incubation period of hepatitis A ranges from 2 to 6 weeks, tracing all the out-of-state cases proved to be a major epidemiological problem. At the time of the report, 17 additional ill persons in 13 states had been identified as having eaten at the incriminated restaurant in Houston at the time of the outbreak. There is no evidence, however, that the HAV replicates in the oyster or clam.

children. The mild or subclinical infections in these early life cases might be expected to lead to a high incidence of immunity in the older children and adults. Therefore the unsanitary environment might be expected to have a lower incidence of clinical hepatitis A than that found in highly sanitary environments in which some aspect of the sanitation suddenly breaks down.

Most epidemics of hepatitis A have been traced to sewage contamination of drinking water. The largest such epidemic thus far reported occurred in New Delhi, India, in 1957, with an estimated 50,000 cases. In this epidemic, the disease in pregnant women (second and third trimester) and in postpartum women resulted in extremely severe symptoms and a high mortality rate. An epidemic of hepatitis A was reported in 1974 involving navy recruits in California (see *MMWR*, 16 November 1974). A total of 113 clinical cases and 19 asymptomatic

HBV Hepatitis—Etiology, Antigenicity, Epidemiology

Although hepatitis following blood transfusion has been known for a long time, there was little understanding of its nature or cause prior to the mid-1960s (see Vyas et al. 1972). In 1963 B. S. Blumberg and his associates in Australia, while searching for ethnic antigens in human blood groups, reported finding a new antigen in the serum of aborigines. They designated the antigen Australia antigen (Au Ag). A few years later Blumberg et al. (1965; 1968) reported correlating the presence of Au Ag in the serum with hepatitis B. They also reported antibody specific for Au Ag in the serum of recovered hepatitis B patients. Subsequent studies indicated that blood containing the Au Ag would transmit hepatitis when inoculated to human volunteers. These observations provided a means of pretesting blood for Au Ag prior to transfusion. Blumberg was awarded a Nobel prize in 1976 (see Blumberg 1977).

Additional studies indicated that Au Ag is polymorphic consisting of (1) spherical core antigen 22 nanometers in diameter, (2) cylindrical tubular antigen 22 nanometers in diameter, and (3) double-shelled spherical particles 42 nanometers in diameter that originally were designated Dane particles. These latter particles are now considered to be the HBV. All these morphological elements share a hepatitis B surface antigen—the Au Ag. Figure 25-2 shows the three forms of antigen.

The WHO Expert Committee on Viral Hepatitis, at an October 1976 meeting in Geneva, advocated the following terminology for hepatitis B virus and its noninfectious antigens:

HBV: the 42-nanometer double-shelled virus (the Dane particles),

HBsAg: hepatitis B surface antigen (Au Ag) found on the virus and on the 22-nanometer spherical and tubular particles,

HBcAg: the hepatitis B core antigen found within the 22-nanometer core of the virus,

HBeAg: the e antigen(s), closely associated with hepatitis B infection.

Antibodies specific for these antigens are designated anti-HBs, anti-HBc, and anti-HBe respectively (see *MMWR*, 7 January 1977).

Krugman and Giles (1970) reported studies on 25,000 sera collected over a 15-year period from 700 hepatitis patients in a school for retarded children. Hepatitis was highly endemic in the school. Using the presence of HBsAg as the indicator of sera from cases of hepatitis B, Krugman and Giles were able to infect susceptible human volunteers by oral administration.

Figure 25–2. Electron micrograph of a serum fraction from a patient severely infected with hepatitis B virus. (A failure of the immune system to counteract the infection allowed extreme levels of the virus.) The three larger spherical particles at the top, (42 nm in diameter) are the complete virus (HBV, Dane particles). The 22 nm diameter spherical and tubular particles both possess the hepatitis B surface antigen (HBsAg), as does the larger 42 nm virion. The 22 nm sphere is the core of the virus and contains the HBcAg. (Courtesy of J. Griffith.)

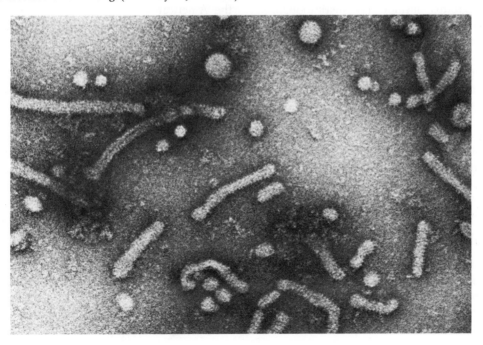

The oral infections resulted in clinically typical hepatitis B in the volunteers after a characteristically long incubation period of around 98 days. There have been reports of accidental oral transmission of hepatitis B by unsterilized dental instruments or by laboratory technologists drawing serum into the mouth while pipetting. Bleeding into the intestinal tract by hepatitis B patients might be expected to result in occasional intestinal excreta transmission of HBV. Other methods whereby blood or serum from hepatitis B patients might get into breaks in the skin or onto mucus membranes also might be expected to cause occasional infection. Kew (1973) described a case of hepatitis B in a nurse who accidentally introduced serum containing HBsAg into her eye.

Although HAV is more likely to be responsible for extensive epidemics of viral hepatitis, type B hepatitis is now recognized as a serious public health problem, especially when considered worldwide. On the basis of 1973 statistics it has been estimated that 150,000 cases of type B hepatitis occur annually in the United States. An increasing proportion of these cases are associated with the use of hard drugs in the 15-to-29-year age group. Other high-risk (nontransfusion) groups include (1) institutionalized patients, (2) patients and staff of hemodialysis units, and (3) clinical laboratory and other paramedical personnel. Many of the HBV infections result in no overt disease, and many of the symptomatic as well as the asymptomatic infections result in chronic carriers of the HBV. These carriers constitute a reservoir of infection estimated to be in the neighborhood of 100 million worldwide. Some of the carriers have been reported to maintain concentrations of 10^{13} to 10^{14} HBsAg particles per milliliter of serum (see Gerin 1976).

Clinical Hepatitis

Except for the considerable differences in the incubation periods of hepatitis A (2–6 weeks) and hepatitis B (7–22 weeks), the two types of viral hepatitis involve essentially the same clinical syndrome. In icteric hepatitis there is a prodromal phase with nausea, vomiting, anorexia, fatigue, low-grade fever, and possibly abdominal pain or tender hepatomegaly. This preicteric period may last several days to a week or more. At this stage the laboratory may be able to demonstrate elevated levels of serum transaminases—glutamic oxaloacetic (SGOT) and glutamic pyruvic (SGPT)—in the blood of the patient. The icteric stage, which generally persists for 1 to 2 weeks, may commence gradually with jaundice first apparent in the conjunctiva and then spreading to the rest of the body. Full recovery may take several months. Subclinical or mild (anicteric) cases of hepatitis A, as indicated above, are common in infants and young children. During epidemics many atypical cases have been reported for each case of typical icteric hepatitis. As mentioned, hepatitis has been reported to be extremely serious in pregnant and postpartum women.

Laboratory Diagnosis of Viral Hepatitis

An immunoradiometric assay designed to differentiate HAV from HBV hepatitis was reported by F. B. Hollinger at a 1976 symposium of the American Society of Clinical Pathologists held in Chicago. The test utilizes HAV antigen obtained from the stools of experimentally infected chimpanzees to assay the anti-HA antibody in the serum of the patient. An adaptation of the test is designed to use known anti-HA antibody to assay the presence of HAV in the stools of the patient. Currently, however, these procedures are restricted to research institutions. Consequently about the only aid that the average clinical laboratory can provide in the diagnosis of hepatitis A is to demonstrate the absence of HBsAg, *Leptospira,* and other potential causes of hepatitis in the patient's blood. If the disease is occurring in epidemic form and no cases show leptospiremia, it probably is hepatitis A.

Since the discovery of hepatitis-B—associated antigen (HBsAg) and the establishment of its presence in the serum as being indicative of current or past infection with HBV, at least five laboratory methods have been developed for routine demonstration of the presence of HBsAg in such sera. (See Hollinger 1974 for a comprehensive discussion.) The tests vary considerably in sensitivity, complexity, speed, and expense. The tests include (1) agarose gel diffusion (AGD), (2) counterimmunoelectrophoresis (CEP), (3) complement fixation (C'F), (4) red blood cell agglutination (RCA), and (5) radioimmunoassay (RIA).

To demonstrate HBsAg in a serum specimen, antiserum (anti-HBs) known to be specific for HBsAg must be available. This can be produced by immunizing animals, such as goats, with highly concentrated HBsAg. Since the test antigen is obtained from human serum (HS), however, there must be little or no contaminating anti-HS antibody in the serotaxonomic anti-HB. The simplest, cheapest, and least sensitive, but frequently adequate, serotaxonomic test for HBsAg in serum is the AGD test (Figure 25-3a). The gel must be prepared from a highly purified agar (agarose or equivalent product). While melted, the agarose must be carefully pipetted onto a horizontal clear-glass slide and allowed to gel in a layer approximately 1/16 inch thick. With the aid of a template, appropriate sized and spaced depots are cut into the gel surround-

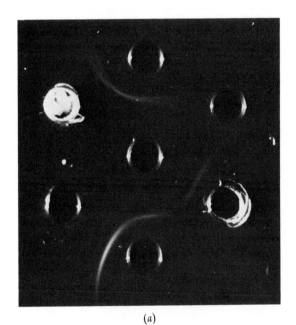

(a)

Figure 25–3. (a) Agar gel diffusion (AGD) test for HBsAg. The top and bottom wells hold known HBsAg. The four side wells hold sera from patients. The central well contains antibody to HBsAg. Note the lines of precipitate: the upper right side well is negative, lower right is positive, and the sera in the two wells on the left contain antibody to HBsAg. (b) Counterimmunoelectrophoresis test for HBsAg. Positive tests are seen between the second, fourth, and sixth pairs of wells from the left. ((a) Courtesy of P. V. Holland; (b) courtesy of Hyland Division Travenol Laboratories, Inc.)

(b)

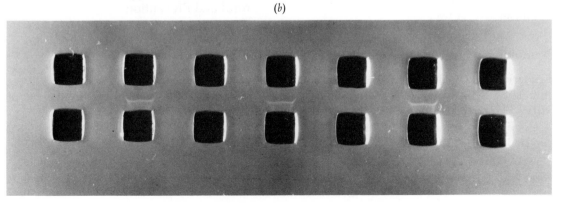

ing a central depot. Alternating peripheral depots are filled with test serum and with a known HBsAg-positive serum (positive control). Two hours later, the central depot is filled with anti-HBs antiserum. This sequence of adding reagents to the depots allows the slow-moving (large) HBsAg particles a chance to diffuse into the gel before the faster-moving (smaller) anti-HBs IgG molecules are added to the central depot. The AGD test must be housed in a moist chamber for 18 to 24 hours before yielding results. Lines of precipitate develop in the agarose gel where the HBsAg and anti-HBs antibody meet in suitable concentrations. Obviously the HBsAg positive control must yield such a line of precipitate. If the anti-HBs antiserum also contains anti-HS antibody, a second line of precipitate may develop nearer the central depot. If the test serum contains HBsAg, a comparable line of precipitate will develop in the gel between it and the central depot.

The most widely used test for detecting HBsAg on a large scale (blood banks) is the counterimmunoelectrophoresis (CEP) test (see Figure 25-3b). It, too, is a test in which precipitation occurs in agarose gel, but the rate of diffusion of both HBsAg and anti-HBs antibody is speeded up by passing an electric current through the gel. Since the HBsAg, in an electrophoretic field, migrates toward the anode, whereas the anti-HBs IgG migrates toward the cathode, the reactants meet in suitable concentrations in the gel and form lines of precipitate much sooner than they do in the unaided agarose gel diffusion (AGD) test. Usually positive or negative test results can be obtained within an hour or two.

Immunity

Recovery from viral hepatitis results in solid immunity to the homologous virus—HAV or HBV—but no cross-immunity. The judicious use of human gamma globulin for passive prophylactic immunization of high-risk individuals (family contacts and pregnant women) during epidemics of hepatitis A has been advocated.

The IgG will not prevent the infection, but it usually reduces the severity of the disease.

A limited amount of HAV for serological or immunological studies is available from infected chimpanzees. However, the possibility of a vaccine for human immunization probably will have to await the successful propagation of the virus in tissue culture.

Fairly extensive immunological studies on type B hepatitis have been made possible by the recovery of HBsAg from human chronic carriers by plasmaphoresis. In this process the plasma, containing the HBsAg, is separated from the cellular elements of the blood. The cells are then returned to the bloodstream of the donor. The different morphological components of the HBsAg (core, tubular, and 42-nanometer HBV) can each be purified by differential centrifugation and electrophoresis (see Gerin et al. 1971; Gerin 1976). Preliminary studies by Purcell and Gerin (1975), using susceptible chimpanzees, have demonstrated the noninfectivity and immunogenicity of the 22-nanometer HBcAg, including resistance of the immunized animals to experimental challenge with live virus.

Passive immunization, using high-titered anti-HBs immune globulin from convalescent patients, also has been proposed to prevent or modify HBV infection and currently is being studied. As in HAV hepatitis, however, propagation of the HBV in tissue culture probably would be the greatest contribution that researchers could make to the future of immunological prevention of viral hepatitis.

Control and Prevention

Control of HBV hepatitis, even in the absence of immunological procedures, has made significant progress during the past decade. The development of sensitive serological assays for HBsAg in sera and the prohibition against the use of HBsAg-positive blood for transfusion has greatly reduced the risk of posttransfusion HBV hepatitis. Moreover, recognition of the danger of HBV infection by laboratory personnel, research workers, and other persons handling human blood specimens has contributed to lowering accidental hepatitis infection.

LEPTOSPIROSIS

Etiology and Epidemiology

Leptospirosis is caused by unique spirochetes belonging to the genus *Leptospira.* The unique characteristic of these spirochetes is the fact that one or both ends are curved back into a characteristic hook (see Figure 25-4). Also contrary to most pathogenic spirochetes, *Leptospira* are easily cultivated in simple broth media, usually supplemented with sterile rabbit serum. The genus includes both saprophytic *Leptospira* (frequently found in water and commonly called *L. biflexa*) and pathogenic *Leptospira.*

The pathogenic *Leptospira* are primarily parasites of rodents and other wild and domestic animals (mice, rats, opossums, raccoons, skunks, dogs, swine, sheep, goats, horses, cattle, and others). At least 130 serotypes of the genus *Leptospira* have been described, and many species designations have been suggested for these pathogens. *Leptospira icterohemorrhagiae,* one of the first species designated, was described in 1915 by Japanese workers as the cause of Weil's disease or infectious jaundice. The species name indicates both the liver damage (icterus or jaundice) and the gastrointestinal hemorrhaging involved in the pathology of severe cases of Weil's disease. It has been estimated, however, that only about 40 percent of cases of leptospirosis show evidence of jaundice. Although a number of other species designations have been suggested for the pathogenic serotypes of *Leptospira,* taxonomic differentiation of these "species" has not been deemed successful. Therefore the eighth edition of *Bergey's Manual of Determinative Bacteriology* recommends that for the time being only one multiserotype species, *L. interrogans,* be recognized.

The pathogenic *Leptospira* invariably involve the kidneys of their hosts and are shed in the urine. Therefore the epidemiology between human cases (which appears to be rare) might well be that illustrated in Figure III-A, but with urine substituted for intestinal excreta as the primary vehicle. Undoubtedly most human

Figure 25–4. (*a*) Darkfield micrograph of *Leptospira interrogans* serotype *illini;* note the hooked ends. 900×. (*b*) Electron micrograph of the same serotype; the sheath surrounding the organism and axial filaments at each end may be seen. 8,960×. (Both courtesy of D. Bromley.)

(*a*)

(*b*)

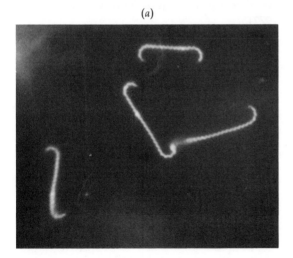

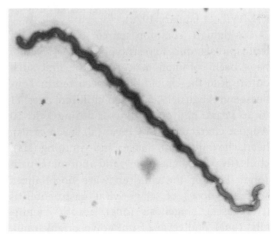

cases of leptospirosis, however, are acquired from infected animal urine contaminating eating utensils and food. It has been established that pathogenic *Leptospira* can penetrate the skin — certainly broken or abraded skin. Therefore skin contact with urine-contaminated moist soil (in mines, farms, and swamps) accounts for cases of leptospirosis in these environments. Infected rats have been reported to excrete up to 10^6 leptospires per milliliter of urine for months after recovery.

Two outbreaks of leptospirosis were reported to CDC in 1975 — one in Florida, the other in Tennessee. Four cases in Florida were discovered as a result of screening suspected arboviral specimens for leptospiral agglutinins. Although leptospira were not isolated from any of the patients, all showed significant antibody titers to *Leptospira* serotypes. One patient showed a rising titer to serotype *L. canicola* with the probable source of infection a pet raccoon. A second patient showed a rising titer to serotype *L. pomona* with cattle the probable source of infection. Two other members of the family of the second patient yielded single high antibody titers (1:400 or greater) to *Leptospira* serotypes. The latter three patients worked on a dairy farm that frequently was flooded after rains. While tending the cattle, these patients often went barefoot. No epidemiological link, other than geographical proximity, could be established between the first patient and the other three. All four were anicteric cases of leptospirosis (see *MMWR*, 24 January 1976).

Although common-source outbreaks of leptospirosis due to serotype *L. grippotyphosa* have been common in Europe, the first such outbreak in the United States occurred in Tennessee in August 1975. Seven children, ages 11 to 16 years, had onset illness, during 1 to 10 August, characterized by fever (all seven cases), headache (all seven), nausea and vomiting (six), chills (five), myalgias (four), and abdominal pain (one). Five of the children were hospitalized with diagnoses of: acute viral gastroenteritis (two cases), shigellosis (one), aseptic meningitis (one), and fever of unknown origin (one). The latter patient was operated on for sus-

pected appendicitis. Although *Leptospira* were not isolated, all patients demonstrated serological evidence of recent infection with serotype *L. grippotyphosa*. The only common-source-infection evidence was the fact that all patients had swum in a local creek. Like the Florida cases, all the Tennessee cases were anicteric (see *MMWR*, 19 March 1976).

More cases of human leptospirosis in the United States were reported in the year 1975 than in any other year since 1964. Although cases were reported from 28 states and Puerto Rico, 6 states — Alabama, California, Florida, Louisiana, Tennessee, and Texas — accounted for 49 percent of the reports. The most probable sources of infection were surface water (ponds, creeks, sewage — 29 percent), dogs (22 percent), rodents (11 percent), and cattle or swine (8 percent). Sixty-four percent of the patients had onset of symptoms during the months of July to October. Of the patients 35 were icteric, 53 were anicteric, and in 31 the presence or absence of jaundice was not reported. These and other observations in the United States during the past 50 years have indicated that occupational exposure is no longer the primary source of infection. Although rats continue to be an important reservoir host, no longer are they the major source of human leptospirosis. And the anicteric form of the disease is more common than the clinically more severe and more easily diagnosed icteric form (see *MMWR*, 28 January 1977).

Clinical Leptospirosis

Leptospirosis can vary considerably in severity of symptoms (from subclinical to fatal). As previously indicated only about 40 percent of such cases develop the clinical evidence of liver damage — jaundice. The incubation period in leptospirosis ranges from 4 to 20 days, followed, in the average acute case, by abrupt onset of headache, chills, muscular aches, prostration, and a rapidly rising temperature. *Leptospira* may be demonstrated in the patient's blood by culture during the first week of symptoms. The onset symptoms may be followed by nausea, vomiting, and abdominal pain. The headache and myalgia may become distressing, and the recurrent chills and high spiking fever may persist for a week or more before defervescence and symptomatic improvement. Because of the clinical similarity of leptospirosis to a variety of other acute, febrile diseases, laboratory aid should be requested in order to arrive at a differential diagnosis.

Laboratory Diagnosis

The diagnosis of leptospirosis, with or without jaundice, usually depends upon demonstrating *Leptospira* in the blood or urine of patients. Blood is the specimen of choice for cultivation, particularly during the first week of symptoms. Since urine specimens usually are contaminated with other bacteria, a selective broth medium containing 5-fluorouracil should be used for urine cultures. Further, a centrifuged urine specimen might reveal the presence of live, motile *Leptospira*. Microscopic examination of blood rarely reveals these organisms even when the cultures yield positive results. Blood cultures are most likely to be positive during the first week of symptoms and should be repeated daily. Thereafter, and possibly for several months, leptospires may be found in the urine. The numbers in the urine of human cases, however, are low and shedding is intermittent.

Because of the ease of recognizing the morphologically unique *Leptospira* in microscopic preparations from positive cultures or from urine, and because of the unsatisfactory serotype differentiation at present, it is recommended that the laboratory merely report the demonstration of *Leptospira* sp. (*interrogans*), serotype unknown. Possibly ongoing studies of *Leptospira* species and serotypes will change this reporting procedure in the future.

During and following clinical leptospirosis, antibodies appear in the serum of patients. These antibodies will yield positive agglutination-lysis test results with live homologous serotype *Leptospira*. Since there are so many serotypes with frequent cross-reactions, however, choosing the homologous serotype for the

test antigen poses a problem for the serodiagnosis of this disease. However, Galton, at the Center for Disease Control (CDC) in Atlanta, after many years studying *Leptospira* serotypes, selected 12 that include the majority of the cross-reacting antigens of the genus. Using these 12 serotype cultures and the agglutination-lysis test, the patient's serum will reveal the presence of antibody stimulated by infection with practically any one of the more than 130 *Leptospira* serotypes. The CDC, the state departments of health, and other public health laboratories maintain cultures of these 12 serotypes for aid in the diagnosis of leptospirosis. For more details see Alexander (1974).

Immunity

Because of the many serotypes of *Leptospira* and the numerous animal sources of infection, it is difficult even to determine whether or not recovery from infection stimulates a lasting immunity to homologous serotypes. Moreover, the multiple serotypes probably rule out the development of effective vaccines for active immunization. None is currently available.

Control and Prevention

Although a number of antibiotics including penicillins, streptomycin, and tetracycline have been advocated for therapy in leptospirosis, the need for early administration of large doses is always emphasized. This complicates the problem of therapy because early diagnosis of leptospirosis is difficult to obtain. If the disease is suspected (which is unusual) and if leptospires are demonstrated in the blood or urine of the patient (which is rare), a diagnosis during the first week of symptoms is possible. More frequently the disease is diagnosed by serological methods that are almost never early diagnoses. Consequently chemotherapy cannot be depended upon to control the incidence of the disease.

About the only effective control measures are these: (1) protect eating utensils and food from contamination with rat and other animal urine, (2) avoid bare skin contact with moist soil contaminated with cattle or other animal urine, (3) avoid bare skin contamination with urine of dogs and other animal pets, and (4) avoid swimming in ponds or creeks known to be contaminated with cattle or other animal urine. Fortunately leptospirosis is rarely a fatal disease.

REFERENCES

Alexander, A. D. 1974. *Leptospira.* Chapter 34 in *Manual of Clinical Microbiology.*

Blumberg, B. S. 1977. Australia antigen and the biology of hepatitis B. *Science* 197:17–25.

Blumberg, B. S., H. J. Alter, and S. Visnich. 1965. A new antigen in leukemia sera. *J. Amer. Med. Ass.* 191:541–546.

Blumberg, B. S., A. I. Sutnich, and W. T. London. 1968. Hepatitis and leukemia antigen. *Bull. N.Y. Acad. Med.* 44:1556–1558.

Gerin, J. L. 1976. Hepatitis, the search for viral and subviral antigens. *Fractions* 1:1–9. Palo Alto: Spinco Div., Beckman Instruments, Inc.

Gerin, J. L., P. V. Holland, and R. H. Purcell. 1971. Australia antigen, large-scale purification from human serum and biochemical studies of its proteins. *J. Virol.* 7:569–576.

Hollinger, F. B. 1974. Hepatitis viruses. Chapter 90 in *Manual of Clinical Microbiology.*

Kew, M. C. 1973. Possible transmission of serum (Australia-antigen positive) hepatitis via the conjunctiva. *Infect. Immunity.* 7:823–824.

Krugman, S., and J. P. Giles. 1970. Viral hepatitis. New light on an old disease. *J. Amer. Med. Ass.* 212:1019–1029.

MMWR Supplement. 1976. Perspectives on the control of viral hepatitis, type B. *MMWR* 25:1–11.

Purcell, R. H., and J. L. Gerin. 1975. Hepatitis B subunit vaccine: a preliminary report of safety and efficacy tests in chimpanzees. *Amer. J. Med. Sci.* 270:395–399.

Vyas, G. N., H. A. Perkins, and R. Schmid (eds.). 1972. *Hepatitis and Blood Transfusion.* New York: Grune & Stratton.

26

Poliomyelitis

Poliomyelitis was first recognized as a clinical entity ("spinal paralysis of children") in 1840. The first described epidemic of the disease occurred in Sweden in 1887. Landsteiner and Popper (1909) showed that monkeys could be infected and that the etiological agent was filterable. Subsequently three antigenic serotypes of the virus were established and designated Brunhilde, Lansing, and Leon. These are now designated serotypes 1, 2, 3 respectively.

ETIOLOGY

Enders et al. (1949) propagated the Lansing strain of poliovirus in a variety of human embryonic tissue cultures, all of which showed evidence of viral cytopathology. Prior to this time it was common belief that the virus required nerve tissue for replication. Subsequently all three serotypes have been propagated in monkey kidney tissue (MKT) cultures and in established cell lines of human tissues. The MKT-cultured virus made possible the development of the Salk and Sabin vaccines (see

the section on immunity) for prophylactic immunization. Tissue cultures also provided a means for isolating and identifying these viruses from fecal excreta, secretions, and tissues of patients and experimental animals. Enders received a Nobel prize for his contributions to the understanding and prevention of poliomyelitis.

Poliovirus (Figure 26-1) belongs to a group of small RNA viruses that have been designated picornaviruses (pico: small; rna: ribonucleic acid). They are members of a large group of viruses found in the intestinal tracts of humans and animals (enteroviruses). The accepted genus, species, and serotype designations for the virus of poliomyelitis are *Poliovirus hominis*, serotypes 1, 2, or 3.

So far as is known, *P. hominis* is found in nature only in humans. In addition to monkeys, chimpanzees can be experimentally infected with *P. hominis* by both the parenteral and oral routes. The experimental disease in chimpanzees is closely similar, if not identical, to the natural human disease. Studies of the distribution of the virus in the tissues of chimpanzees

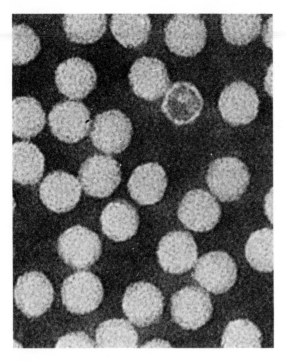

Figure 26–1. Highly-purified, negatively-stained *Poliovirus hominis* Type 1. 395,000×. (Courtesy of B. A. Phillips.)

following experimental oral infections have established the dual primary vehicles involved. They have also provided explanations for a variety of previously poorly understood clinical and epidemiological phenomena in poliomyelitis (see Figure 26-2).

CLINICAL SYMPTOMS AND EPIDEMIOLOGY

Clinically, human poliomyelitis is divisible into major and minor illness. The disease is classified as major illness when symptoms of central nervous system (CNS) pathology are first observed. These symptoms include several but not necessarily all of the following: fever, severe headache, stiffness of the neck and spine, tenderness of the skin, painful muscle or joint motion, tremors, twitching, and exaggerated reflexes. Kernig's and Brudzinski's signs (see Chapter 6) may or may not be present, depend-

ing upon the extent of meningeal damage. This CNS involvement may or may not progress to *paralytic* poliomyelitis, depending upon the sites of viral damage in the central nervous system. If motoneurons of the spinal cord or bulbar region of the brain stem are damaged sufficiently, muscles controlled by those neurons will develop a flaccid paralysis. The time from the first evidence of muscle weakness to the maximum paralysis usually is 2 to 7 days. A case is not considered paralytic poliomyelitis unless the muscle weakness (flaccid state) persists for more than 2 or 3 weeks.

A number of factors have been claimed to predispose a patient to paralytic poliomyelitis: (1) the virulence and dose of the virus, (2) the age of the patient, (3) pregnancy, (4) tonsilectomy, (5) immunogenic injections, and (6) overexertion or fatigue during the early stages of infection. Factors (4) and (5) are the only ones that might normally be avoided—by not having them performed during the hot summer months when epidemic poliomyelitis is more likely to occur. It has been estimated that only 1 or 2 percent of human poliovirus infections progress to the major illness and that only 0.1 to 1 percent develop paralytic poliomyelitis.

Paralytic poliomyelitis may be divided into several types, depending upon the location of the damaged motoneurons:

1. Spinal poliomyelitis may involve motoneurons in the cervical region, as a result of which muscles of the shoulder, arms, chest, intercostal, diaphragm, or upper abdominal region will be paralyzed. If the motoneurons of the lumbar region of the spinal column are damaged, the muscles of the lower abdominal region and legs will be paralyzed.

2. Bulbar poliomyelitis involves motoneurons of the cranial nerves resulting in paralysis of pharyngeal or laryngeal muscles; or the damage may occur in the motoneurons of the respiratory or vasomotor centers in the medulla resulting in heart or respiratory failure.

3. Bulbospinal poliomyelitis usually results in ascending paralyses: first in the legs, then abdominal and thoracic muscles, then shoul-

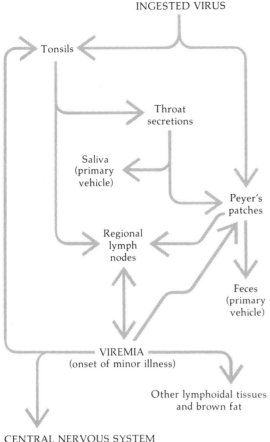

INGESTED VIRUS

Tonsils

Throat
secretions

Saliva
(primary
vehicle)

Peyer's
patches

Regional
lymph
nodes

Feces
(primary
vehicle)

VIREMIA
(onset of minor illness)

Other lymphoidal tissues
and brown fat

CENTRAL NERVOUS SYSTEM
(invasion initiates major illness)

Figure 26–2. The spread of *Poliovirus hominis* in the tissues of orally infected chimpanzees. (After Bodian 1955, 1956.)

ders and arms, and finally the muscles controlled by the cranial and medullary nerves.

Bulbar and bulbospinal poliomyelitis are the most likely to end fatally.

The minor illness commences with the invasion of the virus into the bloodstream (viremia). This type of poliomyelitis involves the same nonspecific prodromal symptoms that precede the onset of the major illness. These symptoms do not progress to those of major illness, however, because the central nervous system is not invaded by the virus. The nonspecific symptoms of the minor illness include some

or all of the following: vomiting, sore throat and possibly other respiratory or gastrointestinal symptoms, sudden onset of fever, mild headache, and listlessness. These symptoms of minor illness have been estimated to occur in only 4 to 8 percent of human poliomyelitis infections. The other 90 to 95 percent of human *P. hominis* infections are asymptomatic (subclinical). The only means whereby the minor illness or subclinical *P. hominis* infections can be established is by isolating and identifying the virus or by demonstrating a rising antibody titer to this virus—and both methods frequently are either not done or are unsatisfactory.

As indicated, Figure 26-2 provides a reasonable explanation for some of the clinical and epidemiological aspects of *P. hominis* infections. Because of the predilection of the virus for lymphoidal tissue the tonsils serve as the first portal of entry for invasion by ingested virus. However, the food or other vehicles might carry the virus past the tonsils without infecting them. The swallowed virus might be expected to invade the lymphoidal tissue (Peyer's patches) in the intestinal tract. Thus the primary infection might be in either or both tonsils and Peyer's patches.

If the tonsils are infected, the virus multiplies there and is shed into the throat secretions, where admixed with saliva it can serve as the primary vehicle for the respiratory modes of transmission of the disease (see Figure II-A). Moreover, the virus in throat secretions will be swallowed and infect previously uninfected Peyer's patches. The virus then multiplies in the latter lymphoidal tissues and is shed into the intestinal tract, thereby involving feces as the second primary vehicle and justifying the inclusion of poliomyelitis in the intestinal group of diseases.

From the tonsils or Peyer's patches the virus travels along the lymph channels to regional lymph nodes where it again multiplies. It then travels lymph channels to other lymph nodes and eventually empties into the bloodstream, thereby initiating the viremic stage and symptoms of the minor illness. In the bloodstream the virus might be carried to and invade any lymphoidal or other susceptible tissues, resulting in further multiplication and antigenic stimulation. If this antigenic stimulation provided by P. hominis in the lymphoidal and other tissues is sufficient, the spread of the virus might be stopped by the immune response before or just after invasion of the bloodstream. This situation would account for the estimated 90 to 95 percent of asymptomatic infections. The 4 to 8 percent of the minor illness infections could be similarly accounted for by the immune response destroying the virus in both the tissues and bloodstream prior to its invasion of the central nervous system. In the remaining 1 to 2 percent of infections that develop symptoms of major illness, the virus must have invaded from the bloodstream into the central nervous system before the immune response neutralized all the virus in the bloodstream. Antibodies in the bloodstream will not pass the blood-CNS barrier; therefore, evidence of CNS pathology— symptoms of the major illness—can commence and progress despite the presence of virus-neutralizing antibody in the blood serum at that time.

Although both throat secretions (saliva) and feces can serve as primary vehicles in poliomyelitis, the presence of the virus in the former appears to be much more transient than in the latter. It is conceivable, moreover, that not all P. hominis infections involve the tonsils. If the tonsils are involved, the Peyer's patches will also be involved either directly or as a result of swallowed saliva. These observations and epidemiological evidence seem to incriminate feces as the more important primary vehicle in poliomyelitis.

Poliomyelitis, when first recognized in 1840, was considered to be a paralytic disease of infants and young children. Due to the inadequate fecal sanitation at that time, one would expect that each newborn child would have been exposed to the disease early in life. If the clinical statistics of the disease were the same then as subsequently determined, one could expect that for each infected infant who developed paralytic poliomyelitis (some of whom would die) 99 to 999 would deveop lifelong immunity. As sanita-

tion improved, however, more and more infants escaped exposure and grew to be susceptible older children and adults. Concurrently, epidemics of poliomyelitis involving these older susceptibles as well as infants began to occur. These epidemics reached their peak in the United States in the 1930s to 1950s. A good example of the change from the infantile to adult disease was the paralytic poliomyelitis that made a cripple of Franklin D. Roosevelt at 30 years of age. Also a good example of the influence of sanitation upon epidemic poliomyelitis was the fact that while Texas from 1930 to 1950 was suffering severe epidemics of late childhood and adult paralytic poliomyelitis, Mexico, with less adequate sanitation, was reporting a low incidence of the disease. Mexico, however, had a higher infant mortality rate from intestinal group diseases in general than did Texas.

Although active immunization with Salk and Sabin vaccines (see the section on immunity) has practically eliminated epidemic poliomyelitis, isolated cases were reported in Connecticut and Texas in 1975 (see *MMWR*, 30 August 1975). Five cases of paralytic poliomyelitis were reported in Freiburg, Germany, in 1976 (see *MMWR*, 22 October 1976).

LABORATORY DIAGNOSIS

The most widely used laboratory procedure for the diagnosis of poliomyelitis is the isolation and identification of the serotype of P. hominis. The procedure depends upon the susceptibility of cultured tissues, mainly monkey kidney (MKT), to infection with P. hominis 1, 2, or 3. The infection results in microscopic morphological changes in the tissue culture cells—the cytopathic effect (CPE) as in Figure 26-3. Since the virus is found in intestinal excreta prior to onset of symptoms of minor illness and persists there for weeks to months, fecal material is the usual specimen for laboratory diagnosis. The specimen should be collected as early as possible in the disease and tested as soon as possible after collection. If the first test is negative a second specimen should be submitted. Some workers

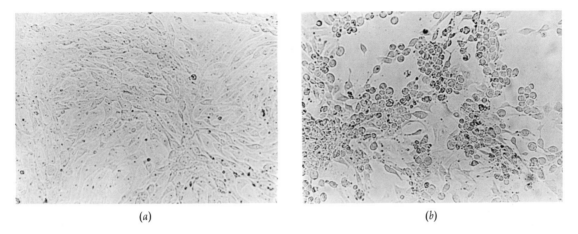

(a)   (b)

Figure 26–3. (*a*) Normal primary rhesus monkey kidney tissue monolayer. (*b*) Cytopathic effect of poliovirus on primary rhesus monkey kidney tissue culture. CPE indicated by rounding and destruction of cells of the monolayer. Both 264×.

advocate inoculating the fecal specimen to a human cell-line tissue culture (HeLa, WI-38, or Hep-2) in addition to the MKT culture. If there is a chance that the clinical symptoms might be caused by another enterovirus sero-type, such as *Coxsackievirus*, a newborn mouse should also be inoculated with the fecal speci-men.

Prior to inoculation to the tissue culture or mouse, the fecal specimen should be suspended in buffered salt solution (BSS) and centrifuged to sediment particulate matter. If there are large numbers of bacteria in the specimen, the super-natant fluid may be centrifuged to sediment these organisms without sedimenting the virus. The supernatant fluid, after either degree of centrifugation, should receive a mixture of anti-biotics (penicillin and streptomycin) designed to kill the residual bacteria present. A suitable aliquot of the treated specimen is then inocu-lated to a vial of MKT culture (and possibly a human tissue culture or a newborn mouse). The cultures are incubated at 37°C and examined for 14 days for evidence of CPE. If CPE develops in the primary culture, it might be due to one of the three serotypes of *P. hominis* or it might be due to some other enterovirus such as *Coxsackievirus* or *Echovirus* serotypes. If the stool virus is *Coxsack-*

ievirus, the infant mouse should develop paraly-sis and die within a few days, whether or not CPE occurs in the MKT culture.

To identify the virus that caused the CPE in the primary tissue culture as *P. hominis* 1, 2, or 3, four additional vials of the same cultured tissue should be inoculated with fluid from the in-fected (CPE) culture. One of the four secondary cultures should have received anti–*P. hominis* 1, a second anti–*P. hominis* 2, and a third anti–*P. hominis* 3. The fourth culture is a control and should receive no antibody. After suitable in-cubation of these secondary cultures they should be examined for CPE, which must occur in the control or the test has no value. Also CPE should occur in any of the three test prepara-tions in which the anti–*P. hominis* is not specific for the virus serotype causing the CPE. If the virus is one of the three serotypes of *P. hominis,* there will be no CPE in the tissue culture receiving the homologous anti–*P. hominis.* If the virus causing CPE in the primary culture and in the control culture was *P. hominis* 2, for example, the test culture containing anti–*P. hominis* 2 (and only that culture) will show *no* CPE. If all four cultures show CPE, the cytopathogenic virus is not *P. hominis* but probably one of the other enteroviruses. This is how the many serotypes of *Echovirus* were discovered while testing for *Poliovirus.*

Antibodies appear in the blood of poliomyelitis patients frequently before the onset of symptoms of the major illness. Since the symptoms of the minor illness are also the prodromal symptoms of the major illness and are nonspecific, collection of a blood specimen for serodiagnosis at the onset of these symptoms is rarely practiced. If a blood specimen is collected at the onset of symptoms of the major illness, the serum antibody titer frequently is so high that a significant (fourfold) rising titer cannot be demonstrated later. Therefore serodiagnosis, using either virus CPE neutralization, complement fixation, or precipitation of known serotypes of *P. hominis,* is rarely practiced.

IMMUNITY

Recovery from a *P. hominis* infection, whether it be asymptomatic or paralytic, results in immunity to the virus serotype involved. Early (ca. 1930) efforts to prepare vaccines using the virus found in the spinal cord of infected monkeys (comparable to Pasteur's rabies vaccine from rabbits) not only did not protect but may have been responsible for some cases of paralytic poliomyelitis in human vaccinees.

After John Enders and his associates in 1949 reported the propagation of *Poliovirus* in human tissue cultures, primary MKT cultures were used as the source of all three serotypes of *P. hominis* for vaccine production. Jonas Salk (1955) and his associates produced the first successful vaccine. It consisted of formalin-inactivated (killed) *P. hominis* serotypes 1, 2, and 3 as a trivalent vaccine. After extensive animal and field trials, which proved it both safe and effective, this vaccine was licensed for general human use in the United States. Shortly thereafter, one or two lots of the vaccine were found to cause paralytic poliomyelitis in the recipients, even though the manufacturer's records indicated compliance with all safety regulations. The safety standards were made more stringent and no further cases have been traced to the killed-virus vaccine. The Salk vaccine is given in two or preferably three injections at monthly intervals followed by a booster injection 6 to 9 months later.

During the first 5 years following the widespread use of the Salk vaccine, the incidence of paralytic poliomyelitis fell precipitously. However, even though the killed-virus vaccine stimulated an immune response that prevented the major illness and the paralytic disease in the vaccinee, it was reported not to prevent intestinal tract infection with, and shedding of, virulent virus into the feces. This immune carrier state could then serve as a source of infection to newborn infants or other nonimmune individuals.

This and other considerations stimulated efforts by Cox, Koprowski, Sabin, and others to spend several years and millions of dollars in efforts to weaken the three serotypes of *P. hominis* to the point where they would infect and multiply in the tissues of monkeys but would not cause significant CNS pathology when administered orally. After extensive study, the Division of Biologic Standards of the U.S. Public Health Service approved Sabin's three strains of *P. hominis* as safe and effective for use as live-virus vaccines in human immunization (see Sabin 1961). Other strains were subsequently approved.

The live-virus vaccine can be produced as monovalent, divalent, or trivalent suspensions of the three serotypes of *P. hominis.* Except for specialized circumstances, the trivalent vaccine is preferred. Because of viral interference, however, wherein infection of tissues by one serotype may prevent infection by other serotypes, even the trivalent vaccine is given in at least two and preferably three initial doses at intervals of 2 months. These doses are followed by a booster dose 8 to 12 months later. One advantage of the trivalent vaccine is that records as to which serotype of virus was previously administered do not have to be kept, as is the case with each dose of monovalent, live vaccine. As a result of the first dose of live trivalent vaccine one, two, or all three serotype viruses might invade simultaneously and stimulate immunity. If only one invades in the first dose, one or both of the other two might invade as a result of the second dose. If only two serotypes invade in the first two doses, the third dose will provide an opportunity for the remaining serotype to invade since the tissues are then immune to the first two serotypes that invaded. If all three serotypes invade simultaneously in the first dose and produce solid immunity, there is no need for the second and third doses, but there is no simple means of determining this situation.

Live-virus poliovaccine has not only proved effective in preventing paralytic poliomyelitis, but has been claimed to provide immunity to the intestinal tract tissues. This local immunity prevents asymptomatic infection with virulent poliovirus and the carrier state reported to occur after immunization with the killed-virus vaccine. And since the live-virus vaccine multiplies in the tissues of the vaccinee, whereas all the virus antigen the tissues will receive must be incorporated in the killed-virus vaccine, the virus dosage of the live-virus vaccine is one-hundredth to one-thousandth that of the killed-virus vaccine. Since primary MKT cultures are required for each batch of vaccine of either type, the strain on the monkey population of the world is serious. On this basis the live-virus vaccine requiring less virus is the choice.

Jonas and Darrell Salk (1977) reviewed the literature dealing with the use of vaccines in the control of poliomyelitis and influenza. Since no live-virus vaccine has been approved for the control of influenza, their discussion of the relative efficacy of killed versus live-virus vaccines was restricted to those approved for use in the control of poliomyelitis. The Salks contend that killed-poliovirus vaccines are safer than the live attenuated vaccine, since the latter causes occasional cases of paralysis and postvaccinal encephalitis. They cite evidence from Finland, where only killed-virus vaccines have been used, to prove that paralytic poliomyelitis can be eliminated by the use of such vaccines (see Figure 26-4). They also indicate that in Canada and European countries the killed-poliovirus

vaccine has been combined with diphtheria and tetanus toxoids and pertussis vaccine to give a quadrivalent (DPTP) vaccine for the immunization of infants. If a rapid immune response is desirable, they advocate the judicious use of an

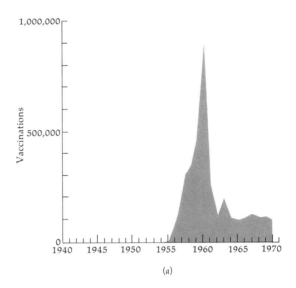

(a)

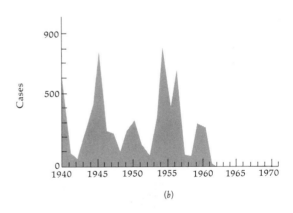

(b)

Figure 26–4. Poliomyelitis in Finland: (*a*) number of vaccinations per year (only killed poliovirus vaccine used); (*b*) number of cases per year. (From Noro, L., *in* Perkins, F. T., 1973.)

adjuvant in the monovalent killed-poliovirus vaccine. Finally, to overcome the drain on the world's monkey population, they advocate the use of other tissue culture cell lines for the propagation of poliovirus.

The live-virus poliovaccine has been advocated as a prophylactic agent to stop an existing epidemic of poliomyelitis. If the serotype of the epidemic strain of P. hominis is known, homologous monovalent vaccine may be administered orally to all members of the area population in a very short time. Because of the speed of the immune response to oral live-virus vaccine, new infections with the epidemic strain may be expected to stop within 2 weeks following administration of the vaccine. If heterologous live-virus vaccine serotypes are administered and invade, it is conceivable that the interference phenomenon might stop invasion by the epidemic strain immediately. Of course invasion by homologous serotype vaccine virus would not result in interference to invasion by the epidemic virus. Therefore trivalent vaccine would not be advocated for this interference type of control of the epidemic.

Again because of the interference phenomenon, immunization with live-virus vaccine is recommended during the winter months when infections with other enteroviruses are less prevalent than in the hot summer months. Since oral administration of live-virus vaccine results in the shedding of one or more of the vaccine serotypes into the intestinal tract, spread of the vaccine strains to susceptible, close (household) contacts can be expected. Although this might limit the need for further immunization of these contacts, there is no practical way for determining whether or not this herd immunization of contacts has occurred.

One of the problems that must be kept in mind in the production of tissue culture vaccines, and especially live-virus vaccines, is that animals frequently have latent infections with viruses that may be pathogenic for humans. Even the Salk killed-virus vaccine encountered this problem when batches of the vaccine were found to harbor live SV-40 virus. Although this simian virus has been proved to be oncogenic in experimental animals, there is no evidence of cancer in humans resulting from use of these batches of *Poliovirus* vaccine. After the discovery of the SV-40 virus contamination, procedures for eliminating it from subsequent batches of vaccine have been established as standard requirements.

A more serious latent virus problem (*Herpesvirus simiae*) was encountered in green monkeys in West Germany in 1967. Seven laboratory workers who removed the kidneys from the animals for vaccine production died as a result of infections with this highly virulent virus. There have been a total of 24 human infections with *H. simiae* reported worldwide with a mortality rate of 75 percent. There have been no reports of human infections with this virus resulting from immunization with poliovaccines, however. After the West German incident, existing green monkey kidney tissue vaccine was taken off the market. Methods were then devised for preventing this and other dangerous latent viruses from being transmitted by tissue culture vaccines.

CONTROL AND PREVENTION

Although, as indicated above, sanitary excreta disposal has had a marked influence on the epidemiology of poliomyelitis, it failed to prevent and even seemed to favor epidemics of this disease. House flies were shown to be capable of harboring and transporting large amounts of *P. hominis* in or on their bodies. Elimination of these insects in a community by DDT, however, did not influence the expected incidence of poliomyelitis during the epidemic years. In fact no control measure tried prior to 1955 influenced the incidence of this disease.

This situation changed spectacularly with the introduction of the Salk vaccine. Thus widespread active prophylactic immunization—first with the Salk killed-virus vaccine and since 1962–1963 with either the Salk or the Sabin live-virus vaccine—has practically eliminated poliomyelitis in the industrialized nations.

Texas, for example, for the first time since medical records were kept, reported no cases of paralytic poliomyelitis during 1973. One case, however, possibly acquired in Mexico, was reported in El Paso in 1975 (see *MMWR*, 30 August 1976). Ongoing immunization programs aimed at infants and young children, if adequate, should completely eliminate this crippling disease.

Not all cases of paralytic poliomyelitis, however, need result in permanent crippling. Following recovery from the symptoms of the major illness, the paralyzed patient should be placed on a physical therapy program designed to nourish and gradually strengthen the flaccid muscles. These programs are frequently carried out with the patient suspended in warm water such as the facilities at the Warm Springs Foundations in Georgia and in central Texas. The paralyzed muscles are first subjected to gentle massage while the patient is immersed in warm water. This regimen is designed to stimulate the flow of blood to nourish the muscles. Gradually the muscles are subjected to gentle exercise, such as the manual movement of the paralyzed limb by the therapist. Too much exercise too early can result in damage leading to permanent crippling. As the muscles become stronger, the exercises may be increased and the patient is instructed to attempt to control the movements of the paralyzed limb. If the motoneurons that controlled the muscles prior to infection have not been completely destroyed, new nerve paths might result from this conscious effort. If so, the patient might regain partial or complete use of the paralyzed muscles. This treatment program frequently is both prolonged and expensive. The March of Dimes program, initiated in honor of President Roosevelt's birthday, was designed to aid in these treatments.

In cases of respiratory muscle paralysis, the patient will require the aid of a mechanical respirator (iron lung). A classic example of this requirement was a young man named Fred Snite. After years in his respirator, with around-the-clock nursing attendants, he regained sufficient voluntary control of his respiratory muscles to enable him to leave the respirator, at least during waking hours. Snite even became a husband and father.

REFERENCES

Bodian, D. 1955. Emerging concept of poliomyelitis infection. *Science* 122:105–108.

———. 1956 . *Poliovirus* in chimpanzee tissues after virus feeding. *Amer. J. Hyg.* 64:181–197.

Enders, J. F., T. H. Weller, and F. C. Robbins. 1949. Cultivation of the Lansing strain of poliomyelitis virus in cultures of various human embryonic tissues. *Science* 109:85–87.

Landsteiner, K., and E. Popper. 1909. Übertragung der Poliomyelitis acuta auf Affen. *Z. Immunitätsforsch.* 2:377–390.

Phillips, C. A. 1974. Enteroviruses. Chapter 78 in *Manual of Clinical Microbiology*.

Sabin, A. B. 1961. Eradication of poliomyelitis. *Ann. Intern. Med.* 55:353–357.

Salk, J. E. 1955. Considerations in the preparation and use of poliomyelitis virus vaccine. *J. Amer. Med. Ass.* 158:1239–1248.

Salk, J. E., and D. Salk. 1977. Control of influenza and poliomyelitis with killed virus vaccines. *Science* 195:834–847.

27

Brucellosis

ETIOLOGY

Brucellosis is the generic designation for diseases of animals and humans caused by small, nonmotile, asporogenous, gram-negative bacilli belonging to the genus *Brucella* (see Figure 27-1). The original clinical entity was described in the 1860s by British medical officers stationed on the island of Malta. It was then called Malta fever or Mediterranean fever. The disease became so extensive in British military personnel stationed on Malta that David Bruce was sent there to attempt to combat it. In 1887 he reported the isolation of the causative organism from the spleen of a dead patient. He named the organism *Micrococcus melitensis*. T. Zammit in 1905 traced the source of the infection to milk from goats. In 1897 B. Bang, in Denmark, isolated a small gram-negative bacillus from the uterine discharges of aborting cows. He named this organism *Bacillus abortus*. J. Traum in 1914 described a similar organism in the discharges from aborting sows and named it *Bacillus suis*.

Alice Evans between 1916 and 1918 published studies, at the National Institutes of Health, on the taxonomic characteristics of *M. melitensis* and *B. abortus* that indicated them to be closely related organisms. The former were observed to be rods that, frequently, were as broad as they were long. This accounted for the mistaken conclusion by Bruce that they were micrococci. Additional studies indicated that *Bacillus suis* was even more closely related to *Bacillus abortus* than was *Bacillus melitensis*. These studies led K. F. Meyer in 1920 to propose the genus designation *Brucella* for these three primary isolates. Subsequently numerous biotypes of the original three species have been described. Three additional species have been added to the genus *Brucella*: *B. ovis*, isolated from sheep; *B. neotomae*, isolated from wood rats; and *B. canis*, isolated from dogs, with beagles being particularly susceptible. Thus it is obvious that all the brucellae are animal parasites. This accounts for the miscellaneous contact (see Chapter 19) aspect of brucellosis epidemiology—that

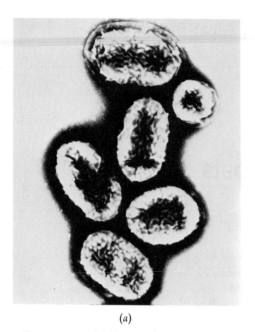

(a)

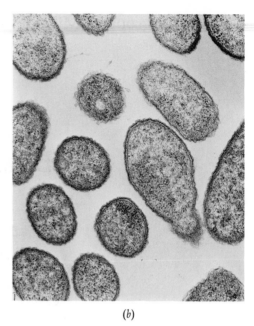

(b)

Figure 27–1.   (a) Negatively-stained cells of Brucella abortus showing short, bacillary morphology. (b) Thin section of B. abortus cells showing gram-negative walls. The shapes may be due as much to the angle of sectioning as to the overall morphology. Both 30,600×. (Courtesy of J. J. Cardamone, Jr.)

is, the high incidence in veterinarians, abattoir workers, and hog farmers. Zammit and others, however, established the milk of infected goats as the primary vehicle responsible for Malta fever. Moreover, the milk and milk products from infected cattle, and inadequately cooked pork and pork sausage from infected hogs, have accounted for many cases of human brucellosis. This is our justification for placing brucellosis in subgroup B of the intestinal group—diseases that involve secretions (milk) or tissue (meat) of infected animals as the primary vehicles, the mouth as the portal of entry, and no secondary vehicles of epidemiological significance.

An early taxonomic study on the original three species of the genus Brucella (which are generally accepted) was reported by Pickett et al. (1953). Biotypes of these species and others (see Table 27-1) are difficult to identify with certainty, however. There still is controversy, for example, as to whether or not the designated species (B. neotomae, B. ovis, and B. canis) should

be accepted as such or be designated different biotypes of the original three species. The latter is advocated particularly for the smooth-colony type of B. neotomae. As indicated in Table 27-1, a significant biotype differential is the requirement of added CO_2 for the isolation of B. abortus. On this basis B. ovis is more closely related to B. abortus than to the other Brucella species. The determination of the requirement for added CO_2 must be made at or shortly after first isolation, because of the rapid tendency of these organisms to adapt to growth in normal atmospheric CO_2 concentrations. Also all biotypes of B. abortus are susceptible to lysis when exposed to bacteriophage Tb. No other Brucella species or biotypes are susceptible to this phage.

Hydrogen sulfide production and dye susceptibility tests are other commonly used taxonomic procedures for Brucella species differentiation. Unfortunately, with the exception of phage lysis, numerous instances of biotype variability have been encountered in the taxonomy of these organisms. Carbohydrate fermentations and other metabolic tests, although advocated, are rarely used in their identification.

The original three *Brucella* species tend to produce smooth (S) colonies on first isolation from hosts, as does *B. neotomae*. The cells share two S-colony surface antigens (A and M) in variable proportions. Therefore all S-colony *Brucella* tend to agglutinate in unabsorbed antisera to any one of the three original species cells. Since the A antigen tends to predominate in *B. abortus* and *B. suis* cells, whereas the M antigen predominates in *B. melitensis* cells, an antiserum specific for *B. abortus* (or *B. suis*) can be carefully absorbed with *B. melitensis* cells to obtain a monospecific anti-A antiserum. Likewise, an antiserum specific for *B. melitensis* can be similarly absorbed with *B. abortus* (or *B. suis*) cells to yield a monospecific anti-M antiserum. Typical S-colony *B. abortus* or *B. suis* cells will agglutinate only in the monospecific anti-A antiserum, whereas typical S-colony *B. melitensis* cells will agglutinate only in monospecific anti-M antiserum. Unfortunately biotypes of all three of the original species occasionally fail to conform to these serotyping results. Smooth-colony *B. neotomae* cells agglutinate only in monospecific anti-A antiserum, and therefore, on this basis, *B. neotomae* is more closely related to *B. abortus* and *B. suis* than to *B. melitensis*. Freeman et al. (1970) reported on the use of soluble antigens to differentiate the brucellae mentioned above, but

Table 27-1. Some differential biotype and serotype characteristics of *Brucella* species.

Taxonomic Characteristics	*B. melitensis*	*B. abortus*	*B. suis*	*B. neotomae*	*B. ovis*†	*B. canis*†
No. of biotypes	4	9	4	1	1	1
CO_2 required (about 10%)	−	(+)	−	−	+	−
H_2S produced	−	(+)	(+)	+	−	−
Growth on dye media						
Basic fuchsin (10^{-5})	+	(+)	(−)	−	+	−
Thionin (2.5×10^{-4})	−	(−)	+	−	+	+
Thionin (5×10^{-4})	+	(−)	+	−	+	+
Thionin (1×10^{-5})	+	(−)	+	+	+	+
Agglutination by:						
Anti-A*	(−)	(+)	+	+	−	−
Anti-M*	(+)	(−)	(−)	−	−	−
Anti-R**	−	−	−	−	+	+
Lysis by phage Tb at RTD	−	+	−	−	−	−

*Monospecific, S-colony antiserum.

†Occur as R colonies only.

**Unabsorbed antiserum to R-colony cells.

( ) = Variable in different biotypes. Predominant reaction is indicated.

RTD = Routine test dilution of phage Tb.

they were unable to differentiate *B. suis* and *B. neotomae* by this means.

    Brucella ovis and *B. canis* produce only R-type colonies, even on first isolation, and do not possess A or M antigens. They do not agglutinate in absorbed or unabsorbed S-type colony antisera. They agglutinate in R-type colony antisera, whether the antisera are produced by immunizing animals with homologous or heterologous R-type colony cells. These observations emphasize the need for careful selection of colony-type antigens for the production of antisera to be used for taxonomic identification of *Brucella* isolates and for the production of serodiagnostic test antigens. Determination of colony type (S or R) is best made using microscopic examination and the oblique illumination described by Henry (1933).

    Cultivation of *Brucella* species generally is not difficult. Since *B. abortus* requires added (10 percent) CO_2 for primary isolation and since other brucellae will grow in the presence of added CO_2, all *Brucella* isolation cultures should be placed in such an environment. For broth cultures, peptones consisting of tryptic digests of casein (Trypticase) or soybean protein (Trypticase-soy) have been advocated. Some peptones have been found to be toxic for small inoculae of *Brucella* species. This toxicity appears to be due to colloidal sulfur liberated by the oxidation of cystine in the peptones (Schuhardt et al. 1949*a*, 1949*b*, 1950, 1952) and can be reversed by activated charcoal, blood serum, or reducing agents in the medium. Brucellae, however, are aerobes and will not grow in a completely anaerobic environment. Solid plating media are prepared by adding 1.5 percent agar to the broth media before sterilization at 121°C for 15 minutes. Some *Brucella* strains may require 7 to 10 percent sterile serum added to the agar media. Brucellae, however, can be grown in chemically defined media (McCullough and Dick 1943; Rode et al. 1950).

CLINICAL SYMPTOMS

Brucellosis is primarily a disease of animals. Contagious abortion (Bang's disease) of cattle illustrates the economic impact of brucellosis on the dairy industry. Not only do the infected animals abort their calves but they frequently are made sterile by the disease. Although Smith et al. (1965) published evidence incriminating erythrotol in the uterine tissues as the factor responsible for the intrauterine localization of the *B. abortus* infection and pathology, other studies failed to confirm this hypothesis. Regardless of the cause of this localization, the damage to the sites of attachment between the blood systems of the cow and calf *in utero* is responsible for both the loss of the calf and the frequent sterilization of the cow. This highly contagious epizootic may decimate an entire herd with resulting loss in both milk production and reproductive capacity. The situation in certain areas of the United States became so serious during the first half of the twentieth century that the federal government initiated "test and slaughter" programs. Dairy cattle were tested by a simple serodiagnostic agglutination test (see the section on laboratory diagnosis) and, if found positive, were slaughtered and sold for the manufacture of dog food or other cooked meat products, not for human consumption. By this means bovine brucellosis has been brought under control in many parts of the United States.

    More recently animal brucellosis in the United States has been a problem of hog farmers and slaughterhouse workers. In Mexico and other areas of the world where goat's milk and milk products (cheese) are common food items for human consumption, infected goats constitute the major problem. It is interesting to note that it is the animals which are bred for milk production, not the range animals, that appear to be selectively attacked by *Brucella* species. Although the hog milk is not a human food, the size of hog litters necessitates that the sow be a prodigious milk producer. Male animals can be infected—*B. ovis* was first isolated from a case of ram epididimitis—but animal brucellosis is relatively rare in males.

    Brucella infection in human beings can result in a variety of clinical syndromes and has been assigned a variety of human disease designations: Mediterranean fever, gastric remittent fever, Malta fever, Neapolitan fever, undulant fever, Rio Grande fever, and Bang's disease. The latter designation, however, is more commonly restricted to the contagious abortion of cattle.

The incubation period, in reported accidental laboratory infections, has varied from 5 to 35 days. In natural infections the incubation period may be weeks to months longer. The onset of clinical disease frequently is difficult to pinpoint. Early symptoms may be malaise, weakness, headache, other aches and joint pains, chills, sweating, and recurrent depression. Some chronic cases lasting for months to a year or more may develop little or no fever. More acute cases may develop remittent fever, or undulating fever, or persistent high, spiking fever. These latter, acute disease symptoms are the ones more likely to be confused with typhoid or other *Salmonella* enteric fevers. The pathogenic mechanism appears to be endotoxic with the possibility that allergy contributes to the overall pathology in some cases. Mortality in human brucellosis has been reduced to the vanishing point by early diagnosis and antibiotic therapy.

The brucellosis patient frequently develops marked hypersensitivity to *Brucella* antigens. Diagnostic skin tests have been advocated, but the frequent severity of skin-test reactions has discouraged their usage. To what extent this hypersensitivity contributes to the clinical syndromes of different cases of brucellosis is not clear. Following bacteremic involvement, the *Brucella* may invade and produce localized pathology in practically any tissues or organs of the body. These localized pathologies can result in symptoms of other diseases, wherein the pathology involves the same tissues or organs. These clinical facts make laboratory aid in the diagnosis of brucellosis practically essential.

LABORATORY DIAGNOSIS

The usual early laboratory diagnostic test for brucellosis is a blood culture. A minimum of 5 milliliters of blood should be used for such cultures. While collecting blood for this early culture an additional 3 to 5 milliliters should be collected for baseline serodiagnostic agglutina-

tion tests (see diagnosis of typhoid, Chapter 24). The blood for serodiagnosis should be placed in a test tube and allowed to clot. After loosening the clot from the wall, the tube is refrigerated at 4–6°C overnight. This allows the clot to contract and squeeze out the serum, which should be transferred to a second tube. If there are residual cells in the serum, it should be clarified by centrifugation. The clear serum, after transfer to a third tube, can be stored at 4–6°C until tested along with a comparable serum specimen collected 7 to 10 or more days later. The two serum specimens will make it possible to determine whether or not a rising antibody titer has occurred during the interim between the blood collections. If the first blood culture is still negative at the time of collecting blood for the rising-titer serodiagnosis, a second blood culture should be inoculated at that time.

The blood/broth ratio in the blood culture should be 1:10 to 1:20 (5 milliliters of blood in 50 to 100 milliliters of broth). If the culture bottle contains 10 percent added CO_2, the blood may be inoculated from the collection syringe through the rubber stopper and, without further treatment, placed in the 37°C incubator. If a loosely covered flask of sterile broth without added CO_2 is used, the blood-inoculated flask should be placed in a desiccator. After partial evacuation of the air, 10 percent CO_2 is added to the desiccator. Any residual vacuum is relieved by allowing air to enter before closing the desiccator airtight and placing it in the 37°C incubator.

The blood culture should be examined daily for evidence of turbidity, indicating bacterial growth. On the third day and at 2–3-day intervals thereafter, a bacteriological loop of the culture should be streaked to the surface of an agar plating medium and the plate incubated in the CO_2 container. The blood culture should not be considered negative before 21 days of incubation and streaking. Since brucellae tend to invade the bloodstream intermittently, repeated blood cultures may be required for isolation.

Castaneda (1947; 1961) devised a blood culture bottle that avoided the need for streaking the surface of agar plates. The bottle had at least one flat side. A sufficient amount of melted agar medium was added to the bottle, which was then plugged with cotton and sterilized at 121°C for 20 minutes. The bottle was placed in a slanted position, allowing the agar to solidify over the entire flat surface. Using aseptic procedures, the bottle was then half-filled with approximately 50 milliliters of sterile broth. The cotton plug was replaced with a rubber stopper through which a hypodermic needle could be inserted. Again using aseptic precautions, the air from the bottle was partially evacuated and 10 percent CO_2 added. Such bottles were incubated at 37°C to be sure they were sterile before use. Blood could then be inoculated to the broth directly from the syringe and the culture incubated and visually examined as previously described. Rather than having to open the bottle or flask at 2–3-day intervals to insert a bacteriological loop for streaking agar plates, the upright bottle in the incubator could be tilted to seed the agar surface in the bottle and then returned to the upright position. If viable *Brucella* cells were present in the broth, frequently within polymorphonuclear leucocytes, they would be deposited on the agar above the broth and would then grow into colonies, which could be fished to agar slants for further study.

If a small, nonmotile, gram-negative bacillus is isolated from blood or other specimens, it can be inoculated to media designed to yield the biotype characteristics indicated in Table 27-1. Also, a suspension of the cells can be tested for agglutination when incubated at 37–40°C for 18 to 24 hours in monovalent anti-A and anti-M antisera. If the cells agglutinate only in anti-M and do not require added CO_2 for growth, they probably are *B. melitensis.* If they agglutinate only in anti-A, however, they could be either *B. abortus* or *B. suis* (you do not expect to isolate *B. neotomae* from humans). Under these circumstances, phage typing of the isolate would constitute the most rapid means of identifying the species. Since all nine biotypes of *B. abortus* are lysed by phage Tb, whereas no other *Brucella* are attacked by this phage, lysis of the isolate by the routine test dose (RTD) of the phage would identify it as *B. abortus.* Failure to obtain lysis by

phage Tb probably would indicate that the isolate which did not agglutinate in monospecific anti-M was *B. suis.* These observations— coupled with the biotype characteristics of CO_2 requirement, H_2S production, and dye susceptibility—should ensure the identification of most *Brucella* isolates. Douglas and Elberg (1976) reported the isolation of a bacteriophage specific for the biotypes of *B. melitensis.* This phage may be expected to supplement phage Tb in the taxonomic differentiation of the brucellae.

Serodiagnosis, involving a rising antibody (agglutinin) titer to *B. abortus,* is a common means of laboratory aid in the diagnosis of human brucellosis, regardless of the species of *Brucella* involved. The single species diagnostic antigen, as indicated above, can be used because all three of the *Brucella* species that commonly cause brucellosis in humans share the same surface antigens A and M. Therefore brucellosis caused by any one of the three species will result in serum antibodies that will react with cells of all three species. The test usually consists of six to eight serial double dilutions (from 1:10), in 0.5-milliliter quantities, of both early and late sera. Then 0.5 milliliter of *B. abortus* antigen is added to each of the serum dilutions and to a saline control. After 18 to 24 hours' incubation at 37–40°C, the highest dilution of each serum that shows visible evidence of agglutination of the *B. abortus* cells constitutes the agglutinin titer of that serum specimen. A threefold to fourfold increase in titer between the first and second serum is highly diagnostic. Of course, rising-titer serodiagnosis is always late diagnosis. However, since blood culture or culture of joint fluids or other laboratory specimens may prove to be negative and because brucellosis frequently is a long-lasting disease, serodiagnosis may be the only positive laboratory aid to diagnosis.

A plate agglutination test usually constitutes the serodiagnostic test in bovine brucellosis (Bang's disease of cattle). A clear glass plate (6 × 12 inches) is etched into 1-inch squares, 11 rows of five squares each. The test antigen is a concentrated and specially treated suspension of *B. abortus,* first reported by Huddleson. To perform the test 0.08 milliliter of serum is pipetted to the bottom square of the first row, followed by 0.04, 0.02, 0.01, and 0.004 milliliter to squares 2, 3, 4, and 5 respectively of row 1. The same amounts of other sera may be pipetted to the squares in other rows. The antigen is dispensed from a calibrated dropper with a rubber bulb attached. The serum in each square receives one drop of the antigen. Positive and negative control sera should be included on each test plate. Using separate toothpicks and beginning with the mixture containing the least amount of serum (0.004 milliliter), the GA mixtures in each row are spread over approximately three-fourths of the area within the squares. The plate is then tilted back and forth for 2 minutes and examined for aggregation of the cells in each mixture. Aggregation in the 0.02-milliliter (1:100 serum dilution equivalent) serum mixture is considered diagnostic for Bang's disease.

IMMUNITY

There are no immunoprophylactic or immunotherapeutic measures applicable to human brucellosis. The Bureau of Animal Industry (BAI), however, has approved the use of a live, weakly virulent strain of *B. abortus* (BAI strain 19) for immunization of calves. The use of this vaccine, coupled with the test and slaughter program, has helped to eradicate Bang's disease from most dairy herds in the United States.

CONTROL AND PREVENTION

The elimination of Bang's disease from most dairy cattle—along with the almost universal pasteurization of milk—has practically eliminated human brucellosis resulting from the consumption of milk or milk products in the United States. Cases of brucellosis transmitted by milk or milk products (butter, cheese, ice cream) are still reported in areas where raw milk is widely used, particularly goat's milk.

Hogs continue to be the major source of human brucellosis in the United States. Most of the recent human cases are contracted as a result of contact with slaughtered hogs in abattoirs.

Between January and December 1970, for example, 53 cases of brucellosis were reported in workers in a large abattoir in Dubuque, Iowa. This was approximately 25 percent of all human cases of brucellosis reported in the United States that year (see *MMWR*, 26 December 1970). After an all-time low of 246 cases of human brucellosis reported in the United States in 1974, an increase to 328 cases was reported in 1975. This was the largest number since 1964. Sixty percent of the cases occurred in persons working in the meat processing industry (see *MMWR*, 24 September 1976).

Practical methods of controlling contact transmission of the disease are difficult to visualize. Adequate cooking of pork, pork sausage, ham, and bacon will prevent brucellosis resulting from consumption of these primary vehicles. There remains the remote possibility of the food preparer handling pork from an infected hog and then transferring the infection from the meat to the fingers and on to the mouth or eyes. Control of such infections could be accomplished by wearing rubber gloves while handling the meat prior to cooking, but I doubt whether butchers or cooks will resort to this precaution.

REFERENCES

Castaneda, M. R. 1947. A practical method for routine blood cultures in brucellosis. *Proc. Soc. Exper. Biol. Med.* 64:114–115.

———. 1961. Laboratory diagnosis of brucellosis in man. *Bull. Wld. Hlth. Org.* 24:73–84.

Douglas, J. T., and S. S. Elberg. 1976. Isolation of *Brucella melitensis* phage of broad biotype and species specificity. *Infect. Immunity* 14:306–308.

Freeman, B. A., J. R. McGhee, and R. E. Baughn. 1970. Some physical, chemical, and taxonomic features of the soluble antigens of Brucellae. *J. Infect. Dis.* 121:522–527.

Henry, B. S. 1933. Dissociation in the genus *Brucella*. *J. Infect. Dis.* 52:574–402.

McCullough, N. B., and L. A. Dick. 1943. Growth of *Brucella* in a simple, chemically defined medium. *Proc. Soc. Exper. Biol. Med.* 52:310–311.

Pickett, M. J., E. L. Nelson, and J. B. Liberman. 1953. Speciation within the genus *Brucella. J. Bacteriol.* 66:210–219.

Rode, L. J., G. Oglesby, and V. T. Schuhardt. 1950. The cultivation of brucellae on chemically defined media. *J. Bacteriol.* 60:661–668.

Schuhardt, V. T., L. J. Rode, J. W. Foster, and G. Oglesby. 1949a. An antibrucella factor in peptones. *J. Bacteriol.* 57:1–8.

Schuhardt, V. T., L. J. Rode, and G. Oglesby. 1949b. The toxicity of certain amino acids for brucellae. *J. Bacteriol.* 58:665–674.

Schuhardt, V. T., L. J. Rode, G. Oglesby, and C. E. Lankford. 1950. The development of peptone toxicity for brucellae with aging and the correlation of this toxicity with the probable oxidation of cystine. *J. Bacteriol.* 60:665–660.

———. 1952. Toxicity of elemental sulfur for brucellae. *J. Bacteriol.* 63:123–128.

Smith, H., A. E. Williams, J. H. Pearce, J. Keppie, P. W. Harris-Smith, R. B. Fitz-George, and K. Witt. 1965. Foetal erythrotol: a cause of localization of *Brucella abortus. Nature.* (London) 193:47–49.

28

Bacterial Food Poisoning

Botulism 301
Staphylococcal Gastroenteritis 304
Other Bacterial Food Poisonings 305

There is a group of human diseases that are caused by the ingestion of preformed toxins (enterotoxins) produced by bacteria growing in foods *prior* to their consumption. The bacterial food poisonings do not involve invasion or multiplication of the toxigenic bacteria in the intestinal tract or tissues, as is the case in cholera, dysentery, *E. coli*, or *Salmonella* gastroenteritis. The enterotoxin, produced in the food, is absorbed into or through the intact gastrointestinal membranes and produces pathological manifestations characteristic of the bacterial species responsible for its production. These toxemias are not infectious diseases, although the bacterial species responsible for the enterotoxin production may occasionally, or in some instances frequently, cause other types of human or animal infection.

BOTULISM

Etiology

The most serious and frequently fatal bacterial food poisoning is botulism, caused by the gram-positive, anaerobic, spore-forming bacilli—*Clostridium botulinum* (see Figure 28-1). There are two biotypes of *C. botulinum*, based on whether or not the isolates are proteolytic (digest casein and other proteins) or nonproteolytic. These biotypes may differ in carbohydrate fermentations and other biochemical characteristics. The biotype characteristics have little, if any, practical significance.

There are seven serotypes (A to G) of *C. botulinum*, based upon the antigenicity of the enterotoxin produced. These differences are extremely significant, because each toxin requires a specific antitoxin for its neutralization. Serotypes A and B have been the most common cause of human botulism. Type E, however, and to a lesser extent type F, have been incriminated in human cases, particularly those resulting from the ingestion of raw, inadequately cooked, or smoked fish. These types have been isolated from the intestinal tracts of both freshwater and saltwater fish. Type E of *C. botulinum* also has been isolated from the meat of blue crabs caught in Chesapeake Bay (see Koutter et al. 1974). Cockey and Tatra (1974) demonstrated the

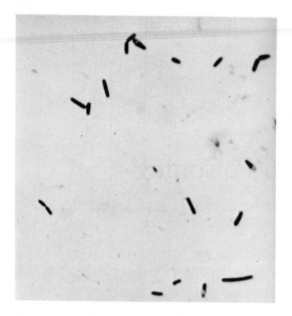

Figure 28–1. Gram stain of *Clostridium botulinum* type A grown for 24 hours on chopped-meat medium. Several subterminal oval spores are in the field. About 3740×. (Courtesy of H. D. Bredthauer.)

presence of *C. botulinum* spores in 21 of 24 bottom mud samples collected from the crabbing areas of Chesapeake Bay. Type C bacilli have been isolated from fly larvae, from forage causing botulism in cattle, and from freshwater pond mud. The latter has caused extensive mortality (limberneck) in ducks feeding in such ponds. Toxins from all the serotypes appear to be capable of causing limberneck in chickens.

Clostridium botulinum enterotoxins are neurotoxins with typical exotoxin characteristics — for example, they are neutralized in multiple proportions by antitoxin. Type A toxin is the most potent poison known, exceeding in this respect the toxins of diphtheria and tetanus. The toxins can be converted to toxoid by treatment with formaldehyde. Such toxoids are used primarily for animal immunization to produce homologous antitoxins.

Type C of *C. botulinum* has been reported to require lysogenization with bacteriophage for toxin production (Eklund et al. 1971). When the bacilli are cured of their lysogenic status they cease to produce toxin. Eklund et al. (1974) reported that the nontoxigenic (nonlysogenized) strains of *C. botulinum* type C can be converted back to toxigenicity by lysogenization with the original type C tox$^+$ phage. Even more remarkable, the nontoxigenic *C. botulinum* type C cells can be transduced to an antigenically distinct toxigenic *Clostridium novyi* type A by lysogenization with another bacteriophage. Thus phage lysogenization can determine not only the toxigenicity but even the taxonomic species identity of this *Clostridium*.

Clostridium botulinum enterotoxin is heat-labile: Its toxicity can be destroyed by heating to 100°C. Boiling contaminated liquid foods for 3 minutes will prevent botulism. It should be emphasized, however, that the detoxifying temperature must penetrate throughout the food. Such foods as cream corn, green beans, and solid foods (ham, sausage, or other meats) are very poor conductors of heat. More prolonged heating is required to raise the temperature throughout these foods to that required for detoxification.

Clostridium botulinum spores are highly resistant to heat and drying. They are found in varying concentrations in soil from farms, ranches, and woodland sites. Some types grow and produce toxin in the mud of bays or in shallow ponds containing decaying vegetation. Others have been isolated from decaying fodder consumed by cattle and horses. Still others are found in the intestinal tracts of fish, crabs, and other animals and in the decaying dead bodies of animals. This widespread distribution of *C. botulinum* spores results in the frequent likelihood of contamination of vegetables, meat, and other foods. The organisms are strict anaerobes and because they must grow and produce toxin in the contaminated foods prior to ingestion, canned, smoked, or otherwise preserved foods constitute the greatest hazard.

The canning industry has based its food processing temperatures and times upon those required to kill *C. botulinum* spores that are experimentally added to such foods. This practice has resulted in very few cases of botulism being traced to commercially canned foods. During 1974, for example, 30 cases of botulism in the United States were reported to the Center for Disease Control (CDC) in Atlanta. Only two of these cases were traced to commercially canned food—a single can of beef stew. Twenty-three cases were traced to home-canned foods including chow-chow, corn, tomatoes, fish, potatoes and peas, mixed vegetables, beets, figs, mushrooms, seal meat in seal oil, and a beef-mushroom mixture. The food sources in three cases in Alaska and one in Ohio were not reported. Thus it is obvious that the major source of human botulism is home-canned foods. Similar canned food sources were noted in the 19 cases of botulism reported in the United States in 1975 (see *MMWR*, 6 March 1976). In 1974, however, 11 cases (3 fatal) of type A botulism were reported in Argentina due to consumption of a commercial cheese spread (*MMWR*, 18 June 1976); and in 1975 a fatal case of botulism in Mexico City was traced to commercially canned tuna distributed only in Mexico.

As this book was being prepared for publication (April 1977), the largest outbreak of human botulism ever reported in the United States was occurring. As of 7 April, newspaper reports indicated 44 confirmed cases. All were traced to a single Mexican restaurant in Pontiac, Michigan, serving home-canned jalapeño peppers. CDC identified the toxin as type B and listed a final count of 46 cases (see *MMWR*, 22 April 1977).

Clinical Symptoms

The incubation period in botulism generally ranges from 20 to 36 hours after consumption of the contaminated food, but occasionally it may be prolonged several days depending upon the amount of toxin consumed. Symptoms include vomiting, diplopia (double or blurred vision), weakness, dysarthria or aphonia (speech aberrations or loss), ptosis (a paralytic drooping of the eyelid), bilateral oculomotor or facial nerve paralyses, pharyngeal or laryngeal paralyses, and respiratory failure. The paralyses are indicative of the neurotoxic pathology involving the autonomic nerves that control these organs.

Although the meninges may be congested at autopsy, there is no evidence that the toxin involves other tissues of the central nervous system. Usually there is no fever except during terminal stages when bronchial pneumonia occurs. The patient remains conscious and retains mental faculties until near the end. There is no tissue invasion by the *C. botulinum* cells responsible for the production of the toxin in the food. Death may occur within 24 hours or may be delayed for up to a week. In patients who survive, complete recovery—particularly recovery of eye movements—may be delayed for several months to a year. For a consideration of wound botulism, see Chapter 37.

Laboratory Diagnosis

Unfortunately, botulism can be so rapidly fatal that there may not be time for laboratory aid in the diagnosis. Once clear symptoms of botulism develop, moreover, the chances of therapeutic efficacy of antitoxin are limited. Consequently early recognition of the *onset* clinical symptoms and relating them to the consumption of a suspect food is usually all that the clinician has time to consider before treatment. When such clinical evidence is established, the patient should be treated with trivalent (A, B, and E) *C. botulinum* antitoxin prior to any efforts to identify the toxin type.

However, laboratory specimens should be submitted for confirmation of the diagnosis and to establish the serotype of the toxin involved. This is important because there may be other batches of the contaminated food to be identified and other patients to be treated—preferably with monospecific antitoxin. The specimens should be kept cold until all laboratory tests are completed. They should include: (1) any residual suspect food; (2) if there is none, the empty food container; (3) vomitus, feces, and blood from the patient. Blood should be collected before the administration of antitoxin. If the food specimen needs homogenization or centrifuging it should be done in the cold (4°C). The empty container should be rinsed with a small amount of sterile saline or glycerine-phosphate-buffer (GPB). Extracts (GPB) of the food or washings from the container, vomitus, and blood serum may be tested for the presence of botulinum toxin by injecting aliquots of each into three test mice individually protected with antitoxin A, B, or E and into an unprotected control mouse. If one antitoxin-protected mouse survives and the other test mice and the control mouse die, the evidence would indicate botulinum toxin of type homologous to the type of antitoxin used in the surviving test mouse. Blood usually does not contain sufficient toxin to kill mice, until the patient approaches fatal termination of the toxemia.

Clostridium botulinum may be isolated from the food, or from the vomitus or feces of the patient, by culturing the specimens in suitable media under anaerobic conditions. Contaminating, asporogenous bacteria may be eliminated from these specimens by heating at 80°C for 30 minutes; the clostridial spores will not be killed by this heat treatment. Failure to isolate *C. botulinum,* particularly from vomitus or fecal specimens, would not rule out botulism in the patient, however.

Food contaminated with *C. botulinum* may or may not demonstrate evidence of spoilage. If the spoilage involves proteolytic digestion, odor evidence of spoilage may be present. If fermentative spoilage occurs in canned foods, the can may be swollen or gas bubbles may be present at the time of opening. Such foods should not be tasted—even a taste may involve sufficient toxin to result in botulism. For additional details see Foster et al. (1974).

Control and Treatment

Adequate heat processing of home-canned foods would eliminate more cases of botulism than any other control measure. Adequate heating of home-canned foods prior to consumption also would help in the control. Acid tends to interfere with toxin production by *C. botulinum.* Consequently neutral or alkaline foods are more likely to cause botulism than comparably contaminated acid foods.

The only treatment of any value in botulism is antitoxin specific for the serotype of *C. botulinum* involved. Since there may be no time for toxin-serotype identification in the initial case, trivalent (A, B, and E) antitoxin should be administered immediately. Others who consumed the suspect food, but show no symptoms of illness, should receive a prophylactic injection of the trivalent antitoxin. As soon as the serotype of the toxin is established, monospecific antitoxin should be used for prophylaxis or therapy.

The Center for Disease Control in Atlanta has emergency telephone numbers to call for *C. botulinum* antitoxin:

(404)633-3311 Monday through Friday
except holidays
8:30 A.M. to 4:30 P.M.:
All other times: (404)633-2176 or (404)633-8673

Note: Serotype A and B antitoxins may be obtained from local commercial sources.

STAPHYLOCOCCAL GASTROENTERITIS

One of the most common types of food poisoning is caused by enterotoxigenic strains of *Staphylococcus aureus* (see Chapter 20). These gram-positive, cluster-forming cocci usually produce golden-yellow colonies although this characteristic may vary. *Staphylococcus aureus* is a common inhabitant of normal human skin and body cavities, particularly the nasal passages.

Coagulase-positive strains of *S. aureus* are the common cause of boils and other skin abscesses. Practically any abrasion of the skin will become infected with these organisms. As indicated in Chapter 20, antibiotic-resistant strains of *S. aureus* were incriminated in many outbreaks of hospital-acquired infections during the 1950s and 1960s.

Hollander (1965) reported that about 10 percent of coagulase-positive *S. aureus* isolates studied by him were enterotoxigenic. There were no other distinguishing characteristics between the enterotoxigenic and the nonenterotoxigenic strains studied. The enterotoxin is relatively heat-stable: Reheating the food in which the staphylococci have grown and produced the toxin will not destroy the toxicity.

Clinical Symptoms

After a brief incubation period of 2 to 4 hours there is onset of nausea followed by vomiting and diarrhea. Dr. O. B. Williams designated this "the two-bucket disease"—the patient sits on one bucket and drapes the head over the other. The abdominal griping and related symptoms may become quite distressing, but they usually subside within 24 to 36 hours after onset.

Monkeys are the only other animals that show symptoms (repeated vomiting) when the staphylococcus enterotoxin is administered by mouth. Kittens may develop similar symptoms when the enterotoxin is injected intraperitoneally.

Diagnosis

Staphylococcal gastroenteritis usually is diagnosed epidemiologically. This is particularly true when a group of people consume moist food such as custards, beef stew, and picnic or banquet food which, after cooking, has been set aside at room temperature for consumption some hours later. If, 2 to 4 hours following the meal, a number of the participants develop the nauseous symptoms of enterotoxemia, the chances are that the patients are suffering from staphylococcal food poisoning.

Finding large numbers of *S. aureus* in the food or in the onset vomitus may confirm the clinical diagnosis. If the food was reheated prior to serving, however, the staphylococci may be killed without destroying the enterotoxin. Consequently failure to isolate staphylococci might not rule out staphylococcal enterotoxemia.

Frequently an epidemiological investigation will reveal that the incriminated food was prepared by someone with a staphylococcal infected sore on the hand. Other outbreaks have been traced to nasal carriers of enterotoxigenic

S. aureus. A most embarrassing outbreak of staphylococcal gastroenteritis occurred a few years back following a noon meal at a national convention of the American Society for Microbiology. Another outbreak involving 277 of 343 passengers on board a commercial aircraft must have been most difficult to cope with—not enough buckets. The aircraft was en route from Tokyo to Copenhagen. At an interim stop in Anchorage, food for breakfasts (cheese omelets with ham slices) was taken aboard. The breakfasts were stored at room temperature in ovens until heated just prior to serving. Breakfast was served about 5 1/2 hours out of Anchorage. First symptoms were noted about 30 minutes later, with an average onset time of 2 1/2 hours. Although 143 passengers and 1 crew member required hospitalization in Copenhagen, all patients recovered with no serious sequelae. Epidemiological investigations incriminated ham as the food responsible for the outbreak, and a cook in Anchorage with an inflamed finger lesion was identified as the source of the staphylococcal contamination (see *MMWR*, 15 February 1975).

Control and Prevention

The only sure way to prevent staphylococcal food poisoning is to keep stored foods that might serve as growth media for the staphylococci refrigerated at 4–6°C from the time of preparation to just prior to consumption. Obviously persons with inflamed or other potential staphylococcal lesions on their hands should not be allowed to prepare foods that might require storage before consumption.

OTHER BACTERIAL FOOD POISONINGS

As indicated in prior chapters *V. cholerae, Shigella* spp., *Salmonella* serotypes, streptococci, *Escherichia coli,* and possibly other bacteria and fungi may be responsible for food-borne gastroenteritis. In most of these, however, the pathological syndrome is the result of true infection with the enterotoxin produced *in situ* as discussed in detail regarding cholera (Chapter 23). During the last quarter century, another bacterial food poisoning due to *Clostridium perfringens* has received increasing attention.

C. perfringens Enteritis

Although *C. perfringens* (formerly *C. welchii*) has long been known as a cause of wound infections of the gas gangrene type (see Chapter 37), it was first reported to be the cause of human food poisoning in Europe in 1943 and in the United States by McClung (1945). When Dische and Elek (1957) fed live *C. perfringens* that had been isolated from food poisoning outbreaks to 48 human volunteers, 42 experienced typical symptoms of abdominal cramps and diarrhea with practically no nausea or vomiting—an enteritis rather than a gastroenteritis. Both bacteria-free culture filtrates and heat-killed whole cultures of the isolate failed to produce such symptoms in volunteers.

Clostridium perfringens is a gram-positive, spore-forming bacillus that is widely distributed in the soil and in human and animal intestinal excreta. Smith and Holderman (1968) consider *C. perfringens* to be more widely spread over the earth than any other pathogenic bacterium.

Nygren (1962) correlated the production of alpha toxin (lecithinase) with the enterotoxigenicity of *C. perfringens*. Also, using media that suppressed spore formation by *C. perfringens* and using asporogenous mutants, Duncan et al. (1972) correlated enterotoxin production with sporulation capacity. Thus it became apparent that there are both enterotoxigenic and nonenterotoxigenic strains of *C. perfringens*. Nakamura and Schulze (1970) reviewed the literature on *C. perfringens* food poisoning and, among other conclusions, expressed the opinion that the mechanism of enterotoxicity was not established at that time.

Stark and Duncan (1971) extracted enterotoxigenic protein from sporulating *C. perfringens* cells and from their culture filtrates. These extracts induced fluid accumulation when inoc-

ulated into ligated ileal loops of the rabbit. Nillo (1974) obtained similar results in ligated intestinal loops of the chicken. These results appear to be analogous to results obtained with *V. cholerae* and *E. coli* enterotoxin in rabbits (see Chapter 23). Comparable mechanisms of action have not been reported, however, and certainly *C. perfringens* enteritis does not involve the serious prognosis of that in either cholera or *E. coli* infections.

Most of the enterotoxigenicity studies have been done on *C. perfringens* type A of the five biotypes (see Chapter 37). However, Skjelkvåle and Duncan (1975) reported the purification and characterization of enterotoxin from *C. perfringens* type C.

Despite all the interesting research on *C. perfringens* enterotoxin—the findings that there is a short incubation period (8 to 12 hours) and that food (chicken and other meats) containing large numbers of *C. perfringens* has been the major vehicle of transmission—the author has failed to find clear-cut evidence that enterotoxin produced in the food prior to ingestion is the etiological agent of *C. perfringens* enteritis. In other words: Is this disease a noninfectious toxemia of the botulism or the *S. aureus* food poisoning type? Or is it an infectious enteritis of the cholera or *E. coli* type? Is the designation "food poisoning" a misnomer in the case of *C. perfringens* enteritis? Or is this syndrome the result of the massive numbers of *C. perfringens* in the meat at the time of ingestion resulting in the rapid synthesis of enterotoxin *in situ* and the short postingestion incubation period? Possibly a reader will research these questions and provide answers—the author is too old to undertake the job.

Control and Prevention

Regardless of the etiology, the only available control measures for *C. perfringens* enteritis are these: (1) clean environments for processing fowl or other meats and (2) refrigeration (4–6°C) particularly after cooking if the meat is to be stored for several hours or longer prior to consumption.

REFERENCES

Cockey, R. R., and M. C. Tatra. 1974. Survival studies with spores of *Clostridium botulinum* type E in pasteurized meat of the blue crab, *Callinectes sapidus*. *Appl. Microbiol.* 27:629–633.

Dische, F. E., and S. D. Elek. 1957. Experimental food-poisoning by *Clostridium welchii*. *Lancet* 2:71–74.

Duncan, C. L., D. H. Strong, and M. Sebald. 1972. Sporulation and enterotoxin production by mutants of *Clostridium perfringens*. *J. Bacteriol.* 110:378–391.

Eklund, M. W., F. T. Poysky, J. A. Meyers, and G. A. Pelroy. 1974. Interspecies conversion of *Clostridium botulinum* type C to *Clostridium novyi* type A by bacteriophage. *Science* 186:456–458.

Eklund, M. W., F. T. Poysky, S. M. Reed, and C. A. Smith. 1971. Bacteriophage and the toxigenicity of *Clostridium botulinum* type C. *Science* 172:480–482.

Foster, E. M., R. H. Deibel, C. L. Duncan, J. M. Goepfert, and H. Suigiyama. 1974. Bacterial food poisoning. Chapter 92 in *Manual of Clinical Microbiology*.

Hollander, H. O. 1965. Production of large quantities of enterotoxin B and other staphylococcal toxins on solid media. *Acta Pathol. Microbiol.* 63:299–305.

Koutter, D. A., T. Lilly, Jr., A. J. LeBlanc, and R. K. Lynt. 1974. Incidence of *Clostridium botulinum* in crab meat from the blue crab. *Appl. Microbiol.* 28:722.

McClung, L. S. 1945. Human food poisoning due to growth of *Clostridium perfringens* in freshly cooked chicken: preliminary note. *J. Bacteriol.* 50:229–231.

Minor, T. E., and E. H. Marth. 1976. *Staphylococci and Their Significance in Foods*. Amsterdam: Elsevier.

Nakamura, M., and J. A. Schulze. 1970. *Clostridium perfringens* food poisoning. *Ann. Rev. Microbiol.* 24:359–372.

Nillo, L. 1974. Response of ligated intestinal loops in chickens to the enterotoxin of *Clostridium perfringens*. *Appl. Microbiol.* 28:889–891.

Nygren, B. 1962. Phospholipase C-producing bacteria and food poisoning. An experimental study on *Clostridium perfringens* and *Bacillus cereus*. *Acta Path. Microbiol. Scand. Suppl.* 160:1–88.

Skjelkvälé, R., and C. L. Duncan. 1975. Characterization of enterotoxin purified from *Clostridium perfringens* type C. *Infect. Immunity* 11:1061–1068.

Smith, L. D., and L. V. Holderman. 1968. *The Pathogenic Anaerobic Bacteria*. Springfield: Charles C. Thomas.

Stark, R. L., and C. L. Duncan. 1971. Biological characteristics of *Clostridium perfringens* type A enterotoxin. *Infect. Immunity* 4:89–96.

PART FOUR

Inoculation Group Diseases

Subgroup A: Arthropod Inoculation

As indicated in Chapter 1, the skin serves as the portal of entry for the disease organisms of the inoculation group. The subgroups of this group are:

A. Arthropod inoculation:
those diseases transmitted from host to host by blood-sucking (hemophagous) insects and other anthropods;

B. Vertebrate inoculation:
those diseases transmitted from host to host by the bite of infected vertebrates;

C. Wound inoculation:
those diseases caused mainly by anaerobic spore-forming bacilli as a result of soil or other inanimate source contamination of traumatic injury or burn lesions.

The primary vehicle of all subgroup A diseases is the blood of the infected host. Therefore, as a general rule, the arthropod must have a blood meal from an infected host before being able to transmit the infection to other hosts. This rule holds true for most insect vectors. An exception, however, was reported by Watts et al. (1973), who demonstrated the transmission of an encephalitis virus (La Crosse) from infected female mosquitoes through the eggs (*transovarial*) to the larval progeny. This transovarial infection then persisted through the larval and pupal stages and on to the adult. The adult progeny were demonstrated capable of transmitting this infection to infant mice and chipmunks during their first blood meals.

Female ticks and possibly mites (both of which taxonomically are arthropods but not insects) can pass infectious agents transovarially to the newly hatched larvae. These agents persist in the nymphal and adult ticks. Thus the transovarially infected larval, nymphal, and adult progeny of the infected female tick may be able to transmit the infection during their first feeding without the necessity of a prior infectious blood meal.

There are many significant host-vector-parasite adaptations in the diseases transmitted by hemophagous arthropods. One of the most interesting examples of such adaptations is found in the protozoan disease malaria. Human malaria parasites have adapted strictly to human hosts. They are transmitted from host to host by female mosquitoes, mainly by those belonging to the genus *Anopheles*. The male *Anopheles* are not hemophagous insects. To become infected the mosquito must feed upon an infected human host and must ingest both male and female sexual forms (gametocytes) of the parasite. In the stomach of the mosquito these gametocytes fuse (the sexual phase of the life cycle) to form amoebalike zygotes. The zygotes burrow into the stomach wall of the mosquito, where they undergo extensive asexual reproduction. The progeny of this phase of the life cycle then rupture into the body cavity of the mosquito where they penetrate the salivary glands. These infectious forms then are inoculated, along with saliva, when the mosquito next feeds upon a host. The parasites in a new human host undergo further asexual cycles of reproduction in the erythrocytes. The simultaneous rupturing of increasing numbers of the infected erythrocytes results in the liberation of toxic products and the intermittent chills and fever of malaria. During these reproductive cycles of the parasite in the human host, new gametocytes are produced that continue to circulate in the bloodstream until picked up by another female mosquito during the act of feeding. With such an ideal series of reproductive and transmission adaptations, it is no wonder that malaria became one of the most prevalent human diseases. Although other protozoal and some helminthic parasites may have adapted to comparably complicated host-vector-parasite life cycles, none of the pathogenic organisms considered in this text has so adapted —even though specific adaptations to hosts and vectors are common and will be cited.

REFERENCES

Watts, D. M., S. Pantuwatana, G. R. DeFoliart, T. M. Yuill, and W. H. Thompson. 1973. Transovarial transmission of La Crosse virus (California encephalitis group) in the mosquito *Aedes triseriatus. Science* 182:1440–1441.

29

Bubonic Plague

Human bubonic plague is caused by the plague bacillus, which is primarily a parasite of wild rodents. In wild rodents the disease is relatively mild. When the organism invades urban rodents (rats), however, its virulence for these hosts frequently has resulted in highly fatal epizootics (animal epidemics). Some of the greatest human pestilences have coincided with these rat epizootics. The term *bubonic* derives from the fact that the human disease frequently results in inflammatory swelling of lymph glands (buboes), particularly those in the inguinal and axillary regions.

Although fatal cases of what is believed to have been human bubonic plague were reported in North Africa and Syria during the third century B.C., the presence of the disease in epidemic form prior to the Christian era is subject to question. The first clearly described epidemic of human bubonic plague, with associated high rat mortality, occurred in the sixth century A.D. during the reign of the Byzantine emperor Justinian (the Justinian plague). This epidemic spread over Byzantium and contiguous Middle Eastern areas resulting in mortality rates ranging from 50 to 90 percent. The Justinian plague has been classified as one of the three greatest pestilences of human history. The second of these (the Black Death), also bubonic plague, began in Europe during the fourteenth century and persisted intermittently for several centuries. During the worst years of the Black Death, an estimated one-fourth of the population of Europe perished as a consequence of the disease. The epidemic in London alone left an estimated 70,000 dead.

The disease then remained enzootic (endemic) in rodents until the last decade of the nineteenth century, when it reappeared in epizootic and epidemic form in Indochina and spread to Hong Kong. From there it spread to India, where millions of deaths were attributed to the disease during the ensuing 20 years. From Hong Kong infected rats carried plague aboard ships, which dispersed the disease to seaports around the world. The disease appeared in San Francisco early in the twentieth century. California health officials, however, refused to admit the presence of the disease until the state was threatened with quarantine by federal officials. In California the disease spread to wild rodents (ground squirrels). By 1975 this wild-rodent (*sylvatic*) plague had spread throughout the western United States and eastward to far western Texas, New Mexico, western Kansas, and North Dakota and from northern Mexico to southwestern Canada. This represents one of the largest areas of sylvatic plague in the world.

The disease also appeared in New Orleans, Galveston, and south Atlantic seaports during the first quarter of the twentieth century. However, prompt rat control measures by the U.S. Public Health Service, under the supervision of Dr. G. W. McCoy, eliminated the disease from these areas with no evidence of spread to wild rodents. As indicated in Chapter 13, the third of the three greatest human pestilences was the 1918 pandemic of influenza.

ETIOLOGY AND HOST-VECTOR BIOLOGY

Alexander Yersin and S. Kitasato in 1894 independently announced the discovery of the plague bacillus. The organism reported by Kitasato, however, was a gram-positive, slightly motile bacillus. The true plague bacillus is a gram-negative, nonmotile, ovoid rod. Although not apparent in gram-stained preparations, plague bacilli yield bipolar staining with modified Giemsa stain or, preferably, with Wayson's stain (see Paik and Suggs 1974). The bipolar staining is much more apparent in smears of infected tissue or bubo aspirates than in smears of cultured cells (see Figure I on the back cover).

For many years the plague bacillus was assigned by American and other taxonomists to the genus *Pasteurella* (*P. pestis*). However, the eighth edition of *Bergey's Manual* lists the organism in the genus *Yersinia*. *Yersinia pestis* is primarily a parasite of wild rodents (about 220 species), with widespread areas of endemicity in

various parts of the world. This sylvatic plague involves a high percentage of latent or asymptomatic infections. When *Y. pestis* infects rats of the genus *Rattus* in urban areas, however, a highly virulent rat epizootic may develop. In the past these rat epizootics, with high rat mortality, have preceded or coexisted with the fatal epidemics of human plague. Historical records, indicating the prevalence of dead rats during the human epidemics, have helped medical historians to recognize the described human disease as bubonic plague.

A number of rat fleas and fleas of other rodents may serve as vectors in the spread of *Y. pestis* among the animal hosts. Many of these fleas will not feed upon humans and, therefore, are not involved in the rodent-to-human transmission. Rat fleas of the genus *Xenopsylla*, however, will feed on human blood and have been incriminated as the major vector in the human disease (see Figure 29-1). The fleas are insects and must have an infectious blood meal before they are capable of transmitting the infection to other hosts. Studies of infected rats have indicated the presence of up to 10^8 plague bacilli per milliliter of rat blood during the acute rat disease. Consequently a single blood meal may result in the ingestion of large numbers of *Y. pestis*.

Figure 29–1. Xenopsylla cheopis, a rat flea that is a major vector of human bubonic plague. An early infection of *Yersinia pestis* is visible in the gut (see text). (Courtesy of Plague Branch, Center for Disease Control, Fort Collins, Colo.)

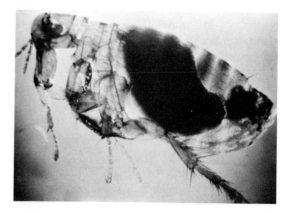

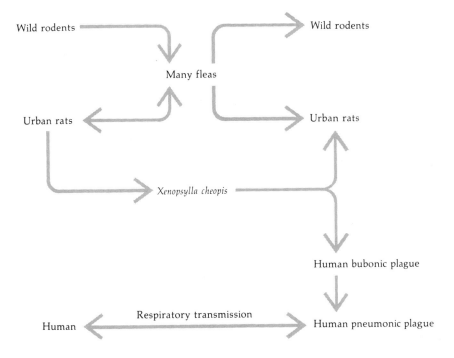

Figure 29–2. Host-vector transmission of *Yersinia pestis.*

In the stomach of the flea, the plague bacilli multiply rapidly without invasion of the flea tissues. The mass of bacilli may become so great that it blocks the valve between the stomach and the suction apparatus (the proventriculus) of the flea. When blood is sucked into the proventriculus of a blocked flea it is seeded with many plague bacilli. Since the proventricular valve is blocked, however, the blood is not passed back to the stomach but is regurgitated into the bite wound, leading to greater certainty of infecting the host. Moreover, since the blocked flea derives no satisfaction from the blood meal, it is more prone to move from host to host for attempted feeding and thereby to spread the disease more widely than would an unblocked flea.

Human bubonic plague is not transmissible from human to human and rarely, if ever, from humans to fleas. If the patient's lungs become involved, however, the resulting pneumonic plague is transmissible to other humans by the respiratory route. Figure 29-2 summarizes the epizootology of sylvatic plague of rodents and the epidemiology of human bubonic and pneumonic plague.

Yersinia pestis can be cultivated in relatively simple liquid media, but the addition of blood to agar media appears to enhance the growth of fresh isolates. The organisms grow better at 25–30°C than at 37°C, although they may grow slowly at either temperature. There are three biotypes of *Y. pestis* with differing geographical distribution and slight epidemiological significance. The biotypes are distinguished on the basis of their ability to ferment glycerol and reduce nitrates to nitrites.

Although *Y. pestis* is antigenically homogeneous, considering the fact that there are no practical serotype distinctions, the bacilli have been shown to possess a number of different antigens (about 16). At least two of these—(1) the F-1 envelope or capsular antigen and (2) the V antigen—are always found in demonstrably virulent isolates. The V antigen is usually in association with a W antigen (the VW complex).

Burrows (1955) described a dark-brown pigmentation (P⁺) of virulent *Y. pestis* colonies when grown on a defined medium containing hemin. The pigmentation factor appears to be due to the absorption of the iron-containing hemin. Cells from colonies that lacked this P⁺ character (P⁻ colonies) were of low virulence regardless of other cell characteristics. *Yersinia pestis* also produces at least two distinct protein toxins, both of which are antigenic (see Montie et al. 1975). Since both virulent and avirulent bacilli produce one or both of these toxins, however, it is clear that toxigenicity is not the only characteristic required for the pathogenicity of *Y. pestis*.

CLINICAL PLAGUE

Human plague may range in severity from practically asymptomatic (plague minor) through typically severe to rapidly fatal disease. Severe cases of flea-transmitted plague show sudden onset of headache, high temperature, and rapid pulse. Nausea and vomiting may occur at this stage also. The symptoms progress rapidly to nervousness, great prostration, bloated appearance, conjunctivitis, apathy, mental confusion, and death. The infection is either bacteremic or septicemic at early stages. As subcutaneous lymph glands (inguinal, axillary, and others) become involved they become inflamed, indurated or swollen, and very painful—the buboes. If the bacteremic or glandular infection spreads to the lungs, pneumonic plague results. In this form of the disease, large numbers of plague bacilli are found in the sputum and the disease is transmissible from person to person by the respiratory mode. Pneumonic plague is the most serious form of the disease. Past epidemics have aproached 100 percent mortality.

Another plague complication is illustrated by a case of bubonic plague in an 11-year-old boy in New Mexico in February 1975. After apparent recovery from the primary symptoms, the boy developed plague meningitis (*MMWR*, 8 March 1975). The primary infection apparently resulted from skinning a dead coyote found in the mountainous area (contact transmission). Fortunately, concentrated intrathecal and intravenous antibiotic and chemotherapy resulted in recovery with no neurological sequelae.

The total number of reported cases of human plague worldwide in 1974 was 2,737 with 164 deaths; in 1975 the incidence was 1,478 cases with 99 fatal. This decrease was mainly attributed to incomplete reporting from the Republic of South Vietnam during 1975 (see *MMWR*, 17 September 1976). In the Americas in 1975 Brazil reported 496 cases and 5 deaths and the United States reported 20 cases and 4 deaths. Five states were involved: Arizona (3), California (1), Colorado (1), New Mexico (14), and Utah (1). Between January and August 1976, some 13 additional cases (2 fatal) were reported from the same states—indicating the persistent and widespread prevalence of sylvatic plague in the western United States. These human plague cases have resulted both from arthropod (flea) inoculation and contact with infected animals.

LABORATORY DIAGNOSIS

The specimen of choice for laboratory diagnosis of plague depends upon the stage of the infection and the clinical manifestations. If plague is suspected in the early febrile stage, blood should be submitted both for culture and to establish baseline antibody titers. If the primary or secondary symptoms are pneumonia (pneumonic plague), then sputum coughed up from the lung area is the specimen of choice, although blood culture also should be performed. Blood cultures should be incubated at 28°C for 24 to 48 hours or until growth turbidity develops.

Direct smears of the sputum on microslides should be fixed with absolute methanol. One smear should be stained by the gram method and the other with Wayson's stain (see Figure I on the back cover). The sputum may also be streaked onto the surface of blood agar and incubated for 24 to 48 hours at 28°C. Smears of the culture growth should be stained as described above. Aspirates from buboes and pus from abscesses may be tested by stained smears and by culture on blood agar. Finding morphologically typical, gram-negative, bipolar staining bacilli in any one or more of these specimens would indicate the possibility of the disease being plague. If the isolated bacilli agglutinate to the titer of a specific anti–*Y. pestis* antiserum, the disease may be considered to be plague. If early and late blood specimens are collected, their sera should show a rising antibody titer to known *Y. pestis* cells if the disease is plague.

Culture isolates of suspected *Y. pestis* should be submitted to the Plague Branch, Vector-Borne Diseases Division, Bureau of Laboratories, CDC, for further study and confirmation. This laboratory maintains fluorescent antibody and bacteriophages specific for *Y. pestis*. It also has other reagents and animal facilities necessary for a thorough study of the isolate. For additional details see Sonnenwirth (1974).

IMMUNITY AND CHEMOTHERAPY

As indicated above, *Y. pestis* cells possess a variety of somatic antigens and produce at least two antigenic toxins. The toxins do not appear to be involved in virulence, and serum antitoxins are not therapeutic in experimental plague. Extensive studies on active immunization in humans using (1) killed, virulent *Y. pestis* vaccines and (2) live attenuated *Y. pestis* vaccines have been reported (see Cavanaugh and Steele 1974). One live vaccine widely used was a P⁻ mutant of an otherwise virulent (F-1, VW) strain of *Y. pestis*. Although there have been reports of reduced morbidity and mortality in those immunized with either killed or live vaccines, the results to date have not been overly encouraging.

Tetracyclines, streptomycin, chloramphenicol, and sulfonamides have proved effective in the treatment of bubonic, septicemic, and pneumonic plague if treatment is instituted early in the disease. Penicillin has no therapeutic value. An excessive initial dose of a bactericidal drug, such as streptomycin, may result in the liberation of large quantities of endotoxin, which may cause a severe to fatal shock reaction (the Jarisch-Herxheimer reaction). Meyer (1965) rec-

ommends an initial 2-gram dose of streptomycin followed by 1 gram per day for 10 days or longer.

CONTROL AND PREVENTION

Rural (sylvatic) plague is almost impossible to control. The wild rodent hosts generally do not suffer the extensive mortality from plague infection that is observed in urban rat infections. Therefore the wild rodent plague enzootics are not as prone to be self-limiting as are the rat epizootics. Furthermore, practical measures for wild rodent control, comparable to those for urban rat control, have not been devised.

Effective urban-rat *control* measures—and note the emphasis on the word control*—must take cognizance of the fact that it is the rat *flea* which is responsible for the transmission of the disease from rat to rat and rat to human. Trapping or poisoning rats without coincident control of their fleas may result in an actual increase of the incidence of human plague as the infected fleas leave the dead bodies of the rats to feed upon other hosts.

Rat-flea control measures in urban areas involve using persistent insecticides (DDT or others) in rat runs and nesting areas. These measures alone have been known to stop epidemic plague and should be instituted prior to rat trapping and poisoning programs. The objective of the flea control program is to get the persistent insecticide into the fur and onto the bodies of the rats to destroy their ectoparasites—especially the fleas.

Both rat-flea and rat control measures should be initiated at the periphery of the urban area to be controlled and should proceed inward to the center of the area. This tends to concentrate, rather than disperse, the infected rats and their ectoparasites. The most effective rat control measures include trapping, poisoning, and starving. For the latter, garbage, grain, house-

---

*I once made the mistake of saying "rat elimination" to Dr. George W. McCoy, the plague expert in the United States. He corrected me, saying: "Rats have never been eliminated, merely controlled within practical limits."

hold, and other potential rat food must be stored in rat-proof containers and buildings. Rat control measures should include preventing rats in known endemic areas of the world from boarding ships. Metal guards 3 feet in diameter are placed on hawsers that tie the ship to the wharf. These are designed to block rats attempting to board the ship, but rats may gain entrance along with cargo being loaded. Therefore ships from endemic areas may be quarantined, inspected, and if need be fumigated while at anchor in the harbor prior to being allowed to proceed to wharves and unload cargo.

The rat population, especially in economically depressed and run-down urban areas, frequently equals or exceeds the human population of the area. The rats may be involved in the transmission of a variety of inoculation group diseases in addition to plague and also a variety of intestinal group diseases. Besides the health hazard, each urban rat has been estimated to consume food and destroy property valued at $4 to $5 annually. Thus their control is justified both on the health and the economic basis.

Bubonic plague generally is not transmissible from human to human whereas pneumonic plague is highly contagious. The clinician should check the patient carefully for the onset of pneumonic symptoms—then clinician, nurses, and other hospital personnel should take strict precautions against the respiratory spread of the infection to themselves and to others.

REFERENCES

Burrows, T. W. 1955. The basis of virulence for mice of *Pasteurella pestis*. In *Mechanisms of Microbial Pathogenicity*. London: Cambridge University Press.

Cavanaugh, D. C., and J. H. Steele (eds.). 1974. Trends in research on plague immunization. *J. Infect. Dis.* 129(Supplement):S1–S120.

Meyer, K. F. 1965. *Pasteurella* and *Francisella*. Chapter 27 in *Bacterial and Mycotic Infections of Man*.

Montie, T. C., D. B. Montie, and D. Wennerstrom. 1975. Aspects of the structure and biological activity of plague murine toxin. In *Microbiology, 1975*, ed. D. Schlessenger. Washington: American Society for Microbiology.

Paik, G., and M. T. Suggs. 1974. Reagents, stains, and miscellaneous test procedures. Chapter 96 in *Manual of Clinical Microbiology*.

Sonnenwirth, A. C. 1974. *Yersinia*. Chapter 19 in *Manual of Clinical Microbiology*.

Watts, D. M., S. Pantuwatana, G. R. DeFoliart, T. M. Yuill, and W. H. Thompson. 1973. Transovarial transmission of La Crosse virus (California encephalitis group) in the mosquito *Aedes triseriatus*. *Science* 182:1440–1441.

30
Relapsing Fever (Spirochetal)

As indicated in Chapter 2, spirochetes in the blood of febrile patients in Berlin were reported by Otto Obermeier in 1873. This was the first report of a microorganism in the tissues of a human patient that later proved to be the etiological agent of the disease. Obermeier could not prove the etiology of his organism because he could not isolate it in pure culture. H. Lebert in 1874 proposed the name *Protomycetum recurrentis* for Obermeier's organism because of the recurrent (relapsing) tendency of the fever. This species designation has persisted, although the genus designation has been changed repeatedly.

ETIOLOGY AND EPIDEMIOLOGY

The relapsing fever studied by Obermeier was the epidemic form; and many extensive epidemics have occurred in various parts of the world during historical times. The vector transmitting this form of the disease is the human body louse—*Pediculus humanus* (see Figure 30-1). This louse feeds on humans only, and the epidemiology therefore is human→louse→human. Obviously, lousy environments are essential to epidemic relapsing fever.

The infected louse does not transmit relapsing fever by the bite. The spirochetes are found only in the body fluid between the gut and body wall and there is no salivary gland involvement comparable to that in the mosquito transmission of malaria. Since these lice feed only on humans, researchers have allowed infected lice to feed upon themselves thousands of times without becoming infected. If the infected louse was either crushed or maimed so that body fluid was deposited on the skin at the site of the bite, however, infection resulted. DDT and other persistent insecticides have eliminated epidemic relapsing fever from the technologically advanced countries of the world.

The eighth edition of *Bergey's Manual* designates the spirochete responsible for louse-borne relapsing fever as *Borrelia recurrentis*. The legitimacy of the generic designation, *Borrelia*, is open to question, however. Claims have been made that the relapsing fever spirochetes differ no more from spirochetes of the genus *Treponema* (syphilis, bejel, yaws, pinto) than spirochetes of the genus *Treponema* differ among themselves. Nevertheless, the genus designation *Borrelia* is widely accepted.

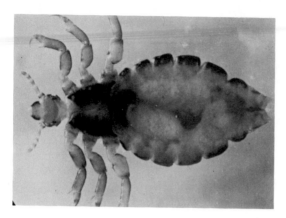

Figure 30–1.   Human body louse *Pediculus humanus* (female), the vector of epidemic, louse-borne relapsing fever. (Courtesy of the Center for Disease Control, Atlanta, GA.)

Borrelia recurrentis, like all other relapsing fever spirochetes, are helical (corkscrew-shaped) organisms (see Figure 30-2) that are highly motile as a result of rotations produced by contractions and relaxations of a springlike axial filament encased in contractile protoplasm. This rotational motion permits the spirochetes to burrow into and through soft tissues. The movements are random, forward or backward. The *Borrelia* are longer and less tightly coiled than are *T. pallidum* and are much more prone to twisting and turning movements.

P. H. Ross and A. D. Milne and J. E. Dutton and J. L. Todd in 1904–1905 independently reported the transmission of spirochetal relapsing fever (African tick fever) by ticks (*Ornithodoros moubata*) in central Africa. This tick-transmitted disease has been classified as endemic in contrast to the louse-borne, epidemic relapsing fever. At least 12 species of the genus *Ornithodoros* have been incriminated in the transmission of the disease to humans (see Figure 30-3). This endemic relapsing fever is distributed worldwide with the possible exception of Australia, New Zealand, and the surrounding South Pacific islands. The *Ornithodoros* (soft-shell) ticks are primarily ectoparasites of burrowing rodents or other animals, but they will feed upon practically any warm-blooded or even cold-blooded animals (snakes).

The designation of species of the tick-transmitted members of the genus *Borrelia* has gone through multiple changes since their discovery in 1905. None has gained complete acceptance by taxonomists. *Bergey's Manual* lists tick-transmitted ralapsing fever spirochete species that have been named after discoverers (*B. duttoni*), geographic locations of endemicity (*B. hispanica, B. persica, B. caucasica, B. venezuelensis*), and after the species designation of the transmitting tick vector. Examples of this latter designation method are represented by the three species of relapsing fever spirochetes found in the United States: *B. hermsi (O. hermsi), B. parkeri (O. parkeri),* and *B. turicatae (O. turicata).* Immunological, serological, and other accepted methods of microbial species taxonomy have not proved effective in differentiating members of the genus *Borrelia.* Until more significant taxa can be established, it would seem preferable, to this author, to designate all relapsing fever spirochetes as *B. recurrentis* and designate the biotypes (or varieties) on the basis of the trans-

Figure 30–2.   Borreliae in the blood of a pine squirrel. This species is one of the causes of relapsing fever in the United States and is considered either a biotype of *Borrelia recurrentis* or a separate species, *B. hermsi* (see text). (Courtesy of W. Burgdorfer.)

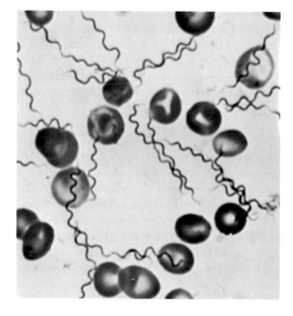

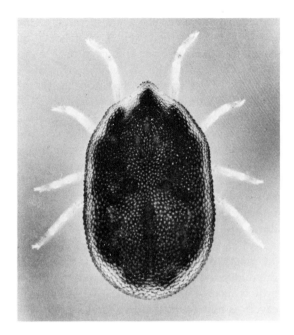

Figure 30–3. Ornithodoros hermsi, the vector of tick-borne relapsing fever in the western United States. (Courtesy of W. Burgdorfer)

mitting vector, if known. To honor Obermeier and Dutton, however, the louse-transmitted spirochetes might be designated *B. recurrentis (obermeieri)*, whereas the *O. moubata*–transmitted spirochetes could be designated *B. recurrentis (duttoni)*. In this scheme other tick-transmitted spirochetes would be given biotype designations denoting the transmitting tick vector, such as *B. recurrentis (turicatae)*, if the tick vector is known.

The *Ornithodoros* ticks tend to secrete themselves in the soil of animal burrows, pig sties, or shallow caverns where larger animals may bed down. In such habitats, the ticks lie in wait for the blood meal to come to them. When this occurs they attack, suck blood voraciously, and detach when engorged. Adults then mate and after approximately 10 days the female begins laying eggs. One large female tick in my "ticktorium" (Schuhardt 1940b) began laying eggs 11 days after engorgement and over the following 31 days laid a total of 1,608 eggs. This is an *Ornithodoros* record, so far as I have been able to ascertain. Usually an engorged female *O. turicata* will lay 300 to 500 eggs.

The infection in female *Ornithodoros* ticks is

passed transovarially to a variable percentage of the newly hatched larvae. These infected larvae then can infect hosts during their first blood meal. Since the bite of the larvum frequently is not detectable and since the larvae feed and detach within 10 minutes, infection from larval bites can occur with no recognition of exposure. Professor O. B. Williams, of the Department of Microbiology, The University of Texas at Austin, apparently was infected by this mode while he was in the vicinity of the tick-infested cavern at Falls Creek on the Colorado River of Texas. The transovarial infection of the larvae then persists during the several nymphal instars, which occur following each blood meal, and on to the adult progeny. Thus many of the progeny of an infected female tick do not require an infectious blood meal prior to transmitting the infection to new hosts.

The shallow limestone cavern (see Figure 30–4) near the mouth of Falls Creek has an interesting history in the annals of relapsing fever in Texas. During the 1930s old-timers in the area related an outbreak of febrile disease in a group of Boy Scouts who traveled by wagon from Gatesville in 1915 to camp beside the clear pool at the base of the 104-foot falls. The falls resulted from a spring-fed creek plunging over a fern-covered cliff to the river bottom. The scouts explored the area including a shallow ledge cavern in the cliff a hundred yards or so from the pool. About a week after arriving, the boys began developing chills, headache, high fever, and other symptoms and were housed at various ranches in the area to recuperate. The disease was not diagnosed.

In 1929 four University of Texas students spent a summer weekend camping and exploring at the Falls Creek pool. A week later, after returning to Austin, three of the four developed the chills and fever syndrome. Dr. Weller, the university physician, and his pathologist colleague, Dr. Graham, found spirochetes in the blood of one of these patients. Dr. Graham went to the cavern and collected some ticks (*O. turicata*) and succeeded in transmitting the spirochetal infection from these ticks to animals. A week after his trip to collect ticks, Dr. Graham developed relapsing fever. Weller and Graham

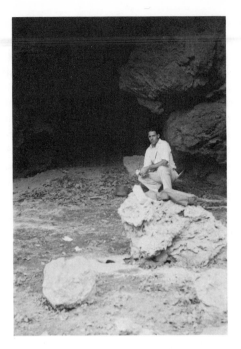

Figure 30–4. Shallow, tick-infested cave near the mouth of Falls Creek where it joined the Colorado River of Texas.

(1930) published their findings as one of the early reports of relapsing fever in Texas.

In 1932 Dr. Graham received a telegram from Dr. E. Brumpt, professor of parasitology at the University of Paris. Brumpt stated that he planned to be in Austin on a certain day and would like to go to the Falls Creek cavern and collect some of the ticks for his laboratory studies. Since I had isolated spirochetes from another patient into white mice at the State Department of Health Laboratory, Dr. Graham asked the director of the laboratory, Dr. Bohls, and me if we would care to go along with Dr. Brumpt and him. We agreed and arranged to pick them up at 8:00 A.M. on the appointed day. Apparently the thought of a noted parasitologist from Europe coming to visit a country-boy doctor from Texas was too much for Dr. Graham. When we picked him up he was pretty well inebriated and continued to nip at his bottle on the way to the cavern.

We proceeded to a spot about 20 yards in front of the mouth of the cavern, where we unfolded a white bed sheet and spread it on the grass. Dr. Brumpt then said, "Dr. Graham, you have had relapsing fever and are probably immune. You go into the cavern and bring out a shovelful of the limestone dust from the floor." Feeling no pain and being most obliging, Dr. Graham crawled farther than need be into the cave, brought out a shovelful of dust, and deposited it on the sheet. We then picked ticks off his clothing along with those that crawled out of the dust onto the sheet. The collected ticks were placed in screw-capped bottles for the return trip. A week later, Dr. Graham was again down with relapsing fever. He proclaimed, with some humor, that he had proved two things: (1) an attack of relapsing fever did not confer immunity and (2) alcohol in the system did not protect against the infection. The Falls Creek cavern is now inundated by the waters of Lake Buchanan.

In 1968 an outbreak of *B. hermsi* relapsing fever occurred in 11 of 42 Boy Scouts who camped in two old and poorly kept log cabins in the mountains about 7 miles out of Spokane, Washington (see *MMWR,* 1 June 1968). In the summer of 1973 an outbreak of *B. hermsi* relapsing fever occurred among park personnel and tourists occupying rustic cabins in the Grand Canyon, Arizona, North Rim Park. No cases were traced to the South Rim Park (see *MMWR,* 24 July 1973). One of the tourist cases came down with the disease in Georgia after returning from the park. On 11 June 1976, the first case of relapsing fever in North Carolina was reported in Durham. Although the patient denied noting ticks or lice on him, he and a friend had spent a great deal of time in wooded areas at Sun River, Oregon, the week prior to flying back to Durham on 4 June. On the evening of 9 June the patient was febrile and unable to walk without falling. Examination of a blood smear for malaria was negative but spirochetes were seen. Approximately 8 hours after receiving oral doxycycline therapy the patient's blood pressure dropped to 90/50 and he became hyperpyrexic with a fever of 105°F. This was believed to be a Jarisch-Herxheimer reaction (*MMWR,* 2 July 1976).

Adult *Ornithodoros* ticks are extremely long-lived. Francis (1938) reported starving infected, adult *O. turicata,* from the Falls Creek cavern, in humidors for 5 years without a blood meal. When these starved ticks were fed on rats they were still capable of transmitting the infection. Larval ticks are hungrier and much more restless than adults and do not survive starvation for more than a few months.

Infected *Ornithodoros* ticks transmit the relapsing fever spirochetes either by the bite, during the extraction of a blood meal from the host, or by contamination of the bite area with coxal fluid secreted from glands at the base of the legs. *Ornithodoros* species vary in the secretion of coxal fluid; for example, adult *O. moubata* and *O. turicata* secrete copious amounts of coxal fluid during the act of feeding, whereas *O. hermsi* secretes little if any.

Since the human body louse feeds upon humans only, natural infections with *B. recurrentis* are observed in humans only. These spirochetes, however, will infect a variety of animals including mice, rats, and monkeys when inoculated along with infected human blood. Tick-transmitted *Borrelia* species also infect a variety of animals, some of which may serve as reservoirs of infection in nature. In our studies at Falls Creek cavern (Schuhardt 1940*a*), we exposed a variety of animals to the ticks (*O. turicata*) in cages placed in the cave for 3 to 4 hours. A cage containing a white rat was exposed along with each group of test animals. Although ticks were observed feeding on all test animals, two vultures and a chicken were not infected as indicated by 15 negative daily microscopic examinations of their blood. The white rats invariably were infected, with an incubation period of 2 to 4 days and one or more relapses. Twelve Mexican free-tailed bats also were not infected. A raccoon, an opossum, an armadillo, and a dog were infected. All the animal infections with the exception of the dog and raccoon tended to show microscopic relapses during a 13-day examination period. The dog was positive on the sixth, seventh, and eighth days after exposure and microscopically negative thereafter. Since the incubation period in the dog was the same as

that in humans, it is conceivable that one or more relapses might have occurred after the examinations were discontinued. The raccoon became microscopically positive on the fourth day after exposure to the ticks and continued to be positive through the thirteenth day, when examinations were discontinued. Thus, as indicated by others, our studies added to the evidence that tick-infected animals can serve as possible reservoir hosts to provide infectious blood meals for ticks that failed to acquire their infections transovarially.

Since louse-borne *B. recurrentis* has never been cultivated on artificial media and since the successful cultivation of a tick-transmitted species (*B. hermsi*) was first reported by Kelly (1971), the only past means of maintaining these spirochetes for laboratory studies has been animal passage, and this continues to be the surest way. White mice and rats, if susceptible, have been the animals of choice. Restraining the animal in a hardware cloth cylinder with the tail protruding from one end permits snipping off the tip of the tail to obtain blood for microscopic examination or for animal-passage inoculation. The spirochetes will also invade the brains of these animals and persist there for months after disappearance from the bloodstream. Thus successful brain passage of the spirochetes can be made at greater intervals of time than those required for blood passage.

CLINICAL SYMPTOMS AND IMMUNOBIOLOGY

After an incubation period of 3 to 10 days (average 7), spirochetal relapsing fever commences suddenly with malaise, headache, myalgia, chilly sensations or hard chills, and nausea followed within 12 to 24 hours by high fever (103°F or higher). There are reports that the louse-borne disease is characterized by two (occasionally three) paroxysms of fever, each lasting 6 to 7 days and separated by a fever-free period lasting 5 to 7 days. Under famine or other stress conditions, louse-borne relapsing fever epidemics in the past have been known to result in high mortality rates.

The tick-transmitted disease is characterized by more febrile paroxysms (2 to 12, averaging 4 + for *B. turicatae*), each separated by 5 to 7 fever-free days. The fever paroxysms generally are shorter (1 to 4 days) than those in the louse-borne disease, and usually the duration of the fever decreases in the late paroxysms. Mortality in tick-transmitted relapsing fever is nil.

Schuhardt and Wilkerson (1951) noted that rats infected with single spirochetes (*B. turicatae*) showed the same microscopic relapsing tendency as rats infected with multiple spirochetes. They also noted a continuously rising antibody titer to first-attack spirochetes (onset passage) throughout the infections. Other workers had reported that prior-attack antigenic varieties of the spirochetes never recur in relapses. However, this continuous rise in antibody titer to first-attack spirochetes in our single-cell-infected rats was interpreted as evidence that mutations back to first-attack antigenic varieties did occur and did exert antigenic stimulation even though the back mutants were destroyed by the prior antibody present in the rat at the time of back mutations.

Many workers have reported antigenic changes in the spirochetes involved in the first and subsequent fever paroxysms. In 1925 J. Cunningham, after studying the spirochetes of Indian relapsing fever, designated the two antigenic strains usually involved as A and B and noted that they were freely reversible (A ⇌ B). If an attack were started with strain A the relapse would be due to strain B and vice versa. However, when Cunningham et al. (1934) studied the spirochetes derived from occasional third paroxysms of fever they reported a total of nine (A to I) distinct antigenic strains. Schuhardt (1942) analyzed the antigenic interrelationships of eight of the nine strains reported by Cunningham et al. (1934) and visualized the complicated set of reversible variations indicated in Figure 30-5. The fact that some tick-transmitted relapsing fever cases have suffered as many as 12 paroxysms of fever indicates that there may be more than the nine antigenic varieties described by Cunningham et al. With the complicated reversible variations in antigenic structure,

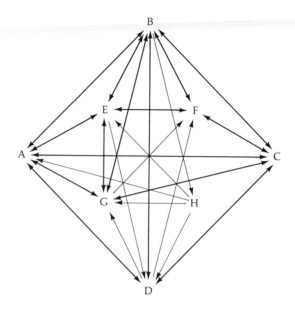

Figure 30–5.   Diagrammatic summary of the demonstrated antigenic phase relationships of the relapsing fever spirochetes studied by Cunningham et al. (1934) as analyzed by Schuhardt (1942). Letters indicate antigenic strains.

illustrated in Figure 30-5, it is easily understandable why serological taxonomy would fail to differentiate species of the genus *Borrelia*. Moreover, this situation explains why an attack of relapsing fever does not provide immunity—particularly in a patient whose infection is terminated by chemotherapy.

These and other studies on the reversible antigenic variability of relapsing fever spirochetes have resulted in the concept that each fever paroxysm is the consequence of a single antigenic type or group of spirochetes. Thus during the first febrile attack antibodies specific for the antigenic varieties involved are produced and destroy these spirochetes, thereby ending the febrile paroxysm. Before these antibodies are produced, however, one or more spirochetes mutate to a new antigenic type not destroyed by the prior-attack antibodies. During the fever-free interval, these antigenic mutants multiply and produce the first relapse paroxysm of fever. This process continues until one of two things happens to terminate the relapses: (1) all possible antigenic types have stimulated their immune responses; or (2) a new antigenic mutation does not occur during the preceding febrile paroxysm.

LABORATORY DIAGNOSIS

Unclotted blood, collected during the early stages of a fever paroxysm, is the specimen of choice for the laboratory diagnosis of spirochetal relapsing fever. The blood may be defibrinated or mixed with an anticoagulant such as sodium citrate, oxalate, or heparin in saline. Thick or thin smears of this blood on microslides may be prepared for staining. A wet mount of the blood, diluted severalfold in isotonic saline, may be examined by dark-field microscopy. If spirochetes are present in the wet mount, the examiner's attention will be drawn to areas where the red blood cells are being disturbed by the movements of the spirochetes. Also a white mouse or rat should be inoculated intraperitoneally with 0.5 milliliter of the blood. Drops of blood from the tail of the animal should be examined for several days beginning 2 or 3 days after inoculation. These examinations may be dark-field microscopy on wet mounts or bright-field microscopy on stained smears.

Thin smears of blood on microslides may be fixed with methyl alcohol and stained with Wright's, Giemsa, or other polychromatic blood stains. The spirochetes in stained smear preparations rarely show the uniform spiral morphology of the live spirochetes. This is due to the fact that, as the blood dries on the slide, one portion of the spirochete becomes attached and the writhing movements of the organism result in fixation in tangled, rather than normal, morphology.

Thick smears of blood (about 3/4 inch in diameter) have the advantage of concentrating the spirochetes in a smaller area on the microslide than do thin smears. However, the red blood cells in the thick smear must be lysed (laked) in distilled water or weak acetic acid before staining with Wright's or any stain that is dissolved in alcohol. Since Giemsa stain is dissolved in water, the thick smear will lake during the staining procedure while the slide is submersed in a stender jar—a jar designed to hold five or more microslides in separate grooves while immersed in staining solution. Experience in recognizing the tangled spirochetes in a thick smear is essential, but once mastered it is preferable to the thin-smear technique. For additional details, see Kelly (1974).

CHEMOTHERAPY

As previously intimated there are no immunoprophylactic or immunotherapeutic procedures applicable to the prevention or treatment of relapsing fever. Prior to the discovery of penicillin and other antibiotics, the organic arsenicals (neoarsphenamine and mapharsen) were the chemotherapeutic drugs of choice, but these were toxic and sometimes not effective. Early studies with penicillin indicated that at least 10^6 units, administered in divided doses every 3 hours over a period of at least 4 days, were effective in the treatment of the human disease (see Schuhardt 1952). Schuhardt and O'Bryan (1944; 1945), however, demonstrated that doses of penicillin adequate to cure the bloodstream involvement in infected rats did not cure the brain involvement in these animals. It is conceivable that some cases of relapse after chemotherapy, which is not uncommon, might be explained on the basis of surviving spirochetes in the brains of human patients. Subsequently oral tetracycline and other broad-spectrum antibiotics have replaced penicillin as the drugs of choice for treating relapsing fever patients. As indicated above, the sudden killing of large numbers of spirochetes by the therapeutic drug may result in a Jarisch-Herxheimer reaction.

CONTROL AND PREVENTION

The prevention and control of louse-borne relapsing fever can be accomplished readily using DDT or other persistent insecticides, to which the louse is susceptible. Control and prevention of tick-borne relapsing fever is more difficult, however, if not impossible. Only when human cases are traced to localized habitats such as shallow caves or log cabins are we likely to learn of the infestation of the site with infected ticks. Such ticks can be killed if coated with lightweight oil, which blocks their breathing pores. Getting the oil onto ticks in cracks or crevices or into the soil where the ticks are secreted is easier said than done, however. Tick poisons are available but, to this author's knowledge, have not been used in efforts to control tick-borne relapsing fever.

REFERENCES

Bohls, S. W., and V. T. Schuhardt. 1933. Relapsing fever in Texas and laboratory methods of diagnosis. *Texas State J. Med.* 29:199–203.

Buchanan, R. E., and N. E. Gibbons. 1974. *Bergey's Manual of Determinative Bacteriology.* 8th ed. Baltimore: Williams & Wilkins.

Cunningham, J., J. H. Theodore, and A. G. L. Fraser. 1934. Further observations on Indian relapsing fever. I. Types of spirochetes found in experimental infections. *Indian J. Med. Res.* 22:105–155.

Felsenfeld, O. 1965. Borreliae, human relapsing fever and parasite-vector-host relationships. *Bacteriol. Rev.* 29:46–74.

Francis, E. 1938. Longevity of the tick *Ornithodoros turicata* and of *Spirochaeta recurrentis* within this tick. *Publ. Hlth. Rep. U.S. Pub. Hlth. Serv.* 53:2220–2241.

Kelly, R. T. 1971. Cultivation of *Borrelia hermsi. Science* 173:443–444.

———. 1974. *Borrelia.* Chapter 35 in *Manual of Clinical Microbiology.*

Schuhardt, V. T. 1940a. Studies of the Falls Creek (Texas) strain of relapsing fever spirochetes. Ph.D. dissertation. Rice University, Houston, Texas.

———. 1940b. A "ticktorium" for the propagation of a colony of infected *Ornithodoros turicata. J. Parasitol.* 26:201–206.

———. 1942. The serology of the relapse phenomenon in relapsing fever. Publication 18, pp. 58–66. Amer. Assn. Adv. Sci.

———. 1952. Treatment of relapsing fever with antibiotics. *Ann. N.Y. Acad. Sci.* 55(Art. 6):1209–1221.

Schuhardt, V. T., and B. E. O'Bryan. 1944. Relationship of penicillin therapy to brain involvement in experimental relapsing fever. *Science* 100:550–552.

———. 1945. Effect of intracranial penicillin therapy on brain involvement in experimental relapsing fever. *J. Bacteriol.* 49:312–313.

Schuhardt, V. T., and M. Wilkerson. 1951. Relapse phenomena in rats infected with single spirochetes (*Borrelia recurrentis* var. *turicatae*). *J. Bacteriol.* 61:299–303.

Weller, B., and M. G. Graham. 1930. Relapsing fever in Central Texas. *J. Amer. Med. Ass.* 95:1834.

31

Spotted Fever

Arthropod-borne rickettsioses occur in animals and humans worldwide (Ormsbee 1969). However, different rickettsia species may be restricted to certain geographical areas. Table 31-1 lists the major arthropod-borne human rickettsioses, their etiological agents, and their arthropod vectors. Although Q fever (see Chapter 19) is a rickettsial disease and can be transmitted from animal to animal by ticks, the etiological agent — *Coxiella burneti* — and its human epidemiology differ sufficiently to justify exclusion from the rickettsioses of Table 31-1. The spotted fever group of tick-borne rickettsioses are transmitted by the bite of hard-shelled, ixodid ticks (*Dermacentor andersoni* and others)—not by the soft-shelled ticks (*Ornithodoros* species) involved in the transmission of relapsing fever. Moreover, only the tick-borne and mite-borne rickettsioses are passed transovarially from the infected adult female to the larval progeny. Of all the tick-borne rickettsioses, we will discuss only the spotted fever of the Rocky Mountain type.

HISTORY, ETIOLOGY, AND EPIDEMIOLOGY

Probably the first cases of spotted fever of the Rocky Mountain type (spotted fever RMT) were described by Idaho physicians along the Snake River as "black measles." At the turn of the century, E. E. Maxey described a serious febrile disease in Montana which he called spotted fever and which "blotched the skin red-purple-black." The exanthem appeared first on the forehead and extremities (including soles of feet and palms of hands) and spread rapidly to the rest of the body. The disease became so serious in the Bitter Root Valley near Hamilton, Montana, that H. T. Ricketts, from the University of Chicago, was sent there in 1906 for an in-depth study. During the next 4 years he was able to infect guinea pigs and monkeys that were inoculated with blood from patients. He demonstrated the transmission of the infection from animal to animal by the ixodid tick *Dermacentor andersoni* (see Figure 31-1). He observed tiny

Table 31-1. Arthropod-borne rickettsial diseases of humans.

Disease	Etiological Agent	Vector
Spotted fever group		
Rocky Mountain type	R. rickettsii	Ixodid ticks
Boutonneuse fever	R. conorii	Ixodid ticks
S. African tick typhus	R. conorii	Ixodid ticks
Indian tick typhus	R. conorii	Ixodid ticks
Siberian tick typhus	R. siberica	Ixodid ticks
Queensland tick typhus	R. australis	Ixodid ticks
Typhus fever		
Epidemic typhus	R. prowazeki	Pediculus humanus (body louse)
Endemic (murine) typhus	R. typhi (mooseri)	Xenopsylla cheopis (rat fleas)
Scrub typhus	R. tsutsugamushi	Trombiculid mites
Rickettsialpox	R. akari	A. sanguineus (mite)

bacterialike organisms in infected tick tissues, but he could not culture them on laboratory media. He noted that the organisms were passed transovarially from infected adult female ticks to a percentage of the progeny. Also he and Wilder demonstrated, by cross-immunity tests, that the clinically similar diseases, spotted fever (RMT) and typhus fever, were etiologically distinct entities. After Ricketts died of an accidental typhus fever infection in Mexico, H. Da Rocha-Lima proposed the genus designation *Rickettsia* for the causative organisms of both spotted fever (RMT) and typhus. As indicated in Table 31-1, the former organisms are now designated *Rickettsia rickettsii.*

Other workers demonstrated the transmission of spotted fever (RMT) from a tick removed from a patient to a human volunteer. The situation continued to be so serious in the Bitter Root Valley area that the U.S. Public Health Service established a national laboratory in Hamilton, Montana, primarily to study the disease. Spencer and Parker (1930) made the significant discovery that ticks collected in the springtime on flannel cloths dragged over the landscape failed to infect guinea pigs. However, ticks collected at the same time from goats, after a blood meal, infected and killed these experimental animals. Also after a blood meal, the cloth-collected ticks became capable of transmitting fatal infections to the experimental animals. Thus the virulence of the rickettsiae in the ticks was lost during the winter hibernation but was restored by a blood meal. They also noted that juice extracted from the cloth-collected ticks, after treatment with phenol, would immunize guinea pigs against a challenge with virulent *R. rickettsii*. This provided a means of immunizing research workers at the laboratory. The reactivation of the rickettsial virulence after a blood meal emphasized the importance of removing attached ticks from the human body as soon as possible after attachment, hopefully to prevent infection. Herald Cox (1938; 1941), while working at the Hamilton laboratory, demonstrated the susceptibility of the yolk-sac tissues of the chick embryo to *R. rickettsii* and thereby provided a better source of the organisms for vaccine production.

Although the disease (recognized human cases) appears to have originated in the Rocky Mountains, it is now known to occur in most, if

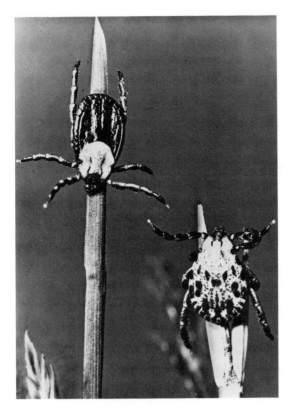

Figure 31–1. Ticks of the species *Dermacentor andersoni* in typical questing positions. Left—female; right—male. (Courtesy of W. Burgdorfer.)

not all, of the continental United States. Currently there are many more cases east of the Rocky Mountains than in the Rocky Mountain states. In 1975, for example, only 10 of the 844 cases of spotted fever (RMT) reported to the CDC occurred in the mountains of the western United States (see Figure 31-2). This is the reason why recommendations have been made to change the name of the disease from Rocky Mountain spotted fever to spotted fever of the Rocky Mountain type.

Whereas both *R. rickettsii* of spotted fever (RMT) and the rickettsiae of typhus fever are intracellular parasites, the former (but not the latter) are found to invade and multiply in the nuclei of the host cells. The typhus fever rickettsiae are found only in the cytoplasm of such cells. *Rickettsia rickettsii* tends to show considerable pleomorphism in infected cells, ranging

from coccoid or diplococcoid to single or paired bacillary forms or short to long chain or filamentous forms. Figure 31-3 shows rickettsiae in the nucleus of a host cell. Whereas spotted fever (RMT) appears to be restricted to North America, other tick-borne rickettsioses are found in other geographical areas of the world.

Spotted fever (RMT) is one of the few serious diseases that has shown a continuously rising incidence in the United States since 1960 (see Figure 31-4). The 844 cases reported in this country in 1975 constitute the highest annual incidence of the disease since before 1950.

CLINICAL SYMPTOMS

After a history of tick bite (in about 80 percent of cases), the incubation period in spotted fever (RMT) varies from 3 to 12 days (average 7). Sudden onset symptoms include severe headache, hard chills, prostration, muscle pains (especially in the back and legs), and fever that frequently reaches 103–104°F within 2 days. In severe cases the fever lasts (with morning partial remissions) for 15 to 20 days. A rash occurs in practically all cases beginning on about the fourth day of fever. The rash appears first on the forehead, wrists, and ankles, extending to the palms and soles. After 6 to 12 hours this exanthem spreads centripetally to all portions of the body. The rash may commence as macular to maculopapular and may persist as petechial (purple spots) in some cases. In severe cases it may change rapidly from macular to purpuric— large reddish-purple to black blotches—over much of the body (see Figure 31-5). Mild to moderately severe cases usually recover within 2 weeks with rapid convalescence. In fatal cases, death usually occurs during the second week. Prior to antibiotic therapy, the overall mortality rate was 20 percent with higher rates (50 + percent) in persons over 40 years of age and lower rates in children. Broad-spectrum antibiotic (chloramphenicol and the tetracyclines) therapy, early in the infection, will prevent most fatalities.

During the early stages of the disease there is a rickettsiemia, with invasion of the endothe-

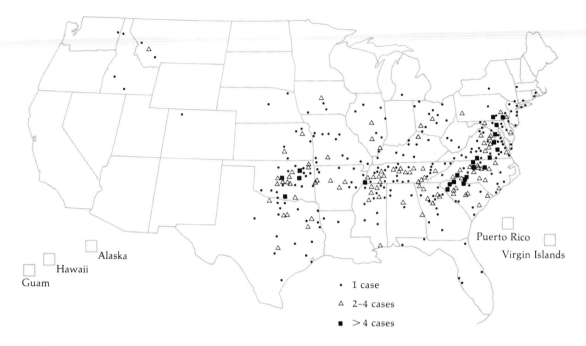

Figure 31–2. Distribution of the 844 cases of spotted fever of the Rocky Mountain type (RMT) reported to CDC during 1975. (From *MMWR* Annual Supplement, August 1976.)

lial cells lining the blood vessels. The rupture of blood capillaries in the skin gives rise to the rash. Thrombosis of larger blood vessels of an extremity may result in gangrene in that area. Pneumonitis may develop, either as an extension of the rickettsiae to lung tissue or as a bacterial complication. Other clinical manifestations are low blood pressure (hypotension), peripheral vascular failure, cyanosis (blue skin due to lack of oxygen), and renal failure.

LABORATORY DIAGNOSIS

The difficulties and danger of working with most rickettsiae preclude attempts at isolation of these organisms into animals or embryonated eggs by personnel in the average clinical laboratory. If such isolations are deemed important, blood samples collected during the early febrile period may be sent to a reference laboratory through the office of the local city or state department of health. For a comprehensive discussion of laboratory diagnostic methods in rickettsioses see Ormsbee (1974).

Guinea pigs, chick embryos (yolk sac), or certain tissue cultures are the animal hosts of choice for the inoculation of a blood specimen to demonstrate the presence of *R. rickettsii.* In the male guinea pig the rickettsiae invade the testicles and recognizable pathological changes in the scrotal tissue provide evidence of infection. Likewise inoculation of the patient's blood into the yolk sac of an embryonated egg results in rickettsial infection of the cells lining the yolk sac. Smears of the infected tissues of the guinea pig or yolk sac can be fixed and stained with polychrome (Giemsa or Giménez) stains for the microscopic demonstration of the presence of morphologically typical rickettsiae and their characteristic intranuclear distribution in the infected cells (see Figure J on the back cover). If specific, fluorescent anti–*R. rickettsii* antiserum is available, the infected tissue smears may be diagnosed by the direct FA technique. Rickettsiae in infected tick tissues can also be demonstrated by these stained smear techniques. The specific anti–*R. rickettsii* antiserum may be obtained from patients who have recovered from spotted fever (RMT) or from rabbits immunized with killed *R. rickettsii* from infected yolk-sac tissues or tissue cultures. A highly specific soluble antigen can be obtained by ether extraction of *R. rickettsii*. This has been advocated for use in complement fixation tests. Again it should be emphasized that these are procedures for reference laboratories, not for inexperienced clinical laboratory personnel.

Serodiagnostic procedures for rickettsioses, however, are available to the average clinical laboratory in the form of the Weil-Felix test. These authors demonstrated that the sera of patients suffering from epidemic or endemic typhus fever or spotted fever (RMT) would agglutinate a suspension of a nonmotile (O) strain of *Proteus* X-19. This nonpathogenic, common intestinal bacterium can be grown on simple culture media to provide a serodiagnostic agglutination test antigen. As in all serodiagnostic tests, a rising antibody titer in paired (early and 7 to 10 days later) blood serum specimens is more significant than the titer of a single specimen. However, antibodies indicated by *Proteus* OX-19 are not as diagnostically specific as are those identified by reactions with *R. rickettsii* cell antigens. The latter antigens, however, may not be commercially available. See Table 32-1 for expected Weil-Felix test results in various human rickettsioses.

Figure 31–3. Rickettsiae in the nucleus of a cell from gut tissue of the tick *D. andersoni* following an experimental infection. In this case the species is *R. canada.* 18,000×. (Courtesy of W. Burgdorfer.)

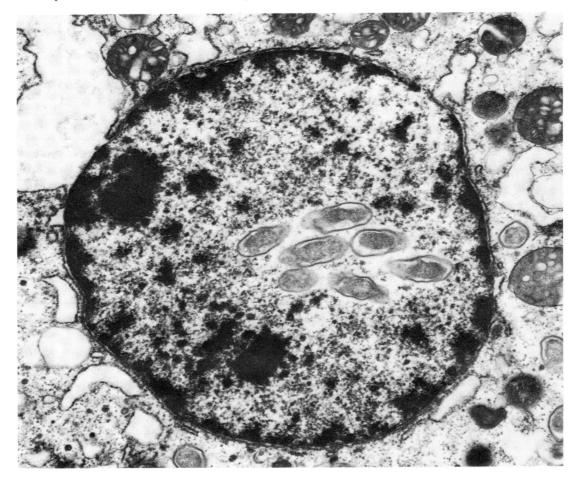

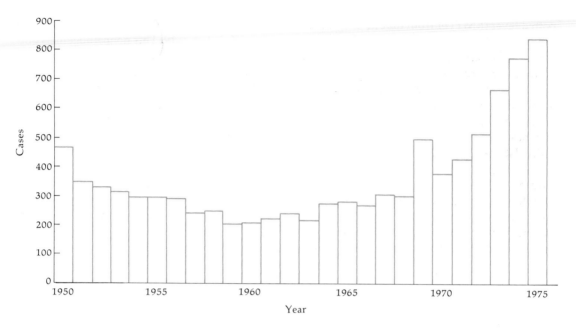

Figure 31–4. Annual cases of spotted fever (RMT) reported to CDC, 1950 through 1975. (From *MMWR* Annual Supplement, August 1976.)

IMMUNITY

Recovery from an attack of spotted fever (RMT) results in solid immunity in experimental animals and apparently in human cases. The Cox vaccine prepared from killed suspensions of *R. rickettsii* from infected yolk-sac tissues of chick embryos has been used extensively for the immunization of high-risk personnel: research and reference laboratory workers, field research workers, and persons who live in or frequent rural areas of known endemicity. Since accidental infections in immunized personnel of research laboratories have been reported, there is justification for continuing efforts to develop better immunogens for this disease. In this regard the report of Kenyon and Pedersen (1975) might be a move in this direction. These workers described an *in vitro,* chick-embryo tissue culture technique for the propagation of *R. rickettsii* and methods for obtaining highly purified suspensions of these organisms. After killing the suspended *R. rickettsii* with formalin, the resulting vaccine was tested for immunogenicity in guinea pigs. The results were claimed to be superior to comparable tests using the yolk-sac-propagated vaccine. Kenyon and Pedersen plan to test their vaccine on monkeys and, if results justify, on human beings. Because of the low incidence of the disease, however, proof of efficacy of their vaccine in human beings will be the most difficult aspect of their problem. There is no evidence of immunotherapeutic efficacy of antirickettsial antiserum in spotted fever (RMT).

CONTROL AND PREVENTION

Tick control measures in large rural areas are either impractical, impossible, or ecologically detrimental. The only hope for preventing spotted fever (RMT) and other tick-borne rickettsioses is active immunoprophylaxis, particularly in high-risk personnel. Since the *R. rickettsii* in an infected tick may be avirulent prior to a blood meal, however, persons in endemic areas are advised to search for and remove attached ticks at least once daily.

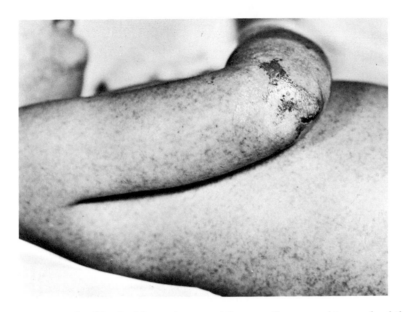

Figure 31–5. Severe rash of Rocky Mountain spotted fever on the arm and torso of a child. A large purpuric region is visible on the elbow. (Courtesy of T. E. Woodward.)

REFERENCES

Cox, H. R. 1938. Use of the yolk sac of the developing chick embryo as a medium for growing rickettsiae of Rocky Mountain spotted fever and typhus groups. *Pub. Health. Rep.* 53:7241–7247.

———. 1941. Cultivation of rickettsiae of the Rocky Mountain spotted fever, typhus, and Q fever groups in the embryonic tissue of developing chicks. *Science* 94:399–403.

Kenyon, R. H., and C. E. Pedersen, Jr. 1975. Preparation of Rocky Mountain spotted fever vaccine suitable for human immunization. *J. Clin. Microbiol.* 1:500–503.

Ormsbee, R. A. 1969. Rickettsiae (as organisms). *Ann. Rev. Microbiol.* 23:275–292.

———. 1974. Rickettsiae. Chapter 88 in *Manual of Clinical Microbiology.*

Spencer, R. R., and R. R. Parker. 1930. Studies on Rocky Mountain spotted fever. *Pub. Hlth. Serv. Hyg. Lab. Bull.* 154. Washington: Governmental Printing Office.

Weiss, E. 1973. Growth and physiology of rickettsiae. *Bacteriol. Rev.* 37:259–283.

Woodward, T. E., and E. B. Jackson. 1965. Spotted fever rickettsiae. Chapter 50 in *Viral and Rickettsial Infections in Man.*

32

Louse-Borne and Flea-Borne Typhus Fevers and Mite-Borne Rickettsioses

TYPHUS FEVERS

As indicated in Table 31-1, a number of different arthropod-borne rickettsial diseases have been designated "typhus." Two (louse-borne and flea-borne typhus) are generally accepted as members of the typhus fever group of human rickettsioses. A third member of this group—Brill's or Brill-Zinsser disease, or recrudescent typhus (see Brill 1910)—is etiologically the same as louse-borne (epidemic) typhus, however. It occurs apparently as a relapse in occasional individuals, years after symptomatic recovery from the primary attack of epidemic typhus fever. Also, as indicated in Table 31-1, epidemic typhus fever is transmitted from human to human by the body louse *Pediculus humanus* (see Ricketts and Wilder 1910), whereas endemic (murine) typhus fever is transmitted from rat to rat by a variety of rat fleas and from rat to humans by the rat flea *Xenopsylla cheopis*. Since P.

humanus feeds only on human blood, research involving the use of this vector necessitates feeding the lice on either the researcher or other human volunteers. If infected lice are involved, this feeding is dangerous because the lice defecate while feeding and rickettsiae are present in the feces. The rickettsiae can then invade the bite wound. To resolve these research problems, Haddon (1956) devised a method of feeding the lice on human blood through an artificial membrane.

The term *typhus* (derived from the Greek word for smoky or hazy) tends to describe the mental state of the patient during the disease. As indicated in Chapter 24 the clinical symptoms of typhus and typhoid fevers during the first week or two cannot be distinguished. As a consequence the former disease, frequently in the past, was designated typhus exanthématique (pertaining to the skin rash) whereas typhoid fever was designated typhus abdominalis. The

Table 32-1. Proteus OX strain agglutination test reactions in different human rickettsioses.

Disease	OX-19	OX-2	OX-K
Spotted fever (RMT)	+ to 4+	+ to 3+	0
Epidemic typhus	4+	+	0
Murine typhus	4+	+	0
Brill-Zinsser typhus	(+, 0)	(+, 0)	0
Scrub typhus (mite-borne)	0	0	(3+)
Rickettsialpox (mite-borne)	0	0	0
Q fever	0	0	0

( ) = Variable results encountered. Approximately 50 percent of scrub typhus patients are positive.

0 = Negative.

+ to 4+ = Degrees of reactivity with different sera.

early clinical symptoms of typhus fever also can be confused with a variety of other infectious diseases.

Hans Zinsser (1935) wrote a natural history of typhus fever entitled *Rats, Lice, and History*. In this he indicated the difficulty of tracing the genealogy of a disease under its various historical designations and clinical descriptions. He also introduced the evolutionary concept of host-parasite mutual toleration correlated with the time of association. He noted, for example, that rat fleas rarely, if ever, show ill effects resulting from their typhus rickettsial infections. This led Zinsser to conclude that this infection originated and persisted for evolutionary time as a flea-to-flea rickettsiosis. After the flea became ectoparasitic on rats, the flea-borne rickettsiae adapted to the rat tissues. The rat shows relatively minor symptoms resulting from its rickettsial infection, which led Zinsser to conclude that the rat was the second host in these evolutionary host-parasite adaptations. Only when certain of the rat fleas chose to ectoparasitize humans were the typhus rickettsiae first transmitted to the human host. Human typhus frequently is a severe to fatal disease. And only after humans became a host to typhus rickettsiae could the body louse become a host to these rickettsiae, because the lice feed only on humans. The body louse invariably dies as a result of its infection, indicating that the louse-rickettsial association has not persisted long enough in evolutionary time for a mutual tolerance between host and parasite to have developed.

Zinsser also discussed the influence of typhus fever upon human history. Epidemic typhus fever has exerted a marked impact, particularly upon the history of military operations prior to the 1940s. The siege of Granada in 1489, for example, was terminated as a result of an estimated 17,000 deaths from typhus exanthèmatique in the Spanish army. Also, an estimated 30,000 deaths from typhus fever in the French army forced the lifting of the siege of Naples, in 1528, at the point of an otherwise decisive victory. The disaster that befell Napoleon's army of half a million men in 1812 was attributed in part to typhus fever. During World War I, campaigning in the Balkans was immobilized by typhus fever. In less than 6 months more than 150,000 Serbians were reported to have died of the disease. Moreover, from 1912 to 1922 an estimated 30 million cases and 3 million deaths from typhus fever were reported in Russia. During World War II typhus fever epidemics occurred in North Africa and Italy. When the allies invaded Italy, an epidemic was in progress in Naples. Although the allied soldiers had been immunized against typhus, their bodies and clothing and those of the entire civilian population were deloused by dusting with the persistent insecticide DDT. Thereby, for the first time in the history of warfare, the progress of an epidemic of typhus fever was stopped with a minimal loss of life and no serious effect on the military operation. For additional details see Snyder (1965).

Etiology and Epidemiology

The etiological agent of epidemic typhus fever (and Brill-Zinsser disease) is *Rickettssia prowazeki*, named after H. T. Ricketts and S. von Prowazek, both of whom died of accidental infections during their studies of the disease. The etiological agent of endemic (murine) typhus, according to *Bergey's Manual*, is *Rickettsia typhi*. However, many texts continue to list the agent by its former designation, *R. mooseri*.

Rickettsia prowazeki and *R. typhi* are closely related taxonomically. Both share certain antigens, one of which stimulates the production of antibodies, in human patients, which react with a carbohydrate antigen of *Proteus* OX-19 in the Weil-Felix test (see Table 32-1). Both species of typhus rickettsiae produce similar symptoms in patients, although the epidemic form of the disease generally is more severe and produces a significantly higher mortality rate. This greater virulence of *R. prowazeki* might be the result of the rapid homologous-animal passage (human→human) of the louse-borne rickettsiae during an epidemic. Both species produce hemolysis of certain red blood cells and both produce toxic factors for experimental animals (see Cox 1953). These toxic factors can be neutralized by antisera, but the two have been reported to be immunologically distinct. This and the fact that the two *Rickettsia* do not stimulate cross-immunities in experimental animals constitute two of the few taxonomic differentials of *R. prowazeki* and *R. typhi*.

Usually the distinction between the two types of typhus fever (epidemic and murine) is based upon the epidemiological features illustrated in Figure 32-1. Thus in a human environment of heavy louse infestation one can expect an outbreak of typhus fever to be epidemic in nature, to be caused by *R. prowazeki*, and to yield a potentially high mortality rate. If there is little or no louse infestation in the human population but rats are prevalent, intermittent (endemic) human cases might be expected to occur and to be caused by *R. typhi* and to yield a low (less than 2 percent) mortality rate. The endemic type of the disease usually is self-limiting, and complete recovery of most cases occurs in 15 days or less.

Figure 32–1.   Diagrammatic summary of the epidemiology of epidemic and endemic typhus fever.

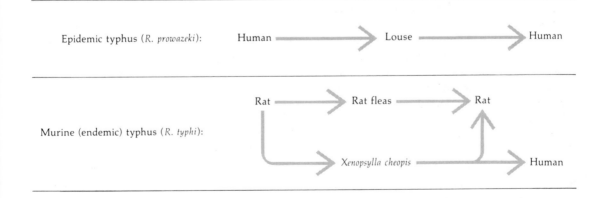

Bozeman et al. (1975) reported the isolation of *R. prowazeki* from flying squirrels captured in Virginia and in Florida. The sera of noninfected squirrels also had antibody specific for these rickettsiae. The epidemiological significance, if any, of this discovery is under investigation.

An example of the endemic status of murine typhus was observed by Dr. G. W. McCoy and the author when we were surveying the prevalence of typhus in south central Texas in the 1930s. In one town, the disease was designated banker's disease because during the preceding few years a number of cases had occurred in the personnel of the local bank. Upon investigation we noted that the bank was located adjacent to a rat-infested feed and grain warehouse. Obviously some of the rat fleas had moved in and fed on the bankers. Moreover, a couple of the warehouse personnel reported having had undiagnosed disease symptoms in the past that could have been due to typhus fever.

Another experience on this trip represents a good example of the old adage—"Ignorance is bliss." One doctor we contacted was greatly agitated by the fact that a colleague in a nearby community had not learned to use the Weil-Felix test to make a differential diagnosis between typhus and typhoid fevers. On the basis of first-week clinical symptoms, the colleague diagnosed all his cases as typhoid fever. Since murine typhus was more prevalent in the area than typhoid, and since even untreated patients recovered from typhus within 2 weeks, the ignorant colleague was making quite a reputation as the physician to see for typhoid therapy. The knowledgeable doctor made the differential diagnosis, and he could not "cure" his cases of typhoid in 2 weeks.

The human body louse, after infection with *R. prowazeki* during a blood meal from a human case of typhus, dies within 1 to 2 weeks; the rat flea, however, infected with *R. typhi* following a blood meal from an infected rat, suffers no ill effects and continues to discharge rickettsiae in its feces during the remainder of its life. Since the rat fleas generally prefer to feed on rats, and since only one species (*Xenopsylla cheopis*) will feed on humans, in the absence of an available rat host, the murine typhus tends to persist as a smouldering, endemic human disease in the area of infected rat infestation.

Clinical Symptoms

As indicated in Chapter 31, the clinical symptoms and severity of epidemic typhus and spotted fever (RMT) are similar. In contrast to spotted fever (RMT), however, the rash of typhus fever appears first on the trunk and then extends to the extremities, but very rarely to the soles of the feet or palms of the hands. Again, except for the severity and mortality rate of epidemic typhus, it and murine (endemic) typhus share almost identical clinical symptoms. After an incubation period of 10 to 14 days, onset usually is abrupt with chilly sensations, weakness, headache, and generalized aches and pains. For the first 2 or 3 days the fever fluctuates with a stepwise rise to 102°F (30°C) to 105°F (41°C) after which it remains high until death (which usually occurs during the second week) or recovery. The uncontrollable headache increases in intensity, as do the muscular pains in the back and legs. Usually between the fourth and seventh day of typhus fever a macular or maculopapular rash appears on the trunk of the patient and during the next day or two spreads to the remainder of the body. During the second week the skin rash may become reddish to reddish-purple or, in severe cases, it may become hemorrhagic. Early in the infection the patient might experience ringing in the ears and in severe cases this may be followed by apparent deafness. The patient frequently shows signs of mental dullness that may progress to apathy or stupor. These symptoms may be interrupted by brief periods of delirium. The symptoms, in those who recover, ameliorate rapidly during or before the third week, with little or no lasting effect.

Laboratory Diagnosis

As indicated in Chapter 31, attempts to demonstrate the presence of *Rickettsia* in a clinical laboratory specimen by inoculation into animals, chick embryos, or tissue cultures should be assigned to reference laboratories with personnel familiar with the dangers involved and specialists in these procedures. For details for submitting specimens and performing tests for this purpose see Ormsbee (1974).

In general, the specimen for suspected typhus fever (usually blood) should be collected early in the febrile stage and either be inoculated within 30 minutes after collection or be quick-frozen in an alcohol-dry ice mixture and packed in sufficient dry ice to maintain the temperature at −70°C for at least 24 hours beyond the expected time of arrival of the specimen at the reference laboratory. The personnel of the reference laboratory should be notified by telephone at the time of shipment and the expected time of arrival of the specimen. The reference laboratory can be expected to have fluorescent antisera for direct FA test identification of the various species of Rickettsia that might be found in the inoculated animal tissues. The reference laboratory will also have known Rickettsia species antigens for serological agglutination, complement fixation, or indirect FA tests to demonstrate specific antibody in patients' sera.

As indicated for spotted fever (RMT), the average clinical laboratory personnel can undertake serodiagnostic (Weil-Felix test) procedures on paired sera (early and late) from the patient using the Proteus OX-19 and related Proteus antigens (OX-2 and OX-K). Table 32-1 lists the relative degrees (titers) of the Weil-Felix agglutination test results expected when sera from different rickettsioses are tested against the three different Proteus antigens. Patients not infected with either epidemic or endemic typhus may demonstrate the presence of serum agglutinins for Proteus OX-19. The agglutinin titers in the paired sera of such patients, however, can be expected to remain stationary rather than showing a significant rise. Some patients with typhus fever may fail to develop Weil-Felix agglutinins prior to the time of death or recovery. Unfortunately the Weil-Felix test usually is the only laboratory aid available to the clinician in attempting to arrive at a differential diagnosis of typhus fever and other infectious diseases including other rickettsioses. Frequently assistance from a rickettsiosis reference laboratory is needed. To obtain this assistance one should consult the state or local public health laboratory for directions.

Control and Prevention

The best preventive measure for epidemic typhus is the elimination of infestation by the human body louse (see Ormsbee 1973). Since the discovery of DDT and other persistent insecticides, this elimination has been accomplished in practically all industrialized nations. Hurlbut et al. (1954) reported DDT-resistant body lice in Egypt, however. When louse infestation is known to be prevalent and DDT and other louse control measures are not immediately available, persons required to enter or live in such environments should be immunized with the Cox-type typhus vaccine (see Cox 1948). Such immunization should also be practiced on special-risk personnel such as typhus research or reference laboratory workers. The Cox-type typhus vaccine is composed of killed R. prowazeki that have been propagated in and extracted from yolk-sac membranes of chick embryos. Millions of doses of this vaccine were administered to armed forces personnel during the early years of World War II. Although the vaccine-induced immunity did not always prevent contracting typhus, it lowered the severity of the disease and prevented serious complications and fatal outcome in those infected.

In view of the incomplete immunization accomplished with the Cox-type vaccine, further research on R. prowazeki immunogens is warranted. Some progress has been made using a spontaneous avirulent mutant of R. prowazeki (designated strain E) that was isolated in Spain during chick embryo yolk-sac passage of the virulent parent strain. As in all live-organism immunogens, the fear of their possible reverse mutation (back to virulence) tends to delay their general acceptance. The principle of live-organism vaccines is well established, however, and generally they tend to stimulate a more solid immunity with small doses than do the killed-organism vaccines.

Although R. prowazeki and R. typhi share certain antigens, these are not mutually immunogenic. The relatively low incidence and severity of murine (endemic) typhus makes immunization against this form of typhus of little consequence, however. For control of murine typhus, see the rat and rat-flea control measures described for bubonic plague in Chapter 29.

Typhus fevers, like other rickettsioses, respond to early chemotherapy with broad-spectrum antibiotics (chloramphenicol and the tetracyclines). In some instances, however, there is a tendency for the patient to relapse after antibiotic treatment unless the therapy is continued beyond the first week. This is particularly true for scrub typhus. In these instances there is indication that the cure of the infection involves a rickettsiostatic, but not a rickettsiocidal, reaction to the antibiotic. This rickettsiostatic suppression, if maintained, is followed by an immune reaction that results in lasting cure of the infection. If the antibiotic therapy is terminated too soon (1 week or less), the surviving rickettsiae are able to multiply and produce the symptomatic relapse after antibiotic therapy.

MITE-BORNE RICKETTSIOSES: RICKETTSIALPOX

There are two mite-borne rickettsioses: rickettsialpox and scrub typhus (tsutsugamushi disease).

Rickettsialpox is caused by *Rickettsia akari*, which shares some antigenicity with *R. rickettsii* and other members of the spotted fever group but does not stimulate the production of Weil-Felix–type antibodies. Also, in contrast to the spotted fevers, rickettsialpox mortality is practically nil. The usual animal host of *R. akari* is the common house mouse, *Mus musculus*, and is transmitted from mouse to mouse and from mouse to humans by the mite *Allodermanyssus sanguineus*. As previously indicated the rickettsial infection is passed transovarially from infected adult female mites to the larvae.

The first known cases of rickettsialpox were reported in New York City. Other cases were reported from urban areas along the Atlantic coast of the United States and from urban areas in Russia. However, the isolation of *R. akari* from wild rodents in Korea and serological evidence

from rural rickettsioses in Africa indicate the possibility of a rural form of the disease that differs from the urban epidemiology in the USA and the USSR.

A prominent symptom of rickettsialpox is a skin lesion (*eschar*) at the site of attachment of the infecting mite. The eschar begins as a firm red papule that after a few days develops vesicles similar to those in chickenpox. The eschar then ulcerates and is covered with a black scab. Fever, headache, backache, and muscle pains usually commence suddenly. A vesiculated skin eruption may develop along with or following the onset of the febrile symptoms. After about a week, the vesicles dry and form scabs that fall off without leaving scars. The clinical symptoms generally are mild and patients recover within 1 to 2 weeks without treatment and with no sequelae.

SCRUB TYPHUS

Etiology and Epidemiology

Scrub typhus (tsutsugamushi, Japanese river fever, mite-borne, rural, or tropical typhus) was first reported in Japan, where human cases frequently followed river flooding that forced wild rodents and other small mammals, with their associated mite parasites, into close association with human habitation. The disease is caused by *Rickettsia tsutsugamushi (R. orientalis)*, and evidence indicates that the rickettsiae are transmitted from infected animal hosts to the larval stage of trombiculid mites (*Trombicula akamushi* and other species). The six-legged larvum is the only *ectoparasitic* stage of the life cycle of the mites. The rickettsiae in the infected larvae persist in the nonparasitic nymphal and adult (eight-legged) stages of the mite. They then pass transovarially from adult females to new larval progeny. Such infected larvae then can infect other rodents and humans during their ectoparasitic feeding. Thus the mite serves as the transmitting vector only in the transovarially infected larval stage. However, along with infected rodents and other small mammals, the infected (but not parasitic) nymphal and adult mites serve as reservoirs of *R. tsutsugamushi* infection in nature. Some authorities disagree with certain aspects of this host-vector-parasite concept of the epidemiology of scrub typhus, but this author is unaware of any generally accepted alternative proposal.

Scrub typhus, by any of its variety of names, is endemic and subject to localized epidemics in a large geographical area bounded by Japan and Korea in the far east, Southern China, Indochina, Bangladesh, and India on the north and west, and by northern Australia on the south. The disease is also found in the Philippines, Malaysia, Indonesia, and the Pacific islands within this large triangular area. As indicated by the names of the disease, the reservoir hosts tend to occupy brushy, scrub, or grassy vegetation in rural areas, particularly along streams or around marshy areas. During World War II scrub typhus posed a serious problem to both the Japanese and the allied armies operating in the Southwest Pacific and the India-Burma-China areas of endemicity.

The virulence of *R. tsutsugamushi* varies considerably. In different epidemic outbreaks the reported mortality rates have varied from a low of 0.6 percent to a high of 60 percent. Comparable strain variations in virulence can be demonstrated experimentally in mice. Moreover, isolated strains of *R. tsutsugamushi* demonstrate a marked degree of antigenic heterogeneity even within small localized areas of endemicity. This antigenic heterogeneity undoubtedly accounts for the frequency of second attacks of scrub typhus and for the failure to develop successful vaccines for this disease.

Clinical Symptoms

Following an incubation period averaging 10 to 12 days, onset symptoms of severe scrub typhus occur suddenly. These consist of chilliness followed by fever that progresses to 104 or 105°F, severe headache, inflamed eyes, and localized or generalized lymphadenitis. A majority of Caucasians develop a skin lesion (the eschar) at the site of infection by the larval mite. This eschar begins as an indurated area about 1 centimeter in diameter that develops a multilocular vesicle comparable to the eschar in rickettsialpox. After ulceration the eschar develops a black scab followed by lymphadenopathy in the regional lymph nodes. A macular rash appears on the trunk after the fifth day of fever and may extend to the extremities or it may disappear after a few hours to several days. Cough and other evidence of lung involvement may develop. Apathy, stupor, muscular twitching, and other signs of central nervous system involvement may develop. Low systolic blood pressure is a common symptom in severe cases. If the untreated patient is to recover, the temperature falls gradually toward the end of the second week. Convalescence in the untreated patient may be more prolonged than is the case in epidemic or endemic typhus described in the first part of this chapter. Death due to scrub typhus usually occurs toward the end of the second week and may be caused by complicating bacterial pneumonia, circulatory failure, or central nervous system involvement. Broad-spectrum antibiotic therapy begun early in the course of the disease will prevent most fatalities.

Laboratory Diagnosis

Although *R. tsutsugamushi* can be demonstrated in tissue smears after inoculation into mice or the chick-embryo yolk sac, their identification even by competent reference laboratory personnel is rendered difficult by the extent of the antigenic heterogeneity of the isolates. Certainly this is no job for the average clinical laboratory. As indicated in Table 32-1, however, about 50 percent of scrub typhus patients will develop significant Weil-Felix test agglutinin titers for *Proteus* OX-K antigen, but not for *Proteus* OX-19 or OX-2. Again paired sera should be tested to demonstrate a significant (threefold or fourfold) rise in antibody titer.

Control and Prevention

Although miticidal and wild-rodent control measures were developed and proved successful in military operations during World War II in the Southwest Pacific, these measures are impractical insofar as civilian control of the disease is concerned. The fact that a successful vaccine has not been developed makes prevention of the disease, even in high-risk personnel, practically impossible. Moreover, the fact that visitors to the endemic areas of scrub typhus and other foreign rickettsioses can, after infection, travel by air to any part of the world during the incubation period makes it important that clinicians and laboratory personnel in nonendemic areas be prepared to recognize symptoms, diagnose, and treat individual cases of these diseases.

REFERENCES

Bozeman, F. M., S. A. Masiello, M. S. Williams, and B. L. Elisberg. 1975. Epidemic typhus rickettsiae isolated from flying squirrels. *Nature* 255: 545–547.

Brill, N. E. 1910. An acute infectious disease of unknown origin. A clinical study based on 221 cases. *Amer. J. Med. Sci.* 139:484–502.

Buchanan, R. E., and N. E. Gibbons. 1974. *Bergey's Manual of Determinative Bacteriology.* 8th ed. Baltimore: Williams & Wilkins.

Cox, H. R. 1948. Method for the preparation and standardization of rickettsial vaccines. *Symposium on Rickettsial Diseases.* Boston: Amer. Assn. Adv. Sci.

———. 1953. Viral and rickettsial toxins. *Ann. Rev. Microbiol.* 7:197–218.

Haddon, W., Jr. 1956. The maintenance of the human body louse *Pediculus humanus corporis* through complete cycles of growth by serial feeding through artifical membranes. *Amer. J. Trop. Med.* 5:326–330.

Hurlbut, H. S., R. L. Peffly, and A. A. Salah. 1954. DDT resistance in Egyptian body lice. *Amer. J. Trop. Med.* 3:922–929.

Ormsbee, R. A. 1969. Rickettsiae (as organisms). *Ann. Rev. Microbiol.* 23:275–292.

———. 1973. The control of lice and louse-borne diseases. *Pan Am. Hlth. Org.* Publication 263: 104–109.

———. 1974. *Rickettsiae.* Chapter 88 in *Manual of Clinical Microbiology.*

Ricketts, H. T., and R. M. Wilder. 1910. The transmission of typhus fever of Mexico (tabardillo) by means of the louse *Pediculus vestamenti. J. Amer. Med. Ass.* 54:1304–1307.

Snyder, J. C. 1965. Typhus fever rickettsiae. Chapter 49 in *Viral and Rickettsial Infections in Man.*

Zinsser, H. 1935. *Rats, Lice, and History.* Boston: Little, Brown.

33

Arbovirus Encephalitides

Approximately 300 viruses have been proved to be transmissible by hemophagous arthropods. This fact justifies the epidemiological grouping of these viruses under the designation of arthropod-borne. It is common practice, moreover, to designate these viruses as arboviruses. As this large group of viruses has been studied more comprehensively by viral taxonomists, however, they have been found to include members of several virus groups—poxviruses, picornaviruses, rhabdoviruses, orbiviruses, arenaviruses, and others. And in addition to arthropod transmission, some of these viruses have been found capable of being transmitted by contact with infected animals or by the ingestion of milk from such animals. As indicated in Table 33-1, a number of the heretofore generally accepted arboviruses of antigenic groups A and B have been designated *togaviruses* (see Pfefferkorn and Shapiro 1974). Since this text is dedicated to the principle of grouping human diseases upon the basis of the adaptations of the etiological agents to modes of transmission from host to host, regardless of their taxonomic classification, we will continue to use the terms *arthropod-borne viruses* and *arbovirus diseases.* The reader will note that we do not use the term *arbovirus* as a genus designation and no species designations are indicated. Nevertheless, the group designation arbovirus diseases is firmly established in the medical literature.

The arboviruses are spherical, enveloped RNA viruses mostly ranging in size from 15 to 70 nanometers, with a few larger members ranging up to 120 nanometers in diameter (see Figure 33-1). The viruses can be propagated in neonatal mice, chick embryos, or tissue cultures. K. R. P. Singh in 1971 reported that tick-borne arboviruses grow best in tick cell cultures, whereas mosquito-borne viruses grow best in mosquito cell cultures. The arboviruses survive for long periods of time when properly frozen and stored at $-70°C$. They frequently cause mild or asymptomatic infections in wild animal hosts even though a persistent viremic stage

Table 33-1. Representative arbovirus diseases transmissible to human beings.

Disease	Antigenic Group	Vector	Major Animal Hosts
Encephalitides			
Eastern equine (EEE)*	A	Mosquito	Equines and birds
Western equine (WEE)*	A	Mosquito	Equines and birds
Venezuelan equine (VEE)*	A	Mosquito	Equines and birds
California (Cal E)	C	Mosquito	Mammals (mice etc.)
Japanese B (JBE)*	B	Mosquito	Birds and pigs
Murray Valley (MVE)	B	Mosquito	Birds
Saint Louis (SLE)*	B	Mosquito	Birds
Russian (SSE)†	B	Ticks	Goats‡
Nonencephalitic			
Colorado tick fever	Ungrouped	Ticks	Rodents
Louping ill	B	Ticks	Sheep
Omsk (HF)**	B	Ticks	—
Dengue fever*	B	Mosquito	—
Dengue (HF)**	B	Mosquito	—
Yellow fever (urban)	B	Mosquito	—
Yellow fever (jungle)	B	Mosquito	Monkeys
Bunyamwera fever	—	Mosquito	Mammals
Rift Valley fever	—	Mosquito	Domestic animals
Phlebotomus fever	—	Sand flies	—

*Togavirus (Pfefferkorn and Shapiro 1974).
†SSE = spring and summer encephalitis.
**HF = hemorrhagic fever.
‡May be transmitted to humans by drinking milk.

may be involved. However, certain of the equine encephalitides, yellow fever, hemorrhagic fevers, and other arbovirus diseases result in high mortality rates in animal and human hosts.

At least 37 antigenic groups of arboviruses have been reported, and other antigenic varieties are known that have not been grouped. There is extensive sharing of antigens both within and between antigenic groups. Specific antisera have been prepared for the serotaxonomic identification of many of the important arboviruses, however, particularly those known to cause human disease. Two of the major antigenic groups, A and B (see Table 33-1), include a number of arboviruses that are neurotropic and tend to cause encephalitis or meningoencephalitis in animal and human hosts. Others are pantropic and cause such human diseases as dengue (pronounced den-gay) fever, yellow fever, and hemorrhagic fevers. Many of the arboviruses possess antigens that cause hemagglutination (HA) of goose or embryonic chick erythrocytes. Other arboviruses cause hemagglutination of human red blood cells of any of the four blood groups—A, B, AB, and O. The relative HA activity, however, is A > AB > O

> B. These arboviruses can be identified by means of the HA-inhibition (HI) test using known specific antisera. Some arboviruses possess antigens that can be demonstrated best by the complement fixation test or by the fluorescein tagged antibody (FA) test. However, many virologists prefer the viral neutralization test using pretitrated dilutions of the unknown virus from infected infant mice and known specific antisera. Neutralization by the homologous antiserum can be demonstrated by inoculating the test mixtures intracerebrally into infant mice or by inoculation to susceptible tissue culture cells. Both positive and negative control mixtures should be included in any of these serotaxonomic tests.

For detailed considerations of the collection, storage, and shipment of clinical specimens and for the isolation and identification of arboviruses, see Shope (1974). Assistance in the laboratory diagnosis of arbovirus diseases in the United States may be obtained from two sources: the World Health Organization (WHO) Regional Reference Center for Arboviruses at the Vector-Borne Diseases Branch of the Center for Disease Control (CDC), P.O. Box 2087, Fort Collins, Colorado 80521; or the Yale Arbovirus Research Unit, 60 College Street, New Haven, Connecticut 06510. These laboratories do special diagnostic tests for the identification of presumed arboviral isolates or serodiagnostic tests on paired sera from patients. Because of the extensive serotype and biotype heterogeneity of the arboviruses, the frequent sharing of antigens, and the frequent similarity of the clinical symptoms in arbovirus diseases, such assistance is essential, particularly in the early cases of an outbreak of arboviral disease. For more details see Casals (1960), Casals and Reeves (1965), and Simpson (1972).

Encephalitis is the idiopathic designation for inflammatory pathology in the encephalon—the brain area within the cranium. This type of pathology can be caused by a variety of infectious organisms, some of which produce the encephalitis only as a complication of their usual systemic infections (for example: mumps, rubella, rubeola, influenza, chickenpox, and smallpox vaccination). In others, as indicated in Table 33-1, the CNS pathology can be caused as

Figure 33–1. Section of infected mouse brain showing spherical virions of California encephalitis virus. 30,000×. (Courtesy of F. A. Murphy.)

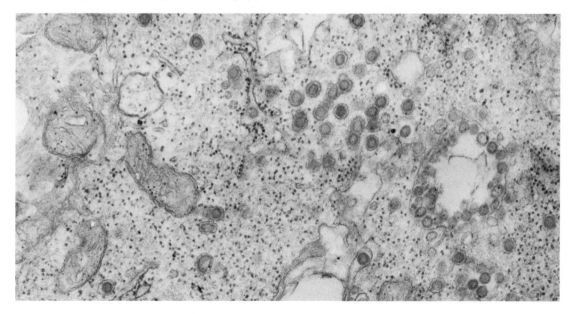

primary infections with neurotropic strains of arboviruses; other strains (pantropic) of these viruses tend to cause primary pathology in tissues other than those of the central nervous system. Since the human encephalitides tend to result in symptoms of drowsiness, stupor, or coma, they have been referred to as sleeping sickness. These viral encephalitides, however, must be distinguished from the protozoal (*Trypanosoma*) sleeping sickness of Africa. For a more comprehensive discussion of the encephalitides and other arbovirus diseases see Casals and Clarke (1965), Clarke and Casals (1965), and Simpson (1972).

ETIOLOGY AND EPIDEMIOLOGY

The morphological, antigenic, epidemiological, and other taxonomic characteristics of the more than 300 arboviruses have been studied extensively. These studies have not, however, resulted in a generally accepted taxonomic classification of the viruses into genera and species. As indicated in Table 33-1, the encephalitic arboviruses are designated in terms of the major animal hosts and the geographic areas wherein the diseases were first recognized or their viral etiology was established (such as Western equine [WEE], Eastern equine [EEE], Venezuelan equine [VEE], Japanese B[JBE], Saint Louis [SLE]). The mosquito-transmitted infections also are differentiated on an epidemiological basis from the tick-borne (TBE) encephalitides, such as Middle European encephalitis and Russian SSE (see Clarke 1964). The spring and summer incidence of the latter is due to early onset of extremely cold weather in the fall in far eastern Russia (Siberia), leading to the early hibernation of the tick vectors in that area. The hibernation of the ticks accounts for the overwintering of the virus in these vectors. The viruses of Middle European encephalitis and Russian SSE are closely related, and the incidence of the human disease overlaps in western Russia. However, the Middle European disease tends to show a higher incidence in autumn than does the far eastern variety. Further, a significant epidemiological aspect of these tick-borne

encephalitis infections in goats is the fact that the virus is shed into the milk and the human disease can be contracted by drinking such milk. For more details, see McGowan et al. (1973).

Most of the encephalitic arboviruses are transmitted by mosquitoes of one or more of a number of different genera. The functional mosquito vector varies from strain to strain of the encephalitic viruses and the region of the disease incidence. Essential factors in the epidemiology of the mosquito-borne encephalitides are (1) climatic and topographic conditions conducive to large populations of mosquitoes and (2) the availability of suitable animal hosts, particularly those that tend to develop prolonged viremias. Occasional additional epizootic vectors in the mosquito-borne encephalitides are birdmites, *Triatoma* species, and possibly other hemophagous arthropods. The arbovirus encephalitides are primarily animal diseases. Humans serve only as incidental hosts with little, if any, significance to the viral life cycle in nature.

As indicated in Table 33-1, several of the encephalitic arboviruses are primarily pathogenic for horses and other equines. With the possible exception of Japanese B encephalitis virus (which has been reported to infect horses), the equine encephalitides appear to be restricted to the western hemisphere. In fact epidemics of all the equine-designated encephalitides have occurred in the United States during this century, although prior to the 1960–1970 decades VEE was restricted to Colombia, Venezuela, and neighboring countries of South and Central America.

The major hosts and vectors of the encephalitic arboviruses listed in Table 33-1 might tend to give a false impression of the complexity of the epidemiological picture of these diseases. For example, Sidwell et al. (1967) listed evidence of infection of cows, pigs, sheep, and dogs as occasional nonequine, domestic animal hosts of VEE. In addition to laboratory mice, rats, rabbits, and monkeys these authors list 14 wild mammalian species as apparent animal hosts to this virus. They also list pigeons and 22 species of wild birds as possible hosts to VEE arbovirus.

As vectors in VEE transmission, these authors report at least 23 species of eight genera of mosquitoes *(Aedes, Anopheles, Anophelina, Culex, Haemogogus, Mansonia, Psorophora,* and *Sabethes)*.

During the 1950s and 1960s extensive outbreaks of VEE occurred in equines in the northern countries of South America and in Panama in Central America. During these epizootics, the first proved cases of human encephalitis involving VEE virus were established. At least 190 fatalities were recorded among the estimated 32,000 human cases reported (Sellers et al. 1965). During these outbreaks, VEE virus isolations from animals were reported in Mexico and from mosquitoes and rodents in Florida (see Chamberlain et al. 1964). Moreover, serological evidence of animal and human (Work 1964) infections were reported from Florida and from migratory birds in Louisiana and Utah. These reports were the first indication that the VEE virus had invaded the United States.

During the spring of 1969 Ecuador experienced an outbreak of VEE in equines and human beings. During May and June 1969, horse encephalitic deaths were reported from Guatemala and El Salvadore. Later that summer VEE virus was isolated from horses, human cases, and mosquitoes in southern Mexico. As the disease spread north in the spring of 1971, the U.S. Public Health Service set up an intensive equine surveillance in south Texas. In late June VEE virus was isolated from human cases just west of Matamoros, Mexico, across the Rio Grande from Brownsville, Texas. During 1970 and early 1971 approximately 2 million equines in Central America and Mexico were immunized with a live attenuated VEE virus vaccine in an effort to stop the spread of the disease. In the first week of July 1971, equine cases and deaths were detected in Cameron County, Texas; on 9 July the Center for Disease Control (CDC) reported that the new epidemic strain of VEE virus had entered the United States. These developments led to a massive escalation of the VEE vaccination program for horses in Cameron and surrounding counties. By 4 July 1971 an estimated 90 percent of the horses in Cameron County had been vaccinated. By 31 December of that year

574,100 horses had been immunized in Texas and the vaccination program had been extended to a total of 19 states ranging across the country from New Jersey south and west to Kentucky and on to California. According to CDC a total of 13,981,941 horses were immunized. Other control measures involved a quarantine on the movement of equines across the Texas border with neighboring states. The U.S. Air Force was requested to start spraying for mosquito control in the lower Rio Grande Valley, and on 11 July, the first day of spraying in the Brownsville area, an estimated 50,000 acres were treated. By mid-August approximately 10 million acres along the Gulf Coast of Texas and Louisiana were sprayed with ultra-low-volume malathion.

These control measures succeeded to the extent that no animal or human VEE was diagnosed in states other than Texas; and the last VEE virus isolation in Texas was from a specimen collected from a nonimmunized horse on 7 November 1971. During the course of the outbreak, however, 88 human cases of VEE were diagnosed by virus isolations or serodiagnosis. No human fatalities were reported. Of the estimated 2,228 equines in Cameron County at the start of the outbreak at least 225 died of VEE—this in spite of the fact that over 90 percent had been immunized by the end of July 1971. Figure 33-2 indicates the 24 Texas counties in which equine encephalitis was confirmed by isolation of VEE virus. No additional cases of VEE have been reported in the United States to date (1977).

During the summer of 1975, however, 82 human cases (6 fatal) of acute febrile CNS disease (suspected to be WEE) were reported in North Dakota and Minnesota. Nine of the cases gave a fourfold or greater rise in HI antibody titers to WEE virus *(MMWR,* 30 August 1975). Also during that summer, 541 confirmed and 496 suspected (serological evidence) human cases of St. Louis encephalitis (41 fatal) occurred in 19 states. The eight states reporting 20 or more confirmed cases of SLE were Alabama (22), Illinois (162), Indiana (75), Kentucky (26), Mississippi (93), New Jersey (20), Ohio (55), and

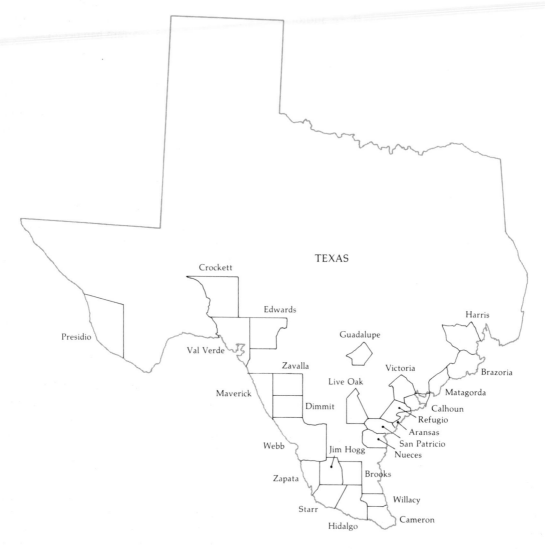

Figure 33–2. Texas counties in which equine encephalitis was diagnosed by the isolation of VEE virus in 1971.

Tennessee (25). Two species of *Culex* mosquitoes appeared to be the responsible vectors of the SLE virus, and sparrows and blackbirds the major animal hosts (*MMWR*, 27 September 1975). Ohio also reported 17 cases of confirmed or suspected cases of California encephalitis (*MMWR*, 18 August 1975).

Although there are reports of exceptions (see Watts et al. 1973; Balfour et al. 1975), mosquito-borne arboviruses generally are not transmitted transovarially from infected females to their progeny. As a rule each newly hatched mosquito must have an infective blood meal before becoming a vector in the disease transmission. In tropical regions a winter die-off of mosquitoes may not occur, but in temperate zones overwintering of mosquito-borne arboviruses is more difficult to explain than is that in tick vectors. The phenomenon probably is best accounted for by prolonged subclinical viremic infections in the bird or wild mammal hosts (see Gebhardt et al. 1964).

CLINICAL SYMPTOMS AND MORTALITY RATES

Different strains of encephalitic arboviruses produce human infections ranging from asymptomatic to severe or even fulminating pathology. The factors involved in this variable pathogenicity are not understood. In fact, there are numerous poorly understood paradoxes in encephalitic and other arbovirus virulence and epidemiology. Since "early" serum specimens from asymptomatic infections are rarely, if ever, tested it is impossible to relate antibodies found in the serum to rising-titer antibody evidence of such infections with encephalitic arboviruses. Since VEE virus had not been present in epidemic form in Texas prior to July 1971, however, it seemed reasonable to conclude that any significant VEE antibody titers in human sera by late August of that year must have resulted from recent VEE virus infection. A survey was conducted at that time in Port Isabel, Texas, involving 1,138 individuals who were questioned about symptoms during the preceding 2 months; and 662 blood specimens (collected from these individuals) were tested for VEE antibodies. Twenty-two of the blood specimens showed significant anti-VEE antibody titers, and 20 of the 22 individuals, from whom the positive bloods were obtained, reported having had symptoms compatible with VEE. On the basis of these results the ratio of asymptomatic/symptomatic infection rates (2/20) would appear to be much lower than generally reported in arbovirus encephalitides. For example, reported ratios of asymptomatic/symptomatic infections on the order of 1,000/1 are commonly found in the literature except for EEE, where a low of 10 to 20 asymptomatic to every clinical case of encephalitis has been reported.

Although EEE outbreaks have occurred only rarely in the United States, the mortality rate in human cases has been reported to be high (60 to 70 percent). Mortality rates in Japanese B, Murray Valley, and Russian SS (Far Eastern) encephalitis have been cited at 20 to 30 percent. Moreover, serious permanent sequelae are prone to develop following recovery from these four types of arboviral encephalitis. In the 1975 outbreaks of SLE in the United States, the mortality rate appeared to have been between 3 and 8 percent, depending upon the acceptance of the serologically diagnosed cases. As of 15 September 1976, some 157 cases of SLE with 8 deaths were reported in the United States. The largest number of cases were reported from Alabama (30), Mississippi (50), and Texas (34)—*MMWR*, 24 September 1976. Deaths due to SLE usually occur in persons over 50 years of age. The 1975 outbreak of WEE in the United States resulted in a mortality rate of around 7 percent. Deaths and serious sequelae due to WEE usually occur in infants under 1 year of age. The mortality rate in human VEE and in California encephalitis appears to be less than 1 percent (190 deaths in some 32,000 cases of VEE in the 1960–1970 outbreaks in South America and no deaths in the 88 proved cases in Texas in 1971). Recovery from these two forms of encephalitis usually is complete with no significant sequelae.

Symptoms of headache and fever are observed in 95 percent or more of the human cases of encephalitis. Muscle aches and vomiting are early symptoms in 80 percent of the cases. These symptoms may constitute the total clinical picture in mild or abortive cases of the disease. In severe cases, evidence of CNS involvement may be preceded by restlessness and irritability in infants and children or by mental confusion and drowsiness in adults. Other evidence of CNS involvement includes muscular pain, tremors, convulsions, delirium, nuchal rigidity, muscular spasticity, speech difficulties, blurred vision, stupor, and coma. Different cases may show any combination or none of these CNS symptoms.

LABORATORY DIAGNOSIS

As indicated in the opening section of this chapter, laboratory aid is essential to the specific diagnosis of these clinical entities, including the arbovirus encephalitides. Unfortunately two factors make this aid difficult to obtain in the average clinical laboratory: (1) the lack of suitable animals (infant mice), stock live viruses, antisera, and facilities for the isolation and identification of the causative viruses and the lack of antigens suitable for serodiagnostic tests; (2) the danger of infection of laboratory personnel with some of the more virulent viruses of the arbovirus groups. Aid in laboratory diagnosis of these diseases can be obtained from WHO and CDC reference laboratories. Public health laboratories with strong virology divisions may also help. See Shope (1974) for detailed considerations of laboratory diagnosis of the arbovirus encephalitides.

The specimens for the isolation of the encephalitic arboviruses from clinical cases are blood, cerebrospinal fluid, and throat washings. From autopsy cases, the specimens are brain and other organ tissues. From vectors, the specimens are pools of suspected mosquitoes or ticks. Tissue and vector specimens should be homogenized in BAPS buffer (0.75 percent bovine albumin, phosphate buffer in physiological saline, pH 7.2) and centrifuged at 2,000 rpm for 10 minutes to sediment larger particles. Throat washings should be collected in BAPS buffer. If immediate inoculation of the specimens to experimental animals (infant mice, newly hatched chicks, or baby hamsters) is impossible, the specimen should be stored at −60°C or colder. If the specimen is contaminated with bacteria, it should be treated with antibiotics prior to inoculation to experimental animals.

Litter-mate infant Swiss mice (1–4 days old) are the animals of choice for isolating encephalitic arboviruses. These should be inoculated intracerebrally with approximately 0.015 milliliter of the undiluted serum, spinal fluid or throat washings, or suitable dilutions of the other specimens. The animals should be observed for 21 days for evidence of illness (lethargy, nonfeeding, tremors, loss of equilibrium, hyperexcitability, or paralysis). Sick animals should be killed by exsanguination (ether and chloroform inactivate arboviruses), and pools of liver and brain from the sacrificed animals should be passed intracerebrally until the passage mice sicken uniformly. Each passage pool should be tested to ensure the absence of bacterial contamination. Virus for taxonomic identification is obtained as a BAPS suspension of homogenized brain tissue from one or more of the passage mice. Precautions must be taken to rule out cross-infections with other laboratory viruses or activation of murine viruses present in the colony of mice.

The virus in the homogenate of the mouse brain tissue should be tested by neutralization, complement fixation, or HI tests using antisera specific for the encephalitic arboviruses known or suspected of being present in the area of isolation or patient infection. Remember, air travel can transport patients long distances during even the short incubation periods (2 to 7 days) of the arbovirus encephalitides.

If the HI test is anticipated, the HA titer of the mouse brain homogenate should be established using chick or goose erythrocytes. Some suitable excess (4 to 8 HA units) of the hemagglutinating virus should be used in the HI test. The specific antisera to be used in the HI tests should be extracted with acetone to remove nonantibody inhibitors of viral hemagglutination and, if need be, absorbed with the test erythrocytes to remove antibody specific for these cells. Known HI concentrations of the treated antisera should be mixed with the 4 to 8 HA units of antigen prior to the addition of the test erythrocytes for the HI tests. The antiserum that inhibits HA by the excess virus tends to identify the virus. This specific antiserum should also give positive complement fixation test results with the mouse brain virus and should neutralize multiple ID/50 of the live virus when inoculated to susceptible mice.

For serological diagnosis, acute and convalescent serum specimens from the patient should be tested to demonstrate a significant (fourfold) rise in antibody titer. Neutralization tests using known live, virulent viruses can be used, but this requires large numbers of susceptible mice. For the complement fixation or HI tests the antigen of choice is a sucrose-acetone extracted brain or liver from individual mice infected with known virulent encephalitic arbovirus strains. For the HI test the patient's sera should be treated as above to remove nonantibody inhibitors of HA and to remove antibody that might react with the test erythrocytes. Serial double dilutions, starting from 1:10, of each of the two treated sera from the patient receive the excess HA antigen specific for one of the known encephalitic arboviruses. Other comparable serum dilutions receive comparable excess HA antigen of each of the other viruses to be tested. Finally, test erythrocytes are added to all virus-antigen + patient-serum preparations. The virus antigen for which the two serum specimens demonstrate a fourfold or greater rise in antibody titer identifies the virus responsible for the type of encephalitis suffered by the now convalescent patient. However, the sharing of antigens by different arboviruses may complicate such serodiagnostic efforts.

CONTROL AND PREVENTION

Because of the large number of wild bird and animal hosts, arbovirus encephalitis is almost impossible to control on a practical basis. Vector (usually mosquito) control measures generally are advocated. If the encephalitic virus produces a frequently fatal disease in domestic animals (horses), a concentrated control program such as that instituted in Texas, Mexico, and the United States in 1971 might be successful. To what extent each of the control measures—mosquito control, horse quarantine, and horse vaccination—contributed to the apparent success in this outbreak is impossible to evaluate. Certainly immunization of economically important animal hosts is a desirable preventive if effective vaccines are available. Usually the only control measure advocated for arbovirus encephalitides is mosquito control.

With few exceptions, vaccines are not available for human encephalitides. Obviously they are needed for the more virulent forms of the disease. If or when they become available, they certainly should be administered to reference laboratory and research personnel.

REFERENCES

Balfour, H. H., Jr., C. K. Edelman, F. E. Cook, W. I. Barton, A. W. Buziky, R. A. Siem, and H. Bauer. 1975. Isolation of California encephalitis (La Crosse) virus from field collected eggs and larvae of *Aedes triseriatus*: identification of overwintering site of California encephalitis. *J. Infect. Dis.* 131:712–716.

Casals, J. 1960. Procedure for the identification of arthropod-borne viruses. *Bull. Wrld. Hlth. Org.* 24:723–734.

Casals, J., and D. H. Clarke. 1965. Chapter 26 in *Viral and Rickettsial Infections in Man*.

Casals, J., and W. C. Reeves. 1965. The Arboviruses. Chapter 25 in *Viral and Rickettsial Infections in Man*.

Casals, J., and L. W. Whitman. 1960. A new antigenic group of arthropod-borne viruses. The Bunyamwera group. *Amer. J. Trop. Med. Hyg.* 9: 73–77.

———. 1961. Group C, a new serological group of hitherto undescribed arthropod-borne viruses. *Amer. J. Trop. Med. Hyg.* 10:250–258.

Chamberlain, R. W., W. D. Sudia, P. H. Coleman, and T. H. Work. 1964. Venezuelan equine encephalitis virus from south Florida. *Science* 145:272–274.

Clarke, D. H. 1964. Further studies on antigenic relationships among the viruses of the group B tick-borne complex. *Bull. Wrld. Hlth. Org.* 31: 45–56.

Clarke, D. H., and J. Casals. 1965. Arboviruses: Group B. Chapter 27 in *Viral and Rickettsial Infections in Man*.

Fraenkel-Conrat, H., and R. R. Wagner. 1974. *Comprehensive Virology*. Vol. 2. New York: Plenum.

Gebhardt, L. P., G. J. Stanton, D. W. Hill, and G. C. Collett. 1964. Natural overwintering hosts of the virus of western equine encephalitis. *New Engl. J. Med.* 271:172–173.

McGowan, J. E., Jr., J. A. Bryan, and M. B. Gregg. 1973. Surveillance of arboviral encephalitis in the United States, 1955–1971. *Amer. J. Epidemiol.* 97:199–207.

Pfefferkorn, E. R., and D. Shapiro. 1974. Togaviruses. In *Comprehensive Virology*, ed. H. Fraenkel-Conrat and R. R. Wagner. New York: Plenum.

Sellers, R. F., G. H. Bergold, O. M. Saurez, and A. Morales. 1965. Investigations during the Venezuelan equine encephalitis outbreaks in Venezuela—1962–1964. *Amer. J. Trop. Med. Hyg.* 14: 460–469.

Shope, R. E. 1974. Arboviruses. Chapter 81 in *Manual of Clinical Microbiology*.

Sidwell, R. W., L. P. Gebhardt, and D. B. Thorpe. 1967. Epidemiological aspects of Venezuelan equine encephalitis virus infections. *Bacteriol. Rev.* 31: 65–81.

Simpson, D. I. H. 1972. Arbovirus diseases. *Brit. Med. Bull.* 28:10–15.

Watts, D. M., S. Pantuwatana, G. R. DeFoliart, T. M. Yuill, and W. H. Thompson. 1973. Transovarial transmission of La Crosse virus (California encephalitis group) in the mosquito *Aedes triseriatus. Science* 182:1440–1441.

Work, T. H. 1964. Serological evidence of arbovirus infections in Seminole Indians of Southern Florida. *Science* 145:270–272.

34

Dengue, Yellow, and Hemorrhagic Fevers

The arboviruses responsible for the diseases considered in this chapter are examples of pantropic viruses, in contrast to the neurotropic viruses involved in the arbovirus encephalitides. (*Pantropic* signifies a predilection for the gastrointestinal tract, blood vessels, the respiratory system, and the viscera; *neurotropic* refers to a predilection of the virus for the central nervous system.) Although each of the pantropic arboviruses has been demonstrated capable of causing severe hemorrhages in human patients, the tendency of this symptom syndrome is greatest in the hemorrhagic fevers, lesser (but common) in yellow fever, and least (and possibly strain-specific) in dengue fever. For a more comprehensive discussion of these and other arbovirus diseases see Simpson (1972).

DENGUE FEVER

Etiology and Epidemiology

Dengue (pronounced den-gay) has occurred in epidemic form around the world in a belt between the 30° and 40° latitudes north and south of the equator. In general the transmitting vector has been *Aedes aegypti* (see Figure 34-1). This is one of the most domesticated of all mosquitoes, with its distribution usually restricted to close association with human habitation. If given the environment, such as indoor plants growing in water, adult *A. aegypti* will feed upon the inhabitants, mate, and lay eggs that hatch into larvae (wiggletails) that grow and metamorphose into pupae that metamorphose into new adults—all without leaving the human habitation. Other common *A. aegypti* breeding sites are rain barrels, cisterns, tin cans, bottles, bamboo stalks, and other containers in which standing water may be available near human habitation. In some parts of the world, however, additional species of the genus *Aedes* may serve as vectors. These may not be as domesticated as *A. aegypti* and, therefore, may complicate control measures in their areas of distribution in brush country or rain forest terrain (see Rao et al. 1967).

There is no evidence of significant animal hosts for dengue fever virus other than humans. Extensive epidemics of the disease have oc-

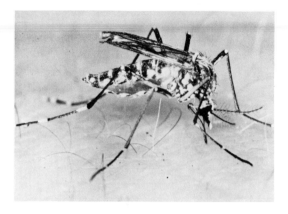

Figure 34–1. The mosquito *Aedes aegypti*, the common vector for dengue fever. (Courtesy of the Center for Disease Control, Atlanta, GA.)

curred repeatedly. One during the early 1920s in the southern United States was estimated to have involved more than a million cases. Although the disease is rarely fatal, it can be extremely debilitating and convalescence may be prolonged. These aspects of the disease caused the American military and government authorities to become concerned about the effects that an epidemic of dengue fever would have on the war-related industries along the Gulf Coast early in World War II. My graduate professor, Dr. Asa C. Chandler of Rice Institute in Houston, was assigned the job of organizing a mosquito control program throughout the area. He enlisted the aid of the news media, boy and girl scouts, and other volunteers to carry out the program. Whether or not their control measures were responsible will never be known, but no epidemic of dengue occurred in the area during the 1940s.

Four serotypes of dengue virus have long been established and two additional serotypes have been recognized. Serotypes 1 and 2 are responsible for most epidemics in the western hemisphere. As indicated in Table 33-1, dengue fever virus belongs to the antigenic group B arboviruses as do the yellow fever virus and several of the mosquito-borne neurotropic viruses and certain of the tick-borne pantropic viruses. Antigens of dengue virus are shared with other group B arboviruses. However, the serotypes of dengue virus are reported to be more closely related to each other antigenically than to the other group B arboviruses.

An epidemic of dengue 2 occurred in Puerto Rico and other Caribbean countries in the 1960s (Shelokov et al. 1962). The disease then persisted as sporadic cases in southwestern Puerto Rico until the summer of 1975. Between 1 September and 14 December 1975, some 679 cases of dengue fever were reported from 30 different municipalities throughout the island. Sixty-five percent of the cases occurred in the San Juan metropolitan area. By February 1976 the number of cases had increased to 1,285 (*MMWR*, 10 January 1976 and 6 March 1976).

Hammon et al. (1960; 1964) were the first to report hemorrhagic fever (HF) syndromes caused by dengue virus. All the serotypes of this virus apparently have been incriminated as capable of causing dengue hemorrhagic fever (DHF). There has been no explanation, however, for the fact that the same dengue virus causes the typical nonfatal dengue fever syndrome in a majority of the patients and the severe DHF (with a 20 to 30 percent mortality) in others. During the 1950s and 1960s extensive epidemics of DHF in children occurred in the Philippines, Thailand, and other Southeast Asian countries. Such epidemics would seem to imply strain differences in the virulence of the virus causing DHF compared to that causing dengue fever. Most if not all of the fatal cases of DHF were in children under 15 years of age. The Southeast Asian locale of the DHF epidemics, however, might indicate ethnic differences in the susceptibility to dengue virus. Only 3 cases of DHF were reported in the 679 cases of dengue fever in Puerto Rico in 1975. Hammon (1973), however, cites evidence that he believes refutes the ethnic-susceptibility hypothesis. He seems to favor a hypothetical modified-virulence of the dengue virus (DV) resulting from (1) synergism between two DV serotypes or between DV and another, unrecognized virus; (2) mutation and selection of a more virulent DV, possibly in a jungle monkey-mosquito cycle; or (3) double virus infections leading to recombination or phenotypic mixing and yielding a more virulent strain of DV. Hammon entitles his article "Dengue Hemorrhagic Fever—Do We Know Its Cause?" and he ends his study on the same questioning note.

Not only is dengue virus restricted to humans as the natural host, but experimental animal hosts rarely show disease symptoms following primary inoculation of specimens, from human patients, containing virulent dengue virus. This includes intracerebral inoculation of the animal of choice—infant mice. If the brains of such mice are subjected to a series of blind passages, however, the mouse-adapted virus eventually will produce fatal pathology. Large amounts of dengue virus may be recovered from such brain tissue. This mouse-adapted brain tissue virus has been used (1) to immunize adult mice to obtain specific antisera for serotaxonomic tests and (2) as known antigen for serodiagnostic tests. The time involved in the blind-passage adaptation of the virus, however, complicates the use of virus isolation as a means of laboratory diagnosis of dengue fever, even when serotaxonomic antisera are already available.

Monkey kidney (LLC-MK$_2$), KB, HeLa, and other tissue culture cells are susceptible to infection by dengue virus. Primary infections of these tissue cells, as is the case with infant mice, do not result in visible evidence of infection— there is no cytopathic effect (CPE). The infected status of the cells, however, can be established indirectly by exposing the primarily inoculated cultures to a virus (such as *Poliovirus*) that will cause CPE in noninfected tissue cells. Cells infected with dengue virus will continue to show no evidence of CPE after exposure to the second virus (the viral interference phenomenon). Mouse-adapted (by brain passage) dengue virus tends to cause visible CPE in certain tissue cultures. Singh and Paul (1969) reported that tissue cultures of *Aedes albopictus* cells show syncytial-type CPE (see Figure 34-2) on primary inoculation with dengue virus. Chappell et al. (1971) compared three methods of isolation of dengue 2 virus from blood specimens of patients in Puerto Rico: (1) IC inoculation of infant mice;

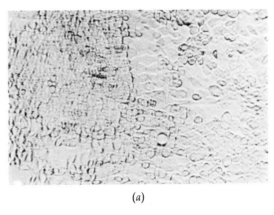

(a)

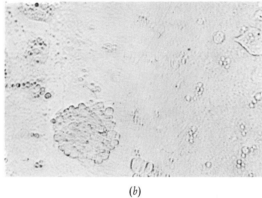

(b)

Figure 34–2. Cultures of *Aedes albopictus* cells. (a) Uninoculated normal cells. (b) Culture inoculated with dengue fever virus showing syncytial cytopathic effect. (Courtesy of W. A. Chappell.)

(2) inoculation of LLC-MK$_2$ cell cultures; and (3) Singh's *A. albopictus* cell cultures. They recommended that the three methods be used in combination; but if only one method is to be used, Singh's method has definite advantages.

Clinical Symptoms

Classic dengue fever is an acute but rarely fatal disease with an incubation period of 5 to 8 days. There usually is a short prodromal period of headache and malaise followed by a sudden rapid rise in temperature and increasingly severe muscular, ocular, and other aches and joint pains. The severity of these aches and pains is such that the disease has been designated "breakbone fever." A maculopapular skin rash frequently occurs on the trunk about the third day and spreads to the extremities and face. The acute symptoms usually terminate suddenly on about the eighth day. However, convalescence from severe attacks may be characterized by marked weakness and prolonged (several weeks) incapacitation. Comparable symptoms have been reported in other arbovirus infections and, like other such infections, asymptomatic and abortive dengue virus infections have been reported to be quite common. The antibodies stimulated by the shared antigens of the non-dengue viral infections further tend to complicate diagnostic procedures. For symptoms of the more severe dengue virus infections (DHF) see the section of this chapter dealing with hemorrhagic fevers.

Laboratory Diagnosis

The only unequivocal diagnosis of dengue fever involves the isolation and identification of the virus. In the past this has been impractical for the average clinical laboratory and was time-consuming and difficult even for the experts in the WHO and other arbovirus reference laboratories. As indicated above, however, the observation of syncytial CPE in primary inoculated cultures of *A. albopictus* cells tends to give a more rapid presumptive evidence of the presence of dengue virus than other methods of isolation.

For laboratories with the various serotype dengue and related group B virus antigens, serodiagnostic tests on paired sera from the patient may provide diagnostic aid. In addition to the usual live-virus neutralization test and the HI, C'F (complement fixation), and indirect FA tests, these laboratories may perform a modified FA test (the FA—C'F test). The antigen for this test consists of impression smears of the dengue-virus-infected mouse brain or smears of a positive tissue culture. Such smears are flooded with a mixture of the patient's serum (heat-inactivated) and guinea pig serum complement (GPC'). After suitable incubation to allow an antigen-antibody C'F reaction, the smear is washed and then exposed to fluorescent rabbit-serum antibody specific for GPC'. Again after a suitable reaction time the smear is washed, dried, and examined with an ultraviolet-light microscope. If the patient's serum has antibody specific for the virus in the mouse brain or tissue smear, this antibody will react with that virus and fix the GPC'. This fixed GPC' will then react with the fluorescent anti-GPC' on the infected cells in the smear. These cells will fluoresce when exposed to the ultraviolet light of the microscope. No fluorescence indicates a negative test.

Control and Prevention

Because of their close association with human habitation, mosquito control measures for *A. aegypti* are more likely to be effective than those for any other mosquito species. See evidence for this control in the following section on yellow fever, which also is transmitted by *A. aegypti*.

Efforts to provide vaccines for the prevention of dengue fever are in progress but, to the author's knowledge, they have not been licensed for use to this date (February 1977). Obviously there is a need for such vaccines—particularly to prevent the serious DHF infections where they tend to occur in epidemic form. Moreover, a vaccine might help solve the epidemiology problem of dengue fever where nonurban *Aedes* species are vectors of the disease. For results of experimental, multiple arbovirus immunizations in monkeys, see Price et al. (1973) under the discussion of yellow fever control and prevention below.

YELLOW FEVER

Introduction and Epidemiology

Yellow fever occupies a unique historical position among the great human pestilences. Its first appearance as an epidemic disease occurred in the mid-seventeenth century in Central America. There is suggestive evidence that the slave trade introduced or helped maintain the disease in the original endemic area in the Caribbean countries. The adult African black slaves appeared to be immune to yellow fever, possibly as a result of having survived childhood infections in Africa. The question of whether the disease originated in the Caribbean area or was brought over from Africa has never been resolved. Regardless of origin, countries in the Caribbean area were heavily infected during the eighteenth and nineteenth centuries. Repeated devastating epidemics of yellow fever spread throughout the tropical and subtropical areas of the world during this 200-year period. Mortality rates in some epidemics were reported as high as 60 percent. The disease was carried along trade routes to metropolitan centers from New York south to Brazil and across the Atlantic to London, Lisbon, and other European port cities. The last of the extensive epidemics in North America occurred in New Orleans and other southern cities in 1905.

In 1900, following the Spanish-American War, the United States sent a commission composed of army medical officers (Reed, Lazear, Carroll, and Agramonte) to study the disease in Havana, Cuba, where morbidity and mortality were high at that time. A physician by the name of Finlay had contended for some 20 years that the disease was transmitted by mosquitoes, but he offered no proof and had few believers. Using naturally infected cases and human volunteers, the commission proved Finlay correct and established the transmitting vector to be *Aedes aegypti*. To become infected, the mosquito had to feed upon a patient during the first 3 or 4 days of the disease. The mosquito then became capable of transmitting the infection about 2 weeks after the blood meal. The commission also noted that the infectious agent was filterable. These observations led to the initiation of *A. aegypti* control measures that soon eradicated the disease from Havana.

During the nineteenth century, French engineers repeatedly attempted to dig a ship canal across the isthmus of Panama. Each effort was defeated by the high morbidity and mortality caused by yellow fever and malaria. When the United States, in the early twentieth century, chose to undertake the canal project, a mosquito control crew under Colonel Gorgas was first sent in to eliminate the mosquitoes from the Canal Zone. This step, coupled with continuous control measures throughout the project, enabled the successful completion of this strategic waterway.

These early successes in the eradication of yellow fever from urban areas by controlling *A. aegypti* infestation raised hopes that the disease would soon be eliminated from the face of the earth. Eradication was in fact successful in practically all urban areas by the late 1920s, but then a wild animal reservoir of yellow fever virus was found in monkeys in the equatorial jungles and rain forests of South America and Africa. Isolated human cases of yellow fever were recognized in persons who entered the jungle areas even though no *A. aegypti* were present. Moreover, epizootics and other evidence of infection of jungle monkeys were observed. In South America the epizootic disease was found to be transmitted from monkey to monkey and occasionally to humans by mosquitoes of the genus *Haemogogus*. These are arboreal mosquitoes living in the forest canopy. They lay their eggs in water holes high in tree trunks and rarely descend to the ground level except at the edges of forest clearings. In Africa the monkey disease was found to be transmitted by arboreal species of *Aedes* mosquitoes. Some of these would feed only on monkeys whereas others fed on both monkeys and humans. Moreover, *A. aegypti* were found in the vicinity of some of the areas involved in the jungle yellow fever (JYF). This wild primate reservoir of yellow fever virus poses a constant threat of reinitiation of epidemic yellow fever where nonimmune human beings and *A. aegypti* live in close association with the jungle disease (see Trapido and Galindo 1956; Jones and Wilson 1972). Two cases of human JYF, both fatal, were reported in Ecuador in January 1975. Subsequent epidemiological investigations in Ecuador yielded reports of several deaths of villagers who had symptoms of fever and black vomitus. Villagers reported seeing dead monkeys in the area.

An outbreak of 16 cases of JYF (all fatal) were reported from central Colombia in November and December 1974, raising the total cases from Colombia for that year to 29. Two

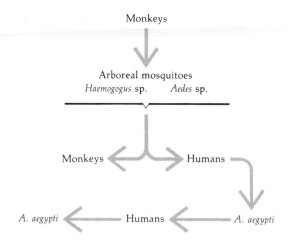

Figure 34–3. The epizootology and epidemiology of jungle yellow fever.

additional fatal cases were reported in January 1975. The Pan American Health Organization reported a total of 335 cases of JYF from 1972 to 1975 in nine countries of South and Central America (*MMWR,* 12 April 1975).

The epizootology and epidemiology of this potential reintroduced urban yellow fever is illustrated in Figure 34-3. Such human outbreaks have been described in Central America and in Ethiopia also. For a more comprehensive discussion of yellow fever see Strode (1951).

Etiology

The yellow fever virus is a typical spherical arbovirus approximately 30 nanometers in diameter. It possesses a lipoprotein envelope and produces viral hemagglutination. A disease similar, if not identical, to yellow fever can be produced by inoculation of the virus to monkeys or other primates. The white mouse is the animal of choice for most laboratory work. Infant mice can be infected by any route of inoculation, whereas adult mice may require intracerebral inoculation. Primary infection results in fatal pathology in both experimental animals. The virus will infect and produce CPE in mouse, chick embryo, KB, HeLa, and mon-key-cell tissue cultures. Virus can be obtained from any of these infected animal or tissue culture sources, and antisera for taxonomic or other studies are available. Although dengue fever and yellow fever viruses are both antigenic group B arboviruses, the latter is much more adaptable to laboratory studies than the former.

Theiler (1930; 1951) noted that continued intracerebral passage of a virulent strain of yellow fever virus in mice resulted in reduced virulence of the virus for monkeys; and additional passage of the virus in chick embryos further reduced its virulence. These observations led to the development of the first attenuated-virus yellow fever vaccine (17D) for successful human immunization. Although several antigenic differences have been reported in yellow fever viruses from different areas of the world, these serotype differences apparently do not include immunogenic heterogeneity—the 17D vaccine appears to be immunogenic around the world.

Clinical Symptoms

Yellow fever infections may vary from asymptomatic to severe to fatal (even fulminating) pathology. Patients who survive the eighth day, however, usually recover completely. Death usually occurs in 5 to 7 days. Following an incubation period averaging 4 to 5 days, there usually is an abrupt onset without prodromal manifestations. In mild cases the symptoms of fever, headache, muscular aches, and pains usually last for less than a week. Severe cases frequently show a diphasic symptomatology. In phase 1 there is an abrupt onset of high fever, headache, generalized aches and pains, dizziness, nausea, and vomiting. A brief remission of these symptoms may occur before the onset of the more toxemic phase 2. The secondary symptoms include, in addition to those of phase 1, marked temperature-pulse aberrations, jaundice, and various hemorrhagic manifestations. Gastric hemorrhages are indicated by black or "coffee-ground" vomitus. Nosebleed, bleeding gums, and intestinal or uterine hemorrhages are common manifestations of severe yellow fever. The patient may become comatose or wildly delirious. Death may occur following any of these severe symptoms or, in fulminating cases, without the diphasic symptomatology. Mortality rates as high as 60 percent have been reported. This and the extent of the devastating epidemics justify the classification of yellow fever as one of mankind's great historical pestilences, even though the *A. aegypti* epidemics persisted for a mere 250 years.

Laboratory Diagnosis

Because of the danger of accidental infection, laboratory diagnosis of yellow fever should be undertaken only by trained virologists in adequately equipped virology laboratories. Yellow fever virus can be isolated from the blood of the patient during the first 3 or 4 days of symptoms. Consequently blood should be collected during this period and 0.015 to 0.02 milliliter inoculated intracerebrally in white mice or to tissue cultures. Serum from the remaining blood should be refrigerated for possible use in subsequent rising-antibody-titer serodiagnosis. When the inoculated mice die or develop symptoms of encephalitis, the brains should be removed and tested for yellow fever virus by neutralization tests using antiserum specific for yellow fever virus. Controls should include antisera specific for other group B arboviruses known to be prevalent in the area of infection. The neutralization tests involve injection of mixtures of the brain-virus + specific-antiserum intracerebrally into white mice. If only the antibody specific for yellow fever virus neutralizes the test virus, this result identifies the virus as yellow fever.

If no virus is isolated from the blood (and the patient survives) a second blood specimen should be collected during convalescence. The serum from this and the first blood specimen should then be tested for antibody titers specific for yellow fever virus. The tests may be neutralization of virus in mice or tissue culture system, HI tests, or a quantitative FA–C'F test. A fourfold or greater rise in antibody titer in the convalescent versus the onset serum is considered significant. Again controls should include other antigenic group B arboviruses indigenous to the area. For more details, see Shope (1974).

Control and Prevention

Success in the eradication of *A. aegypti*–transmitted yellow fever was attained with measures designed to eliminate these mosquitoes from the vicinity of human habitation. These measures included: (1) elimination of standing water from within and surrounding such habitations; (2) treating such water that could not be eliminated with a film of light machine oil to asphyxiate the larval form of the mosquitoes; (3) installation of tight screens on doors, windows, chimneys, and all openings through which mosquitoes might gain entrance to human habitation; and (4) sleeping under mosquito netting as a double indoor precaution. As persistent insecticides (DDT and others) became available they were added to the anti-mosquito armamentarium.

These measures, however, could not be depended upon to prevent the occasional human infections caused by jungle yellow fever mosquitoes. Nor could they prevent the reinitiation of *A. aegypti* outbreaks following such infections in remote areas of the world. Consequently those who must frequent areas of known endemic jungle yellow fever, and all laboratory personnel involved in yellow fever diagnosis, should be immunized with the Theiler 17D or other approved yellow fever vaccine. Such immunization has been reported to yield significant virus-neutralizing antibody titers that have persisted in the vaccinees for 17 to 19 years (Rosenzweig et al. 1963).

Price et al. (1973) reported interesting results of experimental immunization of monkeys with three live-attenuated group B arbovirus vaccines: (1) yellow fever (17D); (2) dengue 2 (a New Guinea isolate); and (3) Langat E5 virus. Monkeys that were immunized sequentially with these three vaccines developed high HI antibody titers for all 21 arboviruses tested and neutralizing antibodies for 20 of these viruses. Immunized monkeys were reported to be protected against subcutaneous challenges with a variety of viruses: yellow fever virus; dengue virus serotypes 1, 2, 3, 4; Kyasanur Forest disease virus; Omsk HF virus; Russian SSE, Japanese B, and Murray Valley encephalitis viruses; and West Nile and Kadam arboviruses.

In prior paragraphs, we have cited the detrimental aspects of the shared antigenicity of the group B arboviruses in taxonomic and serodiagnostic studies. If the results of Price et al. in monkeys can be confirmed and extrapolated to humans, the capacity of these three vaccines to immunize against at least 12 arbovirus diseases would be a real plus for this antigenic heterogeneity. This possibility certainly justifies additional research along these lines.

HEMORRHAGIC FEVERS

The hemorrhagic syndrome of severe yellow fever has been recognized for 200 years. However, there is a group of epidemic hemorrhagic fevers, caused by other arboviruses, all of which have been recognized etiologically only since the 1940s. The delay in this recognition might be attributed to the relative complexity of viral isolation and identification; to the multiplicity and antigenic heterogeneity of the viruses involved; to the lack of adequately trained virologists prior to the twentieth century; and to the frequent occurrence of hemorrhagic fever epidemics in the more remote and undeveloped areas of the world. Undoubtedly, isolated cases of the hemorrhagic syndrome had been noted during past epidemics of dengue fever. However, the dengue virus etiology of these DHF cases was not established prior to the mid-1950s; and, as stated above, the dual pathogenicity of the virus causing DF and DHF still is not comprehended. According to Simpson (1972), nine arboviruses have been established as etiological agents of epidemic hemorrhagic fevers. Many more than nine HF-virus isolates have been given names associated with the geographic area of their isolation. The more these viruses have been studied, however, the more they tend to fit into a relatively limited number of taxonomic groups.

Geographic Distribution and Epidemiology

Only two of the epidemic arbovirus diseases with hemorrhagic syndromes are known to be transmitted by mosquitoes—yellow fever and dengue fever. Although both these arboviruses are transmitted from human to human by *Aedes aegypti,* yellow fever generally is not included among the designated hemorrhagic fevers. For the epidemiology and distribution of these mosquito-borne HF diseases see the prior sections of this chapter. For more comprehensive considerations see Gajdusek (1962) and Hammon (1973).

Tick-borne and possibly mite-borne HF epidemics have been reported in the Crimea and other south central Asian areas. The same virus or one closely related causes hemorrhagic fevers in Manchuria, in Korea, and in the Congo and surrounding areas of Africa (Casals and Tignor 1974). Moreover, the same virus has been reported to be the cause of hemorrhagic fevers in European Russia west of the Ural Mountains, in the Balkans, and in south, central, and western Europe including Scandinavia. *Hyalomma* and *Rhipicephalus* ticks have been incriminated as probable vectors in the Eurasian disease and *Hyalomma, Amblyomma,* and *Boophilus* ticks in the central African disease. Casals et al. (1970) reviewed the results of Russian studies on Soviet hemorrhagic fevers during the 5 years prior to 1969. They reported serological evidence incriminating horses, cows, and rabbits as epizootic hosts. Results of serological studies on human beings indicated that asymptomatic infections in humans were uncommon. Fatal cases frequently suffer a renal syndrome, and some epidemics have involved mortality rates of 10 to 20 percent. The disease was not reported in north central Russia east of the Urals nor in Siberia.

Another epidemic hemorrhagic fever (Omsk) was reported during the 1940s in western Siberia, however. The epizootic hosts appear to be muskrats and other rodents. The arthropod vector has been reported to be tick species of the genus *Dermacentor.* Human cases in trappers have resulted from contact with infected muskrats. The Omsk HF virus appears to be closely related to the Russian SSE virus and to the Kyasanur Forest (KF) disease virus in India. The KF virus has been reported to cause massive hemorrhages in the chest cavity. However, the mortality rate in the Omsk-KF virus hemorrhagic fever has been reported to range from 0.5 to 5 percent—significantly lower than the Crimean and related hemorrhagic fevers that show the renal syndrome. The tick vector in the KF disease appears to be a *Haemaphysalis* species, and small mammals have been reported to be the reservoir hosts.

In 1955 human cases of hemorrhagic fever were reported from near the town of Junin in Argentina. A new virus was isolated from these cases and designated Junin virus (see Figure 34-4). Subsequently 300 to 1,000 cases of this disease were reported annually from the surrounding area (see Shelokov et al. 1965). During a 1958 epidemic, mortality rates reached 20 percent. Additional outbreaks of viral hemorrhagic fever were reported from widely separated areas of South America (including Bolivia) and Trinidad. Although the viruses isolated from these outbreaks were given new name designations, additional studies indicated that they were not significantly different from the Junin virus. Extensive studies of arthropod pools failed to incriminate a vector for either the epizootic or the epidemic transmission of South American HF virus. The principal animal host for the zoonotic virus was established as a mouselike rodent that, mouselike, frequently enters human habitations. Evidence has been cited that "infected houses" continue to serve as sources of infection for other cases of this hemorrhagic fever. The Junin virus was also found in the throat secretions (indicating possible respiratory transmission) and in the blood of infected patients.

Clinical Symptoms

Many infectious diseases include hemorrhagic syndromes of varying degrees in their symptomatology. This results when the disease pathology includes increased permeability or fragility of cutaneous and other capillaries. Small ruptures of these capillaries result in *petechiae* (small purple spots on the skin) and other *exanthemata* (skin rash) or *enanthemata* (mucus membrane rash). In the arbovirus hemorrhagic fevers, however, the bleeding syndrome generally is more extensive and constitutes a major

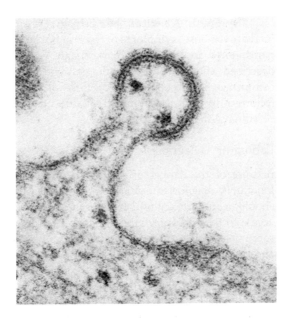

Figure 34–4. Junin virus budding from plasma membrane of a Vero cell. The viral envelope is distinct from the membrane and two (dark) ribosomes are present in the bud. 173,000×. (Courtesy of F. A. Murphy.)

basis for the frequently poor prognosis in these diseases. Early symptoms include fever, headache, vomiting, and abdominal pain. The onset of the hemorrhagic syndrome may involve peripheral vascular congestion, petechiae, or other forms of subcutaneous bleeding. In dengue hemorrhagic fever (DHF) these early symptoms may be followed by abrupt hypotension and collapse. The fourth and fifth days of DHF are critical with vomiting of blood, intestinal bleeding, severe shock, and coma indicating a poor prognosis.

In the European-Crimean-Korean and related hemorrhagic fevers, the onset symptoms of chills, high fever, prostration, severe retroorbital (back of eyes) headache, vomiting, and generalized muscle and joint pains were followed by hemorrhagic manifestations including petechiae and subcutaneous and scleral hemorrhages (see Casals et al. 1970 for illustrations). The renal syndrome of these hemorrhagic fevers includes marked proteinuria or hematuria followed by cardiovascular instability, shock, and renal failure.

The South American hemorrhagic fever includes the onset symptoms of fever, aches, and pains noted in the other hemorrhagic fevers described above. The hemorrhagic syndrome commences with cutaneous petechiae or rash, followed by nasal, gastrointestinal, and uterine bleeding with severe prostration.

Laboratory Diagnosis

Because of the danger of accidental infection, laboratory diagnosis of viral hemorrhagic fever should be undertaken only by experts who have access to the necessary viral antigens and antisera, susceptible animals and tissue cultures, and adequate facilities to limit the dangers to a bare minimum. Isolated virus can be identified by neutralization, C'F, HI, or FA tests. Serodiagnosis, using paired sera (acute and convalescent), can be performed using known HF virus antigens. In the neutralization and HI tests, controls must be included to rule out nonspecific (nonantibody) inhibitors or the sera must be treated (acetone) to eliminate them.

Control and Prevention

If the vector of the HF disease virus is known, control measures are directed at their elimination. This is not easy in the remote areas of the world where these diseases frequently occur. The best hope for control is the development of effective vaccines. Studies such as those reported by Price et al. (1973) hopefully will result in the eventual control of the viral hemorrhagic fevers.

REFERENCES

Casals, J. 1969. Antigenic similarity between the virus causing Crimean hemorrhagic fever and Congo virus. *Proc. Soc. Exper. Biol. Med.* 131:233–236.

Casals, J., B. E. Henderson, and H. Hoogstrall. 1970. A review of Soviet viral hemorrhagic fevers, 1969. *J. Infect. Dis.* 122:437–453.

Casals, J., and G. H. Tignor. 1974. Neutralization and haemagglutination inhibition tests with Crimean hemorrhagic fever–Congo virus. *Proc. Soc. Exper. Biol. Med.* 145:960–966.

Chappell, W. A., C. H. Calisher, R. F. Toole, K. C. Maness, D. R. Sasso, and B. E. Henderson. 1971. Comparison of three methods used to isolate dengue virus type 2. *Appl. Microbiol.* 22:1100–1103.

Gajdusek, D. C. 1962. Virus hemorrhagic fevers. Special reference to hemorrhagic fever with renal syndrome (epidemic hemorrhagic fever). *J. Pediat.* 60:841–857.

Hammon, W. McD. 1973. Dengue hemorrhagic fever—do we know its cause? *Amer. J. Trop. Med. Hyg.* 22:82–91.

Hammon, W. McD., A. Rudnick, and G. E. Sather. 1960. Viruses associated with epidemic hemorrhagic fevers of the Philippines and Thailand. *Science* 131:1102–1103.

Hammon, W. McD., and G. E. Sather. 1964. Virological findings in the 1960 hemorrhagic fever epidemic (dengue) in Thailand. *Amer. J. Trop. Med. Hyg.* 13:629–641.

Jones, E. M., and D. C. Wilson. 1972. Clinical features of yellow fever cases at Vom Christian Hospital during the 1969 epidemic on the Jos Plateau, Nigeria. *Bull. Wld. Hlth. Org.* 46:653–657.

Price, W. H., J. Casals, I. Thind, and W. O'Leary. 1973. Sequential immunization procedure against Group B arboviruses using living attenuated 17D yellow fever virus, living attenuated Langat E5 virus and living attenuated dengue 2 virus (New Guinea C isolate). *Amer. J. Trop. Med. Hyg.* 22:509–523.

Rao, T. R., et al. 1967. A symposium on *Aedes aegypti*, its ecology and relationship to human disease. *Bull. Wld. Hlth. Org.* 36:519–702.

Rosenzweig, E. C., R. W. Babione, and C. L. Wisseman, Jr. 1963. Immunological studies with group B arthropod-borne viruses. IV. Persistence of yellow fever antibodies following vaccination with 17D strain yellow fever vaccine. *Amer. J. Trop. Med. Hyg.* 12:230–235.

Shelokov, A., et al. 1965. Symposium on some aspects of hemorrhagic fevers in the Americas. *Amer. J. Trop. Med. Hyg.* 14:789–818.

Shelokov, A., C. J. Gibbs, and D. Mendez-Casbion. 1962. Arbovirus infection of Puerto Rican children with obscure neurological syndromes. Abstract. *J. Clin. Invest.* 41:1400–1401.

Shope, R. E. 1974. Arboviruses. Chapter 81 in *Manual of Clinical Microbiology*.

Simpson, D. I. 1972. Arbovirus diseases. *Brit. Med. Bull.* 28:10–15.

Singh, K. R. P., and S. D. Paul. 1969. Isolation of dengue virus in *Aedes albopictus* cell cultures. *Bull. Wld. Hlth. Org.* 40:982–983.

Strode, G. K. 1951. *Yellow Fever.* New York: McGraw-Hill.

Theiler, M. 1930. Studies on the action of yellow fever virus in mice. *Ann. Trop. Med. Parasit.* 24:249–272.

———. 1951. See Strode (1951).

Trapido, H., and P. Galindo. 1956. Epidemiology of yellow fever in Middle America. *Exptl. Parasitol.* 5:285–323.

35

Rabies

Rabies is primarily a disease of wild and domestic warm-blooded animals that is generally transmitted to humans by the bite of a rabid animal. The disease is one of great antiquity and worldwide distribution (see Tierkel 1971). Although earlier reports may have been rabies, the disease in dogs was clearly described in the fifth century B.C. and was mentioned in Aristotle's writings in the fourth century B.C. Celsus in the first century A.D. recognized the relationship of rabies in dogs to hydrophobia in humans and advocated cauterizing the bite wound. Galen also recognized the bite-induced disease in humans and advocated surgical excision of the bite area. The experimental transmission of rabies from an infected animal to a normal dog by intramuscular inoculation of saliva was reported during the first decade of the nineteenth century. This demonstration of the mode of transmission of the disease led to the practice of destruction of stray dogs and quarantine of domestic dogs as measures for rabies control. By 1826 these measures had proved effective in the Scandinavian countries, but periodic reintroduction of the disease was reported subsequently.

Although rabies was prevalent in wolves in western Europe during the thirteenth century, the first recorded epizootic of rabies in domestic dogs occurred in Italy in the early eighteenth century. During the following 150 years the disease became increasingly prevalent in dogs, reaching epizootic status in many areas of western Europe by 1860. Since the disease in human beings was invariably fatal once symptoms developed, and since it usually led to a horrible death, rabies became one of the most greatly feared human diseases even though both morbidity and mortality were far lower than in many other infectious diseases.

After the domestic rabbit was established as a suitable experimental animal for rabies research, E. Roux demonstrated that the inoculation of brain tissue from an infected animal intracranially (IC) in rabbits led to paralysis and death much faster than subcutaneous (SC) or intramuscular (IM) inoculations. These observations led to surer means of diagnosis and paved the way for extensive studies of the disease reported by Pasteur et al. (1881). Although Pasteur suspected that the rabies infectious agent was submicroscopic, its passage through a bacterial (Berkefeld) filter—that is, its viral nature—was not established until 1903.

Pasteur et al. noted that after primary IC inoculation of saliva from a rabid dog into a rabbit, the test animal would become paralyzed and die after 2 to 3 weeks, whereas SC or IM inoculation might take months. This salivary virus was designated "street virus." When infected brain tissue from rabbits infected with street virus was passed serially by the IC route from rabbit to rabbit, the time required to produce paralysis and death decreased gradually until it reached 6 or 7 days. Further passage resulted in no further decrease in the incubation time. This virus was designated "fixed virus." After 100 IC passages in rabbits, the fixed virus had little residual pathogenicity for dogs when inoculated subcutaneously.

Since Pasteur had used drying to weaken his fowl cholera organisms (see Chapter 2) to the point where they could be used safely as a live vaccine, he undertook drying the rabbit CNS tissue containing fixed virus to weaken the rabies agent for comparable vaccine production. The CNS tissue he chose was the spinal cord of the paralyzed rabbit. The cord was suspended over sodium hydroxide or other drying agents at room temperature in closed containers. Portions of the cord were tested by daily IC inoculation into rabbits until the fixed virus had lost infectivity both for rabbits and for dogs. Other paralyzed rabbits were sacrificed daily and their spinal cords were subjected to drying. This

procedure gave Pasteur a continuous series of infected spinal cords ranging from fully virulent (no drying) to avirulent (maximum drying).

Pasteur then immunized dogs by daily SC inoculations, starting with an emulsion of avirulent cord and ending with fully virulent cord. The immunized animals resisted SC challenge with fully virulent street virus. Furthermore he demonstrated that the immunization could be started after the inoculation of the street virus and still prevent disease in the test animals. This immunotherapeutic effect was explained by the prolonged incubation time (1–3 or more months) of the disease. Pasteur (1885) published the results of these animal immunization experiments; because of the tremendous fear of rabies, this report received wide publicity.

Shortly after the Pasteur publication a young boy who had been severely bitten by a rabid dog was brought to Pasteur to be treated by his vaccination procedure. Since this treatment had only been tried in dogs and since Pasteur was not a medical doctor, he was loath to undertake the treatment. The severity and extent of the dog bites about the face made it almost certain the boy was infected and would die. Pasteur also realized that if his treatment failed, the boy's death might be blamed on him. The boy's predicament and his mother's pleading finally prevailed, however, and Pasteur agreed. Whether due to the treatment or not, the boy survived. As other dog-bite victims were brought to Pasteur for treatment, the vaccination procedure became accepted and centers for such treatment—Pasteur Institutes—were established around the world.

When the author joined the Texas Department of Health Laboratory in 1931, the Pasteur Institute for Texas was housed in the laboratory building. Texans exposed to rabies came to Austin for the 21-day treatment, which consisted of 21 subcutaneous injections of the Pasteur dried-cord vaccine. Prior to that time, the method of removing the spinal cord from the paralyzed rabbit was something of a mystery to me. The simplicity of the operation, however, was amazing. The paralyzed animal was sacrificed and the body immersed in a disinfectant. After draining off the excess disinfectant, the spinal column was cut through at the neck and hind quarter regions. A sterile cotton swab on a long wire handle was inserted into the posterior end of the spinal canal and used as a ramrod to force the cord out from the anterior end onto a sterile cotton towel. The cord was then suspended on a sterile thread inside the drying container. At least one rabbit was inoculated intracranially every day with virulent fixed virus, and at least one cord was harvested each day from a paralyzed or just dead rabbit. This provided a constant supply of cords, in all necessary stages of drying, for the preparation of the fixed-virus vaccines for patients in the various stages of their treatment.

The preparation and administration of the vaccines was equally simple. An assistant would set up the required number of sterile containers (pedestal wine glasses with aluminum covers) with the required amount of sterile saline for the day's treatments in each. He would then snip off a 0.5-inch or longer segment of the appropriate dried cord and place it in the glass. The cord was emulsified with a sterile glass pestle, and this emulsion constituted the vaccine for those patients who required that strength of virus. Similar vaccines were prepared for other patients who required different strengths (times of drying) of virus. The daily subcutaneous inoculations consisted of 2 milliliters of the appropriate vaccine given in the abdominal region. This site was chosen merely because of the expanse of loose skin for making the 21 injections. If need be, other skin sites could be substituted.

Because of the expense and inconvenience to patients having to spend 21 days for treatment at the Pasteur Institutes, new rabies vaccines were tested. During the 1920s, phenol-inactivated rabbit-brain vaccine was developed by A. B. Semple and proved effective in treating human rabies. An advantage of the Semple vaccine was the fact that, being a killed-virus vaccine, it could be prepared in volume, dispensed into vials (2 milliliters each), and shipped to doctors for administration at the home town of the patient. Moreover, the Semple vaccine treatment generally required only 14 inoculations.

We started production of the Semple vaccine at the Texas Department of Health Laboratory in 1933. The process consisted of harvesting the brains, aseptically, from 30 or more rabbits paralyzed as a result of prior IC inoculations of Pasteur fixed virus. The brains were placed in sterile quart jars containing a small amount of broken Pyrex glass chips. Sufficient sterile saline (0.8 percent NaCl) and phenol were added to give 4 percent brain tissue and 1 percent phenol in the mixture. The jars were mounted on a mechanical (paint-can type) shaker and agitated vigorously for a sufficient time to emulsify the brain tissue. After overnight exposure to the 1 percent phenol to inactivate the virus, the product was diluted with an equal volume of sterile saline to yield a vaccine containing 2 percent brain tissue virus and 0.5 percent phenol preservative. This vaccine was tested for bacterial sterility and noninfectivity prior to bottling in 2-milliliter vials for distribution. Random vials were then submitted to the National Institutes of Health for checking prior to release for treatment of exposed human beings.

Because some individuals gave more or less severe reactions (including occasional encephalitic symptoms) to the rabbit CNS vaccine, other methods of propagating and inactivating the fixed virus were studied. The virus was adapted to duck-egg embryo propagation, and this type of killed-virus vaccine (DEV) displaced the rabbit brain-tissue vaccine. Kissling (1958) adapted the Pasteur fixed virus to propagation in nonneural tissue cultures. Koprowski (1967) and his coworkers at the Wistar Institute propagated rabies virus in WI-38 human diploid cell cultures and used this virus to prepare a killed-virus vaccine that has been reported to produce fewer adverse reactions and to be a much more potent immunogen in humans than the prior rabies vaccines (see Sikes et al. 1971). For results of the use of this vaccine in human rabies, see the discussion of post exposure treatment below. For review of the literature on rabies, see

Nagano and Davenport (1971), Debbie (1974a), and Baer (1975).

ETIOLOGY

Rabies virus probably is the best-known example of an obligately neurotropic infectious agent. When inoculated through the skin either experimentally or by animal bite, the street virus invades regional nerve tissue and travels slowly along the neural pathway to the central nervous system. After reaching the CNS the virus may travel centrifugally along nerve paths to the salivary glands and other tissues. Although the extent of involvement of the salivary glands may vary, there are reports of higher concentrations of the virus in the salivary glands and in lung tissues than in the CNS tissue in some animals. This appears to indicate that the street virus might be able to multiply in glandular and possibly other nonneural tissues. Additional evidence that rabies virus can multiply in nonneural tissues is the fact that it has been propagated in serial passages in hamster kidney, human carcinoma, and other tissue cultures. Rabies virus produces a complement-fixing (C'F) soluble (S) antigen. Antibody specific for this S antigen, however, will not neutralize rabies virus. The particulate virus (V) antigen is a weak C'F antigen, but anti-V antibody neutralizes the rabies virus. The Pasteur fixed virus can also be propagated in human fibroblast tissue cultures. There is, however, little or no evidence of viremia in either animal or human rabies, which might indicate that the virus must travel neural pathways to arrive at nonneural tissues in which it can multiply.

Until the mid-twentieth century rabies virus was considered to be a single immunogenic entity throughout the world; the efficacy of the Pasteur vaccine seems to justify that conclusion, at least from a practical standpoint. The

Figure 35–1. Bullet-shaped virions of rabies virus surrounding an inclusion body in a section of hamster brain. There is speculation that such bodies are the sites of viral assembly. 70,000×. (Courtesy of F. A. Murphy.)

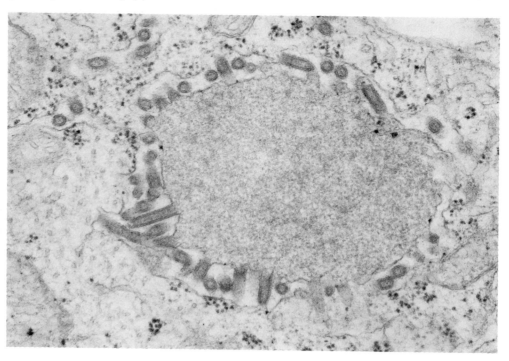

virus is a member of the rhabdovirus group, which are bullet-shaped viruses—cylindrical with one end flattened and the other rounded (see Figure 35-1). Boulger and Porterfield (1958) isolated a rhabdovirus from African fruit bats (the Lagos bat virus) that was morphologically and serologically related to rabies virus. This and another serologically and morphologically related rhabdovirus, isolated from African shrews (IbAn 27377 virus), were studied by Shope et al. (1970). Tignor and Shope (1972) conducted immunological studies on the classic Pasteur fixed virus, a recently isolated rabies (street) virus, and the two related African viruses. Mice individually immunized with the fixed and street rabies viruses resisted homologous challenge and challenge with the Lagos bat virus. However, they were only slightly resistant to challenge with the shrew (IbAn 27377) virus. Mice immunized with the African viruses resisted homologous, but not heterologous, challenge. Thus there appears to be a remote possibility of one or more heterogeneous serotypes of rabies virus to contend with in the future. Nevertheless, the classic Pasteur street virus continues to be the rabies virus of worldwide concern.

EPIDEMIOLOGY

As previously indicated rabies is primarily a disease of warm-blooded wild animals. Those of major concern in the transmission of rabies to domestic animals (dogs, cats, cattle) and to humans are wolves, foxes, and other wild canine species; skunks, raccoons, and vampire and other bats; and members of the mongoose and weasel families (see *MMWR*, 2 April 1976). Although most infected animals die as a result of rabies, there is evidence that bats may harbor the virus in brown fat for long periods of time (Allen et al. 1964a and 1964b). There is also evidence that skunks and weasels may serve as permanent hosts to rabies virus.

Enright (1962) published evidence of the widespread distribution of bat rabies in the United States; and Bigler et al. (1975) published an analysis of bat rabies in Florida during the 20

years from 1954 to 1973. During the first 8 years of the study, multiple impression smears of the brain of each bat were stained and examined for Negri bodies. Only 0.85 percent (55 of 6,447) of bats so studied were found positive. During the remaining 12 years of the study the bat-brain impression smears also were tested by the fluorescent antirabies antibody (FRA) technique (see the section on laboratory diagnosis). These combined tests yielded 10.3 percent positive (236 of 2,293) among bats so examined. Constantine et al. (1972) reported the presence of rabies virus in the nasal mucosa of naturally infected bats, indicating that the virus might be transmitted from these animals by the respiratory route. Moreover, when susceptible animals were exposed (in bat-proof and arthropod-proof screened cages) in a Texas cave known to harbor infected bats, the animals contracted rabies with no chance for bite transmission of the virus.

A member of a Texas Health Department bat-rabies research team, George Menzes, contracted rabies and died. Prior to death, he reported that he had not been bitten, although while wearing rubber gloves he had handled tremendous numbers of bats in several bat caves in Texas and had bled some 75 for serological studies (Irons et al. 1957). A fatal case of apparent airborne rabies in Texas was also reported by Winkler et al. (1973). The victim, a laboratory worker, was exposed to an aerosol of fixed virus during homogenization of rabid goat brains in the preparation of rabies vaccine for veterinary use.

In spite of these examples of nonbite transmission of rabies virus, the major epidemiology of the disease continues to be bite or abraded skin exposure to the buccal secretions of a rabid animal. During 1974, a total of 3,123 rabid animals were reported in the United States. These included 240 dogs, 250 cattle, 425 other domestic animals, 298 foxes, 1,157 skunks, 512 bats, 188 raccoons, and 53 other wild animals. Texas had the dubious distinction of leading the nation with 383 rabid animal reports; California finished a close second with 349 such infections (*MMWR* 1974 Supplement, 15 July 1975). In certain areas of South America vampire bats have transmitted rabies to cattle in such numbers as to necessitate the immunization of entire herds to prevent economic loss to ranchers.

In the past dogs have constituted the major source of human exposure to rabies, and these animals, because of their close association with humans, continue to be a significant source of such exposure. The incidence of rabies in dogs has been greatly reduced, however, by community ordinances requiring the destruction of stray dogs and the immunization of pet dogs. Neither of these ordinances is as rigidly enforced as it should be. An extensive outbreak of rabies in dogs was in progress in Laredo, Texas, in 1976–1977.

SYMPTOMS IN ANIMALS

Because of the tendency toward involvement of the central nervous system, any aberrant activity of domestic or wild animals should be considered as possibly due to rabies. If nocturnal animals (skunks, foxes, bats, raccoons) are observed in more or less active states in the daytime, the possibility of rabies should be considered. This activity becomes more indicative of rabies if the wild animals, which normally fear and avoid human beings, appear unduly bold or aggressive in their approaches. Bats that are found in broad daylight or that flutter about in a partially paralyzed state should not be handled. The incubation period in animals has been reported to vary between 10 and 209 days.

Likewise, if normally docile or friendly pets suddenly become irritable, or run about in an erratic manner, or attack their owners, rabies should be considered. Rabies in dogs may take either or both of two possible symptom syndromes. In the *furious* form (mad dog rabies) the dog may jump fences and run about attacking other dogs or anything that moves. If you wave a stick in front of a chained rabid dog, he will attack it viciously. Such a rabid dog will chew a restraining rope in two in a matter of minutes. Such dogs may travel for miles before becoming paralyzed and then die as a result of the CNS pathology. In other rabid dogs, the CNS pathol-

ogy may be so fulminating that the first observable symptom may be weakness in the hindquarters (and even this symptom may be missed) followed by total body paralysis (*dumb rabies*). Rabid dogs frequently develop an inability to swallow and may appear to be choking. Many nonbite exposures to rabies have resulted from the owner's attempts to determine whether or not the pet is choking on a bone or other object in the throat.

SYMPTOMS IN HUMANS

Documented incubation periods in human rabies have varied between 2 weeks and 6 months. Longer incubation periods (to 8 years) have been reported but are difficult to document; if true, they certainly are rare. Prodromal symptoms of headache, malaise, fever, nausea, and sore throat frequently are associated with abnormal sensations at the site of the bite wound. Varying degrees of hypo- and hypersensitivity of the skin may develop. In the case of Menzes, who suffered no bite wound, the first symptoms were vision difficulties followed by a night of fitful sleep interrupted by nightmares. When he awoke and attempted to take a drink of water he suffered two convulsive seizures. Such spasms of the throat muscles may be precipitated by the mere sight or sound of water. These fearful reactions to water are responsible for designating the human disease "hydrophobia." When a physician was called, Menzes was perfectly coherent and volunteered the information that he had rabies.

Additional convulsive seizures may lead to respiratory difficulties, which may be accompanied by maniacal behavior. Such periods of intense excitement may be interspersed with periods of relative quiet, at which times the patient appears normal and may be perfectly coherent. Usually the patient expires during one of the acute seizures. If these are survived, the patient may sink gradually into a progressive state of apathy, stupor, and coma prior to death. Menzes died on the fourth day following onset of his clinical symptoms. Autopsy specimens yielded unequivocal evidence that the diagnosis of rabies was correct.

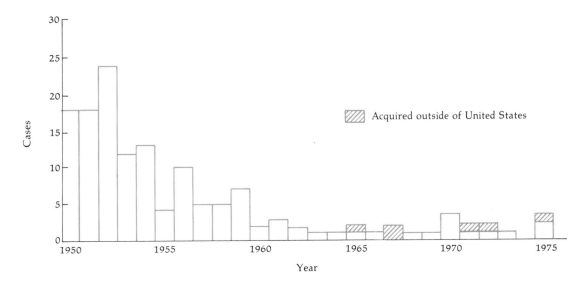

Figure 35–2. The number of human cases of rabies reported in the United States from 1950 to 1975 (From *MMWR,* 15 October 1976.)

Although patients with clinical rabies have been known to survive for up to 133 days, all such cases prior to 1970 eventually terminated fatally. Post facto proof of clinical rabies in survivors is difficult to establish, however. One such case in a 6-year-old boy in Lima, Ohio, in October 1970 appears to be an exception to the rule of fatal termination. While sleeping the boy was bitten by a bat that was later captured and proved rabid by the Ohio Health Department. Although given a 14-day course of duck embryo vaccine, the boy developed typical symptoms of rabies including respiratory difficulties that necessitated a tracheostomy. He was in and out of coma before he began to improve and finally to recover. During 2 months of convalescence, serum antibody titrations ruled out encephalitides and leptospirosis. His antirabies neutralizing antibody titer during this period climbed from 1:5,900 to 1:78,000 (*MMWR,* 19 December 1970). The boy was reported to be well and happy in December 1975.

Single cases of human rabies, all fatal, have been reported from Puerto Rico in 1975 (*MMWR,* 2 April 1976), California in 1975 (*MMWR,* 11 October 1975), England in 1976 (*MMWR,* 21 January 1977), Texas in 1976 (*MMWR,* 4 February 1977), and Maryland in

1976 (*MMWR,* 30 July 1976). Figure 35-2 (from *MMWR,* 15 October 1976) illustrates the annual numbers of human rabies cases reported in the United States from 1950 to 1975. All but one were fatal. Although there were no deaths from the disease in the United States in 1974, there were 412 deaths from rabies reported worldwide that year (*MMWR,* 15 October 1976).

LABORATORY DIAGNOSIS

Efforts to obtain laboratory aid in diagnosing clinical rabies in human patients are rarely attempted. In general such diagnosis depends upon the demonstration of rabies virus in secretions or tissues of the patient. For postmortem diagnosis, brain tissue is examined. Such efforts usually are restricted to public health or research virology laboratories. Negative results in these efforts, however, do not rule out the disease.

Because at least one clinical case of rabies has survived, there have been recommendations that more intensive therapeutic and supportive treatment measures be practiced in the future, in the hope that other lives may be saved. Since currently recommended postexposure treatment involves both passive (antirabies IgG) and active (vaccine) immunotherapy, part of the treatment regimen includes monitoring the antirabies antibody (ARA) in the patient's serum. To be able to establish a baseline for this monitoring, a blood serum specimen should be collected by the clinician prior to beginning antirabies treatment. The serum should be refrigerated and held for submission to the laboratory responsible for monitoring the ARA titers during and following treatment (see the section on treatment below).

Most laboratory diagnosis in rabies is directed at determining the infection status of animals that have bitten or otherwise exposed humans. After Negri in 1903 described the intracytoplasmic inclusion (Negri) bodies in CNS cells of infected animals and fatal cases of human rabies, the demonstration of these bodies in CNS tissue became the diagnostic method of choice. For the diagnosis of animal rabies, either the whole body or the intact head of the suspected animal should be packed in a closed container surrounded by ice and sent to the diagnostic laboratory. Damage to the head should be avoided in sacrificing the live animals suspected of being rabid.

If the suspect animal is a normal-appearing dog or other pet, the best procedure is to have the animal caged by a veterinarian for a 10-day examination period. The longer the animal survives, the less the danger of rabies. If the animal was infected and capable of transmitting rabies at the time of exposure, it can be expected to develop typical symptoms and die in less than 10 days. This is due to the fact that the virus has already invaded the brain before it travels the neural pathway to the salivary glands. Only after this migration can the animal transmit the infection. If not caged, the animal may break loose, jump fences, and disappear prior to dying—in which case the exposed person must be treated for rabies, whether or not the animal was infected.

For the demonstration of Negri bodies, the brain of the animal is removed. The cylindrical Ammon's horn of the hippocampus at the base of the brain is the best tissue for searching for Negri bodies. Thin cross-section segments of the Ammon's horn are placed on a tongue depressor or other disposable support, and five or six impression smears are prepared on each of two or more microslides. The smears are fixed and stained with a polychrome (Sellers) stain. The round or oval intracytoplasmic Negri bodies stain differentially from the cytoplasm and nucleus of the large nerve cells in the impression smears. Although 90 percent of rabid dogs develop Negri bodies, a variable percentage of other animals and a very low percentage of rabid skunks develop these inclusion bodies.

Other tests for demonstrating rabies virus in infected animal tissues are (1) intracranial inoculation of antibiotic-treated brain tissue from the suspect animal into highly susceptible Swiss white mice and (2) treatment of tissue (Ammon's horn) impression smears with fluorescent antirabies antiserum (FRA), introduced by Goldwasser and Kissling (1958) and advocated by Kaplan et al (1960). Lennette et al. (1965) compared the three methods of diagnosing animal rabies on several thousand specimens, 363 of which were considered positive. In this study only 65.8 percent of the 363 were positive by the Negri body test, 98.3 percent were positive by the mouse inoculation test, and 99.4 percent were positive by the FRA test (see Figure 35-3). The low percentage (65.8) of Negri body test positives was explained by the large number of skunks included in this study. For the FRA test, fluorescein-conjugated antirabies IgG from hyperimmunized hamsters was recommended. Positive and negative mouse brain controls should be included along with the test impression smears. Because of the speed of obtaining test results and the almost 100 percent positive results, the FRA test should be performed on all suspect animals.

Although rabies virus produces hemagglutination of goose and other erythrocytes, Halonen et al. (1968) reported that nonantibody ("nonspecific") inhibitors (HI) of this activity were found in normal human, burro, and goat sera. Since this "nonspecific" HI was difficult to remove from the normal animal sera, the simple serotaxonomic and serodiagnostic HI tests for rabies are not recommended. As indicated above, the soluble (S) antigen of rabies virus in

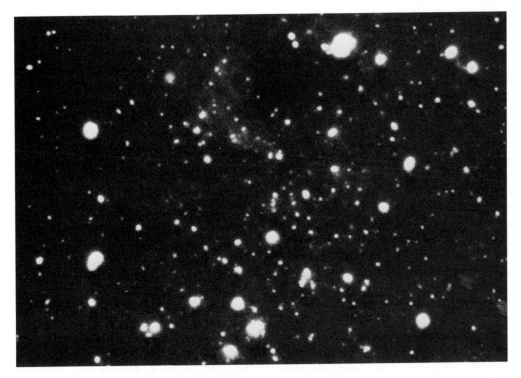

Figure 35–3. The light spots (actually light green in color) are fluorescing rabies antigen in a slip-smear slide of rabid skunk brain. The preparation was stained with fluorescein isothiocyanate-tagged anti-rabies IgG. Only the largest few spots would have been identified as Negri bodies if this fairly typical preparation had been stained by Seller's method, demonstrating the greater sensitivity of FA staining mentioned in the text. About 1175×. (Photo by J. D. Woodie, courtesy of R. W. Emmons.)

mouse brain or tissue cultures can be demonstrated by complement fixation and other serological tests, but these tests have little practical value.

For monitoring the serum antirabies antibody titers of patients undergoing postexposure treatment, the indirect fluorescent antibody (IFA) test is the method of choice. This test involves multiple impression smears of brains from mice that have been infected with a standard strain of rabies virus. Each smear is treated with a separate dilution of the patient's serum. Following a suitable reaction time, the excess serum is washed from the preparations and all are exposed to fluorescent antihuman IgG antibody (FAHA). Following this secondary reaction, the preparations are examined with the ultraviolet-light microscope. The highest dilu-

tion of the patient's serum that yields significant fluorescence of the infected mouse brain smear constitutes the titer of the antirabies antibody in the patient's serum. If the patient's therapy involves both equine antirabies antiserum and rabies vaccine, the IFA test will measure only antibody resulting from the vaccine therapy, because the FAHA will not react with the equine antibody attached to the impression smears. If human-antirabies-immune globulin (HRIG) is used, however, the IFA test will measure the combined concentration of both the passively administered antibody and the actively (vaccine) stimulated antirabies antibody. A pretreatment blood serum should be included in monitoring the antirabies antibody concentration in the patient. For more details, see Kaplan and Koprowski (1973) and Johnson (1974).

POSTEXPOSURE TREATMENT

Bites by rabid animals involving deep lacerations on the face or head are particularly dangerous. The rabbit CNS-propagated fixed-virus rabies vaccine, first proposed by Pasteur and modified by Semple and others, constituted the only specific antirabies treatment until it was displaced during the 1940s by the duck-embryo-propagated virus vaccine (DEV). Active (vaccine) immunotherapy constituted the sole specific postexposure treatment until after the mid-twentieth century. Koprowski and Cox (1951) were among the first to report immediate treatment of persons exposed to rabid dog bites with antirabies horse serum (ARHS) antibody followed by 14 doses of phenolized rabies vaccine. All 29 of their patients survived. Baltazard and Bahmanyar (1955) and Habel and Koprowski (1955) reported results of treating 46 patients bitten by rabid wolves in Iran including many with head lacerations. Their reports indicated that ARHS plus vaccine lowered the mortality rate significantly when compared to vaccine alone. Subsequently many workers have advocated this combined immunotherapy for postexposure rabies treatment. The equine antibody posed two problems: not being able to use the ARHS in patients who were hypersensitive to horse serum; and sensitizing and causing serum sickness in patients not previously hypersensitive to this serum. K. Habel in 1968 reported results of using homologous versus heterologous animal antiserum in the treatment of experimental rabies; Winkler et al. (1969) applied this approach to the treatment of humans exposed to rabies. During the 1970s, human-rabies-immune globulin (HRIG) became available for the passive immunotherapy aspect of postexposure rabies treatment.

Habel (1957) reported that prior administration of rabies-immune globulin to mice interfered with the antigenicity of subsequently administered rabies vaccine. This interference has been confirmed in humans, and Hattwick et al. (1974) studied the problem using HRIG and DEV in 205 healthy human volunteers. They monitored the serum antirabies antibody concentrations for 70 days in volunteers receiving 10, 15, or 40 international units (IU) of HRIG per kilogram of body weight administered either alone or in combination with injections of DEV for 16 or 23 days. Two groups of volunteers received no HRIG and either 16 or 23 injections of DEV. Based on the immediate antirabies serum antibody (ARA) titers obtained and the level of ARA titers over a 70-day period, Hattwick et al. recommended the administration of between 15 and 40 IU per kilogram of HRIG followed by a 23-dose course of DEV.

Bahmanyar et al. (1976) reported the successful use of the human diploid cell cultured rabies virus vaccine (HDCV) of Koprowski et al. in 45 severely exposed humans in Iran. The virus in the vaccine was killed by treatment with beta-propriolactone prior to lyophilization. The lyophilized vaccine was dispensed in single-dose aliquots along with 1 milliliter of diluent in a sterile disposable syringe. The treatment schedule consisted of one dose (40 IU/kilogram body weight) of mule antirabies antiserum (MARA) on day 0, followed by single HDCV injections on days 0, 3, 7, 14, and 30. A 1-milliliter booster injection of HDCV was given on day 90. Blood was collected from each individual just prior to each injection of HDCV, and the sera were monitored for ARA titers by virus neutralization tests in mice. The titers in the 45 individuals on day 30 averaged 48.9; in those tested on day 100 they averaged 320+ IU/kilogram body weight per milliliter of serum. All the exposed individuals survived, although prior experience in Iran with CNS and duck egg vaccines would have predicted a significant fatality rate. Unless unexpected complications develop in future testing, the HDCV and treatment regimen developed by Koprowski et al. can be expected to displace the currently (1977) recommended DEV postexposure rabies treatment.

Immediately following an animal bite, the wound should be thoroughly cleansed with soap and disinfected, preferably by a physician. Corey and Hattwick (1975) listed the questions and answers necessary to determine whether or not treatment is needed and, if needed, the type of postexposure treatment to administer to persons possibly exposed to rabies. Table 35-1

Table 35-1. Postexposure antirabies treatment guide.*

Species	Condition at Time of Attack	Treatment† Bite	Nonbite
Wild			
Skunk	Regard as rabid	S,V,1	S,V,1
Fox, wolf	Regard as rabid	S,V,1	S,V,1
Raccoon	Regard as rabid	S,V,1	S,V,1
Bat	Regard as rabid	S,V,1	S,V,1
Domestic dog and cat	Healthy	None,2	None,2
	Rabid	S,V,1	S,V,1
	Unknown (escaped)	S,V	V,3

*These recommendations are only a guide. They should be used in conjunction with knowledge of the animal species involved, circumstances of the bite or other exposure, vaccination status of the animal, and presence of rabies in the region. Animals not listed here are to be considered individually.

† V = rabies vaccine; S = 30–40 IU/kg HRIG; 1 = discontinue vaccine if fluorescent antibody tests of animal killed at the time of attack are negative; 2 = begin HRIG and vaccine at first sign of rabies in biting dog or cat during holding period (10 days); 3 = 23 doses of duck embryo vaccine. As indicated in the text, the 6-dose HDCV of Koprowski et al. may soon displace the 23-dose DEV.

(slightly modified) is taken from their report and summarizes the recommendations of the U.S. Public Health Service Committee on Immunization Practices as published in *MMWR* Report 21 (Supplement 25, 24 June 1972).

CONTROL AND PREVENTION

The control of rabies in wild animals is impossible; and this reservoir of infection frequently introduces the disease into susceptible domestic animals. Certainly dogs and possibly other domestic animals (such as cattle exposed to vampire bats) should be immunized with rabies vaccine.

Since a modified-virulence, live-virus rabies vaccine is available for animal immunization, Debbie et al. (1972), Debbie (1974b), and Winkler et al. (1975) have reported efforts to immunize foxes and other wild animals by the ingestion of vaccine-treated baits (dog biscuits or eggs). Although experimental administration of such vaccine to captured animals has indicated an antirabies antibody response, there is little hope that this approach will affect the wild animal reservoir significantly.

The only generally successful antirabies programs to date have been strict enforcement of ordinances requiring the immunization of pet dogs and the destruction of stray dogs, along with the immunization of cattle in areas of vampire bat rabies.

REFERENCES

Allen, R., R. A. Sims, and S. E. Sulkin. 1964a. Studies with cultured brown adipose tissue. I. Persistence of rabies virus in bat brown fat. *Amer, J. Hyg.* 80:11–24.

———. 1964b. Studies with cultured brown adipose tissue. II. Influence of low temperature on rabies virus infection in bat brown fat. *Amer. J. Hyg.* 80:25–32.

Baer, G. M. (ed.). 1975. *Natural History of Rabies.* 2 vols. New York: Academic Press.

Bahmanyar, M., A. Fayaz, S. Noursalchi, M. Mohammadi, and H. Koprowski. 1976. Successful protection of humans exposed to rabies infection. Postexposure treatment with the new human diploid cell rabies vaccine and human antirabies serum. *J. Amer. Med. Ass.* 236:2751–2754.

Baltazard, M., and M. Bahmanyar. 1955. Essai pratique du sérum antirabique chez les mordus par loups enragés. *Bull. Wld. Hlth. Org.* 13:747–772.

Bigler, W. J., G. L. Hoff, and E. E. Buff. 1975. Chiroptean rabies in Florida: a twenty-year analysis, 1954 to 1973. *Amer. J. Trop. Med. Hyg.* 24:347–352.

Boulger, L. R., and J. S. Porterfield. 1958. Isolation of a virus from Nigerian fruit bats. *Trans. Roy. Soc. Trop. Med. Hyg.* 52:421–424.

Constantine, D. G., R. W. Emmons, and J. D. Woodie. 1972. Rabies virus in nasal mucosa of naturally infected bats. *Science* 75:1255–1256.

Corey, L., and M. H. W. Hattwick. 1975. Treatment of persons exposed to rabies. *J. Amer. Med. Ass.* 232:272–276.

Debbie, J. G. 1974a. Rabies. *Prog. Med. Virol.* 18:241–256.

———. 1974b. Use of inoculated eggs as a vehicle for the oral vaccination of red foxes (*Vulpes fulva*). *Infect. Immunity* 4:681–683.

Debbie, J. G., M. K. Abelseth, and G. M. Baer. 1972. The use of commercially available vaccines for the oral vaccination of foxes against rabies. *Amer. J. Epid.* 96:231–235.

Enright, J. B. 1962. Geographic distribution of bat rabies in the United States, 1953–1960. *Amer. J. Pub. Health* 52:484–488.

Goldwasser, R. A., and R. F. Kissling. 1958. Fluorescent antibody staining of street and fixed rabies virus antigen. *Proc. Soc. Exper. Biol. Med.* 98:219–223.

Habel, K. 1957. Rabies antiserum interference with antigenicity of vaccine in mice. *Bull. Wld. Hlth. Org.* 17:932–936.

Habel, K., and H. Koprowski. 1955. Laboratory data supporting clinical use of ARS in persons bitten by a rabid wolf. *Bull. Wld. Hlth. Org.* 13:773–779.

Halonen, P. E., F. A. Murphy, B. N. Fields, and D. R. Reese. 1968. Hemagglutinin of rabies and some other bullet-shaped viruses. *Proc. Soc. Exper. Biol. Med.* 127:1037–1042.

Hattwick, M. H. W., R. H. Rubin, S. Music, R. K. Sikes, J. S. Smith, and M. B. Gregg. 1974. Postexposure rabies prophylaxis with human rabies immune globulin. *J. Amer. Med. Ass.* 227:407–410.

Irons, J. V., R. B. Eads, J. E. Grimes, and A. Conklin. 1957. The public health importance of bats. *Texas Rep. Biol. Med.* 15:292–298.

Johnson, H. R. 1974. Rabiesvirus. Chapter 82 in *Manual of Clinical Microbiology.*

Kaplan, M., Z. Forsek, and H. Koprowski. 1960. Demonstration of rabies virus in tissue culture with fluorescent antibody technique. *Bull. Wld. Hlth. Org.* 22:434–435.

Kaplan, M., and H. Koprowski. 1973. *Laboratory Techniques in Rabies.* 3rd ed. Geneva: World Health Organization.

Kissling, R. E. 1958. Growth of rabies virus in non-nervous tissue cultures. *Proc. Soc. Exper. Biol. Med.* 98:223–225.

Koprowski, H. 1967. Vaccines against rabies: present and future. *Proceedings of First International Conference on Vaccines against Viral and Rickettsial Diseases of Man.* Washington: Pan American Health Organization.

Koprowski, H., and H. R. Cox. 1951. Recent developments in the prophylaxis of rabies. *Amer. J. Pub. Health* 41:1483–1489.

Lennette, E. H., J. D. Woodie, K. Nabamura, and R. L. Magoffin. 1965. The diagnosis of rabies by fluorescent antibody method (FRA) employing immune hamster serum. *Health Lab. Sci.* 2:24–34.

Nagano, Y., and F. M. Davenport (eds.). 1971. *Rabies.* Baltimore: University Park Press.

Pasteur, L. 1885. Méthode pour prévenir la rage après morsure. *Compt. Rend. Acad. Sci.* 101:765–772.

Pasteur, L., C. Chamberland, E. Roux, and Thuillier. 1881. Sur la rage. *Compt. Rend. Acad. Sci.* 92:1259–1260.

Shope, R. E., F. A. Murphy, A. K. Harrison, O. R. Causey, G. E. Kemp, D. I. H. Simpson, and D. L. Moore. 1970. Two African viruses serologically and morphologically related to rabies virus. *J. Virol.* 6:690–692.

Sikes, R. K., W. F. Cleary, and H. Koprowski. 1971. Effective protection of monkeys against death from street virus by post-exposure administration of tissue culture rabies vaccine. *Bull. Wrld. Hlth. Org.* 45:1–11.

Tierkel, E. S. 1971. *Rabies—Historical Review.* Baltimore: University Park Press.

Tignor, G. H., and R. E. Shope. 1972. Vaccination and challenge of mice with viruses of the rabies serogroup. *J. Infect. Dis.* 125:322–324.

Winkler, W. G., T. R. Fashinell, L. Leffingwell, H. Paxton, and J. P. Conomy. 1973. Airborne rabies transmission in a laboratory worker. *J. Amer. Med. Ass.* 226:1219–1221.

Winkler, W. G., R. G. McLean, and J. C. Cowart. 1975. Vaccination of foxes against rabies using ingested baits. *J. Wildlife Dis.* 11:383–388.

Winkler, W. G., R. Schmidt, and R. K. Sikes. 1969. Evaluation of human rabies immune globulin and homologous and heterologous antibody. *J. Immunol.* 102:1314–1321.

36

Rat-Bite and Related Fevers

There are at least two etiologically distinct diseases commonly transmitted by the bite of apparently normal rats, including wild and laboratory animals. Both diseases have been designated "rat-bite fever," although this designation may be a misnomer in instances of each disease.

Febrile human disease of unknown etiology, following the bite of a rat, was described in the early nineteenth century. In the early twentieth century, a rat-bite fever designated soduka (sodoku) was described in Japan; the etiological agent was reported to be a short spiral organism—a spirillum. The taxonomic designation for this organism has undergone a variety of both genus and species changes over the years with the most generally accepted current designation being *Spirillum minus*. The eighth edition of *Bergey's Manual* lists the species as *minor* instead of *minus*, however. It appears to this author that this minor change is one of those confusing and unnecessary modifications of a widely accepted taxonomic designation frequently perpetrated by overzealous bacterial taxonomists. It is comforting to know that the change has not been accepted by many authorities, including those of the sixth edition of Wilson and Miles (1975).

Therefore we will continue to designate the etiological agent of this form of rat-bite fever as *S. minus.*

The second etiologically distinct form of rat-bite fever is caused by an actinomycete. Although the genus and species designations for this organism, like *S. minus*, have undergone numerous changes, the generally accepted and still current designation is *Streptobacillus moniliformis.*

As indicated above, the designation rat-bite fever may be a misnomer for instances of both etiological forms of the disease. The clinical disease sodoku, for example, may result from the bites of rats but also from the bites of mice and animals that frequently feed upon rats and mice: cats, ferrets, weasels, pigs, and others. Consequently we will use the Japanese designation of sodoku for the spirillosis form of rat-bite fever.

The rat-bite fever symptomatology caused by *S. moniliformis* has occurred in epidemic form in persons drinking contaminated milk. Such a clinical entity hardly should be called "rat-bite fever," even though the *S. moniliformis* contamination of the milk probably came from a rat. It is conceivable that other foods also might be similarly contaminated and account for the rat → food → human transmission of the disease. Although the first milk-borne epidemic of this disease, which occurred in Haverhill, Massachusetts, was designated Haverhill fever, it would be an equal misnomer to so designate the rat-bite-transmitted form of the disease. Also, as indicated for sodoku, other animals might be contaminated by feeding on infected rats and transmit the disease. Consequently we will designate this clinical entity as a streptobacilliosis whether or not rat bite is involved in its transmission.

ETIOLOGY AND EPIDEMIOLOGY

Spirillum minus is a gram-negative, short (2 to 5 microns), spiral organism (two to six spirals); each end has a polar tuft of flagella. Although actively motile, *S. minus* does not show the flexible and twisting type of motility characteristic of spirochetes such as *Borrelia*, *Leptospira*, and *Treponema*. The organism has been found in the nasobuccal secretions of normal rats and appears to be an obligate parasite, since it has not been cultivated on nonliving media. However, this was the situation for *Borrelia* spirochetes until 1971 (see Chapter 30). It is the author's opinion that systematic efforts will provide a suitable medium for future cultivation of *S. minus*. The organism will infect guinea pigs, rats, mice, and monkeys. Guinea pigs and mice are the animals of choice for laboratory diagnostic use. The epidemiology usually involves the bite of a rat or an animal that feeds on rats.

Streptobacillus moniliformis is a polymorphic organism with cell shapes varying from small bacillus or coccobacillary forms to long (100 to 300 microns) homogeneous or fragmented filaments. The filaments may develop numerous spindle-shaped or spherical swellings (1 to 3 microns in diameter). Some of this morphological variation appears to depend upon the medium in or on which the organism is cultivated (see Figure 36-1a and b). Culture media (broth or agar) must be supplemented with 10 to 15 percent (v/v) horse or rabbit serum or ascitic

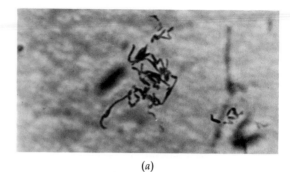

(a)

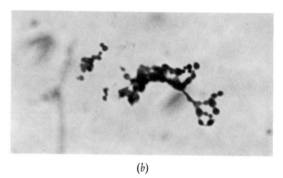

(b)

Figure 36–1. Two forms of *Streptobacillus moniliformis.* (a) Early culture showing rods developing into filaments. (b) L form; note rounded cells. Both about 3000×. ((b) Courtesy of J. Dyckman.)

fluid. The bacterial phase of *S. moniliformis* is a gram-negative, facultative anaerobe.

L-phase variants of *S. moniliformis* have been demonstrated in agar culture. They produce small, subsurface colonies on semisolid agar media. These colonies demonstrate the characteristic "fried egg" appearance of other bacterial L forms (a dark center surrounded by a light periphery). Since the L-phase cells are fragile and tend to grow into, rather than on, the surface of the agar, they are best transplanted by the aseptic transfer of a small block of the agar containing the colony, to the surface of a fresh plate of the agar medium. The upper surface of the block should be placed face down and carefully pushed over the surface and pressed into the surface of the transplant medium. The L-phase cells do not possess normal cell walls. This accounts for both their osmotic fragility and their resistance to penicillin, cephalosporins, and other drugs that depend upon their capacity to interfere with cell-wall synthesis for their antibiotic effect.

CLINICAL SYMPTOMS

Two easily recognized clinical differences between rat-bite fevers caused by *S. minus* and *S. moniliformis* are (1) the duration of the incubation period—10 to 23 days for the former and usually 3 to 10 days for the latter—and (2) the inflammatory or ulcerative recrudescence at the site of the previously healed bite wound that occurs coincident with the onset of symptoms in the former but not in the latter. In addition to the recrudescent inflammation, pain, and possible ulceration at the site of the bite wound, sodoku is characterized by a relapsing-type fever, lymphadenitis, and a maculopapular or purpuric rash spreading from the bite lesion. Failure to cultivate the causative organism from blood or involved tissue fluids might also be indicative of sodoku rather than streptobacilliosis. Gracheva (1974) described clinical aspects of sodoku in Russia. This spirillosis has been treated successfully with penicillin and streptomycin. In untreated cases the mortality rate has ranged from 5 to 10 percent (see Kowal 1961).

Streptobacilliosis, whether contracted by animal bite or the ingestion of contaminated food, usually commences with chills followed by a prostrating, remittent-type fever (to 104°F), severe headache, and myalgias. A cutaneous macular rash may progress to a measles-type or petechial eruption. Migratory arthritic symptoms are common, with joint pains and swelling. This joint syndrome led Place et al. (1926) and Hazard and Goodkind (1932) to designate the Haverhill fever, which they studied, as erythema arthriticum epidemicum. Untreated the symptoms may persist for weeks to months with fatal terminations ranging up to 10 percent. Serious complications or sequelae of streptobacilliosis are pneumonia and endocarditis.

Savage (1972) studied experimental streptobacilliosis in mice. He noted that intravenous inoculation of *S. moniliformis* produced progressive bacteremia and polyarthritis, whereas sub-cutaneous inoculation in a hind foot produced intermittent bacteremia and arthritis in that limb only. He also noted that cells grown in serum broth were more virulent than those grown on serum-agar medium.

Rat-bite streptobacilliosis has been cured by large doses of penicillin continued over a period of 1 to 3 weeks (see Roughgarden 1965). However, because of the likely presence of penicillin-resistant transitional and L forms of *S. moniliformis,* it has been recommended that the penicillin (10^6 units/day) be combined with streptomycin (1 gram/day). A case in Texas in 1974, however, because it was first misdiagnosed as Rocky Mountain spotted fever and because the patient was allergic to penicillin, was treated with chloramphenicol (50 milligrams/kilogram/day) for 10 days. The patient's temperature returned to normal on the second day of treatment and recovery was uneventful (see *MMWR,* 19 October 1974). Lambe et al. (1973) studied five isolates of *S. moniliformis* from a patient who apparently was infected by contact with rats he had killed in his yard. The isolated *S. moniliformis* were susceptible to chloramphenicol, kanamycin, tetracycline, erythromycin, lincomycin and gentamycin. At 24 hours, they were susceptible to ampicillin and cephalothin, but at 48 hours they were resistant to these cell-wall antibiotics. The antibiotic susceptibility testing, however, could not be performed on standard Mueller-Hinton agar because the isolates would not grow on this medium. For a more comphrehensive discussion of both varieties of rat-bite fever see Jellison (1963).

LABORATORY DIAGNOSIS

Sodoku

Since *S. minus* cannot be cultivated on nonliving media, the organism must be demonstrated either (1) in wet mounts or stained smears of blood, lymph, or lesion exudates from the patient or (2) in the blood or heart tissue of a guinea pig or mouse after intraperitoneal inoculation of a specimen from the patient. In the latter procedure the blood of the test animals should be examined microscopically (dark field), prior to inoculation of the specimen, to rule out natural infections with spiral organisms. Specimens that fail to reveal the presence of typical spirilla by microscopic examination should be inoculated to at least one guinea pig and four mice. Control animals should be inoculated with comparable aliquots of the specimens that have been heated at 52°C for 1 hour to rule out natural infections during the 3-week examination period.

In addition to direct microscopic examination of wet mounts of the patient's blood, lymph, or lesion exudates for *S. minus*; smears of these specimens on microslides should be stained with gram stain and with a polychromatic stain (Wright or Giemsa) and examined with a light microscope. Comparable preparations from the test and control animals also should be examined over a period of 3 weeks before considering the results negative. If the blood or peritoneal exudate of the test animals fails to reveal typical spirilla, their hearts may be sliced in half, and impression smears of the cut surface may be fixed and stained as described above. The infected heart tissues have been reported to yield large numbers of *S. minus* even in the absence of these organisms in blood smears.

Streptobacilliosis

Since *S. moniliformis* can be cultivated in suitable broth and agar media, laboratory specimens from the patient usually are inoculated to such media rather than to experimental animals. The specimens for laboratory diagnosis include blood plasma, fluid from arthritic joints, and exudate from suppurative lesions. Aseptically collected and citrated blood or joint fluid may be inoculated directly to broth media. A commonly advocated medium is composed of fresh or dehydrated heart infusion broth, supplemented with 10 percent sterile horse or rabbit serum or ascitic fluid and 0.5 percent yeast extract. The broth should be sterilized by filtration and incubated for 24 hours to ensure sterility prior to inoculation. After inoculation both broth and agar plate cultures should be incubated at 35 to

37°C for 2 or 3 days in a candle jar to provide CO_2 and prevent drying.

In broth culture, *S. moniliformis* tends to grow as "fluff ball" or "bread crumb" aggregates on the bottom of the tube or on the surface of sedimented blood cells. The cultures should not be shaken during examinations and transferring. In transplanting the growth to fresh medium or transferring for the preparation of smears for staining, an entire fluff-ball or breadcrumb aggregate should be carefully drawn into a sterile pipette for the transfer. The use of bacteriological loops is not recommended for manipulations of *S. moniliformis* cultures. Daily transfers of broth cultures may be required to maintain the viability of the organism.

Both the bacterial and the L forms of *S. moniliformis* can be grown on a plating medium composed of fresh or dehydrated heart infusion agar (0.5 to 1.0 percent) which, after sterilization at 121°C for 15 minutes and being cooled to approximately 50°C, is supplemented with 10 percent sterile rabbit or horse serum and sufficient sterile yeast extract solution to yield a final 0.5 percent (v/v) concentration. The supplemented agar medium, while still fluid at 45 to 50°C, should be dispensed into sterile petri plates and allowed to solidify into a semisolid gel.

The patient's blood plasma, joint fluid, or diluted exudate should be pipetted to the agar and distributed over the surface by carefully tilting the plates back and forth. After inoculation the plates should be incubated as indicated above, but in an upright position.

On agar media, *S. moniliformis* develops raised, granular colonies that may range up to 5 millimeters in diameter. The cells of these colonies are viable for longer periods (around 7 days) than those of broth cultures. Microscopic L-form colonies may be observed beneath or adjacent to the bacterial-phase colonies. The L-phase organisms may be isolated in pure culture and transplanted to fresh agar medium by the agar-block technique described above. There is evidence that the L phase may regenerate the bacterial phase of *S. moniliformis*.

Since L forms of other bacterial species may be present in the specimens from the patient, it may become important to identify them as *S. moniliformis* L forms. Biochemical tests are available for the identification of both the bacterial-phase and the L-phase cells. The bacillary forms of the bacterial phase can also be identified by serotaxonomic agglutination or FA tests using specific antiserum. Likewise the bacillary forms of *S. moniliformis* may be used as a specific antigen for serodiagnostic agglutination tests on a patient's sera. For a more comprehensive discussion of the laboratory diagnosis of rat-bite fevers see Lambe et al. (1973) and Rogosa (1974).

CONTROL AND PREVENTION

There is little that can be done to prevent rat-bite fevers beyond the exclusion of rats from the vicinity of human habitation. Since the two cases reported from Texas and Virginia (*MMWR*, 19 October 1974) were both laboratory persons, bitten by normal laboratory rats, such personnel should take precautions against this type of exposure.

REFERENCES

Buchanan, R. E., and N. E. Gibbons. 1974. *Bergey's Manual of Determinative Bacteriology.* 8th ed. Baltimore: Williams & Wilkins.

Gracheva, N. M. 1974. Clinical aspects of sodoku disease. *Sov. Med.* 37:150–151.

Hazard, J. B., and R. Goodkind. 1932. Haverhill fever (erythema arthriticum epidemicum): a case report and bacteriologic study. *J. Amer. Med. Ass.* 99:534–538.

Jellison, W. L. 1963. Rat-bite fever (Sodoku and Haverhill fever). In *Diseases Transmitted from Animals to Man,* ed. T. G. Hull. 5th ed. Springfield: Charles C. Thomas.

Kowal, J. 1961. *Spirillum* fever. Report of a case and review of the literature. *New Eng. J. Med.* 264:123–128.

Lambe, D. W., Jr., A. M. McPhedran, J. A. Mertz, and P. Stewart. 1973. *Streptobacillus moniliformis* isolated from a case of Haverhill fever: biochemical characterization and the inhibitory effect of sodium polyanethol sulfonate. *Amer. J. Clin. Path.* 60:854–860.

Place, E. H., L. E. Sutton, and O. Willner. 1926. Erythema arthriticum epidemicum. *Boston Med. and Surg. J.* 194:285–287.

Rogosa, M. 1974. *Streptobacillus moniliformis* and *Spirillum minor.* Chapter 31 in *Manual of Clinical Microbiology.*

Roughgarden, J. W. 1965. Antimicrobial therapy of rat-bite fever. A review. *Arch. Intern. Med.* 116:39–54.

Savage, N. L. 1972. Host-parasite relationships in experimental *Streptobacillus moniliformis* arthritis in mice. *Infect. Immunity* 5:183–190.

Wilson, G. S., and A. A. Miles. 1975. *Topley and Wilson's Principles of Bacteriology and Immunity.* 6th ed. Baltimore: Williams & Wilkins.

37

Wound Infections

Broken skin can serve as the portal of entry for a variety of bacterial infections. Staphylococci (see Chapter 20), for example, are almost invariably present on human skin, and they tend to invade abrasions, cuts, or penetrating wounds. Usually they cause self-limited inflammatory and pyogenic infections.

AEROBIC BACTERIA

Aerobic streptococci, particularly *S. pyogenes* (see Chapter 8), although less frequently present on normal human skin than staphylococci, are found on nasobuccal membranes. These streptococci can infect wounds and are more invasive than staphylococci. They may cause localized pyogenic abscesses or they may spread along lymph channels (lymphangitis) to involve regional lymph nodes (lymphadenitis) and on to the invasion of the bloodstream (septicemia).

Also, as indicated in Chapter 9, aerobic mycobacteria (*M. ulcerans* and *M. marinum*) in swimming pools and seawater can invade skin abrasions and cause localized skin lesions (Daphne sores). A more severe wound infection, associated with exposure to seawater, was reported by Rubin and Tilton (1975). An aerobic vibrio (*V. alginolyticus*) was isolated from the infected deep muscle wounds. Even the common saprophytic intestinal bacterium *Escherichia coli* has been known to invade deep muscle wounds and cause gas-gangrene type infections. An unusual aerobic bacterial infection of a wound involving *Shigella flexneri* (a dysentery bacillus of Chapter 23) was reported by Gregory et al. (1974). For examples of mycotic (fungal) infections in subgroup C, see Chapter 21.

ANAEROBIC BACTERIA

The major anaerobic bacteria, which invade human wounds and cause disease ranging in severity from mild to fulminating, are (1) anaerobic streptococci (see Martin 1974) and sev-

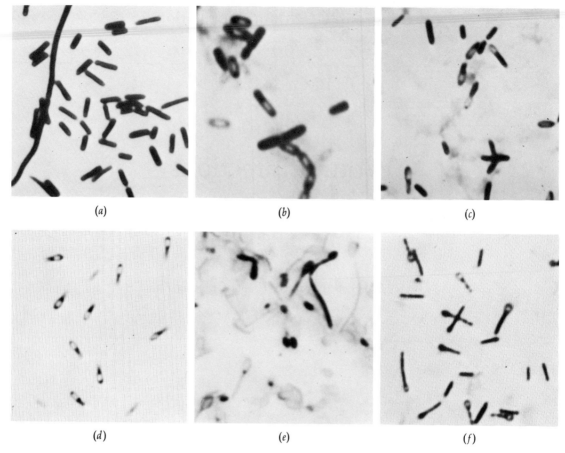

(a)   (b)   (c)

(d)   (e)   (f)

Figure 37–1. Examples of vegetative cell and spore morphologies of species of *Clostridium.* (a) *Clostridium perfringens* type A; thioglycollate medium, 24 hrs. No spores are seen here and are rare under most conditions. (b) *C. bifermentans;* cooked-meat glucose medium, 24 hrs; central to subterminal oval spores. (c) *C. novyi* type A; cooked-meat glucose medium, 24 hrs; subterminal oval spores. (d) *C. subterminale;* blood agar medium, 48 hrs, 35°C; subterminal oval spores. (e) *C. tertium;* blood agar medium, 48 hrs, 35°C, anaerobic conditions; terminal oval spores. (f) *C. tetani;* cooked-meat glucose medium, 24 hrs; terminal spherical spores. All about 4500×. (Courtesy of V. R. Dowell, Center for Disease Control, Atlanta, GA.)

eral other genera of non-spore-forming an-aerobes including *Bacteroides fragilis* and (2) members of the genus *Clostridium,* all of which are spore-forming bacilli. Smith and Hobbs (1974) list 61 species of this genus, but many have not been isolated from human disease. These spore-forming bacilli are frequently found in soil and in human and animal intestinal excreta, especially in that of horses. All stain gram-positive in young cultures but tend to become gram-negative within 24 hours. Most vegetative clostridia are motile by means of peritrichous flagella. The spores are either spherical or oval and tend to be broader than the vegetative cell. They may be located terminally, subterminally, or centrally (see Figure 37-1). The spores are highly resistant to heat, to drying, and to disinfectants. Conditions required for spore formation, however, may vary for different species of clostridia and consequently spores may not always appear in a given laboratory specimen.

Rode et al. (1967) and Rode (1970) described a number of unique spore appendages produced by both saprophytic and pathogenic (*C. bifermentans* and *C. botulinum*) clostridial species. The appendages are demonstrable only by electron microscopy (see Figure 37-2). Rode and Smith (1970) studied the spore appendages of 35 isolates of *C. bifermentans*. On the basis of the presence or absence of spore appendages and the morphology of the appendages when present, the 35 isolates were divided into the following five biotypes illustrated in Figure 37-2: (1) no spore appendages; (2) appendages designated "pinlike"—such appendages also were reported by Hodgkiss et al. (1966) on *C. botulinum* spores; (3) appendages designated "smooth tubular"; (4) appendages designated "hirsute tubular"; and (5) appendages designated "featherlike." Beyond the possibility of taxonomic significance, no functional aspects of these appendages have been suggested.

Most of the pathogenic clostridia produce toxins or enzymes that are involved in their pathology. At least two of the clostridia, *C. botulinum* and certain strains of *C. perfringens*, produce enterotoxins that cause food poisoning (see Chapter 28). *Clostridium perfringens*, however, is a common cause of myonecrotic (gas gangrene) wound infections. Also *C. botulinum* occasionally has been reported as the etiological agent of human wound disease. In 1974, for example, *MMWR* described five cases of wound botulism: one each in Pennsylvania, Texas, and Utah and two in California. Most of the *Clostridium* species, however, are saprophytes and one, *C. acetobutylicum*, has been used commercially to produce butyl alcohol and acetone in the fermentation of sweet potatoes and other substrates.

Smith and Hobbs (1974) subdivided the 61 species of the genus *Clostridium* into the following five biotype groups on the basis of spore location and gelatin hydrolysis or on the basis of special growth requirements:

1. Spores subterminal (or central)
   (a) Gelatin not hydrolyzed: Group I, Species 1–11
   (b) Gelatin hydrolyzed: Group II, Species 12–31
2. Spores terminal
   (a) Gelatin not hydrolyzed: Group III, Species 32–50
   (b) Gelatin hydrolyzed: Group IV, Species 51–56
3. Species with special growth requirements: Group V, Species 57–61

Table 37-1 lists the results of fermentation tests, toxin, enzyme, or hemolysin production, and other biotype characteristics of nine of the more important *Clostridium* species responsible for human wound infections. These and other clostridia and anaerobic organisms may be involved individually or in mixed infections, particularly in the myonecrotic (gas gangrene) pathology.

As indicated above the clostridia are anaerobic bacilli, some species even to the extent that a brief exposure of the vegetative cells to atmospheric oxygen may result in their death (Smith 1974). This fact is important in terms of collecting and submitting specimens for laboratory diagnosis. Although some clostridia will grow in the presence of slight amounts of atmospheric oxygen (are microaerophilic), all will grow under strict anaerobic culture conditions. Therefore all specimens suspected of containing a *Clostridium* or other anaerobic species should be collected, transported to the laboratory, and cultured under strict anaerobiosis. The two major clostridial wound diseases are tetanus and gas gangrene (myonecrosis), the latter being caused by one or more of some 17 different *Clostridium* or other microbial species.

TETANUS

Etiology

Tetanus is a disease known to the early medical writers (Hippocrates, Galen, and others). Because the human disease tends to cause spastic paralysis of the masseter muscles of the jaw, it became known as "lockjaw" long before its etiology was established. Kitasato in 1889 iso-

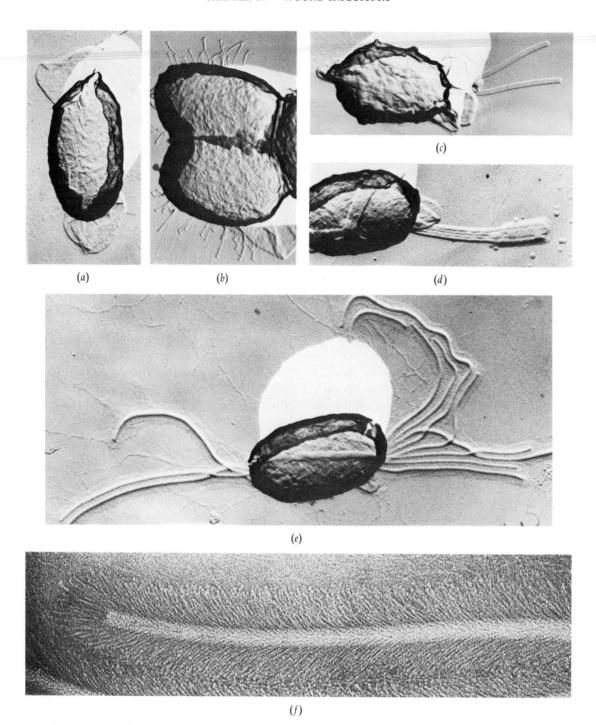

Figure 37–2.   Electron micrographs showing spore appendages of *Clostridium bifermentans*: (a) none, 28,160×; (b) pinlike, 30,800×; (c) smooth tubular, 22,100×; (d) hirsute tubular, 29,750×; (e) feather-like, 25,000×; (f) enlargement from *e*, 220,000×. (Courtesy of L. J. Rode and L. DS. Smith.)

Table 37-1. Biotype characteristics of selected species of the genus *Clostridium.*

Fermentation and Other Tests	*C. tetani* 55	*C. perfringens* 26	*C. histolyticum* 23	*C. novyi A* 25	*C. septicum* 30	*C. tertium* 36	*C. sporogenes* 19	*C. bifermentans* 13	*C. fallax* 7
Milk	C	ACG†	CD	CG	ACG	ACG	CD	CD	−
Casein digested	−	−	+	−	−	−	+	+	−
Lecithinase	−	+	−	+	−	−	+	±	−
Glucose	−	+	−	+	+	+	+	+	+
Maltose	−	+	−	+	+	+	+	+	+
Lactose	−	+	−	−	+	+	−	−	−
Sucrose	−	+	−	−	−	+	−	−	−
Salicin	−	V	−	−	+	+	±	−	−
Indole produced	+	−	−	−	−	−	+	+	±
Nitrate reduced	+	+	−	−	+	+	−	−	−
Blood hemolyzed	+	±	+	+	+	−	+	V	−
Toxin produced	+	+	+	+	+	−	−	−	−
Spore shape	S	O	O	O	O	O	O	O	O

*Species numbers (see Smith and Hobbs 1974 for group characteristics).
†Stormy fermentation.
Milk: A = acid; C = clotted; D = clot digested; G = gas.
Spores: S = spherical; O = oval.
V = variable; ± = positive or negative; + = positive; − = negative.

lated an anaerobic, spore-forming bacillus from a human case of lockjaw. Later he and Von Behring reported that the toxin produced by this isolate could be neutralized by specific tetanus antitoxin. This toxin appears to be antigenically homogeneous throughout the world. It is second only to *C. botulinum* toxin in toxic potency. The tetanus neurotoxin is not histolytic. However, the hemolysin produced by the tetanus bacillus has a supplemental necrotizing effect (see Table 37-1). This hemolysin appears to be the factor responsible for lowering the oxidation-reduction potential (O/R) of the tissues, thereby aiding the germination of the tetanus spores. The generally accepted designation for the etiological agent of tetanus is *Clostridium tetani.*

The spores of *C. tetani* survive heating at 80°C for 45 minutes to 1 hour. Although experimental animals (mice, guinea pigs, monkeys) can be fatally infected by the intramuscular inoculation of exudates from patients or with unwashed spores, culture spores that have been washed free of the neurotoxin and necrotoxic hemolysin may not produce infection when inoculated intramuscularly. This discovery led to the concept that, in addition to an anaerobic environment, the spores require the presence of dead tissue to initiate infection. The dead tissue might result from the presence of preformed necrotoxin on the surface of the spores or, in natural wounds, from tissue destroyed by the injury. The deeper and dirtier the wound (the more foreign matter), the greater the amount of dead tissue and the greater the likelihood of infection by *C. tetani.* This discovery led to recognition of the need for thorough cleansing and surgical debridement (removal of foreign matter and dead tissue) of the wound as one of the first steps in the therapy of potential tetanus. For the cultural requirements of *C. tetani* see Laboratory Diagnosis.

Clinical Symptoms and Treatment

Although clinical tetanus has been greatly reduced (from that of the horse and buggy days) in the more technologically developed countries, it continues to be a serious morbidity and mortality problem of worldwide scope. Bytchenko (1966), after a comprehensive study of the geographic distribution, estimated the number of tetanus cases during the 1950–1960 decade at more than a million with a mortality rate of approximately 50 percent. The incubation period following injury usually ranges from 2 to 8 days, although in some infections the spores may remain dormant in the tissues for longer periods before germination and toxin production. Clinical tetanus has been classified as (1) neonatal, in newborn infants in whom the cut surface of the umbilical cord serves as the site of infection; (2) postpartum or puerperal, when the ruptured tissues of the genital tract of the mother, after childbirth, become infected; (3) cephalic, when head wounds become infected; and (4) visceral, when infections of intestinal tract tissue occur. Although *C. tetani* is commonly found in human intestinal excreta, type 4 tetanus is uncommon.

Smyth et al. (1974) reported that the mortality in neonatal tetanus prior to 1958 was over 90 percent and gradually decreased to 79 percent by 1967. Between 1967 and 1972 they treated 283 cases of neonatal tetanus using intermittent positive pressure respiratory ventilation with tracheostomy and muscle relaxants. They reported that the mortality rate in their first 186 cases was lowered from 79 percent to 21 percent and down to 10 percent in the subsequent 97 cases.

There were 94 cases of tetanus reported to CDC in the United States in 1973 and again in 1974. Two of these 1974 cases were in Houston women, one 81 years of age who died and one 50 years of age who survived. Neither had had a primary course of toxoid immunization, but both were given a "booster" injection of toxoid—which, of course, did no good. Fortunately, the second woman was given 4,500 units of tetanus immune globulin, which may have saved her life (R. A. MacLean, M.D., Houston Health Department, personal communication). The 16 cases reported in Texas during 1975 showed an interesting age distribution: 5 cases, one a neonate, were in infants under 5 years of age and the other 11 cases were in adults more than 40 years of age. Eight of the adult cases (50 percent of all cases) were in the 60+ age group. Seven of the 16 Texas cases in 1975 were fatal.

Garnier (1975) reported on the treatment of 230 cases of tetanus in patients over 3 years of age in the Albert Schweitzer hospital in Haiti between 1969 and 1973. During the same period the pediatric service of the hospital treated 193 neonates (under 1 month of age) and 42 patients aged 1 month to 3 years. Garnier classified 96 of his cases of tetanus as severe, 82 as moderate, and 61 as mild. Clinical symptoms in the severe cases included marked trismus (lockjaw), marked hypertonicity of the spinal musculature resulting in the backward bending of the head and legs (opisthotonos), long frequent or continuous convulsive seizures accompanied by respiratory distress, proceeding to periods of cardiopulmonary arrest. Mortality in the severe cases, in spite of modern therapy, was 36.8 percent. The moderate cases presented trismus, opisthotonos of varying degrees, and spontaneous fairly severe convulsive spasms, but without respiratory distress. Mortality in the moderate cases was 4.88 percent. The mild cases presented trismus and moderate spinal spasms. Convulsive seizures either did not occur or were rare and of short duration. All mild cases survived.

Treatment in the Garnier cases consisted of intravenous (IV) feeding (nothing by mouth); Diazepam injected either intravenously or intramuscularly (IM) for sedation and spasm control; a single dose (10,000 units) of equine antitoxin or 250–500 units of hyperimmune-human tetanus immune globulin—TIG(H); a booster dose of toxoid; surgical care of the wound; penicillin; humidified oxygen as required; tracheostomy if needed; gastrostomy if required after 3 or 4 days for oral intake of calories and protein.

Masawe (1975) reported studies on 509 cases of tetanus between 1963 and 1969 with a mortality rate of 51.2 percent. Some 224 of the 263 deaths (85.2 percent) occurred during the first 7 days of symptoms. Only 39 (14.8 percent) died after 7 days. Masawe contends that good nursing care and constant observation during the first week of hospitalization are most critical. He considers 10,000 units of tetanus antitoxin inadequate. He used 25,000 to 50,000 units in children under 10 and 100,000 to 200,000 units in older cases.

Nourmand (1973) reported studies on 42 cases of tetanus in Iran. The average incubation period for the fatal cases was 8.2 days and for the nonfatal cases 11.5 days. The case fatality rate for children was 38 percent and for adults 20 percent. Symptoms reported were:

Lockjaw	100%
Convulsions	72.3%
Neck rigidity	59.2%
Opisthotonos	50.0%
Generalized hypertonicity	39.1%
Cyanosis	23.5%
Spasms	23.0%
Respiratory distress	20.7%
Coma	6.9%

Unusual portals of entry of C. tetani were ears (otitis); cutaneous leishmaniasis of face or lips; smallpox vaccination (3-week) sore; and severe chickenpox lesions. Two uterine cases occurred after illegal abortions.

Since simple immunization with two to three doses of alum (adjuvant) tetanus toxoid, followed by a booster injection every 10 years and at the time of injury, will give lifetime protection against tetanus, a case of tetanus reported by Larkin and Maylan (1975) illustrates the tragic consequences of failure to be so immunized, even when the patient finally survives the attack. The patient was a 77-year-old farmer who suffered a deep burn on the plantar surface of his right foot when it came in contact with a heater. Two days after the injury, the patient noticed stiffness of the neck and jaw and progressive difficulty in swallowing. On entrance into a hospital he presented a small (4 × 6 centimeters) full-thickness burn, inability to open his mouth wider than 1 centimeter, and mild neck rigidity.

Treatment consisted of wound debridement, 2,000 units of TIG(H) injected around the burn site, 3,000 units injected intramuscularly in the right thigh, and a booster injection of 0.5 milliliter of adsorbed toxoid in the left deltoid. Since he had not been immunized previously, this "booster" injection had no therapeutic immunological effect, of course. The wound was treated topically with sulfadiazine. Diazepam sedation was employed and 3,000,000 units of aqueous penicillin was administered intravenously every 6 hours for 3 weeks. The patient required endotrachial (tube-ventilation) respiratory support for 50 days. He had two cardiac arrests—successfully resuscitated. Renal failure required dialysis during the seventh week. Other complications were congestive heart failure with pulmonary edema and later a staphylococcal pneumonia. Skin grafting of the granulating wound was accomplished. Renal function slowly improved and the patient was discharged after 113 days in hospital to a convalescent center. Imagine, if you will, the pain, anxiety, and expense of this patient, all of which could have been prevented, even at his age, by a few prior injections of tetanus toxoid at a maximum cost of a few dollars.

Results such as those reported above led Furste (1975) to editorialize: "At present we physicians have the means to eliminate tetanus. We must educate the nonphysicians—the public—about how easily tetanus can be eliminated so that they will come to us of their own free will for adequate tetanus prophylaxis. Then and only then will tetanus become a disease of only historical significance."

Laboratory Diagnosis

Anaerobic microbiology has received increasing importance in clinical diagnostic laboratories during the 1950–1970 decades. As indicated above, both spore-forming and non-spore-forming anaerobes constitute a significant portion of the microflora of the normal human intestinal tract and buccal and genital mucus membranes. This, and the fact that these organisms are potential opportunistic pathogens, makes it doubly important that laboratory specimens be chosen carefully to avoid contamination with anaerobes unrelated to the pathological process in the patient. For a comprehensive coverage of the pathogenic anaerobic bacteria see Smith (1975).

Tetanus, like diphtheria, is a rapidly developing toxemia requiring immediate prophylaxis or therapy. Moreover, relatively few *C. tetani* are required to cause serious to fatal pathology. Thus the clinical laboratory plays a minor role in the diagnosis of this disease. This is even more true in severe tetanus (and gas gangrene) than in diphtheria. The usual clinical practice in nonimmunized, potential tetanus patients is to administer prophylactic tetanus antitoxin (or, in the previously immunized, a booster injection of toxoid) immediately following a traumatic injury. Laboratory tests should be performed to confirm or to alter the clinical diagnosis, but they should not be allowed to delay onset of therapy.

Finegold et al. (1974) list 14 clinical hints that suggest possible infection with anaerobic microorganisms. Among these are: (1) foul-smelling discharges—not always true in cases of gas gangrene; (2) necrosis and/or gas in the tissues and exudates; (3) infection associated with impaired circulation—thrombophlebitis; (4) black discoloration of blood-containing exudates; (5) presence of yellowish ("sulfur") granules in exudates—actinomycosis; (6) septic abortion (puerperal sepsis); (7) infection following human or animal bites or gastrointestinal surgery; (8) infection of the umbilical cord in neonates; (9) chronic middle ear infection (otitis media) or sinusitis; and (10) aspiration pneumonia.

The collection and transport of the laboratory specimen may be critical. Many authorities advocate collecting fluid specimens (such as exudates) by aspiration with a needle and syringe rather than on a cotton swab. During this collection, no air should be trapped within the syringe and after collection a drop of the specimen should be discarded from the needle into a disinfectant. If the specimen in the syringe is to be hand-carried to the laboratory for immediate testing, the point of the needle should be inserted into a sterile rubber stopper. If more distant transport of the specimen is necessary, it may be inoculated through the rubber stopper of an oxygen-free transport tube containing a small amount of a soft agar base or a reducing broth and an indicator of anaerobiosis.

Frequently tissue specimens are preferable to fluid specimens for the demonstration or isolation of anaerobic microorganisms, particularly in gas gangrene. Finegold et al. (1974) described a "mini-jar" anaerobic transporter for tissue or other laboratory specimens that will fit into a 1-dram vial. The mini-jar is an airtight, aluminum 35-millimeter film container. The specimen is put in the loosely capped 1-dram vial, which is placed in the mini-jar along with a tuft of steel wool that has been immersed in acidified copper sulfate solution, and the jar lid is closed airtight. Oxygen in the specimen vial and in the closed mini-jar is removed by the tuft of treated steel wool. See Finegold et al. (1974) and Smith and Dowell (1974) for additional suggestions for the collection and transport of anaerobic disease specimens.

Most species of the genus *Clostridium* will grow on relatively simple culture media provided strict anaerobiosis is maintained during collection, transport, inoculation, and incubation. Upon arrival at the laboratory a portion of the specimen should be smeared on a microslide for gram staining and another portion should be prepared as a wet mount for either phase-contrast or dark-field microscopic examination.

These preparations may yield almost immediate critical information for the clinician in fulminating cases and may yield suggestive information for the technologist concerning media to be used for the cultivation of fastidious anaerobes. The relative numbers of different types of organisms present, their motility, spore formation, and gram-stain reaction may be significant in subsequent test procedures.

Inoculation of both broth culture and agar plate media should be performed as soon as possible after arrival of the specimen. If more than 2 hours is to elapse before the inoculation of media, the specimen (still under anaerobiosis) should be refrigerated. Culture media should be inoculated for aerobic, microaerophilic (10 percent CO_2), and anaerobic incubation. Commonly used anaerobic broth media are (1) a good peptone–meat-infusion broth (brain-heart infusion—BHI—Difco or equivalent), which may be supplemented with a small amount of precooked, chopped lean meat prior to sterilization; or (2) thioglycolate broth. Broth media should be heated to boiling, and cooled rapidly just prior to inoculation, to remove dissolved O_2. Agar plating media may be one of the foregoing (isotonic) broth media (without chopped meat) to which 1.5 percent agar is added prior to sterilization. The agar media, while fluid at 50°C, usually are supplemented with whole sheep blood or with laked sheep red blood cells just prior to pouring into sterile petri plates. Additional supplements may be needed for fastidious anaerobes (see Sutter et al. 1972). Prior to inoculation, all media should be held under strict anaerobiosis. During inoculation of a tubed medium (broth or rolled agar) a sterile glass canula (V-shaped capillary attached to rubber tubing) delivering a stream of oxygen-free CO_2 should be inserted 2 to 3 inches into the culture tube (to prevent the entrance of air).

For maintenance of anaerobiosis during incubation of plate or tube cultures, anaerobic jars are advocated (Rosenblatt et al. 1973). The first commercial anaerobic jars were the McIntosh-Fildes jar in England and the J. H. Brown jar in America. John Brewer, a former colleague of mine at the Texas Department of Health Laboratory, designed a widely used modification of the Brown jar in 1939. These original anaerobic jars depended upon evacuation of the air from the tightly sealed jar and replacement of the vacuum with hydrogen (H_2) or methane (CH_4). The airtight lid of the jar, held in place by a screw clamp, contained a copper wire grid that housed a platinum or palladium catalyst. Electrical heating then catalyzed a reaction between the H_2 and O_2 in the jar to yield H_2O and anaerobiosis, which could be visualized by an O/R indicator within the jar. These jars worked well—unless a spark from the electric connections exploded the contained H_2 or CH_4. It was considered a judicious precaution to house such jars in a strong box constructed of loosely fitted 2×4 planks before plugging in the electric current.

During the 1960s two improvements in the anaerobic jars (Figure 37-3) were developed: (1) a catalyst that functions at room temperature (platinum or palladium-coated alumina pellets); and (2) a disposable envelope containing chemicals that upon addition of a small quantity of water liberates the necessary CO_2 and H_2 inside the jar (the GasPak). The cold catalyst after each use can be reactivated by heating at 160°C for 2 hours (see Brewer and Allgeier 1966; Rosenblatt et al. 1973).

Martin (1971) and Collee et al. (1972) discuss practical suggestions for the isolation of anaerobic bacteria in the clinical laboratory using the anaerobic jar and Gaspak procedures. A miniaturized system (Minitek) has been advocated by Stargel et al. (1976). Among the most frequent nontetanus *Clostridium* species isolated by Smith and Dowell (1974) from clinical specimens, three species not listed in Table 37-1 (*C. ramnosum, C. inoccuum,* and *C. sordellii*) constituted 29 percent of the isolates. In their studies *C. perfringens* was the most frequent isolate (27 percent).

Tetanus Immunology

Although the neurotoxin of *C. tetani* is antigenically homogeneous, a number of serotypes of the organism, based on antigenic differences in

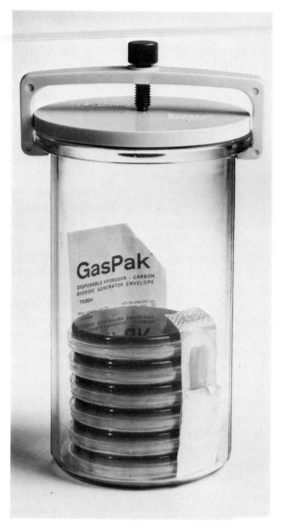

Figure 37–3. A modern anaerobic jar (BBL GasPak Anaerobic System) with GasPak envelope for generation of CO_2 and H_2. (BBL and GasPak are trademarks of Becton, Dickinson and Company.)

the flagellar and somatic antigens, have been described. These serotypes, however, have no practical significance. If a morphologically typical, spore-forming anaerobe is isolated it could be subjected to the biotype tests listed in Table 37-1, but its identification as a toxigenic *C. tetani* can be established most quickly by the mouse protection test, using tetanus antitoxin to protect the control mice.

After Kitasato and Von Behring demonstrated the presence of antitoxin in animals immunized with sublethal doses of tetanus toxin, equine antitoxin became the agent of choice for both prophylactic and therapeutic treatment of human tetanus. The efficacy of passive immunoprophylaxis, in preventing tetanus in wounded soldiers, was demonstrated in the British army during World War I. After the introduction of this prophylaxis late in 1914, the incidence of tetanus fell dramatically from $650/10^5$ wounded in 1914 to $100/10^5$ wounded during the 1915–1918 years. Frequent delay in the administration of antitoxin to the wounded, necessitated by battle conditions, undoubtedly was responsible for many of those who developed the disease after 1914.

Ramon in 1925 reported the detoxification of tetanus toxin, by treatment with formaldehyde, without affecting its antigenicity—tetanus toxoid. This toxoid proved to be a safe and excellent immunogen for both horses and humans. As indicated in Chapter 5, the tetanus toxoid can be combined with diphtheria toxoid and killed *B. pertussis* cells to give a trivalent (DPT) immunogen for infants. Moreover, the *B. pertussis* cells exert an adjuvant effect on the two toxoids. For booster immunization or for primary immunization in adults, monovalent alum-precipitated (adsorbed) tetanus toxoid is the immunogen of choice. The efficacy of active (toxoid) immunization against tetanus was dramatically demonstrated during World War II when practically no cases occurred in the wounded. This resulted from the fact that all personnel were immunized with tetanus toxoid prior to going into battle.

After an adequate primary immunizing course of tetanus toxoid (two to three injections of adjuvant toxoid), antitoxin can be demonstrated in the immunee's serum for long periods (Gottlieb et al. 1964). Thereafter booster injections (0.5 milliliter of adsorbed toxoid) every 10 to 20 years will maintain an immune status. Edsall et al. (1967) and Trinca (1974) confirmed the long-lasting immunity following primary tetanus toxoid immunization (three doses at intervals of 6 weeks between doses 1 and 2, and 6 months between doses 2 and 3). They cited evidence that unnecessarily frequent booster injections of the toxoid tended to produce undesirable hypersensitivity to the toxoid in the recipients. Also the antibody response to booster injections in those with prior primary immunization is so rapid that this procedure has replaced the passive immunoprophylaxis with tetanus antitoxin, previously practiced following wounds or other potential exposures to tetanus. *Warning:* This prophylaxis is effective only in those individuals who have a prior history of a complete primary immunization with three doses of adjuvant toxoid.

Human blood donors can be hyperimmunized with tetanus toxoid and their antitoxic serum processed to yield human tetanus immune globulin—TIG(H). This is particularly valuable to patients who are hypersensitive to horse serum. As indicated in the section on treatment, the therapeutic dosage and sites of injection of antitoxin advocated by different authorities vary considerably. All agree, however, that once the tetanus toxin is absorbed by nerve tissue, no amount of antitoxin will neutralize it. This accounts for the necessity for the immediate injection of adequate antitoxin following the onset of tetanic symptoms. If laboratory aid is requested for these patients, the maximum immediate aid should consist of microscopic examination of a stained smear and a wet mount of the specimen. Culture of the specimen should be performed for confirmation or alteration of the clinical diagnosis.

Control and Prevention

Tetanus, except for the neonatal form, can best be prevented by active immunization of infants with adjuvant tetanus toxoid, preferably with DPT, followed by booster injections at 10-year intervals. Miller (1972) advocated maternal immunization, either primary or booster toxoid, to prevent neonatal tetanus. This, of course, would also prevent possible puerperal tetanus in the mother.

GAS GANGRENE (MYONECROSIS) AND CELLULITIS

Etiology

Gas gangrene and other clostridial or anaerobic bacterial diseases, worldwide, have always been a problem in deep lacerating wounds—particularly those with dirt-contaminated compound fractures or those contracted during warfare. With the prevention of tetanus in the military personnel of technologically advanced countries by prophylactic immunization with tetanus toxoid, infection of wounded individuals by other *Clostridium* species has replaced tetanus as a serious cause of morbidity and mortality. Mac-Lennan (1962) reviewed the literature on the histotoxic clostridial human infections including publications during and following World War II. Of the 17 *Clostridium* species that have been considered the etiological agents of human traumatic infections, MacLennan reported that only 6—*C. perfringens, C. novyi, C. septicum, C. bifermentans, C. histolyticum,* and *C. fallax*—are capable of causing gas gangrene. Of these six, he considers the first three to be of overriding importance in human traumatic disease. However, gas gangrene lesions following dirty, ragged wounds frequently house a variety of other clostridia and other obligate or facultative anaerobic bacteria. Even aerobic or microaerophilic organisms may invade the wound and exhaust the available oxygen, thereby helping to lower the O/R potential of the tissues to that necessary for the germination and multiplication of the spore-forming bacilli present. Thus the etiology and the microflora of both gaseous and nongaseous anaerobic myonecroses and cellulitis infections can be quite complex following traumatic injury.

It is beyond the scope of this text to present a detailed discussion of the numerous anaerobic microorganisms isolated from wound infections. However, a brief consideration of the toxic products of *C. perfringens* and *C. novyi* will tend to illustrate the complexity of the etiology and pathology of the anaerobic wound diseases. For more details see Duncan (1975).

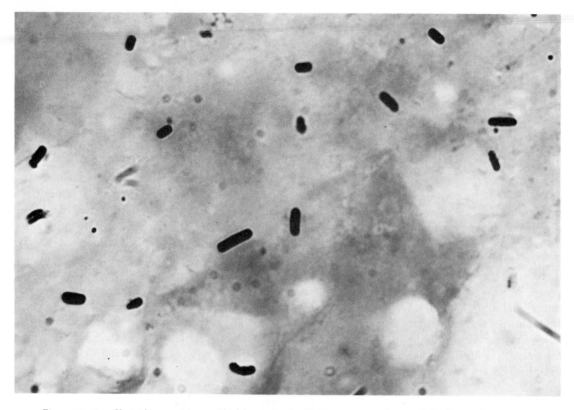

Figure 37–4. *Clostridium perfringens* (darkly-stained cells) in a smear of wound discharge from a case of myonecrosis. (Courtesy of R. W. Jackson.)

Clostridium perfringens (formerly *C. welchii*) has been divided into five biotypes designated A, B, C, D, and E *(Bergey's Manual).* All five biotypes are composed of large, encapsulated, gram-positive bacilli that rarely develop spores in infected tissues or exudates (see Figure 37-4). Type A is most commonly associated with human myonecrosis. The other biotypes cause a variety of animal and occasionally human diseases. Table 37-2 lists the designations for and the nature of the 11 toxic products shared by two or more members of the five biotypes of *C. perfringens.* Although all five biotypes produce alpha toxins, the lecithinases involved in the different alpha toxins tend to be immunologically heterogeneous. Immunological heterogeneity has been reported in the other toxic products also. Certain type A strains have been claimed to produce the enterotoxin responsible for the *C. perfringens* food poisoning discussed in

Chapter 28; these claims, however, have been questioned. *Clostridium perfringens* type C, in addition to its frequent animal pathogenicity, has been established as the etiological agent of cases of a frequently fatal necrotic enteritis of humans.

Bergey's Manual divides *C. novyi* into three biotypes, A, B, and C, on the basis of differences in the production of six toxic products. Many of these products involve the same types of activity (lethal, necrotic, hemolytic, lecithinase, and so on) as those of *C. perfringens* but are immunologically distinct from the latter. Whereas all lecithinases are alike in their enzymatic activity, for example, those produced by *C. novyi* A and B are antigenically distinct from each other and both differ antigenically from the lecithinases involved in the alpha toxins of *C. perfringens.* The lethal alpha toxin of *C. novyi* type A has been reported to be 40 to 50 times more toxic for experimental animals than that of *C. perfringens* type A. Although some of these myonecrotic exotoxins have been converted to toxoids, such immunogens have not been advocated for general immunoprophylaxis.

Pathology and Clinical Symptoms

Although human cases of nontraumatic, anaerobic myonecrosis have been reported, the great majority of such infections follow severe lacerating trauma, particularly that associated with dirt-contaminated compound fractures and high-velocity gunshot wounds. The pathogenic mechanisms involved in anaerobic myonecroses are complex, variable, and poorly understood. Given a suitable O/R potential, dead tissue, or foreign objects in a traumatic area, spores of the myonecrotic clostridia will germinate and the vegetative cells will multiply rapidly and invade surrounding healthy tissue. If the spread to

healthy muscle tissue is not stopped immediately, in cases due to the more virulent myonecrotic clostridial infections such as *C. perfringens*, *C. novyi*, and *C. septicum*, the patient will lose either a limb or life. This fact minimizes the use of the clinical laboratory as an aid to diagnosis prior to therapy.

Among the numerous toxic products of these clostridia (see Table 37-2) lecithinase appears to be one of the more important in destroying muscle tissue. This enzyme attacks the lecithin in the cell membranes, thereby destroying the integrity of the tissues and liberating nutritious fluids for further bacterial growth. The collagenases and proteinases could be expected to participate in the digestion of damaged tissues and tissue fluids also. And it is tempting to speculate, as many others have done, on the possible role of hyaluronidase on the rapid spread and metabolism of the myonecrotic clostridia. This enzyme hydrolyzes hyal-

Table 37-2. Toxins and enzymes involved in *Clostridium perfringens* pathology.

Designation	Nature of Toxic Products	C. perfringens Type[6]				
		A	B	C	D	E
Alpha	Lethal[1], necrotic[2], hemolytic, lecithinase	+	+	+	+	+
Beta	Lethal, necrotic	−	+	+	−	−
Gamma	Lethal	−	+	+	−	−
Delta	Hemolytic	−	+	+	−	−
Epsilon	Lethal, necrotic	−	+	−	+	−
Theta	Lethal, hemolytic, oxygen-labile[3]	±	+	+	+	+
Iota	Lethal[4]	−	−	−	−	+
Kappa	Lethal and necrotic[5], collagenase	+	−	+	±	+
Lambda	Protease	−	+	−	±	+
Mu	Hyaluronidase	±	+	−	±	−
Upsilon	Deoxyribonuclease	+	+	+	+	+

[1]Lethal to mice on intravenous injection.

[2]Necrotic on intradermal injection in guinea pig.

[3]Similar but not identical to streptolysin O (see Chapter 8).

[4]A protoxin activated by a protease.

[5]In rabbits.

[6]One or more of the toxic products produced by types indicated by +. ± = variable; − = negative.

Table 37-3. Differential clinical aspects of certain anaerobic wound infections. (Modified from MacLennan, 1962.)

Clinical Aspect	Myonecrosis: C. perfringens	C. novyi	Cellulitis: C. sporogenes	Streptococcus (anaerobic)
Incubation period	18–24 hr	3–6 days	3 days	3–4 days
Onset	Acute	Sudden	Gradual	Insidious
Toxemia	Moderate	Severe	Nil	Severe (late)
Pain	Extreme	Severe	Nil	Variable (usually severe)
Swelling	Moderate	Marked	Slight	Marked
Skin reaction	Tense, blanched white	Pallid	Little change	Tense, coppery tinge
Gas	Moderate	Slight	Abundant	Slight
Exudate	Moderate, hemorrhagic	Marked, yellowish	Slight	Marked, seropurulent
Smell	Slight, sweetish to foul	Nil	Foul	Slight, often sour
Muscle tissue	Soft, soggy, slate blue	Pale-pink, edematous	No change	Red, streaked purple
Mortality (untreated)	50–70+ %	60–80+ %	Nil	?

uronic acid, the interstitial ground substance of muscles. This activity would appear to be capable of aiding the spread of the clostridia through the tissues. The hyaluronic acid also contains a carbohydrate moiety that upon liberation should enhance the nutritive quality of the liberated tissue fluids for the anaerobes. Unfortunately for this speculation, no one has been able to prove a correlation between the *in vitro* production of hyaluronidase and the invasiveness or virulence of the myonecrotic clostridia.

The pathology and clinical symptoms in myonecrotic wound infections vary from relatively mild to fulminating—with the latter frequently being the case in improperly or inadequately treated cases of gas gangrene. Table 37-3 summarizes the clinical aspects of (1) two myonecrotic infections—*C. perfringens* and *C. novyi;* (2) one clostridial cellulitis infection—*C. sporogenes;* and (3) an anaerobic *Streptococcus* infection. The *C. perfringens* myonecrosis is characterized by a short incubation period and rapid

onset of excessively severe pain—localized in but out of proportion to the extent of the area of involvement. The pain is not relieved by the usual analgesics. Jackson and Waddell (1973) reported coincident fever in 22 of the 24 cases in their report. Gas in the lesion may or may not be obvious—certainly less obvious than the designation gas gangrene would imply. MacLennan (1962) reported little, if any, putrefactive odor in the 300 cases of gas gangrene in his experience, whereas Jackson and Waddell reported a thin, dark-brown, foul-smelling exudate occurring late in 15 of their 24 patients.

Laboratory Diagnosis

The procedures described above for the laboratory diagnosis of tetanus are applicable to the diagnosis of clostridial myonecrosis and other anaerobic wound infections (see Dowell and Hawkins 1974). As in tetanus, treatment of the myonecroses must be based on clinical judgment and should not be delayed more than a few minutes to obtain laboratory diagnostic assistance. Microscopic examination of a gram-stained smear of a freshly obtained clinical specimen should be the maximum pretreatment diagnostic aid expected. This immediate aid is more important in the diagnosis of myonecroses than in tetanus. Finding predominant numbers of morphologically typical, gram-positive bacilli would indicate the probability of a clostridial myonecrosis or cellulitis. Predominant numbers of gram-positive streptococci would tend to incriminate these organisms as the etiological agent. Finding predominant numbers of gram-negative bacilli would suggest the possibilities of an E. coli or Bacteroides fragilis or other species as the etiological agent. Since part of the early treatment and prognosis might depend upon the predominant organism in the wound specimen, this immediate information should be helpful to the clinician.

For confirmation of the clinical diagnosis, the laboratory specimen should be cultured on blood agar (and possibly other media) under aerobic, microaerophilic (10 percent CO_2), and anaerobic conditions. Since antibiotics constitute an important part of the therapy, the susceptibility of the causative organism to these drugs poses an important problem (see Sutter and Washington 1974). Unfortunately, routine isolation and susceptibility testing procedures require a minimum of 48 to 72 hours. It appears to the author that a modification of the procedures designed for testing antibiotic susceptibilities of Mycobacterium tuberculosis in sputum (see Chapter 9) might be applicable to such testing of myonecrotic organisms. Under ideal conditions this procedure could be expected to give results within 18 to 24 hours. The four-quadrant blood-agar plates (three antibiotic test quadrants and one no-antibiotic control) should be prepared and inoculated in triplicate, one for each of the three types of incubation required.

Prophylaxis and Therapy

Since prophylactic immunization is rarely practiced, the prevention of anaerobic myonecrosis or cellulitis, following a ragged wound, depends upon immediate and thorough surgical debridement and the administration of adequate dosages of antibiotics. Final closure of the wound should be delayed for 2 to 3 days while thorough drainage is provided. Tourniquets and tight plaster casts should be avoided when possible. Rigid application of these prophylactic procedures reduced the incidence of myonecrosis in wounded personnel spectacularly during the Viet Nam War.

Once symptoms of myonecrosis commence, immediate therapy again consists of the administration of antibiotics and thorough surgical debridement, making sure that *all* involved muscle tissue is removed. MacLennan (1962) stated that "in over 300 cases of gas gangrene, none recovered unless the whole pathological lesion had been extirpated. If necessary, long exploratory incisions are in order to identify and remove all gangrenous muscle." Amputation of the involved limb may be necessary to save the patient's life.

Brummelkamp et al. (1963) were the first to advocate the administration of hyperbaric oxygen in the treatment of clostridial infections. This treatment consists of having the patient breathe pure oxygen while housed in a pressure chamber under several atmospheres of increased pressure.

Jackson and Waddell (1973) reported results of treating 24 cases of myonecrosis (gas gangrene). Prior to the installation of a hyperbaric chamber in the hospital (see Figure 37-5), 9 patients received only the surgical and antibiotic therapy indicated above. The mortality rate in this group was 56 percent (5 of 9 patients), and 3 of the 4 survivors required amputation to control the disease. Four patients received gas gangrene antitoxin and 2 of the 4 died. The following 15 patients received the same basic therapy as the first 9, but their treatment was supplemented with exposure to hyperbaric oxygen. While still undergoing surgical debridement, the patient was prepared for the first 90-minute exposure ("dive") to 3 atmospheres of pressure. If the patient was unconscious or very ill, the eardrums were punctured to avoid painful middle ear reactions. The patient, while breathing 100 percent oxygen, was attended by a

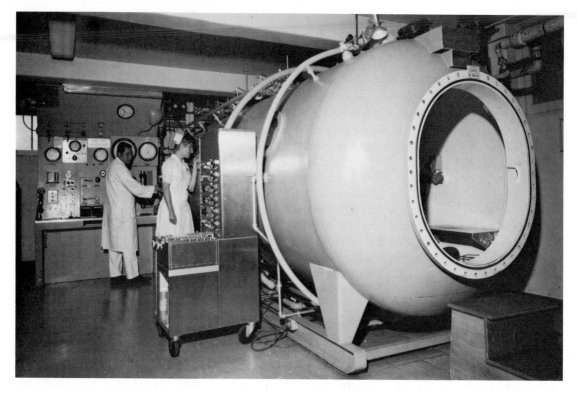

Figure 37–5.   Hyperbaric oxygen chamber capable of housing two patients plus attendants. (Courtesy of R. W. Jackson.)

doctor or nurse in the pressure chamber to care for possible emergencies. The 90-minute dive was repeated four times during the first 30 hours of treatment. Breathing 100 percent oxygen while exposed to 3 atmospheres of pressure has been estimated to force approximately 17 times more oxygen into solution in the tissue fluids than that supplied by ordinary respiration. This could be expected to raise the O/R potential of the tissues and thereby help to halt the progress of an obligate anaerobic infection.

The mortality rate in the 15 patients who received the hyperbaric oxygen treatment was 27 percent (4 of 15). Only 6 of the 15 patients required early or late amputation. All 4 of the patients who died did so after amputation of the affected extremity. Seven of the patients in this group received gas gangrene antitoxin and 4 of the 7 died. Jackson and Waddell concluded that hyperbaric oxygen not only lowers the mortality rate, but also decreases the amount of excision or amputation necessary to control gas gangrene. They also concluded that gas gangrene antiserum had no beneficial effect on the outcome of the disease.

REFERENCES

Brewer, J. H., and D. L. Allgeier. 1966. Safe, self-contained carbon dioxide–hydrogen anaerobic system. *Appl. Microbiol.* 14:985–988.

Brummelkamp, W. H., I. Boeream, and J. Hogendyk. 1963. Treatment of clostridial infections with hyperbaric oxygen. A report of 26 cases. *Lancet* i:235–238.

Bytchenko, B. 1966. Geographical distribution of tetanus throughout the world: 1951–1960. *Bull. Wld. Hlth. Org.* 34:71–104.

Collee, J. G., B. Watt, E. B. Fowler, and R. Brown. 1972. An evaluation of the Gaspak system in the culture of anaerobic bacteria. *J. Appl. Bacteriol.* 35:71–82.

Dowell, V. R., Jr., and T. M. Hawkins. 1974. Laboratory methods in anaerobic bacteriology. *CDC Laboratory Manual.* HEW Publication 74-8272. Atlanta: Center for Disease Control.

Duncan, C. L. 1975. Role of clostridial toxins in pathogenesis. In *Microbiology, 1975,* ed. D. Schlessenger. Washington: American Society for Microbiology.

Edsall, G., M. W. Elliott, T. C. Peebles, L. Levine, and M. C. Eldred. 1967. Excessive use of tetanus toxoid boosters. *J. Amer. Med. Ass.* 202:17–19.

Finegold, S. M. 1977. *Anaerobic Bacteria in Human Disease.* New York: Academic Press.

Finegold, S. M., L. Sutter, H. R. Attebery, and J. E. Rosenblatt. 1974. Isolation of anaerobic bacteria. Chapter 38 in *Manual of Clinical Microbiology.*

Furste, W. 1975. Editorial: Tetanus, the continuing problem of physicians and nonphysicians. *J. Trauma* 15:549–550.

Garnier, M. J. 1975. Tetanus in patients three years of age and up. A personal series of 230 consecutive patients. *Amer. J. Surg.* 129:459–463.

Gottlieb, S., F. X. Laughlin, L. Levine, W. C. Latham, and G. Edsall. 1964. Long term immunity to tetanus—a statistical evaluation and its clinical implications. *Amer. J. Pub. Health* 54:961–971.

Gregory, J. E., S. P. Starr, and C. Omdal. 1974. Wound infection with *Shigella flexneri. J. Infect. Dis.* 129:602–604.

Hodgkiss, W., Z. J. Ordal, and D. C. Cann. 1966. The comparative morphology of spores of *Clostridium botulinum* type E and the "OS mutant." *Canad. J. Microbiol.* 12:1283–1284.

Jackson, R. W., and J. P. Waddell. 1973. Hyperbaric oxygen in the management of clostridial myonecrosis. *Clin. Orthop.* 96:271–276.

Larkin, J. M., and J. A. Maylan. 1975. Tetanus following a minor burn. *J. Trauma* 15:546–548.

MacLennan, J. D. 1962. The histotoxic clostridial infections of man. *Bacteriol. Rev.* 26:177–276.

Martin, W. J. 1971. Practical method for isolation of anaerobic bacteria in the clinical laboratory. *Appl. Microbiol.* 22:1168–1171.

————. 1974. Anaerobic cocci. Chapter 40 in *Manual of Clinical Microbiology.*

Masawe, A. E. 1975. Letter: Management of tetanus. *Lancet* i:932.

Miller, J. K. 1972. The prevention of neonatal tetanus by maternal immunization. *J. Trop. Pediatr.* 18:159–167.

Nourmand, A. 1973. Clinical studies on tetanus. Notes on 42 cases in southern Iran with special emphasis on portal of entry. *Clin. Pediatr.* 12:652–653.

Rode, L. J. 1971. Bacterial spore appendages. *Critical Rev. in Microbiol.* 1:1–27.

Rode, L. J., M. A. Crawford, and M. G. Williams. 1967. *Clostridium* spores with ribbon-like appendages. *J. Bacteriol.* 93:1160–1173.

Rode, L. J., and L. DS. Smith. 1970. Taxonomic implications of spore fine structure in *Clostridium bifermentans. J. Bacteriol.* 105:349–354.

Rosenblatt, J. E., A. Fallon, and S. M. Finegold. 1973. Comparison of methods for isolation of anaerobic bacteria from clinical specimens. *Appl. Microbiol.* 25:77–85.

Rubin, S. J., and R. C. Tilton. 1975. Isolation of *Vibrio alginolyticus* from wound infections. *J. Clin. Microbiol.* 2:556–558.

Smith, L. DS. 1974. Introduction to anaerobic bacteria. Chapter 37 in *Manual of Clinical Microbiology.*

————. 1975. *The Pathogenic Anaerobic Bacteria.* 2nd ed. Springfield: Charles C. Thomas.

Smith, L. DS., and V. R. Dowell, Jr. 1974. Clostridium. Chapter 39 in *Manual of Clinical Microbiology.*

Smith, L. DS., and G. Hobbs. 1974. Genus III *Clostridium.* In *Bergey's Manual of Determinative Bacteriology.* 8th ed. Baltimore: Williams & Wilkins.

Smyth, P. M., M. D. Bowie, and T. J. V. Voss. 1974. Treatment of tetanus neonatorum with muscle relaxants and intermittent positive pressure ventilation. *Brit. Med. J.* 1:223–226.

Stargel, M. D., F. S. Thompson, S. E. Phillips, G. L. Lombard, and V. R. Dowell, Jr. 1976. Modification of the Minitek miniaturized differentiation system for characterization of anaerobic bacteria. *J. Clin. Microbiol.* 3:291–301.

Sutter, V. L., H. R. Attebery, J. E. Rosenblatt, K. Bricknell, and S. M. Finegold. 1972. *Anaerobic Bacteriology Manual.* Los Angeles: Extension Division, University of California.

Sutter, V. L., and J. A. Washington, II. 1974. Susceptibility testing of anaerobes. Chapter 49 in *Manual of Clinical Microbiology.*

Trinca, J. C. 1974. Antibody response to successive booster doses of tetanus toxoid in adults. *Infect. Immunity* 10:1–5.

Figure and Table Credits

Front and Back Cover Credits

A and B. Cultures provided by L. M. Pope, Dept. of Microbiology, the Univ. of Texas at Austin.

C. L. J. LeBeau, Dept. of Pathology, Univ. of Illinois at the Medical Center, Chicago.

D1 and D2. S. M. Gibson, General Bacteriology Lab., Texas Dept. of Health Resources, Austin.

E1. A. M. Gordon, C. Hoke, and N. Vedros, Neisseria Repository, Naval Biosciences Lab., Univ. of California, Berkeley.

E2. A. N. James and R. P. Williams, Dept. of Microbiology and Immunology, Baylor College of Medicine, Houston.

F1 and F2. L. M. Pope and D. R. Grote, Dept. of Microbiology, the Univ. of Texas at Austin.

G1. R. W. Smithwick, Mycobacteriology Branch, Center for Disease Control, Atlanta, Ga.

G2. J. E. Steadham, Mycobacteriology and Mycology Lab., Texas Dept. of Health Resources, Austin.

H and J. Photo-Art Resource Library, Instructional Media Div., Center for Disease Control, Atlanta, Ga.

I. T. H. Chen, School of Public Health, Univ. of California, Berkeley.

Figure Credits

2–2. (*a*) Bausch and Lomb, Rochester, N.Y. (*c*) The Bettmann Archive, Inc. (*d*) Forgflo Corporation, Sunbury, Pa.

3–1, 8–1, 18–1, 18–2, 19–3, 21–2(*b*–*e*), 21–4, 21–6, 21–8, 21–11, 30–1, 34–1. Photo-Art Resource Library, Instructional Media Division, Center for Disease Control, Atlanta, Ga.

3–2. The Upjohn Company, Kalamazoo, Mich.

4–1. N. M. Green, National Institute for Medical Research, London.

4–3. T. A. Barber, Dept. of Pathology, School of Medicine, Univ. of Wisconsin, Madison.

4–7. R. M. Albrecht and S. D. Horowitz, Div. of Immunology, Dept. of Pediatrics, Univ. of Wisconsin, Madison.

5–2. Photo by D. R. Grote, Dept. of Microbiology, the Univ. of Texas at Austin.

7–2. R. Austrian. 1953. *J. Exp. Med.* 98:21.

8–2. (*a*) After J. A. Bellanti. 1971. *Immunology.* Philadelphia: W. B. Saunders. (*b*) H. Bauer, Dept. of Pathology, Georgetown Univ. Medical Center.

9–1. R. B. Morrison, M. D., Austin, Texas.

10–1. After W. Burrows. 1973. *Textbook of Microbiology,* 20th ed. Philadelphia: W. B. Saunders.

11–1, 16–2(*a*) J. J. Cardamone, Jr., and J. S. Youngner, Dept. of Microbiology, Univ. of Pittsburgh School of Medicine.

11–2(*a*), 25–2. J. Griffith, Dept. of Biochemistry, Stanford Univ. School of Medicine.

11–2(*b*), 19–1(*b*), 19–2(inset). S. C. Holt, Dept. of Microbiology, Univ. of Massachusetts, Amherst.

11–3. B. Roizman, Committee on Virology, The Univ. of Chicago.

11–4. (*a*) N. Sharon, Depts. of Pathology and Lab. Med., Evanston Hosp., Evanston, Ill. (*b*) S. Dales and S. L. Wilton, Dept. of Bacteriology and Immunology, Health Scis. Centre, The Univ. of Western Ontario.

12–1. J. H. Schieble, Viral and Rickettsial Disease Lab., California State Dept. of Health, Berkeley. *In*: Lennette, E. H., et al. 1974. *Manual of Clinical Microbiology,* 2nd ed. Washington D. C.: Am. Soc. for Microbiology.

13–2(*a*) R. C. Williams, Virus Laboratory, Univ. of California, Berkeley.

15–1. B. Wolanski, Merck Sharp and Dohme Research Labs., West Point, Pa.

16–2(*b*), 33–1, 35–1. F. A. Murphy, Viral Pathology Branch, Center for Disease Control, Atlanta, Ga.

16–3. World Heath Organization, Geneva, Switzerland.

17–1. J. L. Swanson, Depts. of Pathology and Microbiology, College of Medicine, The Univ. of Utah.

17–2. *MMWR,* Jan. 14, 1977.

19–1(*a*), 19–2. P. S. Brachman, Bureau of Epidemiology, Center for Disease Control, Atlanta, Ga.

19–4. W. Burgdorfer, Rickettsial Diseases Section, Rocky Mountain Lab., Hamilton, Mont.

19–5, 34–4. F. A. Murphy and S. G. Whitfield. 1975. *Bull. World Health Organ.* 52:409–419.

19–6. Viral Pathology Branch and Special Pathogens Branch, Center for Disease Control, Atlanta, Ga. *Via* A. Mather, Managing Editor, *MMWR.*

20–1. P. B. Smith. 1972. *In*: Cohen, J. O. (ed.). *The Staphylococci.* New York: Wiley Interscience.

20–2. P. B. Smith, Clinical Bacteriology, Center for Disease Control, Atlanta, Ga.

20–3, 23–1. L. M. Pope, Dept. of Microbiology, the Univ. of Texas at Austin.

21–1. M. A. Gerencser and J. M. Slack, Dept. of Microbiology, West Virginia Univ. Medical Center.

21–2(*a*). J. T. Sinski. 1974. *Dermatophytes in Human Skin, Hair and Nails.* Springfield, Ill.: Charles C. Thomas.

21–5, 21–7, 21–9, 21–12, 21–15. J. E. Steadham, Mycobacteriology and Mycology Lab., Texas Dept. of Health Resources, Austin.

21–10. R. J. Schlegel, Dept. of Pediatrics, Charles R. Drew Postgraduate Medical School, Los Angeles, Ca. *In*: *Pediatrics.* 1970. 45:926.

21–13. C. T. Dolan, J. W. Funkhouser, E. W. Koneman, N. G. Miller and G. D. Roberts. 1976. *Atlas of Clinical Mycology* V: *Subcutaneous Mycoses.* Chicago: American Soc. of Clinical Pathologists.

21–14. G. D. Roberts, Dept. of Lab. Medicine, Mayo Clinic, Rochester, Minn.

23–2. R. A. Finkelstein, Dept. of Microbiology, the Univ. of Texas Health Science Center at Dallas.

23–3. *MMWR*, Sept. 20, 1975.

24–1. W. L. Dentler, Dept. of Physiology and Cell Biology, Univ. of Kansas, Lawrence.

24–3. E. A. Edwards and R. L. Hilderbrand. 1976. *J. Clin. Microbiol.* 3:339–343.

25–1. E. H. Cook, Jr., and C. R. Gravelle, Bureau of Epidemiology, Phoenix Laboratories, Center for Disease Control, Phoenix, Ariz.

25–3. (*a*) P. V. Holland, Blood Bank Dept., Clinical Center, National Institutes of Health, Bethesda, Md. (*b*) Hyland Division Travenol Labs., Inc., Los Angeles, Ca.

25–4. D. Bromley, Dept. of Microbiology, West Virginia Univ. Medical Center.

26–1. B. A. Phillips, Dept. of Microbiology, Univ. of Pittsburgh School of Medicine.

26–2. D. Bodian. 1955. *Science.* 122:105–108.

26–4. L. Noro. 1973. *In*: Perkins, F. T. (acting ed.). *International Symposium on Vaccination Against Communicable Diseases.* Basel: S. Karger AG.

27–1. J. J. Cardamone, Jr., Dept. of Microbiology, Univ. of Pittsburgh School of Medicine.

28–1. H. D. Bredthauer, Texas Dept. of Health Resources, Austin.

29–1. Plague Branch, Bureau of Labs., Center for Disease Control, Fort Collins, Colo.

30–2, 31–3. W. Burgdorfer. 1970. *Infect. Immun.* 2: 256–259.

30–3. R. S. Thompson, W. Burgdorfer, R. Russell, and B. J. Francis. 1969. *JAMA* 210:1045–1050.

31–1. W. Burgdorfer. 1977. *Acta Tropica* 34(2): 103–126.

31–2, 31–4. *MMWR*, Annual Supplement, Aug. 1976.

31–5. T. E. Woodward, Univ. of Maryland School of Medicine, Baltimore.

34–2. W. A. Chappell, Viral and Rickettsial Products Branch, Center for Disease Control, Atlanta, Ga.

35–2. *MMWR*, Oct. 15, 1976.

35–3. J. D. Woodie and R. W. Emmons, Viral and Rickettsial Disease Lab., California State Dept. of Health, Berkeley.

36–1. J. D. Dyckman, Houston Health Dept. Lab., Houston, Texas.

37–1. V. R. Dowell, Enterobacteriology Branch, Center for Disease Control, Atlanta, Ga.

37–2. L. J. Rode and L. DS. Smith. 1971. *J. Bacteriol.* 105: 349–354.

37–3. BioQuest, Div. of Becton, Dickinson and Company, Cockeysville, Md.

37–4, 37–5. R. W. Jackson, Toronto Western Medical Bldg., Toronto, Ont.

Table Credits

24–1. L. Le Minor, R. Rohde, and S. T. Cowan. 1974. *In*: *Bergey's Manual of Determinative Bacteriology,* 8th ed., Part 8. Baltimore: © 1974 The Williams and Wilkins Co.

37–3. J. D. MacLennan. 1962. *Bacteriol. Rev.* 26: 177–276.

Index